New Challenges in Ocular Drug Delivery

New Challenges in Ocular Drug Delivery

Editors

Rosario Pignatello
Hugo Almeida
Debora Santonocito
Carmelo Puglia

MDPI

Basel • Beijing • Wuhan • Barcelona • Belgrade • Novi Sad • Cluj • Manchester

Editors
Rosario Pignatello
University of Catania
Catania
Italy

Hugo Almeida
Mesosystem, SA
Porto
Portugal

Debora Santonocito
University of Catania
Catania
Italy

Carmelo Puglia
University of Catania
Catania
Italy

Editorial Office
MDPI AG
Grosspeteranlage 5
4052 Basel, Switzerland

This is a reprint of articles from the Topic published online in the open access journals *Journal of Nanotheranostics* (ISSN 2624-845X), *Nanomaterials* (ISSN 2079-4991), *Pharmaceuticals* (ISSN 1424-8247), *Pharmaceutics* (ISSN 1999-4923), and *Journal of Functional Biomaterials* (ISSN 2079-4983) (available at: https://www.mdpi.com/topics/ocular_drug_delivery).

For citation purposes, cite each article independently as indicated on the article page online and as indicated below:

Lastname, A.A.; Lastname, B.B. Article Title. *Journal Name* **Year**, *Volume Number*, Page Range.

ISBN 978-3-7258-1581-4 (Hbk)
ISBN 978-3-7258-1582-1 (PDF)
doi.org/10.3390/books978-3-7258-1582-1

Contents

About the Editors vii

Rosario Pignatello, Hugo Almeida, Debora Santonocito and Carmelo Puglia
New Challenges in Ocular Drug Delivery
Reprinted from: *pharmaceutics* **2024**, *16*, 794, doi:10.3390/pharmaceutics16060794 1

Kevin Y. Wu, Jamie K. Fujioka, Tara Gholamian, Marian Zaharia and Simon D. Tran
Suprachoroidal Injection: A Novel Approach for Targeted Drug Delivery
Reprinted from: *Pharmaceuticals* **2023**, *16*, 1241, doi:10.3390/ph16091241 3

Andrea Gabai, Marco Zeppieri, Lucia Finocchio and Carlo Salati
Innovative Strategies for Drug Delivery to the Ocular Posterior Segment
Reprinted from: *Pharmaceutics* **2023**, *15*, 1862, doi:10.3390/pharmaceutics15071862 76

Julia Prinz, Nicola Maffulli, Matthias Fuest, Peter Walter, Frank Hildebrand and Filippo Migliorini
Honey-Related Treatment Strategies in Dry Eye Disease
Reprinted from: *Pharmaceuticals* **2023**, *16*, 762, doi:10.3390/ph16050762 114

Federica De Gaetano, Martina Pastorello, Venerando Pistarà, Antonio Rescifina, Fatima Margani, Vincenzina Barbera, et al.
Rutin/Sulfobutylether-β-Cyclodextrin as a Promising Therapeutic Formulation for Ocular Infection
Reprinted from: *Pharmaceutics* **2024**, *16*, 233, doi:10.3390/pharmaceutics16020233 127

Elide Zingale, Angela Bonaccorso, Agata Grazia D'Amico, Rosamaria Lombardo, Velia D'Agata, Jarkko Rautio and Rosario Pignatello
Formulating Resveratrol and Melatonin Self-Nanoemulsifying Drug Delivery Systems (SNEDDS) for Ocular Administration Using Design of Experiments
Reprinted from: *Pharmaceutics* **2024**, *16*, 125, doi:10.3390/pharmaceutics16010125 146

Susmita Bose, Chau-Minh Phan, Muhammad Rizwan, John Waylon Tse, Evelyn Yim and Lyndon Jones
Fabrication and Characterization of an Enzyme-Triggered, Therapeutic-Releasing Hydrogel Bandage Contact Lens Material
Reprinted from: *Pharmaceutics* **2024**, *16*, 26, doi:10.3390/pharmaceutics16010026 173

Phatsawee Jansook, Hay Man Saung Hnin Soe, Rathapon Asasutjarit, Theingi Tun, Hay Marn Hnin, Phyo Darli Maw, et al.
Celecoxib/Cyclodextrin Eye Drop Microsuspensions: Evaluation of In Vitro Cytotoxicity and Anti-VEGF Efficacy for Retinal Diseases
Reprinted from: *Pharmaceutics* **2023**, *15*, 2689, doi:10.3390/pharmaceutics15122689 189

Brandon Ho, Chau-Minh Phan, Piyush Garg, Parvin Shokrollahi and Lyndon Jones
A Rapid Screening Platform for Simultaneous Evaluation of Biodegradation and Therapeutic Release of an Ocular Hydrogel
Reprinted from: *Pharmaceutics* **2023**, *15*, 2625, doi:10.3390/pharmaceutics15112625 203

Simona Sapino, Giulia Chindamo, Elena Peira, Daniela Chirio, Federica Foglietta, Loredana Serpe, et al.
Development of ARPE-19-Equipped Ocular Cell Model for In Vitro Investigation on Ophthalmic Formulations
Reprinted from: *Pharmaceutics* **2023**, *15*, 2472, doi:10.3390/pharmaceutics15102472 215

Natallia V. Dubashynskaya, Anton N. Bokatyi, Andrey S. Trulioff, Artem A. Rubinstein, Igor V. Kudryavtsev and Yury A. Skorik
Development and Bioactivity of Zinc Sulfate Cross-Linked Polysaccharide Delivery System of Dexamethasone Phosphate
Reprinted from: *Pharmaceutics* **2023**, *15*, 2396, doi:10.3390/pharmaceutics15102396 . . . . **230**

Yali Zhang, Jingjing Yang, Yinjian Ji, Zhen Liang, Yuwei Wang and Junjie Zhang
Development of Osthole-Loaded Microemulsions as a Prospective Ocular Delivery System for the Treatment of Corneal Neovascularization: In Vitro and In Vivo Assessments
Reprinted from: *Pharmaceuticals* **2023**, *16*, 1342, doi:10.3390/ph16101342 . . . . **245**

Weizhen (Jenny) Wang and Nonna Snider
Discovery and Potential Utility of a Novel Non-Invasive Ocular Delivery Platform
Reprinted from: *Pharmaceutics* **2023**, *15*, 2344, doi:10.3390/pharmaceutics15092344 . . . . **266**

Mohamed A. El-Gendy, Mai Mansour, Mona I. A. El-Assal, Rania A. H. Ishak and Nahed D. Mortada
Travoprost Liquid Nanocrystals: An Innovative Armamentarium for Effective Glaucoma Therapy
Reprinted from: *Pharmaceutics* **2023**, *15*, 954, doi:10.3390/pharmaceutics15030954 . . . . **284**

About the Editors

Rosario Pignatello

Prof. Rosario Pignatello received a master's degree in pharmacy in 1985 at the University of Catania (Italy). He is a Full Professor of pharmaceutical technology and legislation at the University of Catania and the Director of the Department of Drug and Health Sciences (DSFS). His main teaching tasks concern pharmaceutical technology and pharmaceutics, drug delivery and targeting, pharmaceutical and health legislation, and environmental legislation. He is a member of the Council of the Research Doctorate (PhD) in 'Neuroscience' (University of Catania). He acted as an Independent Expert for the European Commission in the evaluation of research project applications within the 6th and 7th Framework and the Horizon2020 Programmes. He is a member of Controlled Release Society (CRS—Italian Chapter) and of SITELF (Italian Society of Pharmaceutical Technology and Legislation). He acts as a Scientific Consultant of several companies operating in the fields of medicine and health products (medical devices, food supplements).

Prof. Pignatello is Co-Author of 190 scientific publications in international journals and about 200 among invited lectures and oral and poster contributions to scientific congresses.

His main research interests at present include the following:

(1) The preparation, physico-chemical characterization and biological evaluation of polymer micro- and nanoparticles as controlled drug delivery systems (nanomedicine).
(2) Supramolecular lipid-based drug carrier systems: liposomes, solid lipid nanoparticles (SLN), nanostructured lipid carriers (NLC) and drug–lipid conjugates for pharmaceutical and cosmetic applications.
(3) Synthesis and pharmaceutical applications of novel polymeric biomaterials.

His specific areas of research include ocular drug delivery, brain drug targeting, and ileo-colonic controlled release of drugs and nutraceutical ingredients.

Hugo Almeida

Hugo Almeida received his degree in pharmaceutical sciences from the Faculty of Pharmacy, University of Coimbra (Portugal) in 2006, and a master's degree in quality control (branch: drug substances and medicinal plants) from the Faculty of Pharmacy, University of Porto (Portugal) in 2009. In 2016, he received his PhD degree in pharmaceutical sciences (branch: pharmaceutical technology) from the Faculty of Pharmacy, University of Porto (Portugal).

He has more than 18 years of experience in the medical device industry, as Technical Director and Head of the Quality Control Department in a medical device company, as well as one year of experience in the pharmaceutical industry. At present, he is a production manager in a medical device and cosmetic company.

He is also a Researcher at UCIBIO, REQUIMTE, MEDTECH, Department of Drug Sciences, Laboratory of Pharmaceutical Technology, Faculty of Pharmacy, University of Porto, Portugal. He develops his research in the application of stimuli-responsive polymers in controlled and self-regulated drug delivery systems and also in developing lipid-based nanosystems to improve drug delivery. He is the Author of several scientific articles, Editor of one book, Author of one book chapter, Invited Editor of two Special Issues in the journals Pharmaceutics and Current Pharmaceutical Design, and an Invited Editor of two Topics for MDPI.

Debora Santonocito

Debora Santonocito is a Researcher at the Department of Pharmaceutical and Health Sciences of the University of Catania. She is a teacher of Herbal product technology and co-teacher of Pharmaceutical technology, socioeconomics and pharmaceutical legislation at the University of Catania and the co-author of numerous publications (H index: 14). She was a Visiting Researcher at the Departamento de Farmacia y Tecnología Farmacéutica-University of Santiago de Compostela (Spain), where she acquired expertise on toxicity and ophthalmology studies. Her main scientific interests are focused on the formulation and characterization of nanoparticles and the extraction and delivery of natural biocompounds.

Carmelo Puglia

Prof. Carmelo Puglia is Associate Professor at the Department of Drug and Health Sciences, University of Catania. He is a teacher of Pharmaceutical technology, socioeconomics and legislation for the undergraduate course in Pharmaceutical Chemistry and Technology of the University of Catania. Prof. Puglia has authored and co-authored more than 100 scientific publications on peer-reviewed international journals and about 60 conference papers (H index: 39). The research theme carried out by Prof. Puglia concerns the formulation and the evaluation of nanocarriers as drug delivery systems to increase the bioavailability and stability of active pharmaceutical ingredients (APIs) through different routes of administration.

pharmaceutics

MDPI

Editorial

New Challenges in Ocular Drug Delivery

Rosario Pignatello [1,2,*], Hugo Almeida [3,4,5], Debora Santonocito [1,2] and Carmelo Puglia [1,2]

1 Laboratory of Drug Delivery Technology, Department of Drug and Health Sciences, University of Catania, Viale A. Doria 6, 95125 Catania, Italy; debora.santonocito@unict.it (D.S.); carmelo.puglia@unict.it (C.P.)
2 NANOMED—Research Centre for Nanomedicine and Pharmaceutical Nanotechnology, Department of Drug and Health Sciences, University of Catania, 95125 Catania, Italy
3 UCIBIO (Research Unit on Applied Molecular Biosciences), REQUIMTE (Rede de Química e Tecnologia), MEDTECH (Medicines and Healthcare Products), Laboratory of Pharmaceutical Technology, Department of Drug Sciences, Faculty of Pharmacy, University of Porto, 4050-313 Porto, Portugal; hperas5@hotmail.com
4 Associate Laboratory i4HB-Institute for Health and Bioeconomy, Faculty of Pharmacy, University of Porto, 4050-313 Porto, Portugal
5 Mesosystem Investigação & Investimentos by Spinpark, Barco, 4805-017 Guimarães, Portugal
* Correspondence: r.pignatello@unict.it

The clinical treatment of diseases affecting the eye globe, and specifically the retina and posterior eye segment, is often hindered by the physiological protection structures and mechanisms of the organ, as well as by the unsuitable physico-chemical features of the active molecules. Intravitreal injection of drugs and monoclonal antibodies is at present the most common therapeutic procedure to reach the retinal area; however, it is associated with a high risk of side effects and requires the intervention of a physician. One of the 'dream goals' in this field is to reach the retinal area using a simple topically applied eye-drop formulation. Research in recent years has progressively made new strategies and technologies available in order to overcome the problems that hinder an efficacious ocular drug bioavailability, leading to even more safe, easy-to-use, and highly compliant therapeutic means. Controlled release as well as nanomedicine approaches, mainly based on polymeric or lipid matrices, are among the most largely explored strategies to pursue this aim. This Topic is aimed at collecting the most recent studies from worldwide laboratories to make an update of the state of the art and open new perspectives toward innovative and effective ocular therapies. In particular, studies dealing with biotech products and gene material will be welcomed, since the association of new therapeutic means with personalized treatments is set to become the most exciting objective for the future of ophthalmology.

We are extremely delighted to present the latest research, and review works that demonstrate the new challenges to achieving an effective ocular drug delivery to increase bioavailability and therapeutic efficacy, while at the same time reducing the risk of side effects. The articles selected for this Topic include the following:

1. "Suprachoroidal Injection: A Novel Approach for Targeted Drug Delivery".
2. "Innovative Strategies for Drug Delivery to the Ocular Posterior Segment".
3. "Honey-Related Treatment Strategies in Dry Eye Disease".
4. "Rutin/Sulfobutylether-β-Cyclodextrin as a Promising Therapeutic Formulation for Ocular Infection".
5. "Formulating Resveratrol and Melatonin Self-Nanoemulsifying Drug Delivery Systems (SNEDDS) for Ocular Administration Using Design of Experiments".
6. "Fabrication and Characterization of an Enzyme-Triggered, Therapeutic-Releasing Hydrogel Bandage Contact Lens Material".
7. "Celecoxib/Cyclodextrin Eye Drop Microsuspensions: Evaluation of In Vitro Cytotoxicity and Anti-VEGF Efficacy for Retinal Diseases".
8. "A Rapid Screening Platform for Simultaneous Evaluation of Biodegradation and Therapeutic Release of an Ocular Hydrogel".

Citation: Pignatello, R.; Almeida, H.; Santonocito, D.; Puglia, C. New Challenges in Ocular Drug Delivery. *Pharmaceutics* **2024**, *16*, 794. https://doi.org/10.3390/pharmaceutics16060794

Received: 5 June 2024
Accepted: 6 June 2024
Published: 11 June 2024

9. "Development of ARPE-19-Equipped Ocular Cell Model for In Vitro Investigation on Ophthalmic Formulations".
10. "Development and Bioactivity of Zinc Sulfate Cross-Linked Polysaccharide Delivery System of Dexamethasone Phosphate".
11. "Development of Osthole-Loaded Microemulsions as a Prospective Ocular Delivery System for the Treatment of Corneal Neovascularization: In Vitro and In Vivo Assessments".
12. "Discovery and Potential Utility of a Novel Non-Invasive Ocular Delivery Platform".
13. "Travoprost Liquid Nanocrystals: An Innovative Armamentarium for Effective Glaucoma Therapy".

In this way, readers will have the opportunity to read three excellent review articles on different topics, including the use of suprachoroidal injection for drug delivery. The second article covers different innovative strategies for drug delivery to the ocular posterior segment, namely, the use of nanomedicine, liposomes, nanomicelles, dendrimers, organic nanopolymers, ocular inserts, hydrogels, and contact lenses, among others. Finally, the last article covers the use of honey in the treatment of dry eye disease.

As far as the research articles are concerned, several examples of targeted and controlled release of ocular drugs are presented, namely, rutin/sulfobutylether-β-cyclodextrin for ocular injection, resveratrol and melatonin self-nanoemulsifying drug delivery systems (SNEDDS) for ocular administration, enzyme-triggered, therapeutic-releasing hydrogel bandage contact lens material, celecoxib/cyclodextrin eye drop microsuspensions, zinc sulfate cross-linked polysaccharide delivery system of dexamethasone phosphate, osthole-loaded microemulsions for the treatment of corneal neovascularization, and finally, travoprost liquid nanocrystals for the treatment of glaucoma.

We would like to take this opportunity to thank all the authors who have made an exemplary contribution with their valuable literature reviews and scientific research in the field of the ocular drug delivery.

We also believe that the works carried out by everyone and presented in this excellent Topic are exceptional contributions to the continued and future scientific progress in the field of ophthalmic modified drug release.

Conflicts of Interest: The authors declare no conflicts of interest.

pharmaceuticals

MDPI

Review

Suprachoroidal Injection: A Novel Approach for Targeted Drug Delivery

Kevin Y. Wu [1], Jamie K. Fujioka [2], Tara Gholamian [3], Marian Zaharia [1] and Simon D. Tran [4,*]

1 Department of Surgery, Division of Ophthalmology, University of Sherbrooke, Sherbrooke, QC J1G 2E8, Canada; yang.wu@usherbrooke.ca (K.Y.W.)
2 Faculty of Medicine, Queen's University, Kingston, ON K7L 3N6, Canada
3 Faculty of Medicine, University of Ottawa, Ottawa, ON K1H 8M5, Canada
4 Faculty of Dental Medicine and Oral Health Sciences, McGill University, Montreal, QC H3A 1G1, Canada
* Correspondence: simon.tran@mcgill.ca

Abstract: Treating posterior segment and retinal diseases poses challenges due to the complex structures in the eye that act as robust barriers, limiting medication delivery and bioavailability. This necessitates frequent dosing, typically via eye drops or intravitreal injections, to manage diseases, often leading to side effects with long-term use. Suprachoroidal injection is a novel approach for targeted drug delivery to the posterior segment. The suprachoroidal space is the region between the sclera and the choroid and provides a potential route for minimally invasive medication delivery. Through a more targeted delivery to the posterior segment, this method offers advantages over other routes of administration, such as higher drug concentrations, increased bioavailability, and prolonged duration of action. Additionally, this approach minimizes the risk of corticosteroid-related adverse events such as cataracts and intraocular pressure elevation via compartmentalization. This review focuses on preclinical and clinical studies published between 2019 and 2023, highlighting the potential of suprachoroidal injection in treating a variety of posterior segment diseases. However, to fully harness its potential, more research is needed to address current challenges and limitations, such as the need for technological advancements, refinement of injection techniques, and consideration of cost and accessibility factors. Future studies exploring its use in conjunction with biotech products, gene therapies, and cell-based therapies can lead to personalized treatments that can revolutionize the field of ophthalmology.

Keywords: ophthalmology; ocular diseases; drug delivery; controlled drug release; retina; posterior segment diseases; ocular drug bioavailability; suprachoroidal injection

Citation: Wu, K.Y.; Fujioka, J.K.; Gholamian, T.; Zaharia, M.; Tran, S.D. Suprachoroidal Injection: A Novel Approach for Targeted Drug Delivery. *Pharmaceuticals* **2023**, *16*, 1241. https://doi.org/10.3390/ph16091241

Academic Editors: Rosario Pignatello, Hugo Almeida, Carmelo Puglia and Debora Santonocito

Received: 29 July 2023
Revised: 22 August 2023
Accepted: 28 August 2023
Published: 1 September 2023

1. Introduction

The landscape of ocular drug delivery is in constant evolution, presenting new challenges and opportunities in the field of ophthalmology. Treating posterior segment and retinal diseases is particularly challenging due to the eye's complex structures that act as barriers to drug delivery and bioavailability [1]. Traditional administration methods, such as eye drops, periocular and intravitreal (IV) injections, and systemic medications, often require frequent dosing and can result in substantial side effects with long-term use [2]. Recently, suprachoroidal (SC) injection has emerged as a novel strategy for targeted drug delivery to the posterior segment of the eye, offering an innovative approach to address these challenges [3].

The suprachoroidal space (SCS), an anatomical niche nestled between the sclera and the choroid, provides a minimally invasive conduit for precise medication delivery. This approach not only enhances drug concentrations in the posterior segment, increasing drug bioavailability and duration of action but also minimizes the risk of corticosteroid-related adverse events through compartmentalization [4]. The potential of SC injection has been highlighted by promising results from recent preclinical and clinical studies.

This review offers a comprehensive overview of SC injection, covering its rationale, techniques, biomechanics, and implications in treating diverse ocular diseases, particularly those affecting the posterior segment. We also explore the current challenges and future prospects of this technique.

While prior review articles have mainly addressed the use of SC injection for macular edema secondary to conditions such as uveitis, diabetic retinopathy, or CRVO [5–7], our review uniquely extends beyond existing clinical data. We explore not only the application of this technique in clinical settings but also delve into preclinical studies for other ocular conditions such as glaucoma, retinitis pigmentosa, and various chorioretinal diseases. This review goes beyond simply informing clinicians about existing indications as we shed light on new therapeutic possibilities emerging from preclinical studies yet to be applied to human subjects. Furthermore, our examination of the biomechanics of SC injection serves to bridge the gap between theoretical understanding and clinical practice by exploring how alterations in various physical parameters of the injection can influence its applicability.

To achieve this, we performed an extensive literature review, mainly focusing on articles published post-2020, to ensure the inclusion of the latest advancements and insights. Through this exploration, we aspire to capture the current state of this technique, elucidate potential avenues for improvement and innovation, and provide a reference point for further research and clinical applications in this rapidly evolving field.

2. Anatomy and Physiology

2.1. Choroid

The choroid, a layer in the eye, is nourished by blood from the posterior ciliary arteries. This blood flows through two key sub-layers of choroidal vessels, the Haller and Sattler layers, to reach the choriocapillaris, where arterial pressure reduces to a lower level. The choroid's thickness varies across its expanse, being thickest in the central macular region and thinnest at the ora serrata. Typically, in most 50-year-olds, the choroid measures about 287 μm subfoveally, though thickness can vary with age and ocular disease conditions [8].

Located in the posterior pole, the choriocapillaries feature an intricate capillary network that is more irregular toward the periphery. The choroid's composition also includes loose connective tissue, fibroblasts, and melanocytes. In the post-choriocapillaris, blood is gathered in venules, followed by larger channels, to drain into the superior and inferior ophthalmic veins through the vortex veins [9].

The choroid plays a crucial role in supplying nutrients, particularly oxygen, to the retina, one of the body's most metabolically active tissues (Figure 1). Approximately 90% of the oxygen consumed by the outer retina, housing photoreceptors, and retinal pigment epithelium (RPE), is provided by choroidal circulation. Furthermore, the choroid features the highest blood flow rate of any tissue in the body. Despite the high metabolic demand of these tissues, the exiting venous blood maintains high oxygen tension, reflecting the choroid's efficient function in nutrient delivery and metabolic waste removal [9].

2.2. Sclera

The sclera consists of collagen and a small number of elastic fibers embedded in a proteoglycan matrix. Its thickness varies, being the thinnest near the muscle insertion sites and thicker posterior to the limbus, where it terminates [10].

An essential characteristic of the sclera is its permeability, facilitating bidirectional molecular transport. Its permeability enables drug delivery via injections into the sub-Tenon space. However, the sclera's hydrophilic nature means that its permeability to hydrophobic or amphiphilic substances, including certain medications, can vary. This property is a crucial factor to consider when planning periocular injections of pharmacological agents [11].

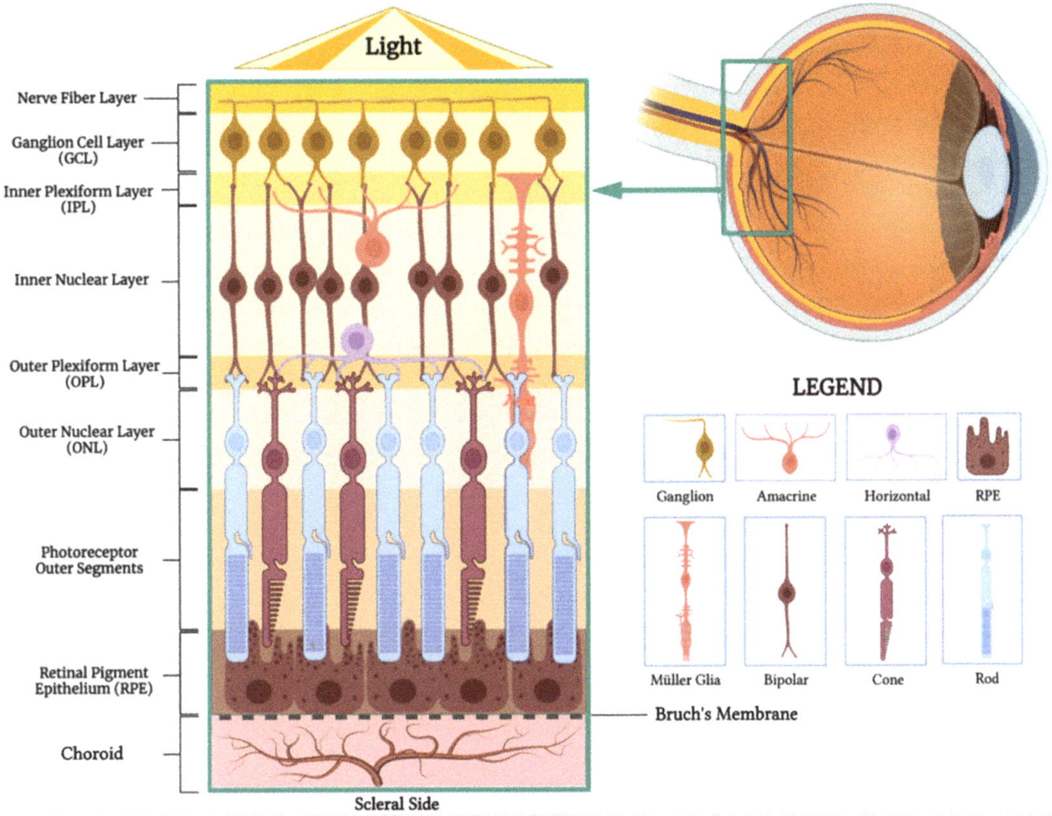

Figure 1. Anatomy of the Retina and Choroid. Critical Role of the Choroid in Nutrient Supply to the Retina.

The thickness of the human sclera varies between individuals and across different regions of the eye. A histomorphometric study conducted by Vurgese, Panda-Jonas, and Jonas on 238 human eyes found that in non-axially elongated eyes (axial length $\leq$ 26 mm, with the average axial length usually being around 23 mm), the sclera was thickest at the posterior pole (0.94 $\pm$ 0.18 mm), followed by the peri-optic nerve region (0.86 $\pm$ 0.21 mm), and the midpoint between the posterior pole and equator (0.65 $\pm$ 0.15 mm). The thickness decreases toward the limbus (0.50 $\pm$ 0.11 mm), the ora serrata (0.43 $\pm$ 0.14 mm), and the equator (0.42 $\pm$ 0.15 mm) and is the thinnest at the peripapillary scleral flange (0.39 $\pm$ 0.09 mm) [11]. The relatively small inter-individual variability in scleral thickness supports a standardized approach to injections, allowing clinicians to use a uniform microneedle length. For most cases, a 0.9 mm microneedle suffices, while certain scenarios may require a slightly longer 1.1 mm microneedle [12,13]. This finding simplifies the suprachoroidal injection procedure, as it reduces the need for individualized microneedle length adjustments based on patient-specific ocular characteristics.

For axially elongated eyes (i.e., myopic eyes, axial length > 26 mm), scleral thinning is more pronounced at and posterior to the equator, with a greater thinning as it nears the posterior pole [11]. Interestingly, the inter-individual variability in scleral thickness is found to be different in high myopia. However, despite this regional scleral thinning, it does not necessitate alterations in the needle length for suprachoroidal injections. This is due to the fact that these injections are typically administered at an anterior location where the thickness of the sclera is relatively consistent among individuals [14].

2.3. Suprachoroidal Space

The SCS is a potential area nestled between the sclera and the choroid (Figure 2) [15]. This space is often in close contact due to the intraocular pressure (IOP) [16] and the presence of attaching fibers [17]. However, the introduction of fluid, whether internally or externally, can transform this potential space into a more defined one.

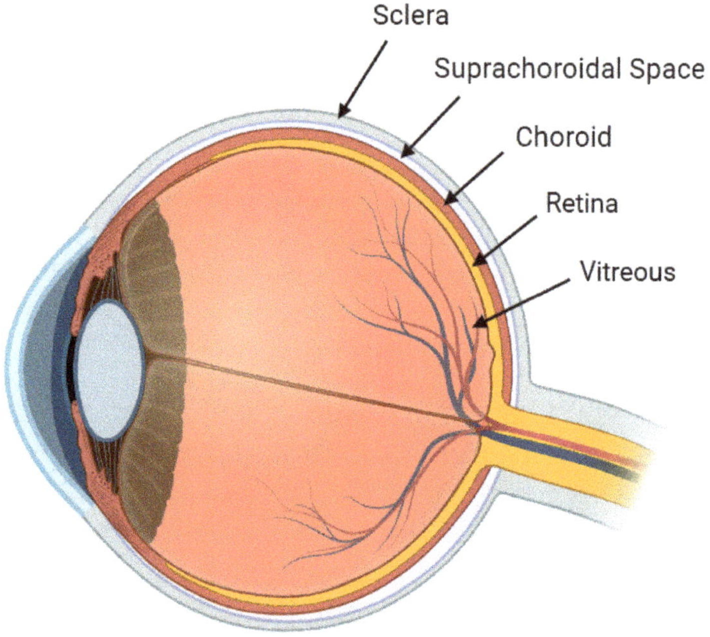

Figure 2. Anatomy of the Suprachoroidal Space and Posterior Segment.

The SCS has shown considerable expansion following the injection of certain drugs in this area. A study involving the injection of triamcinolone acetonide in the SCS demonstrated a notable increase in mean SCS width, from 9.9 μm to 75.1 μm [4]. This expansion proved the influence of SC injection in manipulating the SCS's physical attributes. However, the increase was temporary, with the SCS width returning to approximately 14.9 μm a month after the final injection, revealing no lasting impact on the SCS's anatomy [4].

The SCS, located between the sclera and choroid, has boundaries that are anatomically distinct. Anteriorly, the SCS extends up to the scleral spur, a pivotal landmark that marks the juncture of scleral attachment to the ciliary body. Posteriorly, the SCS is situated near the optic nerve and short posterior ciliary arteries [3,12,18,19]. It is essential to recognize the anatomical placement of the SCS when considering pharmacological interventions, such as SC injections. Distinguishing the SCS from the subretinal space is crucial, as the former lacks the immune privilege characteristic due to its position outside the blood–retinal barrier. For clarity, it is worth revisiting the structure of the blood–ocular barrier. This barrier consists of the vascular endothelium of the retina, which is non-fenestrated and bound by tight junctions. Although the choroidal vessels are fenestrated, the barrier is maintained through the presence of tight junctions within the retinal pigment epithelium (RPE) [3,12,18,19].

3. Route of Administration

Numerous routes are available for administering ocular medications, each with unique strengths and weaknesses. Standard methods include systemic delivery (e.g., oral, intravenous, and subcutaneous routes) and local delivery methods (e.g., topical eye drops, periocular or IV injections, and IV implants). While these methods can be effective, they can also come with certain limitations [20]. An overview of the advantages and disadvantages associated with each ocular drug administration method is summarized in Table 1: Comparison of Different Ocular Drug Administration Methods and Figure 3 [2,21].

Table 1. Comparison of Different Ocular Drug Administration Methods [2,20,21].

Injection Method	Advantages	Disadvantages
Topical Eye Drops [22]	Prevalent, well-known method	Low bioavailability to posterior segment tissues
	Non-invasive method for ocular drug delivery	Short duration of action, requiring frequent administration
		Relies on patient's compliance
		Local complications (ocular surface irritation, cataracts, ocular hypertension, periocular aesthetic issues)
Systemic Drug Administration	Noninvasive and potentially patient-preferred	High doses often required due to reduced accessibility to targeted ocular tissues
	Usable as standalone or in combination with topical delivery	Potential systemic side effects due to high dosage, necessitating safety and toxicity considerations
		Effective bioavailability is challenging due to blood–ocular barriers
Intravitreal Injection [23]	Office-based, outpatient procedure	Requires frequent in-office visits
	High bioavailability (bypass corneal and blood–retinal barriers)	Potential for severe complications (Endophthalmitis, retinal detachment, vitreous hemorrhage)
	Fewer systemic side effects compared to oral or IV administration	Local complications (increased IOP, cataract formation)
	Rapid therapeutic onset	Possible post-injection floaters
		Systemic absorption and side effects can still occur
Subretinal Injection [24]	Targeted treatment for the RPE and outer retina	Invasive procedure, requires vitrectomy
	Reduced immune reactions for gene therapy using viral vectors (due to injection in an immune-privileged site)	Limited distribution of injectate within subretinal space; effects confined to injection site

3.1. Topical Administration

Topical administration, often in the form of eye drops, is a prevalent non-invasive method for ocular drug delivery. However, it is associated with several challenges as a consequence of the anatomy and physiology of the eye.

First, the concentration gradient from the tear reservoir to the cornea or conjunctiva drives passive absorption, but only approximately 20% of a drop (about 10 μL of the 50 μL drop) is retained in the eye [25]. Within 3–4 min, half of the administered medication has typically left the eye, with a turnover rate of roughly 15% per minute. Factors such as reflex tearing, consecutive dosing, and the small cul-de-sac of the eye contribute to a fast tear turnover time, further accelerating drug clearance and challenging the effective drug absorption [2,21].

Second, medications need to travel through the dual barriers posed by the hydrophobic tight junctions formed by the epithelium and endothelium, as well as the hydrophilic stroma layer of the cornea (Figure 3) [26]. The inherent low permeability of the cornea and sclera impedes this process, diminishing the bioavailability of the topically administered drug.

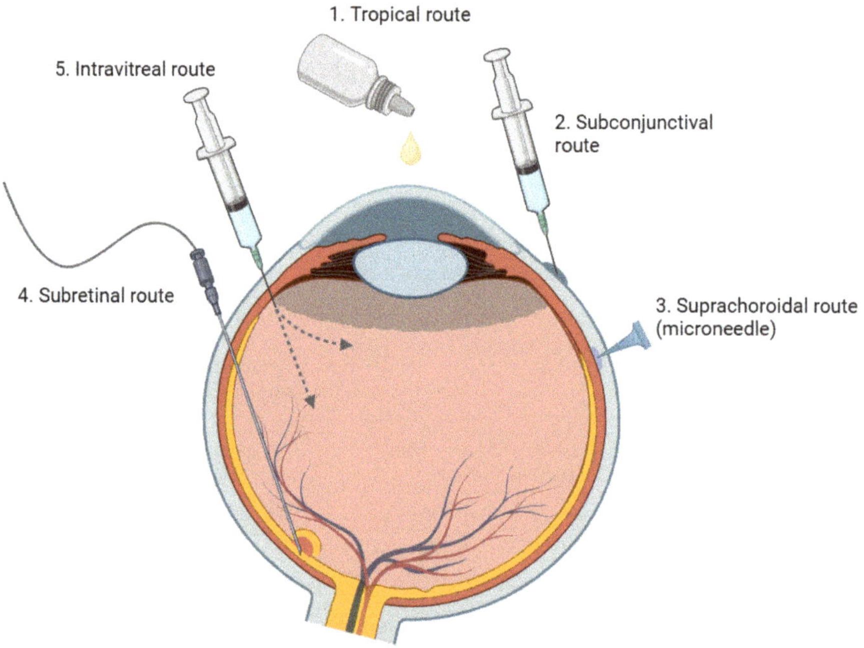

Figure 3. An Overview of Various Ophthalmic Medication Delivery Routes. This figure illustrates the range of administration methods used in ophthalmic medicine, including topical, subconjunctival, intravitreal, suprachoroidal, and subretinal techniques.

Due to the relatively impermeable corneal barriers and high tear turnover rates, topical administration often necessitates frequent, high-dose applications. This approach can cause local and systemic side effects, potentially reducing patient compliance [27]. Remarkably, studies have indicated that the rate of medication non-compliance in the general population is approximately 80% [28]. Such challenges are often exacerbated in certain populations, such as the elderly and those with physical disabilities.

Additionally, the exposure of unaffected tissue to drugs may lead to certain side effects. For instance, chronic usage of topical steroids can result in complications such as cataracts and ocular hypertension [22]. Similarly, topical prostaglandins can lead to undesirable periocular aesthetic concerns [29].

Overall, while topical application serves as a primary mode of ocular drug delivery, these complexities underline the need for advancements in methods of drug delivery.

3.2. Systemic Administration

Oral delivery has been explored as a potential drug administration route for ocular conditions, either standalone or in combination with topical delivery [30–33]. Although it could be a noninvasive, patient-preferred method for managing chronic retinal diseases, the limitations of oral administration include its reduced accessibility to many targeted ocular tissues, necessitating high doses for therapeutic efficacy. However, high dosage can result in systemic side effects, making safety and toxicity critical considerations [34,35].

For the oral route to be effective in ocular applications, high oral bioavailability is a key requirement. Furthermore, following oral absorption, molecules must navigate through systemic circulation and across the blood–ocular barriers, notably the blood–aqueous and blood–retinal barriers (Figure 4). The blood–retinal barrier is further stratified into an inner barrier, protected by the fenestrated endothelium of retinal vasculature, and an outer barrier, upheld by tight junctions within the RPE. The functional properties and inherent barriers posed by these protective ocular structures represent significant challenges for the systemic drug administration [34,35].

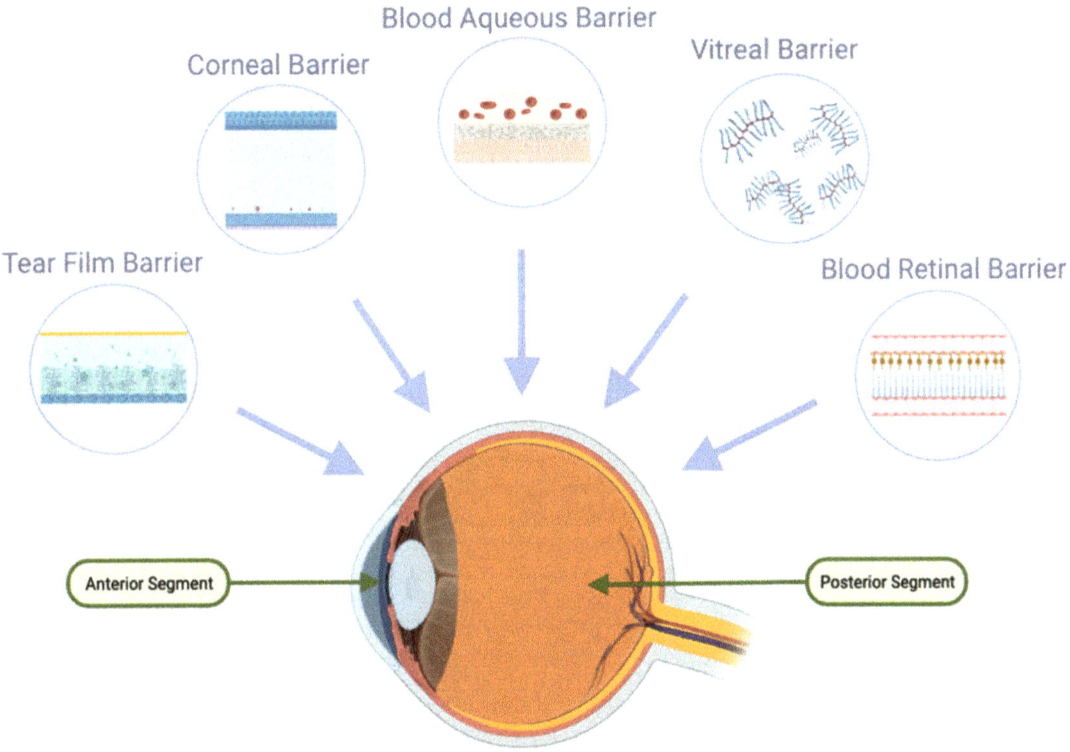

Figure 4. Anatomical and Physiological Barriers in the Eye Impacting Drug Delivery.

For instance, systemic medications, such as steroidal and nonsteroidal anti-inflammato ry drugs and biologic and nonbiologic immunomodulatory agents, can effectively treat uveitic macular edema (UME) but are often recommended for bilateral disease or cases resistant to local therapy due to AEs such as infections and GI disturbances [20,36,37]. Furthermore, nonsteroidal anti-inflammatory drugs and systemic immunomodulatory agents may increase the risk of GI disturbances when used alone or combined with steroids [20,36,37].

3.3. Periocular Injection

Periocular drug administration is employed to address the inefficiencies of topical and systemic dosing, both of which struggle to deliver therapeutic drug concentrations to the posterior segment [2]. The periocular route, including subconjunctival, subtenon, retrobulbar, and peribulbar administrations, is comparatively less invasive than IV drug administration [2].

Subconjunctival injections can improve water-soluble drug absorption by bypassing the conjunctival epithelial barrier. However, drug access to the posterior eye segment is still restricted due to various barriers, including dynamic ones such as conjunctival blood and lymphatic circulation [38–40]. These dynamic barriers often result in rapid drug elimination, reducing ocular bioavailability and vitreous drug levels post-administration [38–40]. While the permeable sclera allows for some molecules to reach the neural retina and photoreceptor cells [20,41], the choroid's high blood flow can remove a significant drug fraction before it reaches its target. Further limitations are posed by the blood–retinal barriers formed by the tight junction within the RPE, restricting drug availability to the photoreceptor cells.

3.4. Intravitreal Injection

In the realm of ocular drug delivery, IV administration offers numerous advantages and has been widely adopted as a first-line therapy for conditions such as neovascular age-related macular degeneration (nAMD) [42], diabetic macular edema (DME) [43], and macular edema secondary to retinal vein occlusion (RVO) [44]. It has been well-accepted due to its proven safety and efficacy alongside the convenience of application in an office setting. Its popularity arises from its salient advantages, such as direct medication delivery to the retina and vitreous by bypassing corneal and scleral barriers (as compared to topical eyedrops) and the ability to circumvent the blood–retinal barrier (unlike systemic medications). This ensures high bioavailability in the target area, triggering rapid therapeutic effects. This method also addresses issues with patient non-compliance typically associated with topical eyedrops, as the administration is under the direct control of an ophthalmologist. The versatility of IV administration covers a spectrum of therapeutics, including anti-VEGF agents and corticosteroids, rendering it highly effective for a wide range of retinal diseases [45].

However, IV injections are not without certain drawbacks and potential complications. Severe complications can occur, which include the risk of endophthalmitis, retinal detachment, and vitreous hemorrhage. Furthermore, IV steroids specifically have associated complications such as increased intraocular pressure and cataract development [43]. These complexities not only challenge the treatment process but also hinder achieving optimal visual outcomes [43]. Minor side effects and inconveniences, such as floaters post-injection and the potential for systemic absorption and resultant side effects, can also adversely affect patient satisfaction and treatment adherence [43].

Another hindrance to optimal IV injection outcomes lies in the necessity for a frequent injection regimen due to the short half-life of these drugs [46–48]. After the IV injection, the drug is primarily expelled either anteriorly or posteriorly. Anterior elimination entails drug diffusion through the vitreous to the aqueous humor and then removal via aqueous turnover and uveal blood flow. Posterior elimination involves the drug permeating the blood–retinal barrier, necessitating either effective passive permeability or active transport mechanisms. Consequently, compounds with hydrophilic properties and large molecular weights tend to have longer half-lives within the vitreous humor [20]. In contrast, hydrophobic drugs with smaller molecular weights tend to have a shorter half-life, implying the need for frequent injections. Regular in-office visits can be burdensome for individuals residing in rural areas or managing chronic conditions, leading to patient non-compliance, which inevitably reduces the overall effectiveness of the treatment [48]. Furthermore, the clearance rate can vary based on patient-specific factors, such as age and whether the patient has undergone a vitrectomy, which adds another layer of complexity to the treatment regimen [49].

To address the challenges of short treatment duration and frequent in-office visits, intraocular implants have been strategically designed. For instance, the Multicenter Uveitis Steroid Treatment (MUST) randomized controlled trial (RCT) (NCT00132691) evaluated the efficacy and safety of a 0.59 mg fluocinolone acetonide (FA) intraocular implant, which releases the drug over approximately 30 months [50]. The study found that the FA implant improved uveitic inflammation control and reduced macular edema (ME) more effectively than systemic corticosteroids in the short term, although the differences diminished by 24 months [51]. Additionally, the FA implant was linked to a fourfold increase in the risk of elevated intraocular pressure (IOP) requiring intervention [51]. After seven years of extended follow-up, patients who received systemic therapy demonstrated better visual acuity than those with IV FA implants [51].

In the field of gene therapy, while early trials on an anti-VEGF transgene product (Adverum Biotechnologies) have shown promise, concerns arise due to the significant inflammatory responses of injecting it intravitreally [52–55]. The vitreous poses an additional hurdle for retinal gene delivery due to its component, particularly hyaluronan, which can interact with cationic lipid, polymeric, and liposomal DNA complexes, leading to severe aggregation and immobilization of DNA/liposome complexes [56,57]. Moreover, the inner limiting membrane (ILM), which separates the retina and vitreous, serves as a barrier to the retinal delivery of gene-based therapies [58]. For choroidal diseases, drug transport from the vitreous to the choroid is difficult due to the presence of the RPE, which serves as a barrier (i.e., outer blood–retinal barrier formed by the tight junction within RPE) [9].

Emerging alternatives, such as subretinal and SC drug delivery, could potentially offer longer-lasting effects, reducing injection frequency and limiting side effects, including gene therapy-induced inflammation [59].

3.5. Subretinal Injection

Subretinal delivery presents a compelling avenue for retinal gene therapy, especially for the treatment of retinal degeneration and vascular diseases. This approach involves the direct introduction of viral vectors into the subretinal space—an immune-privileged site—thus allowing targeted treatment for the RPE and outer retina while reducing the likelihood of immune reactions [24].

The first FDA-approved gene therapy for RPE65-associated inherited retinal dystrophy, Voretigene neparvovec-rzyl (Luxturna), has provided promising outcomes [60,61]. The potential of gene therapy also extends to conditions such as diabetic retinopathy (DR) and age-related macular degeneration (AMD), suggesting the possibility of a single-dose treatment for these chronic diseases. Early data from studies using subretinal adenoviral vector anti-VEGF gene therapy point toward a significant decrease in treatment burden and an encouraging safety profile for nAMD [62].

However, it is important to note that subretinal delivery does have its own set of challenges. It is invasive in nature, requiring a vitrectomy for administration. Moreover, the localized nature of the injectate can limit its distribution within the subretinal space, potentially confining the therapeutic effects to the area surrounding the injection site [59].

4. Suprachoroidal Injection: Rationale

SC injection offers a treatment pathway that is both minimally invasive and potentially long-lasting, effectively combining the advantages of IV and subretinal injections [59,63]. Notably, the SCS can be accessed using a variety of tools, including catheters, needles, and microneedles. The use of a microneedle provides more precise targeting and control during in-office deliveries to the SCS compared to traditional hypodermic needles [59].

4.1. Advantages over the Intravitreal Injection

SC injection stands out as a method that enables precise and targeted delivery to the retina, RPE, and choroid. By bypassing barriers such as the ILM and vitreous, which are commonly encountered in the IV drug administration [64], this method achieves broader bioavailability across the diseased retina and choroid [59,63].

The unique compartmentalization provided by SC injection within the SCS plays a pivotal role in its advantages. This containment restricts drug exposure to target tissues, minimizing unnecessary contact with the anterior segment [59,64], which, in turn, reduces the risk of complications such as cataract formation and elevated intraocular pressure [24]. Furthermore, this compartmentalization minimizes systemic absorption, leading to fewer systemic side effects [24]. Supporting these benefits, a 2022 study involving rabbits demonstrated that SC delivery of TRIESENCE provided a 12-fold greater exposure to the RPE, choroid, sclera, and retina compared to IV delivery [24]. Remarkably, the same study found that SC delivery resulted in a 460-, 34-, and 22-fold reduction in drug exposure to anterior chamber structures, specifically the lens, iris ciliary body, and the vitreous humor, respectively [24]. This decreased exposure highlights the enhanced safety profile of SC drug delivery [24].

Moreover, SC injection offers a sustained-release mechanism, reducing the frequency of injections and, consequently, the number of patient appointments [59]. Unlike the IV space, the SCS is not immune-privileged, thereby theoretically posing a lower risk of endophthalmitis, although further studies are required to substantiate this claim [24]. Furthermore, by avoiding injections directly into the vitreous cavity, risks associated with this method, such as traumatic cataracts and retinal tears with their subsequent potential for detachments, might also be diminished. Further enhancing the patient experience, SC injection mitigates the risk of visual axis obstruction, leading to fewer incidences of post-injection floaters, a common side effect with IV methods [59].

4.2. Advantages over Subretinal Injection

When compared to subretinal injection, the SC method can be administered in an outpatient setting, reducing the need for complex surgical procedures such as vitrectomy [59,63]. Furthermore, it offers the potential to provide a broader distribution of drugs across the posterior segment [64].

4.3. Drug Suspension Size and Formulation Viscosity

Current research is exploring the potential to alter drug suspension size and formulation viscosity in order to adjust the duration and distribution of the injected drugs. This flexibility could allow precise tailoring of drug delivery, ensuring that the right amount of medication reaches the target location.

4.4. Cost-Effectiveness

Over a 10-year horizon, a simulated US adult patient-level model evaluated the cost-effectiveness of suprachoroidal triamcinolone acetonide (SC-TA) compared to the best supportive care for UME derived from the PEACHTREE trial. The authors determined that, at willingness-to-pay thresholds of $50,000 or more (2020 US dollars) per quality-adjusted life-year gained, SCTA was a cost-effective procedure [5].

The combined practicality, enhanced safety profile, proven efficacy, targeted delivery, and durability offered by SC drug delivery have made SC injections an innovative treatment modality for diverse ocular conditions. This underlines the imperative for more extensive research into this therapeutic strategy, which is also the focus of this review article.

5. Suprachoroidal Injection Techniques

Access to the SCS is typically achieved using the following three methods: microcatheters; needles; and microneedles. Catheter-based technology, such as the iTrack microcatheter, involves the insertion of a 250 A microcatheter into the SCS [65]. Using an incision site in the sclera, the microcatheter is carefully advanced through the SCS toward the designated treatment zone. The placement of the microcatheter can be confirmed and adjusted as needed using indirect ophthalmoscopy to ensure accurate positioning. Advantages of this technique include precise targeting and visualization, as the catheter can be guided with a flashing diode [7]. However, drawbacks of using this method include the fact that it is an invasive procedure that typically requires an operating room, and the success of the injection relies on the skills of the administrator. As with all procedures, there are risks of adverse events and complications such as vitreous penetration, SC hemorrhage, choroidal tears, irregularities in choroidal blood flow, post-operative inflammation, scleral ectasia, retinal detachment, wound abscess, and endophthalmitis among others.

Injection into the SCS can also be achieved by a free-hand technique using a standard hypodermic needle attached to a Hamilton syringe or insulin syringe [7,66,67]. In this approach, the needle is inserted through the sclera behind the limbus, with or without sclerotomy. Slow and controlled advancement of the needle is performed by applying gentle pressure on the plunger, and the injection is administered gradually upon experiencing a loss of resistance. The use of standard hypodermic needles offers the advantage of readily available materials and a less invasive procedure, making it more accessible and convenient. However, this technique lacks visualization capabilities and, thus, requires a high level of training and skill to ensure precise injection. There is a risk of inadvertently injecting into unintended structures, which can lead to complications such as choroidal hemorrhage and retinal detachment. The difficulty in controlling the insertion depth and angle further increases the likelihood of unintentional IV or subretinal injections.

Hollow microneedles are miniature devices used primarily for transdermal drug delivery [7,13]. These microneedles possess a hollow internal compartment filled with drug dispersion or solution and tips with small holes. Recent advancements in microneedle technology have revolutionized the accessibility of the SCS without the need for surgical procedures. The SCS microinjector is a manual piston syringe used for accessing the SCS non-surgically. It is designed to be used with varying microneedle lengths (900 μm or 1100 μm) depending on the scleral thickness, which is penetrated until a loss of resistance is felt [68]. In order to minimize the risk of vitreous perforation, the microneedle is slightly longer than the scleral and conjunctival layers. Drug administration with the SCS microinjector involves several steps. First, under local anesthesia, a 900 μm microneedle is positioned perpendicularly 4.5 mm posterior to the limbus at the pars plana (the flat area of the ciliary body). Gentle pressure is applied to the ocular surface to create a sealing gasket between the needle hub and conjunctiva, preventing the backflow of the injectate. The injection into the SCS occurs over 5–10 s while maintaining the perpendicular position and compressing the conjunctiva. After the injection, upon reaching the SCS, the needle hub should be kept in place for 3 to 5 s. If scleral resistance is still felt, an 1100 μm microneedle should be used instead [69].

Microneedle technology offers precise control in reaching the SCS, unlike standard hypodermic needles [7,13]. Short microneedles limit penetration into the SCS by penetrating the sclera consistently and facilitating drug delivery to the intended site. Once inside the SCS, the injectate spreads posteriorly and circumferentially, ensuring broad coverage. In contrast to catheter-based procedures, microneedle-based SC injections can be performed in an office setting under aseptic conditions without requiring vitrectomy or sclerotomy. These SCS microneedles are specifically designed to match the approximate thickness of the sclera and offer several advantages, including ease of use, minimal pain, affordability, minimal invasiveness, low training requirements, outpatient suitability, and improved safety profile. As a result, they represent the most promising route for drug administration.

6. Biomechanics of Suprachoroidal Injection

6.1. Injection Forces

SC injections performed with a microinjector only require the mechanical force applied by a physician's hand to deliver the therapeutic formulation into the SCS. An average glide force of 2.07 N was recorded as the mechanical pressure necessary to administer suprachoroidal triamcinolone acetonide (SCTA) into the SCS of in vivo porcine eyes [70,71]. An SCTA prototype, X-TA, was specifically formulated by Muya and collaborators for SC injections aiming to reduce friction, minimize foaming, and prevent microbubble formation. The glide force of X-TA was compared to Triesence TA (TRI) formulated for IV injections, as well as water and air, which served as control measurements. Interestingly, they found that the injection of X-TA required a smaller glide force (0.73 N) with lower variability than TRI (1.31 N), closer to that of air (0.19 N) and water (0.23 N). This discrepancy could be attributed to the larger size of TRI particles, which likely contributed to the higher and more inconsistent glide force required for its delivery. Adapting formulations specifically for SC injections has the potential to reduce the required glide force and improve the stability of the procedure. This is important for achieving higher success rates of therapeutic injections into the SCS for the treatment of various ocular diseases [72].

6.2. Volume and Injections into Multiple Quadrants

Optimizing SC surface coverage is crucial for the effective treatment of posterior segment pathologies such as AMD, DR, and RVOs. The volume of injectate has a significant role in drug distribution, directly influencing therapeutic coverage and, as a result, outcomes.

In an animal study by Gu and collaborators, it was found that injecting 20 μL of saline and TA expanded the SCS by 130% to 200% more than a 10 μL injection, highlighting the effect of the volume of injectate [73]. However, ex vivo experiments using rabbit eyes demonstrated that larger volumes injected in the SCS primarily increased circumferential coverage rather than thickness [19]. Quantitatively, injecting ≥75 μL of fluorescein covered at least 50% of the choroidal surface, while 100 μL covered approximately 75% of the posterior globe [74,75]. At smaller volumes, thickness expansion appeared to be influenced by the volume of injectate, whereas at larger volumes, circumferential distribution played a more significant role. This discrepancy could be attributed to the presence of lamellae structures between the choroid and the sclera, which restrict expansion of the SCS and direct the flow of fluid posteriorly with larger volumes [75]. One potential solution to overcome this restriction is to degrade the fibrils using collagenase, as adding a 0.5 mg/mL collagenase preparation to the formulation of 1 μm latex microparticles resulted in a 20% to 45% increase in SCS coverage during ex vivo experiments with rabbit eyes [76]. Simultaneous injection of collagenase and latex particles in a single injection yielded better outcomes than subsequent injections. However, this approach is not suitable for individuals with a latex allergy. Non-uniform fluid distribution of injectate in the SCS occurs partially due to anatomical barriers, such as the scleral spur, optic nerve, and short ciliary arteries. To enhance coverage and achieve even more fluid distribution, Nork and collaborators performed injections in multiple eye quadrants in a rabbit study [77]. They were able to demonstrate that injecting 50 μL of sodium fluorescein in the superior-temporal and inferonasal quadrants was sufficient to cover the entire choroid, suggesting that multiple injections in opposing quadrants could be an effective strategy to maximize SCS coverage [77]. This comprehensive coverage of the entire choroid surface can be particularly important in the treatment of certain generalized choroidal–retinal dystrophies, such as retinitis pigmentosa. In these cases, it is beneficial to deliver the therapeutic agent across all affected areas, making the approach of multiple injections in opposing quadrants particularly valuable.

6.3. Viscosity and Polymeric Solution Formulations

Viscosity is another modifiable characteristic of formulations that can be adjusted to optimize the treatment of specific posterior segment conditions. The behavior of fluids with different viscosities, such as Hank's Balanced salt solution (HBSS, viscosity of ≈75,000 ± 35,000 cPs), DisCoVisc (viscosity of ≈75,000 ± 35,000 cPs), and 5% carboxymethyl cellulose (CMC, viscosity of ≈200,000 cPs) has been analyzed [75,78]. The size of the injection site opening was found to be 0.43 ± 0.06 mm for HBSS and 2.1 ± 0.1 mm for 5% CMC. The SCS collapse rate after injection was 19 min for HBSS and 9 days for CMC. HBSS was no longer detectable after 0.33 ± 0.05 days, whereas it took 1.7 ± 0.7 days for the 5% CMC to be cleared. Higher viscosity agents tend to induce greater expansion and slower SCS collapse rates due to their low aqueous solubility and slow dissolution rate [68].

The shear-thinning (S-T) property is the non-Newtonian behavior of fluids, characterized by lower viscosity as the shear rate increases. Kim and collaborators investigated the following fluids with different behaviors: HBSS (lower S-T fluid); DisCoVisc, 2.2 wt% 950 kDa hyaluronic acid (HA) (moderate S-T fluids); and 1.7 wt% 700 kDa CMC and 3 wt% 90 kDa methylcellulose (higher S-T fluids) [79]. These fluids were mixed with fluorescent particles, injected, and analyzed. HBSS spread more rapidly compared to moderate and high S-T fluids. After 14 days, circumferential spread increased more for moderate S-T fluids and remained relatively unchanged for high S-T fluids [79]. In addition to these results, Jung and collaborators developed an in situ-forming hydrogel of Bevacizumab and HA cross-linked with poly (ethylene glycol) diacrylate. When liquid Bevacizumab was used alone, it was cleared from the SCS within 5 days. However, when formulated with a high molecular weight (MW) HA or cross-linked to poly (ethylene glycol) diacrylate, it took 1 month and 6 months, respectively, for clearance [80]. These studies demonstrate that viscosity is an important property of fluids and that polymeric solutions can be manipulated to optimize SC injections. The utilization of polymers extends the duration of drug retention within the suprachoroidal space (SCS) and assists in managing its dispersion. Polymers with elevated molecular weight (MW) and a moderate degree of non-Newtonian behavior, such as hyaluronic acid (HA), have been demonstrated to promote the dispersion of particles. Conversely, polymer solutions with pronounced non-Newtonian characteristics, such as methylcellulose (MC) and carboxymethylcellulose (CMC), tend to remain stationary at the injection site. This approach potentially enhances the efficiency of the treatment by maintaining a higher and more sustained concentration of the drug at the target site, thereby reducing the rate of systemic absorption.

6.4. Particle Suspensions

Particle suspensions, which gradually dissolve over time, can be beneficial in achieving prolonged therapeutic effects on ocular tissues. The clearance kinetics of these suspensions are significantly influenced by the MW of the particles. In order to investigate this relationship, Chiang and collaborators conducted experiments using injections of fluorescein and HBSS containing fluorescent polymeric particles. While fluorescein was detectable for only 1 day, the fluorescent particles in the HBSS suspension were detected for up to 21 days post-injection [81]. Similarly, another experiment comparing fluorescein (detectable for 12 h) with fluorescent dextran (higher MW and hydrodynamic radius than fluorescein, detectable up to 4 days) observed that MW influences the duration of detection [82,83].

Particle size is another factor that significantly affects the clearance kinetics of particle suspensions. Clearance routes include diffusion into the sclera and choroid, transscleral leakage, and choroidal blood flow. The fenestrations of the choriocapillaris allow particles with an estimated size range of 6 to 12 nm to be cleared through choriocapillaris circulation. Larger particles ranging from 20 nm to 10 μm were found to remain in the SCS for several months [79]. In an experiment conducted by Hackett and collaborators using polymeric microparticles of poly (lacto-co-glycolic acid) (PLGA) loaded with acriflavine (ACF) of size 7 μm in Brown Norway rats, the particles were present in the SCS throughout the 16-weeks of the study [84].

However, larger particles may encounter injection difficulties due to their potential blockage by collagen fibers within the sclera, especially when using short microneedles. The spacing between collagen fibers is estimated to be around 300 nm, making injections of particles sized 500–1000 nm more challenging. Therefore, glide force becomes an important parameter for successful SCS delivery when injecting formulations of larger particles [85]. Patel and colleagues observed a significant difference in the distribution of small particles (20–100 nm) and large particles (500–1000 nm) with shorter needles. However, for longer microneedles (1000 μm), all particles behaved similarly, suggesting successful reach of the SCS [3].

Manual injections of particle suspensions ranging from 20 nm to 10 μm were performed by Kim and collaborators and Chiang and collaborators, who both reported similar findings, with particles remaining in the SCS for up to 3 months and consistent fluorescence levels for all particle sizes. This indicates that particle size does not substantially affect SCS distribution but can influence clearance kinetics within a specific size range determined by the choriocapillaris and scleral extracellular matrix pore size [19,79]. The results of these two studies indicate that particle suspensions can be adapted to suit therapeutic needs.

6.5. Osmotic Characteristics and Ionic Charges of Formulation

Osmotic power and ionic charge are additional factors that appear to impact drug distribution within the SCS. In a study by Jung and collaborators, osmotic power was demonstrated through the use of highly concentrated HA solution injection, following a less concentrated HA solution containing fluorescent particles. The highly concentrated HA solution was able to attract fluid, leading to greater expansion of the SCS and displacement of the fluorescent particles toward the posterior pole [86].

Regarding the influence of ionic charge on drug distribution, negatively charged nanoparticles were injected into the SCS, and their concentration in the posterior pole of the eye increased significantly when exposed to a positively charged cathodal current in the same study [87]. Touchard and collaborators obtained similar results with non-viral negatively charged DNA particles exposed to electric current in a rat model [88]. Hence, osmotic power and ionic charge are fluid properties that can be leveraged to optimize drug spread in SC injections.

6.6. Compartmentalization and Duration of Injectates in the SCS

SC injection offers an advantage in terms of injectate compartmentalization and prolonged drug effect, thereby minimizing side effects by avoiding exposure to distal ocular tissues. Microscopic analysis of the compartmentalization of SC injections in porcine eyes with red fluorescent sulforhodamine injectate was conducted by Patel and collaborators [3]. Using in vivo studies on rabbit models, the degree of choroid and retina targeting by SC and IV injections was further quantified. SC injection of fluorescein resulted in the detection of 10 to 100 times more content in the choroid and retina compared to IV injections, where the signals produced were more uniformly distributed throughout the visual axis [12]. Tyagi and collaborators performed SC injections of NaF and found peak concentrations in the choroid retina that were 36 times higher than subconjunctival injections and 25 times higher than IV injections. The SC route provided a 6-fold higher choroid and retina NaF exposure compared to the posterior subconjunctival route and 2-fold higher exposure compared to the IV route [23].

Similar compartmentalization was observed in studies involving TA injections in rabbit models. Negligible amounts of TA were detected in the anterior segment of the eye after 91 days, while the sclera, choroid, and RPE displayed the highest concentrations [89]. SCTA led to scleral, choroidal, and retinal concentrations 12 times higher than IV injections, while concentrations in the lens, iris-ciliary body, and vitreous humor were 460, 32, and 22 folds lower, respectively. Aqueous humor levels were negligible, and plasma levels were undetectable [90]. Similar observations were made with other molecules, such as Axitinib and A01017, showing maximal concentrations in the SCR at 67 days and 90 days, respectively [91,92]. Compartmentalization was further demonstrated in another study on SCTA, which showed plasma levels below 1 ng/L for up to 24 weeks [93].

6.7. Tailoring Suprachoroidal Drug Delivery

In summary, SC injections are a valuable strategy for ocular drug delivery. Its effectiveness is dependent on numerous parameters such as injection force, volume of injectate, formulation characteristics, and compartmentalization. A critical factor is viscosity, with higher viscosity agents favoring drug localization more anterior to the ocular equator and lower viscosity enabling greater posterior delivery. Furthermore, higher viscosity formulations slow clearance rates, thereby prolonging the drug's duration of action. In addition to viscosity, the size of particle suspensions is key [64]. Larger particles tend to stay longer in the SCS and are less subject to washout by the choroidal circulation, thus extending the therapeutic effect [82,83]. By skillfully manipulating these parameters, researchers and clinicians can tailor drug delivery to individual patients' needs, depending on the specific location and chronicity of the ocular disease being treated [1–3]. This personalization could significantly enhance treatment outcomes and patient satisfaction, marking an important step toward precision medicine in ophthalmology.

7. Suprachoroidal Injection in Ocular Diseases

This section presents a detailed overview of the application of SC injection in the treatment of various ocular diseases, encompassing a spectrum of studies from preclinical to clinical stages. We encourage readers to consult Table A1 in Appendix A for a more in-depth understanding of each individual study referenced in our analysis.

7.1. *Macular Edema*

7.1.1. Suprachoroidal Injection for Macular Edema Secondary to Non-Infectious Uveitis

Favorable results from preclinical studies, where SCTA injection effectively concentrated corticosteroid levels in the retina, RPE, and choroid while minimizing exposure to anterior chamber structures, paved the way for subsequent clinical trials [5]. The PEACHTREE clinical trial, led by Yeh and colleagues, demonstrated the effectiveness and safety of SCTA in treating ME secondary to non-infectious uveitis (NIU). This randomized, double-masked study encompassed 160 eyes assigned to receive either 4.0 mg SCTA at two time points (day 0 and week 12) or a sham injection in a 3:2 ratio. Remarkably, by week 24, nearly half (46.9%) of the eyes treated with SCTA exhibited significant visual improvement, gaining 15 or more early treatment diabetic retinopathy study (ETDRS) letters from baseline, compared to only 15.6% in the control group. This improvement was observed as early as 4 weeks and was maintained through week 24. Similarly, a difference of more than 100 μm in mean central subfield thickness (CST) was observed between the two groups at week 4 (−148 μm in the SCTA group vs. −4 μm in the control group) and maintained by week 24. Moreover, ME resolution (CST < 300 μm) was substantially higher in the SCTA group (53% vs. 2% in controls) as early as week 4 until the study's end. SCTA was also effective in reducing the need for rescue therapy (13.5% vs. 72% in controls) and in extending the median time to the first rescue to 89 days versus 36 days. While treatment-related AEs were noted in both groups at rates of 29% (SCTA) and 8% (control), the incidence of cataracts and elevated IOP were comparable with no treatment related serious AEs. Thus, the PEACHTREE trial demonstrated the robust potential of SCTA as a therapeutic approach to managing ocular diseases, showing clinically significant vision improvement and suggesting that further exploration in this domain is both warranted and promising [94].

Henry and collaborators confirmed that patients undergoing SCTA injection for the treatment of ME due to NIU experienced improved visual and anatomical outcomes alongside comparable rates of AEs, regardless of age at 24 weeks [95]. A post-hoc analysis by Merrill and colleagues also found that benefits demonstrated in the PEACHTREE remained consistent regardless of concurrent systemic corticosteroid use or steroid-sparing therapy. The only difference was that among patients receiving steroid therapy, the mean best corrected visual acuity (BCVA) change was statistically significant, while the mean CST change was not statistically significant between the SCTA and control groups. Among patients who did not receive steroid therapy at baseline, 14.7% of those treated with SCTA versus 69.4% in the control group received rescue therapy. In contrast, for patients who received steroid therapy at baseline, the need for rescue therapy was 10.7% versus 80.0% in the SCTA and control groups, respectively. These results showed a statistically significant difference between the groups that received no steroid therapy and those that received it [96]. These post-hoc analyses reaffirm that SCTA outperforms sham treatment in terms of both functional and anatomical outcomes. Notably, the use of SCTA did not result in a statistically significant improvement in CST for patients who received concurrent steroid therapy. This finding highlights the need for additional studies that identify the suitability of SCTA therapy for patients on different concurrent treatment regimens. Certain factors, such as prior steroid therapy, may have the potential to impact treatment outcomes.

Khurana and colleagues conducted MAGNOLIA, an extension safety study of the PEACHTREE trial in 2022. Their results revealed that the statistically significant improvement in BCVA and CST reduction was maintained for the 28 eyes that received treatment versus the 5 eyes in the control group until 48 weeks. While the need for rescue treatment was not statistically different between each group, the median time to rescue therapy was significantly longer in the SCTA group compared to the control group (257 days versus 55.5 days). The proportion of individuals with at least one ocular AE was 64.3% for SCTA eyes and 60% in the control group, with the most common AE being subcapsular cataract. In the 48-week duration study period, eight patients (seven in the SCTA and one in the control group) had a cataract-related AE, with two of them requiring surgery (both in the SCTA group). In total, 14.3% of SCTA patients had at least 1 elevated IOP reading >10 mmHg, versus 0% in the control group, with no one requiring surgical management [97]. In addition to MAGNOLIA, Henry and colleagues (2022) conducted a safety clinical trial called AZALEA. The study involved 38 eyes, with 53% of them having ME, who received two 4.0 mg SCTA injections spaced 12 weeks apart. The results demonstrated that SCTA was well tolerated and safe for a duration of over 24 weeks in these patients. The mean BCVA, CST, and excess retinal thickness improved at all visits until week 24; however, there were no statistical analyses to determine the significance of this improvement. The proportion of individuals with a treatment-related AE was 18.4%, with pain (7.9%), IOP rise >10 mmHg (15.8%), and IOP >30 mmHg (5.3%) being the most common. No one required surgery for their elevated IOP, but 87.5% required treatment with IOP lowering drops. The formation or worsening of a cataract was experienced by 10.5%, with none requiring surgery [93]. As seen in both AZALEA and MAGNOLIA, the efficacy of SCTA treatment for ME due to NIU was maintained for up to 48 weeks. Few experienced treatment-related AEs, most notably, cataract progression and IOP elevation.

Prior to their pivotal clinical trial, PEACHTREE, Yeh and collaborators conducted DOGWOOD, a randomized, masked study in 2019. They concluded that a 4.0 mg injection of SCTA in patients with ME secondary to NIU was efficacious and well-tolerated. A total of 22 eyes received 4.0 mg or 0.8 mg SCTA in a 4:1 ratio and were assessed at 1 and 2 months. In the group that received 4.0 mg, CST and BCVA were both statistically significantly improved at 1 and 2 months. Of the 10 subjects in the 4.0 mg SCTA treatment group with an anterior cell grade >0 cells at baseline, all subjects showed improvement at month 2 with a 60% resolution (change to score of 0). The remaining seven patients had an anterior cell grade of 0, with 85.7% maintaining this grade status at 2 months. Among 10 subjects in the 4.0 mg SCTA treatment arm that had a vitreous haze score >0 at baseline, 80% showed improvement. Patients with a vitreous haze score of 0 at baseline maintained their grade in the second month. At least one AE was reported by 47% and 100% of the 4.0 mg SCTA and 0.8 mg SCTA groups, respectively, with the most common events being eye or injection site pain (18%), conjunctival hemorrhage (13.6%) and ME (13.6%) that all resolved without treatment. No significant elevation in IOP nor serious treatment-related AEs were reported [98]. Hanif and colleagues (2021) found that 4.0 mg SCTA was safe and efficacious for the treatment of ME secondary to NIU, supporting the initiation of larger-scale studies. Their single-arm study involving 30 eyes with ME secondary to NIU found statistically significant differences in CMT and BCVA from baseline to 1 and 3 months. While five patients were found to have lenticular changes, none of these changes had an effect on patient-reported vision, and there was no statistically significant change in IOP at 3 months [99]. Munir and colleagues, using a similar methodology to Hanif and colleagues, found that the mean BCVA improved as early as 1 week for up to 6 months in 50 patients with ME, of which 30 of them were secondary to NIU (other diagnoses included vascular disorders, diabetic ME, sarcoidosis, and pseudophakic edema). In terms of AEs, IOP was highest at 6 months in cases with baseline IOPs of 11–15 mmHg up to 35 mmHg and highest at 1 month in the baseline IOP group of 16–20 mmHg up to 30 mmHg [100].

The functional and anatomic improvement experienced post-SCTA injection for the treatment of ME due to NIU has been repeatedly shown in multiple clinical studies. The improvement in BCVA, CST, and longer time to rescue therapy was present regardless of patient age or concurrent use of systemic corticosteroid or steroid-sparing therapy. The sustained drug effect, as evidenced by patients not requiring rescue treatment for a mean time of 257 days, has the potential to reduce the treatment burden in comparison to current therapeutic regimens. Safety studies, such as MAGNOLIA, confirm that these benefits are longstanding for up to 48 weeks with minimal AEs.

Due to the unique compartmentalization and ocular distribution provided by SC injection, these studies found a low incidence of AEs. The MAGNOLIA and AZALEA trials demonstrate that the rates of AEs, such as increased IOP and cataract progression, were low. However, cataract progression and elevated IOP occurred and sometimes necessitated surgical or medical management, respectively. There were uniformly no reports of serious AEs, such as retinal detachment (RD) or increased IOP requiring surgery. The studies reported varied rates of AEs ranging from 18.4% to 64.3% and described different occurrence rates of IOP elevation, cataract formation, and cataract progression. This variability underscores the importance of conducting larger-scale, masked, and randomized studies with a larger number of enrolled participants. Such studies would provide more reliable and generalizable results, reduce the impact of potential confounders, and increase the overall robustness of the findings. Additionally, the efficacy and safety of SCTA cannot be compared to other therapeutics, injected either suprachoroidally or intravitreally, as all the studies to date have been single-arm interventional trials of SCTA or in comparison to sham injection.

Nevertheless, these studies collectively reinforce SCTA's potential as an efficacious and safe therapeutic approach. As such, SCTA has been the first and only FDA-approved therapy leveraging the SCS for the treatment of ME secondary to NIU. The findings of these studies have paved the way for the study of additional therapeutics administered in the SCS, such as anti-VEGF and viral gene agents.

7.1.2. Suprachoroidal Injection for Diabetic Macular Edema

DME is a common complication of diabetic retinopathy and a leading cause of vision loss. Its current first-line treatment involves IV injections of anti-VEGF agents (Ranibizumab, Aflibercept, and Bevacizumab), which have shown significant efficacy in improving vision [101]. However, these treatments have limitations, including the need for frequent injections and potential AEs related to the IV application. As an alternative, corticosteroids, such as triamcinolone acetonide (TA), have been applied as a second-line treatment due to their anti-inflammatory properties. Intravitreal triamcinolone acetonide (IVTA) has been shown to effectively reduce DME and improve vision but is associated with ocular AEs, such as increased IOP and cataract progression [45].

In this landscape, SCTA has emerged as an alternative for DME treatment. SCTA offers the potential to limit anterior exposure and possibly decrease ocular AEs. The HULK trial by Wykoff and colleagues (2018) evaluated the safety and efficacy of SCTA for the treatment of DME. They administered SCTA (4.0 mg/0.1 mL) alone or combined with IV Aflibercept (2.0 mg/0.05 mL). The combination group (10 treatment-naïve participants) received IV Aflibercept followed by SCTA, with an average of 2.6 injections. The monotherapy group (10 participants who had received previous treatment) had an average of 3.3 SCTA injections. After 6 months, the monotherapy group had a greater reduction in CMT (128 μm) compared to the combination group (91 μm), while the combination group exhibited better visual acuity gains (8.5 ETDRS letters) compared to the monotherapy group (1.1 letters). No serious or systemic ocular AEs were observed, indicating the safety of SCTA in treating DME [102]. A post-hoc analysis of the HULK trial showed that SCTA caused a measurable increase in the SCS, which returned to baseline levels 1 month following injection with no lasting anatomical impacts [4]. Similarly, the TYBEE trial by Barakat and collaborators (2021) compared SCTA with IV Aflibercept versus IV Aflibercept alone in treatment-naïve DME patients among 36 versus 35 participants, respectively. After 24 weeks, the difference in BCVA improvement was not statistically significant between groups. The combination group showed a notable advantage in that they exhibited a greater reduction in CMT and necessitated fewer prn injections compared to the monotherapy group [103].

Studies have also compared the efficacy and safety of SCTA in combination with IV Bevacizumab versus IV Bevacizumab alone. In a phase II/III randomized controlled pilot trial, Fazel and colleagues (2023) randomly assigned 66 eyes with untreated DME to receive SCTA in combination with IV Bevacizumab or IV Bevacizumab alone. They found that adding a single dose of SCTA prior to IV Bevacizumab led to significant improvements in BCVA and reductions in CMT without major ocular AEs. After 3 months, there was a significant improvement in mean BVCA, a significant reduction in mean CST, and no significant change in mean IOP, which remained at around 15 mmHg [104]. They also determined that SCTA with IV Bevacizumab was more effective in reducing CMT compared to IV Bevacizumab alone. However, BCVA changes were not directly assessed in this study, which assumed a correlation between CMT decline and BCVA improvements based on other trials [105]. After randomly assigning 136 participants to receive either SCTA or IV Bevacizumab, Anwar and colleagues (2022) determined that a single dose of SCTA resulted in greater improvements in visual acuity and a more significant reduction in CMT [106].

Comparisons have also been made between SC and IV administration of corticosteroids. In their prospective interventional study, Zakaria and collaborators (2022) randomized 45 eyes in 32 patients to receive IVTA alone or with two different doses of SCTA (4.0 mg/0.1 mL or 2.0 mg/0.1 mL). Significant improvements in visual acuity and CMT were observed in both treatment arms after 1 and 3 months. However, after 3 months, CMT started to increase, and the reduction was not significantly different compared to baseline except in the 4.0 mg SCTA group which sustained a reduction of 60.16 μm. The 4.0 mg SCTA group demonstrated the most substantial improvement in visual acuity and sustained its effect for a longer duration, thereby confirming the effectiveness of this dosage in clinical practice. The incidence of AEs, such as IOP elevation and cataract progression, did not significantly differ between the two routes. Given that CMT had nearly returned to baseline values in most patients, they recommended considering reinjection before 6 months [107].

Other research has identified that SCTA and IVTA are similarly effective at reducing CMT and BCVA at 3 months. However, IVTA has been associated with significantly higher IOP levels and a shorter duration of effect, suggesting SCTA may be a more beneficial treatment option. For instance, Shaikh and colleagues (2023) observed comparable efficacy of SCTA and IVTA in improving BCVA and CMT at 3 months. Their study included 34 patients randomly assigned to each treatment group, with a second injection administered at 6 weeks. After 1 and 6 months, both groups demonstrated statistically significant improvements in BCVA and CMT compared to baseline, but no significant differences were observed between the groups. At 3 and 6 months, there was a significant increase in IOP in the IVTA group compared to the SCTA group. Thus, both routes were equally effective, but the SC route maintained a more favorable effect on IOP. Cataract progression was also found to be slower in eyes that received SCTA [108].

SCTA has also shown promising results in DME post-vitrectomy, with improved visual acuity and reduced macular thickness. In a study by Marashi and Zaza (2022), it was observed that among 11 (1 phakic and 10 pseudophakic) eyes treated with SCTA, significant vision improvement and a 45.74% reduction in CMT from baseline was noted after 8 weeks. Importantly, no IOP elevation or cataract progression was observed [109].

Several nonrandomized, single-arm studies have also provided evidence supporting the effectiveness of SCTA in improving BCVA and reducing CST with minimal AEs [110–115]. However, a study by Tharwat and colleagues (2022) suggests that formulated posterior subtenon TA (PSTA) injection may offer better outcomes for managing rDME with reduced risk of IOP elevation. In their prospective study, 75 patients were randomly assigned to three treatment groups (SCTA (4.0 mg/0.1 mL) alone, a combination of PSTA (40 mg) formulated with VISCOAT containing sodium chondroitin sulfate (20 mg) and sodium hyaluronate (15 mg), or unformulated PSTA (40 mg)). All groups showed a significant increase in BCVA and a significant decrease in CMT at months 1, 3, and 6. However, the group receiving formulated PSTA exhibited the highest BCVA and the lowest CST 6 months post-procedure, suggesting that this may be more therapeutic due to its prolonged contact and increased diffusion through the scleral barrier [116].

There is also emerging research investigating the application of SC-administered gene therapy for DME. RGX-314 is a gene therapy product that contains an AAV8 vector encoding an antibody fragment designed to inhibit anti-VEGF. The ALTITUDE trial, an ongoing industry-sponsored, phase II, randomized, dose-escalation study, is currently exploring the efficacy, safety, and tolerability of delivering this suprachoroidally in patients with center-involved DME [117]. Approximately 100 participants will be enrolled into one of five cohorts containing different dosages of RGX-314 with or without post-procedure steroid injection. While the trial is currently recruiting participants, interim 3-month data suggest that 33% of participants in the treatment arm had a ≥2 improvement in their diabetic retinopathy severity score compared with 0% in the control arm.

Overall, the available data suggest that SCTA at a 4.0 mg/mL dose offers numerous advantages over conventional therapies for both primary and rDME. SCTA used in combination with IV anti-VEGF agents has consistently shown effectiveness in reducing macular thickness, improving visual acuity, and providing a longer duration of action compared to IV anti-VEGF treatments alone. Notably, SCTA was found to be beneficial for patients with rDME despite prior anti-VEGF injections, potentially reducing the need for multiple injections and their associated costs. TA acts as an anti-inflammatory agent, inhibiting factors, such as VEGF, that are involved in DME pathogenesis. Previous studies combining IV corticosteroids with anti-VEGF agents for rDME have demonstrated improved functional and anatomical outcomes at the expense of ocular AEs related to diffuse corticosteroid delivery [118]. In contrast, SCTA combined with anti-VEGF agents addresses both the vascular and inflammatory aspects of DME with targeted delivery and reduced anterior segment exposure. Data comparing SCTA and IVTA have shown that both routes of administration result in significant CMT and BVCA improvement. However, SCTA is associated with fewer IOP-related AEs and a longer duration of effect, indicating SCTA may be more efficacious in resolving DME through corticosteroids.

Despite promising evidence, further research is needed to explore the long-term efficacy, optimal dosing strategies, and comparative effectiveness of SCTA for the treatment of DME, including its impact on visual outcomes, durability of effect, and potential AEs. Most studies have reported significant functional and anatomical improvements in BCVA and CST after SCTA administration within a 3-month timeframe. However, ocular AEs, such as increased IOP and cataract progression, can still occur, although they may have a lower incidence compared to IV administration. Further, comparative studies examining the efficacy and safety of SCTA with other therapeutic approaches, such as PSTA, would be valuable. Additionally, larger multicenter studies with longer follow-up periods are needed to determine whether the improvements in BCVA and CMT are transient or long-lasting.

7.1.3. Suprachoroidal Injection for Macular Edema Secondary to Retina Vein Occlusion

The treatment of ME resulting from RVO has been the focus of several industry-sponsored clinical trials assessing the effectiveness of combined SCTA with IV anti-VEGF agents versus IV anti-VEGF monotherapy alone. For instance, the TANZANITE trial, a phase II, multicenter, masked, industry-sponsored RCT conducted by Campochiaro and colleagues (2018), compared the combination of SCTA (4.0 mg/0.1 mL) with IV Aflibercept (2.0 mg/0.05 mL) to IV Aflibercept monotherapy. Forty-six patients were randomized to either treatment arm and received IV Aflibercept as needed over a 3 month study period. Results showed that the combination therapy significantly reduced the need for retreatment, with 23 retreatments in the combination group versus 9 in the monotherapy group. Moreover, a higher percentage of patients did not require retreatments (78% versus 30%, respectively). The combination group also led to greater visual acuity improvement (18.9 versus 11.3 ETDRS letters in month 3) and a decrease in CST from baseline (731.1 μm to 284.7 μm at month one, stable at 2 and 3 months). In contrast, the IV Aflibercept group had an increase in CST at 2 and 3 months. Additionally, the combination group exhibited a higher percentage of edema resolution (78.3% versus 47.8%) at month 3. Although four patients in the combination group experienced elevated IOP, that was resolved with topical anti-glaucoma agents [119]. Extension data from the study indicated that 74% of patients in the combination group did not require retreatments over a 9-month period compared to 17% in the control arm [120].

Another noteworthy study, the phase III SAPPHIRE study, also compared the combination of SCTA (4.0 mg/0.1 mL) with IV Aflibercept therapy (2 mg/0.05 mL) to IV Aflibercept monotherapy in 460 eyes with RVO. After 8 weeks, approximately 50.0% of patients in both groups reported a significant improvement of ≥15 ETDRS letters in BCVA.

However, no other benefits were observed in the combination arm, leading to the study's discontinuation. Nevertheless, preliminary data from 128 patients in the combination group and 127 patients in the control group revealed that the combination procedure had a favourable safety profile, as only one case of RD and one case of vitreous hemorrhage were reported. These findings indicate that SCTA and IV Aflibercept combination therapy was well-tolerated, without significant ocular AEs [121].

A phase III, randomized, masked RCT (TOPAZ) was designed to investigate if SCTA in combination with IV Ranibizumab or IV Bevacizumab was superior to IV Ranibizumab or IV Bevacizumab alone. Treatment groups received either a combination therapy of IV Ranibizumab (0.5 mg/0.05 mL) with SCTA (4.0 mg/0.10 mL) or IV Bevacizumab (1.25 mg/0.05 mL) with SCTA (4.0 mg/0.10 mL). The control arms received either IV Ranibizumab or IV Bevacizumab, followed by a sham SC procedure. However, the trial was prematurely stopped due to the results of the SAPPHIRE trial findings [122].

In addition to industry-sponsored trials, independent studies have also examined the effectiveness and safety of combining SCTA administration with IV anti-VEGF agents. Nawar (2022) conducted a prospective randomized study on 60 patients with branch retinal vein occlusion (BRVO) to explore this treatment approach. The patients were divided into two groups, one receiving combined IV Ranibizumab with SCTA and the other receiving IV Ranibizumab alone. Both groups received monthly Ranibizumab injections as needed during the 12-month study period. Participants in the combination arm required fewer injections (2.47 ± 1.2) compared to those in the monotherapy arm (4.4 ± 1.5). At 12 months, both groups demonstrated significant reductions in CMT, along with significant improvements in BVCA. The combination group showed more significant BVCA improvement at 6 and 12 months [123].

Studies investigating SCTA as a monotherapy for RVO-associated ME have also shown promising results in terms of BCVA improvement and CST reduction. Recent research conducted by Ali and colleagues (2023) investigated SCTA as a standalone treatment in 16 patients with ME secondary to RVO. Their findings demonstrated that 68.7% of patients had a BCVA improvement of $\geq$15 letters by week 1 and a range of 50% to 62.5% showing this improvement during months 1 to 3. There was also a notable CST reduction throughout the follow-up period. One patient experienced elevated IOP of $\geq$20 mmHg in the first month, but their IOP decreased by the second month [124]. Similarly, Muslim and colleagues (2022) studied the application of SCTA (4.0 mg/0.1 mL) in 45 patients with unilateral RVO-associated ME. A statistically significant improvement in BCVA was observed after 1 month and with further improvement at 3 months. There was also a significant reduction in central retinal thickness (CRT) after 3 months [125].

Stanislao and colleagues (2012) conducted a prospective study of six eyes of six patients with central retinal vein occlusion (CRVO), BRVO, or diffuse DME accompanied by severe refractory subfoveal hard exudates (SHE). Participants received a single SC infusion of Bevacizumab and TA administered into the submacular SCS using a microcatheter at the pars plana. Four eyes showed an improvement of $\geq$2 lines in BCVA, while two eyes remained stable. By 1 to 2 months, SHE was almost completely resolved in all eyes, and ME was significantly reduced with no surgical or post-injection complications reported [126].

Based on these findings, the benefits of a combination of SCTA and IV anti-VEGF therapy for RVO-associated ME include fewer retreatment needs, improved visual acuity, anatomical improvements, and resolution of subretinal exudates. Corticosteroids have shown efficacy in addressing inflammation associated with RVO by targeting molecules that affect vascular permeability and inflammation. The SCS offers a targeted pathway for drug delivery to manage ME secondary to RVO. However, given the lack of large-scale, independent, and multicenter studies examining the application of SCTA in the context of ME secondary to RVO, additional research is required to confirm the optimal combination therapies, most effective drug combinations, and long-term efficacy and safety of SCTA. To address this knowledge gap, an ongoing clinical trial is taking place in Egypt that is investigating the long-term effects of SC injection, including ocular hypertension, cataract progression, and ME resolution, in the treatment of RVO alongside other retinal diseases such as Vogt Koyanagi Harada disease and DME. The trial is still in the recruitment phase, with results pending study completion [127].

7.1.4. Suprachoroidal Injection for Post-Operative/Pseudophakic Cystoid Macular Edema

SCTA has also shown promise as a potential treatment for pseudophakic cystoid macular edema (PCME), a common post-operative complication of cataract surgery. A study by Tabl and colleagues (2022) demonstrated the efficacy of SCTA and IVTA in reducing CFT and improving visual acuity in pseudophakic patients with rDME caused by the epiretinal membrane. They injected SCTA (4.0 mg/0.1 mL, in 13 eyes) or IVTA (4.0 mg/0.1 mL, in 10 eyes) with results consistent with Zakaria and collaborator's findings on the significant improvements in CFT (see Figure 5) and BCVA with a 4.0 mg dose of SCTA. The IVTA group had significantly higher elevations in IOP in the first month (15 mmHg) compared to the SCTA group (12 mmHg). Furthermore, by the third month, the IVTA group still exhibited significantly higher IOP levels (18 mmHg) compared to the SCTA group (14 mmHg), indicating a sustained difference between the two groups [128]. Similarly, Zhang and colleagues (2022) injected SCTA (0.2 mL of 40 mg/mL) in 20 eyes of 20 patients with CME and PCME, resulting from various conditions such as BRVO, CRVO, DME and previous epiretinal membrane (ERM) peeling surgery. Optical coherence tomography (OCT) examination confirmed drug delivery as determined by SCS expansion near the injection site. The injections led to significant improvements in BCVA and CST without significant differences in IOP. No complications, such as cataract induction, hemorrhage, retinal detachment, or endophthalmitis, were observed during the 3-month study period. The authors proposed that the anterior SCS is the most accessible location for injection, in alignment with previous animal and human studies. However, the long-term efficacy and safety of SCTA for CME could not be established due to the lack of participant follow-up [129].

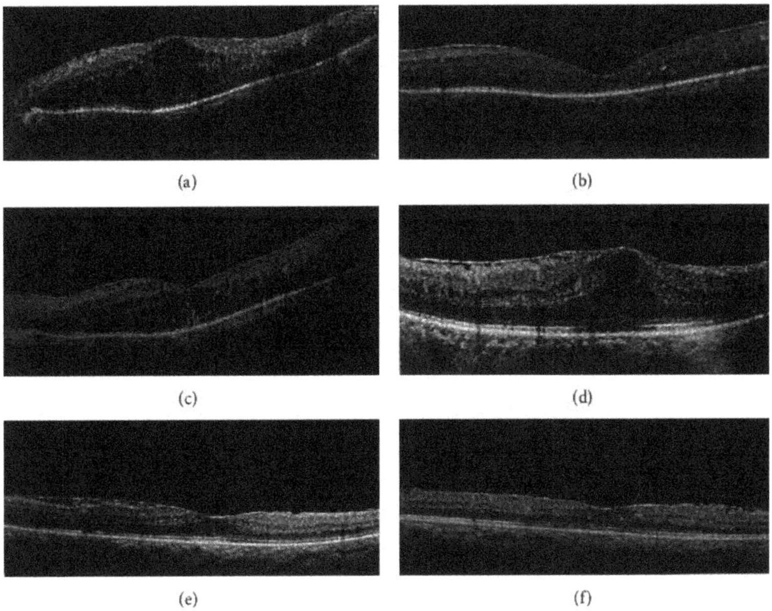

Figure 5. Example of CFT changes measured by OCT after IVTA and SCTA injection at baseline, 1, and 3 months. IVTA group (**a**–**c**). SCTA group (**d**–**f**). Reprinted with permission from Ref. [128]. 2023, Ahmed Abdelshafy Tabl et al.

Other case studies by Oli and Waikar (2021) and Marashi and Zazo (2022) also reported positive outcomes with SCTA for PCME, including improved BCVA and decreased CMT [130,131]. Additionally, a clinical trial is currently investigating the impact of SCTA on CME caused by Irving-Gass syndrome following cataract surgery [132].

Overall, preliminary research suggests that SCTA could be effective for managing PCME. The results align with previous investigations that treated ME secondary to uveitis, DME, or RVO with SCTA using a microinjector approach. However, more extensive randomized studies are needed to evaluate the long-term efficacy and safety of SCTA for post-operative complications such as PCME.

7.2. Photoreceptor Loss

7.2.1. Suprachoroidal Injection of AAV Vectors for the Treatment of Inherited and Acquired Retinal Disorders

Preclinical studies have shown that SC delivery of adeno-associated vectors (AAV) is a promising technique for treating inherited and acquired retinal diseases. Peden and collaborators (2011) conducted a pioneering study using a microcatheter to deliver AAV5 (100 μL of sc-AAV5-smCBA-hGFP vector at a concentration of 4.5×10^{13} vector genomes/mL) into the SCS of eight healthy rabbits. The treatment was well tolerated, with no reports of serious AEs. Analysis of whole-mounted treated eyes 6 weeks post-injection revealed robust transfection, evidenced by the presence of GFP expression in the choroid, the RPE, photoreceptors, and retinal ganglion cells. In contrast, the control group did not exhibit any GFP expression. The authors concluded that the microcatheter approach for SC AAV delivery demonstrated safety, tolerability, and effective gene transfer to target areas [65]. Similarly, Martorana and colleagues (2012) compared the gene transfer of AAV2, AAV5, and AAV2, containing three tyrosine-phenylalanine mutations on the capsid surface [AAV2(triple)]. The efficiency of SC and subretinal transduction was further compared in rabbits. Immunostaining showed that GFP expression was observed in all eyes that received vitrectomy/subretinal or SC injections, with AAV2 producing the strongest GFP expression. There was intermediate expression with AAV2 treatment and minimal expression with AAV5 treatment, unlike Peden's findings. Transduction profiles were not affected significantly by the vector concentration [133]. Both studies demonstrated the feasibility of delivering AAV vectors through SC injection, although outcomes varied depending on the serotypes used. Importantly, this approach reduced the surgical risks associated with the current approach of conventional 3-port PPV followed by subretinal treatment.

Woodard and colleagues (2016) compared different routes of AAV2 administration in mice, including intrastromal, intracameral, IV, subretinal, and SC injections. In their mouse model, AAV2 was used to deliver a genetic construct containing a promoter region derived from cytomegalovirus (CMV) alongside a GFP reporter gene. Examination with fundoscopy and OCT assessed the anatomical impact of the injections at the time of administration, and transduction was evaluated after 6 weeks using fundoscopy and histological analysis of whole globes. Transduction was observed in multiple ocular structures, including the stroma, ciliary body, retinal ganglion cells, outer retina, and the RPE, irrespective of delivery route. Notably, SC injections demonstrated transduction across multiple retinal layers throughout the entire retina. This ability to transduce retinal layers without inducing a temporary RD led the authors to conclude that SC delivery may offer unique advantages over subretinal delivery [134].

Recent studies have investigated the effectiveness of SC AAV delivery in animal models using a conventional hypodermic needle and free-hand method. Ding and colleagues (2020) used this method to inject a GFP-reporter gene with RGX-314, an AAV8 vector expressing a VEGF-neutralizing protein, into the SCS in animal models. India ink injection into the SCS confirmed its spread throughout the posterior segment without entering the RPE or retina. Two weeks later, treated eyes displayed robust fluorescence in the RPE and outer retina on the injected side, extending to the opposite side of the eye. Immunohistochemical staining confirmed GFP presence in the RPE, photoreceptor cell bodies, inner segments, and outer segments, with stronger staining near the injection site. Conversely, subretinal injection resulted in strong fluorescence and GFP staining only on the injected side, with minimal staining in remote quadrants. Rats that received a second SC injection of AAV8 showed increased GFP expression compared to a single injection. The study also compared SC delivery of AAV8, AAV9, and AAV2 serotypes, with AAV8 and AAV9 displaying strong GFP expression in the injected eye quadrant, while AAV2 exhibited limited fluorescence in the far periphery. Serum albumin, an endogenous marker for vascular leakage, was used to assess retinal vascular permeability. Eyes treated with SC or subretinal delivery of RGX-314 showed significantly lower vitreous albumin levels compared to control eyes injected with AAV8, indicating the suppression of VEGF-induced vasodilation and vascular permeability by RGX-314. Additionally, the study confirmed similar levels of anti-VEGF Fab protein in the retina, the RPE, and the choroid between SC and subretinal routes [135].

Ding and colleagues (2020) also conducted a study comparing SC delivery of AAV2tYF-CBA-hGFP, AAV2tYF-GRK1-hGFP, AAV5-GRK1-hGFP, or AAV2-CBA-hGFP in 65 Norway brown rats. Peak GFP expression was achieved by each vector at 2 weeks, with AAV2tYF showing further increase between weeks 2 and 4. AAV2tYF exhibited stronger and more widespread GFP expression, extending approximately $\frac{1}{4}$ of the circumference of the eye in the RPE and all layers of the retina. Significant transduction of photoreceptors and inner retinal cells was also observed with AAV2tYF-GRK1-GFP and AAV5tYF-GRK1-GFP via the SC route. AAV2tYF-CBA provided significantly greater transduction than AAV2-CBA after SC injection. While not as extensive as AAV8 and AAV9, AAV2tYF-CBA resulted in more transduction of inner retinal cells. AAV2tYF-GRK1 demonstrated superior and more extensive transduction of photoreceptors compared to AAV5-GRK1. These findings support the potential of SC injection of AAV2tYF-CBA and AAV2tYF-GRK1 for efficient transduction of retinal cells, particularly photoreceptors [136].

Yiu and colleagues (2020) conducted a study on non-human primates to compare the efficacy of SC, subretinal, and IV gene delivery using AAV8 carrying an enhanced GFP sequence. SC injection resulted in widespread transgene expression in the RPE, while subretinal delivery showed focal transduction in the RPE, photoreceptors, and some ganglion cells near the injection site. IV injection led to scant peripapillary GFP expression in cells, potentially astrocytes or Müller glia. Other studies comparing SC delivery of AAV serotypes with other routes of transmission in animal models have confirmed that SC administration may be preferable due to their widespread transduction and lack of associated retinal complications. However, Han and colleagues (2020) and Tian and colleagues (2021) investigated the use of different AAV serotypes for gene transfer in animal models, which showed that transduction, estimated by GFP expression, varied among serotypes [59,137].

Further, the initial enthusiasm for gene therapy may be tempered by emerging evidence of AAV-associated inflammation. For instance, Yiu and colleagues discovered that SC AAV8 delivery resulted in transient expression, peaking at month 1 with a subsequent decline by months 2 and 3. This decline was attributed to cellular damage and the phagocytic activity of local inflammatory cells. In contrast, subretinal and IV delivery showed lower localized chorioretinitis, although IV administration produced a stronger systemic humoral immune response [24]. A subsequent study by Ching and collaborators (2021) demonstrated that SC delivery induced a lower systemic immune response compared to IV delivery but higher elevations in IOP compared to subretinal delivery. These results were anticipated due to the SCS being located outside the blood–retinal barrier, rendering it susceptible to immune surveillance cells. While the study refrained from extensive immunosuppression to assess the natural immune response to SC AAV8 delivery, future research could explore the influence of corticosteroids. The authors also observed reduced transgene expression after 2 and 3 months, likely due to phagocytic activity of infiltrated macrophages and leukocytes observed at 1 month [138]. In a separate study, Wiley and collaborators (2023) examined the extent and retinal pattern of AAV-associated inflammation in rats following the administration of five distinct AAV vectors (AAV1, AAV2, AAV6,

AAV8, and AAV9). AAV2 and AAV6 consistently induced higher levels of inflammation levels compared to control groups across all delivery routes. Specifically, AAV6 triggered the highest inflammation when delivered using the SC route. AAV1 exhibited significant inflammation with SC delivery but minimal inflammation with IV delivery. AAV1, AAV2, and AAV6 also activated adaptive immune cells. AAV8 and AAV9 caused the least inflammation regardless of the delivery route. Interestingly, the amount of inflammation was not correlated with transduction and GFP expression [139].

Over the past decade, gene therapy using AAV vectors has shown promising results in animal trials, but delivery methods need further investigation to reduce risks and for optimal targeting. By enabling the transduction of multiple retinal layers without the risk of complications such as RD, this route may enhance the efficacy and distribution of gene therapy in the retina. However, translating these findings into clinical practice presents several challenges. First, the precise targeting of specific retinal regions using the SC approach remains unclear. These studies demonstrate that SC injections can treat larger peripheral areas affected by retinal diseases. However, some studies have indicated that SC delivery may result in less exposure to the inner retinal layer, minimizing transduction of retinal ganglion cells in comparison to IV administration. Thus, SC gene delivery using a microneedle may lack regional specificity and require optimization for macular targeting. Strategies such as using a "pushing" formulation that exerts pressure to facilitate movement of therapeutics, iontophoresis, collagenase to expand the SCS, higher injection volume, or catheter-based delivery could improve SC targeting [140]. Another challenge is the potential for immune responses and inflammation associated with AAV gene therapy. Although research suggests that SC AAV injections are associated with reduced systemic inflammation, they can potentially induce local inflammation. For instance, Yiu and colleagues found that persistent transgene expression in scleral cells following SC AAV administration may decrease over time due to the presence of inflammatory cells, leading to disruption of the RPE and photoreceptor segments [24]. Interestingly, IV AAV injections resulted in a stronger systemic immune response compared to subretinal or SC gene delivery, highlighting the different immune consequences of AAV exposure in different compartments surrounding the outer blood–retinal barrier. Further research is needed to explore local inflammatory responses associated with SC gene administration. Additionally, advances in AAV technology, such as the application of multiple AAV vectors simultaneously and intein-mediated protein trans-splicing, should be evaluated for SC delivery.

7.2.2. Suprachoroidal Injection of DNPs for the Treatment of Inherited and Acquired Retinal Disorders

SC injection of nanoparticles is an emerging approach for ocular gene therapy. DNA nanoparticles (DNPs), composed of DNA molecules, can be used to deliver therapeutic genes or gene-editing tools into target cells [59]. Researchers commonly use DNPs carrying a luciferase gene to measure luciferase activity and assess gene delivery efficiency. Kansara and colleagues (2019) performed SC injection of ellipsoid-shaped DNPs, rod-shaped DNPs, or saline in non-human primates, alongside SC injection of analogous DNPs and subretinal injection of rod-shaped DNPs in rabbits. Luciferase activity was observed in the retina, choroid, and the RPE. Ellipsoid-shaped DNPs showed persistent luciferase activity up to day 22, while rod-shaped DNPs declined in non-human primates. In rabbits, both SC-injected rod and ellipsoid-shaped DNPs showed similar luciferase activity after 1 week. The study demonstrated successful transfection of chorioretinal cells using SC-delivered DNPs [137].

In a follow-up study, Kansara and collaborators (2020) compared SC and subretinal injections of DNPs in rabbits. Microneedle-based SC administration of DNPs was also well-tolerated and effective in transfected chorioretinal tissues. SC injection provided greater surface area coverage and aided in the transfection of the peripheral retina. DNPs injected into the SCS showed minimal intraocular toxicity, while subretinal injections displayed ocular toxicity. The study established the potential of nonviral-based gene delivery to the chorioretina via the SC administration [139].

SC delivery of poly (β-amino ester)s nanoparticles (PBAE NPs), a biodegradable polymer used for gene delivery, has also been explored. In a study involving Brown Norway rats, performed by Shen and colleagues, SC injections of PBAE NPs containing various plasmids showed widespread GFP expression throughout the retina. However, this was less intense in the RPE and photoreceptors compared to AAV8 injections. Widespread lateral and radial penetration of polymeric NPs via SC delivery was attributed to a transient pressure increase induced by the injected volume into the SCS space. However, SC injection of PBAE NPs containing a VEGF expression plasmid caused severe subretinal neovascularization, similar to AMD. Conversely, SC injection of PBAE NPs containing a VEGF-binding protein suppressed VEGF-induced retinal vascular leakage and neovascularization, demonstrating therapeutic potential. Expression was quite strong 2 weeks after injection and was maintained for at least 8 months. Compared to a single SC injection of NPs containing pEGFP-N1, three injections resulted in a five-fold increase in ocular expression of GFP, demonstrating the feasibility of increasing expression using repeated injections [140].

Overall, SC injection of nanoparticles holds promise for treating various retinal diseases. Unlike AAVs, nanoparticles offer a nonviral-based gene therapy option that can be repeated over time, allowing for multiple treatments if needed. They can also transfer large genes common in inherited retinal disorders, such as Stargart's macular dystrophy (SMD) [59]. However, they may result in variable gene expression intensity and neovascularization risk. AAVs, on the other hand, may trigger elevated immune responses due to pre-existing antibodies against AAV capsid antigens. As research progresses, SC injection of nanoparticles may become a valuable therapeutic strategy to address the underlying genetic causes of retinal diseases.

7.2.3. Suprachoroidal Injection for the Treatment Dry-Aged Macular Degeneration and Stargardt's Macular Dystrophy

Ongoing research is exploring the use of non-retinal-derived stem cells, specifically mesenchymal stem cells, for the treatment of degenerative retinal diseases. These stem cells secrete various factors that have anti-apoptotic, anti-inflammatory, immunomodulatory, and angiogenic effects, providing trophic support for damaged retinal cells [141]. Recent studies have explored SC delivery of mesenchymal stem cells for dry AMD and SMD. In a prospective study conducted by Kahraman and colleagues (2021), eight patients with advanced-stage dry-type AMD and SMD underwent SC implantation of adipose tissue-derived mesenchymal stem cells (ADMSCs) in their worst eye. All patients experienced improvements in visual acuity, visual field, and multifocal electroretinography (mfERG) with no serious complications. These improvements persisted throughout the 1-year follow-up period, accompanied by choroidal thickening, indicating increased choroidal perfusion. The proximity of SC implantation allows the produced growth factors to enter into the choroidal flow, enhancing interactions with retinal cells. However, the study included only patients with severe visual loss [142]. Thus, future research should focus on larger patient cohorts at earlier stages of the disease to refine treatment timing, graft replacement strategies, and delivery methods. Nevertheless, these findings offer promising evidence for effective treatment of degenerative retinal diseases.

7.2.4. Suprachoroidal Injection for the Treatment of Retinitis Pigmentosa

Retinitis pigmentosa (RP), a collection of inherited retinal disorders, is characterized by progressive photoreceptor loss, leading to significant visual impairment. A wide spectrum of genetic mutations challenge the development of efficacious treatments for RP. Expanding our understanding of potential therapeutic strategies, as demonstrated in Figure 6, remains a critical objective. We have previously highlighted the potential of SC injection as a delivery mechanism for gene therapy in the management of RP. The focus of the current section is to extend this discussion to illustrate the application of SC injections in cell therapy, specifically the use of umbilical cord-derived mesenchymal stem cells (UCMSCs).

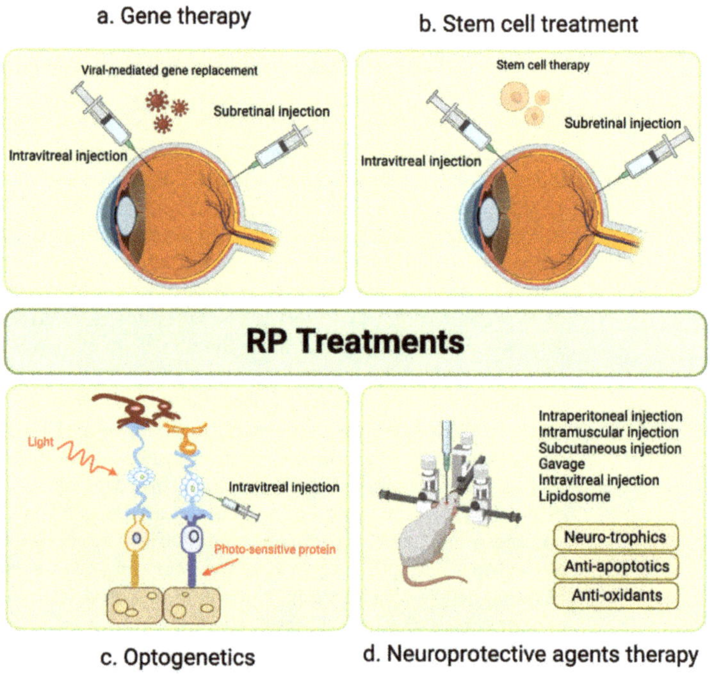

Figure 6. Emerging Therapeutic Modalities for Retinitis Pigmentosa.

Oner and colleagues conducted two studies assessing the effects of UCMSC implantation on RP patients. In their first study, significant improvements were observed in mean BCVA and visual field scores over a 12-month period. Notably, the treatment also led to an improvement in disease score and grade [143]. In their second study, which focused on pediatric RP patients, UCMSC implantation resulted in significant enhancements in BCVA, visual field examination, and mfERG measurements in all 46 eyes of patients. No systemic or ocular complications were reported [144]. However, the use of SC mesenchymal spheroidal stem cell implantation is still being evaluated, and study results are pending [145]. Further research is required to gain a comprehensive understanding of the potential advantages and limitations of this treatment approach for RP.

7.2.5. Suprachoroidal Injection for Solar Retinopathy

Marashi et al. (2021) published a case report describing a 17-year-old female with a sudden scotoma due to solar retinopathy. The patient received a single SCTA (4.0 mg/0.1 mL) injection with a custom-made needle. After 1 week, the patient's BCVA improved from 0.1 to 1.0, and her scotoma disappeared. A mild elevation in IOP to 28 mmHg was observed at 7 weeks, which resolved to normal limits with topical anti-glaucoma agents. After 4 weeks, there was a full recovery in her BCVA, and OCT demonstrated anatomical improvement in the ellipsoid zone layer. No serious AEs were reported [146]. Overall, the implications of this case suggest SCTA may be a promising therapeutic option for solar retinopathy, leading to significant improvements in visual acuity and anatomical changes without serious or unmanageable AEs. However, further research is needed to establish the efficacy, safety, and long-term outcomes of this approach in larger patient cohorts.

7.3. Choroidal Neovascularization

7.3.1. Suprachoroidal Injection for Solar Retinopathy

In individuals with choroidal neovascularization (CNV), the production of VEGF triggers abnormal and chronic angiogenesis. Consequently, sustained suppression of VEGF is required to effectively manage CNV. For this purpose, VEGF inhibitors such as Ranibizumab, Aflibercept, and Bevacizumab are typically intravitreally injected for CNV treatment. However, the need for frequent injections, as often as monthly, can be burdensome for patients and impose substantial costs on the healthcare system [147,148]. Additionally, IV injections of anti-VEGF agents are associated with AEs such as endophthalmitis, cataract, or RD [149,150]. This situation has driven research toward newer delivery methods and longer-lasting alternative medications.

To optimize drug delivery to the macula, Tran and colleagues conducted a preclinical study in 2017. A total of 39 surgical pig models with surgically induced CNV were injected with either 2.5 mg IV Bevacizumab, 1 mg IV Pazopanib, 300 µg IV hI-con1, or 1 mg SC Pazopanib, with comparable SC and IV vehicle controls. This study used novel anti-VEGF agents, such as Pazopanib and ghI-con1, to evaluate their efficacy. IV Pazopanib resulted in smaller mean height measurements of CNV type 2 lesions compared to the SC Pazopanib, and these measurements were statistically smaller than controls. For eyes treated with IV Bevacizumab, there was only a small decrease in the height of the lesions in comparison to controls. There were no significant differences between the surface area of CNV lesions between the three treatment groups. While IV-injected hI-con1 resulted in lesions that were thinner than controls, these results were not statistically significant. Their study concluded that IV Pazopanib, and, to a lesser extent, hI-con1, inhibits induced CNV lesions in pig models [151]. Given the similar properties between Pazopanib and TA, Tran and colleagues hypothesized that this medication would be a well-suited SC injection. Surprisingly, they found that IV injections yielded more significant inhibition of CNV lesions than SC injection. This could be due to Pazopanib's limited solubility, potentially resulting in adequate distribution to the posterior segment. Additionally, the low solubility might lead to a slower drug distribution, causing an insufficient amount to reach the posterior eye. Additionally, there could have been underdosing if some material remained in the syringe, in addition to dosing variations per injection. Consequently, comprehensive studies measuring the precise amount of Pazopanib injected into the SCS and analyzing its pharmacokinetics and distribution in animal models are necessary before advancing to human trials [151].

On the other hand, Mansoor and collaborators (2012) concluded that Bevacizumab (Avastin, 1250 µg/50 µL) injected into the SCS reached excellent levels in the choroid, sclera, and retina but exhibited a rapid decline in the choroid after only 1 day. They attributed this outcome to the suboptimal formulation of SC Bevacizumab, which failed to effectively target the posterior eye segments in a sustained-release matter [152]. Earlier studies of porcine models also demonstrated the rapid clearance of Bevacizumab when injected suprachoroidally in comparison to intravitreally [153]. These findings emphasize the need for optimizing drug formulations for SC injection, potentially through methods such as increasing injectate viscosity and particle size or using novel vehicles to create sustained-release formulations. Interestingly, Tyagi and colleagues (2013) successfully formulated a gel network using light-activated polycaprolactone dimethacrylate and hydroxyethyl methacrylate. This network enabled the sustained release of Bevacizumab for over 4 months when injected into the SCS in animal models. This sustained release approach did not compromise the mechanism of action of Bevacizumab [66]. Similarly, Jung and colleagues (2022) demonstrated that an in-situ forming hydrogel comprised Bevacizumab and HA crosslinked within 1 h of injection into the SCS of a rabbit allowed for slower release as the hydrogel underwent biodegradation. The degradation happened for over 6 months, and ophthalmological examination, fundoscopy, imaging, histological analysis, and IOP assessments confirmed it was well-tolerated [80].

Acriflavine is recognized for its ability to suppress neovascularization by reducing the transcriptional activities of hypoxia-inducible factor-1 and factor-2 involved in pathogenesis. Zeng and colleagues conducted a study using a laser-induced rat model of CNV in 2017 and found that 300 ng of SC Acriflavine spread throughout the retina and choroid by day 1 and was maintained for 5 days. Additionally, this treatment caused a CNV reduction 14 days after Bruch's membrane rupture. They also examined intraocular injection of 100 ng and extraocular 0.5% drops, but there was no formal comparison between different routes of administration. They concluded that various modes of Acriflavine delivery have the potential to be used for CNV treatment pending further research [154]. Building on this, Hackett and collaborators (2020) developed a sustained delivery method that increased the delivery time of Acriflavine into the SCS using poly (lactic-co-glycolic acid) microparticles for up to 60 days. They found IV and SC injections of Acriflavine using this microparticle suppressed CNV for 9 weeks in mice and 18 weeks in rats, respectively. Notably, IV injection of 38 μg Acriflavine resulted in a modest reduction in full field electroretinogram function, while SC injection resulted in no electroretinogram functional, IOP, or retinal changes over 28 days [84].

Emerging methods, such as SC electrotransfer, present alternatives for drug delivery into the SCS. Touchard and colleagues (2012) found that SC electrotransfer of a VEGFR-1 (sFlt-1)-encoding plasmid significantly inhibited laser-induced CNV in rats at 15 days. No retinal or vascular AEs were observed, suggesting that this minimally invasive method opens the door for novel research in the retinal disease treatment [88].

Animal studies have demonstrated the efficacy of established and novel anti-VEGF agents in the SCS for the treatment of CNV, including Bevacizumab, Pazopanib, and Acriflavine. Notably, sustained-release formulations have prolonged the efficacy of SC Bevacizumab and Acriflavine without compromising their safety. However, human trials are essential to confirm their safety and effectiveness, with further comparative studies needed to assess the suitability of various drugs. It is also crucial to recognize that animal studies have limitations, particularly their inability to replicate aging-related CNV lesions driven by VEGF, which are typically type 1 lesions seen in humans, unlike the type 2 lesions induced by Tran and colleagues [151]. Resultantly, clinical studies are imperative to bridge this gap [80]. Nonetheless, the relevance of porcine models should not be underestimated due to their anatomic similarities to humans, including comparable scleral thickness size, ocular blood flow, and RPE characteristics [155].

7.3.2. Suprachoroidal Injection for Choroidal Neovascularization Secondary to Neovascular Age-Related Macular Degeneration

Gene therapy is a promising treatment for inherited and acquired retinal diseases, with its use being explored for CNV. In a 2022 phase II clinical trial of 50 patients, Khanani used an AAV8 vector to deliver anti-VEGF fab transgene with the goal of creating continuous therapy in the eye. Patients were randomized to receive SC RGX-314 at levels of 2.5×10^{11} and 5×10^{11} genomic copies/eye or monthly 0.5 mg IV Ranibizumab. Patients were found to have stable BCVA and CRT at 6 months, with a meaningful reduction in anti-VEGF treatment burden (>70%). In both groups, 29% and 40%, respectively, received no anti-VEGF injections over 6 months following RGX-314 administration. Treatment-related AEs were mild, with 23% of participants experiencing mild intraocular inflammation at similar rates for both dose levels that resolved with topical corticosteroids. While the full results of this study remain unpublished, this approach could transform the landscape of nAMD treatment by offering an alternative regimen with reduced injection frequency [156,157].

Another area of investigation centers on the safety of SC Bevacizumab and TA for resolving treatment-resistant nAMD. Using a new microcatheter, Tetz and collaborators injected a combination of Bevacizumab and TA in the SCS in 21 eyes. After 6 months, they observed no serious intraoperative or postoperative complications. IOP elevation was experienced by 4.76% of participants at 3 months that normalized with medical treatment, and an increase in nuclear sclerotic cataracts was noted in 10.5% [158]. Similarly, a phase I clinical trial by Morales-Canton and colleagues (2013) injected four patients with CNV secondary to wet AMD with 100 μL of Bevacizumab. While patients reported moderate pain, there were no serious AEs, IOP elevation, nor need for rescue therapy at 2 months [159].

Patel and colleagues compared the effects of SC saline to 40 mg/mL SC Aflibercept in a laser-induced CNV rat model. The study revealed a notable and significant reduction in the neovascular leak area on fluorescein angiography at 21 days in those treated with SC Aflibercept [160]. Another molecule, CLS011A, has anti-VEGFR and anti-PDGFR binding properties, making it a promising new candidate for CNV treatment [92]. Kissner and colleagues (2016) injected 4 mg SC CLS011A into the eyes of rabbits and found this to be well tolerated until day 91. Over 60% of the molecule remained in the sclera, choroid, and RPE at this time point. There were no signs of toxicity and no detectable drug levels in the plasma or aqueous humor. The drug was present for the full study duration in the following areas in order from the highest concentration to the lowest: sclera; choroid; RPE; retina; and vitreous humor [161].

The safety of Axitinib, a protein kinase inhibitor that also acts as an anti-VEGF agent, is currently being assessed in a multi-center study for the treatment of nAMD at doses of 0.03, 0.10, 0.50, and 1.0 mg injected into the SCS following IV 2 mg Aflibercept in 27 eyes for 12 weeks. Preliminary safety data show that all doses were well-tolerated with no treatment-related serious AEs. Final safety data are anticipated to be released later in 2023 [162]. Further, an ongoing extension study is underway, which aims to evaluate long-term outcomes for an additional 12 weeks [163]. Before these human clinical trials, Axitinib's safety and drug characteristics were tested in laser-induced CNV animal models by two separate studies. Both studies revealed favorable tolerance and no detectable presence of the drug in plasma or aqueous humor. Moreover, sustained high levels of Axitinib were observed in the sclera, choroid, RPE, and vitreous humor for an extended period. In a rat CNV model, 40% of eyes showed improvement by day 21 in contrast to the saline-injected group. Meanwhile, in the pig CNV model, a statistically significant reduction in fluorescein leakage was observed at weeks 1 and 2 when compared to the saline-injected group [90,92].

Given the successful outcomes of SC therapeutic agents in treating ME secondary to NIU, DME, and CNV, it is unsurprising that well-established corticosteroids and anti-VEGF agents also offer promise for SC treatment of nAMD with minimal AEs. To advance our understanding, larger and longer multicenter trials are needed to assess the safety and feasibility of SC Bevacizumab and TA. While animal studies have demonstrated Aflibercept's efficacy and CLS011A's favorable pharmacokinetic profile, clinical trials are required to confirm their safety and effectiveness. As discussed, a multi-center phase I/II study for the treatment of nAMD with SC Axitinib was initiated based on encouraging data from animal studies. While the preliminary safety results of this clinical trial are promising, the final efficacy and safety results, along with the extension safety study data, are critical to determine if SC Axitinib is a viable treatment option for nAMD in the long term [162,163]. In addition, novel research assessing the anatomical and functional effects of SC RGX-314 for nAMD highlights exciting new advancements that may reduce the need for frequent injections [156,157]. After the results of these clinical trials are released, comparative studies should be leveraged to identify the safest and most efficacious pharmacological agent for long-term nAMD treatment. Emerging research is also exploring novel therapeutic agents. For instance, an ongoing phase I clinical trial aims to assess the use of an integration-deficient lentiviral vector, BD311, to deliver a VEGF antibody gene for the treatment of ocular diseases characterized by CNV, such as nAMD, DME, and ME following RVO. The goal of this study is to achieve constant anti-VEGF activity by delivering the gene to the posterior segment of the eye, suppressing CNV [164].

The separation between the RPE and the innermost part of Bruch's membrane is known as retinal pigment epithelial detachment. Many chorioretinal diseases, such as nAMD, can lead to this pathology alongside idiopathic causes. Recently, Datta and colleagues studied the efficacy and safety of two 0.1 mL SC injections of Bevacizumab administered

1 month apart in 30 patients with serous pigment epithelial detachment for 8 weeks. BCVA improved for all patients 1 week after the first injection, which was maintained and statistically significant at 8 weeks post-injection. There was an objective decrease in pigment epithelium detachment at 2 weeks post-injection, with a statistically significant decrease in mean height of the pigment epithelium detachment at 6 weeks. IOP rose transiently after injection, and patients were treated with 500 mg oral acetazolamide. Patients noted more pain in comparison to IV injections, but no other AEs were reported [165]. Considering the absence of established treatment guidelines for serous pigment epithelial detachment, as well as its limited response to existing treatment options, the findings of this study offer promising prospects for the management of this condition pending larger studies of longer duration.

7.4. Suprachoroidal Injection for Retinal Detachment

The safety and efficacy of SCTA have been well-established in preclinical and clinical studies for ocular diseases, such as ME, secondary to NIU and DME, leading to further investigation of its application for RD. Traditionally, surgical intervention has been the cornerstone for managing rhegmatogenous RD, but addressing the underlying inflammatory process associated with this approach has been deemed beneficial. Systemic steroid therapy may not be universally applicable due to patients' medical comorbidities, such as uncontrolled diabetes and hypertension. Topical steroids pose an increased risk of globe perforation and result in inconsistent drug bioavailability. Likewise, IV corticosteroids can raise IOP and increase the risk of cataract formation and progression [166].

Given these challenges, the utilization of SCTA injections has emerged as a potential alternative to address the limitations associated with other treatment options. Tabl and collaborators (2022) conducted the first clinical trial assessing the use of SC injection for the treatment of RD via injection of SCTA. The study encompassed six eyes with serous retinal detachment caused by Vogt–Koyanagi disease, with untreated eyes serving as controls. Notably, all patients were in the acute phase of the disease and concurrently receiving systemic steroids. The trial demonstrated significant improvements in BCVA and central foveal thickness (CFT) in eyes treated with SCTA at both 1 and 3 months, with no significant difference in IOP between the treated and untreated eyes. These findings confirm the potential of SCTA as an effective adjunctive treatment, along with oral steroids, for managing serous RD due to Vogt–Koyanagi disease [167]. Similarly, another study by Kohli and collaborators (2022) showcased the success of using 4.0 mg SCTA prior to vitrectomy and scleral buckle surgery in 10 patients with serous choroidal detachment associated with rhegmatogenous RD. This prospective, non-comparative study revealed that SCTA resulted in 50% of eyes having >50% reduction in fluid by day 3 and 20% by day 5. In total, only 30% of eyes required surgical drainage before proceeding with vitrectomy. While one eye (10%) experienced a transient increase in IOP to 30 mmHg, which was managed with topical anti-glaucoma medications, no other treatment-related AEs were reported [166].

While preliminary studies show that SCTA may be a promising adjuvant treatment for two types of RD, larger comparative studies are needed to assess if the long-term outcomes of this additional procedure are worth the extra cost and time required to perform it. Currently, clinical research on SCTA is limited to serous RD due to Vogt–Koyanagi disease and serous choroidal detachment associated with rhegmatogenous RD. Expanding research to other RD could shed light on responsive cases warranting SCTA alongside corticosteroid use. Furthermore, longer-term safety studies are required to assess for common AEs known to SCTA use, including cataract progression and IOP elevation.

Several studies have investigated the injection of non-pharmacological substances into the SCS as a medical alternative to scleral buckling procedures for improving outcomes in patients with RD. Gao and colleagues (2019) explored sodium hyaluronate injection into the SCS, followed by retinal hole scleral freezing and laser photocoagulation for rhegmatogenous RD. Remarkably, 50% of the eyes achieved complete reattachment, 33.33%

were partially reattached with subsequent reabsorption of subretinal fluid, and 16.67% did not reattach and required further intervention [168]. The concept of sodium hyaluronate acting as an internal buckle through SCS injection was initially explored in rabbit models by Mittl and collaborators (1987). They demonstrated that, while the buckling effect was short-lived (between 12 and 72 h), sodium hyaluronate remained in the SCS for 10 and 14 days, regardless of the concentration or formulation used [169]. Earlier, Smith (1952) reported a series of five RD cases in which air was injected into the SCS to act as an internal buckle. Satisfactory repositioning of the retina was achieved in all five retinas. However, one case experienced vitreous hemorrhage, two cases had relapsed at 2 and 3 months that required surgical management, and one case required further diathermy [170]. The injection of sodium hyaluronate has shown efficacy in the treatment of rhegmatogenous RD in combination with current standards of treatment in one small clinical study. Larger comparative studies are needed to assess if SC sodium hyaluronate results in improved efficacy compared to the current treatment alone. Additionally, further optimization of the formulation of sodium hyaluronate could result in sustained treatment levels that induce buckling via the SCS for a longer duration. While sodium hyaluronate injection has shown promise in small-scale studies, the scarcity of follow-up research since 2019 may be attributed to advancements achieved through SCTA. Moreover, examining the functional and anatomical changes associated with anatomical improvements is crucial. Comparative clinical trials comparing SC sodium hyaluronate and SCTA versus placebo could lead to new treatment regimens that yield better outcomes for patients with various types of RD.

7.5. Suprachoroidal Injection for Uveitis

SCTA has demonstrated positive effects on visual and anatomical outcomes with minimal AEs in the treatment of ME secondary to NIU, as previously discussed. Moreover, the literature has provided insights regarding its potential role in managing uveitis. Goldstein and colleagues (2016) were the first to explore the use of 4.0 mg SCTA for eight eyes with NIU to assess the preliminary efficacy and safety of this approach. All treated eyes showed improvements in BCVA by 26 weeks. Among the 38 AEs reported, 89% were mild or moderate in severity, and 58% affected the ocular domain. Notably, 18% were related to uveitis progression, 3% were associated with cataract progression requiring extraction, and 16% were attributed to ocular pain with no cases of increased IOP [171].

Prior to human studies, Noronha and colleagues (2015) examined the use of SCTA in a porcine model of acute uveitis induced by lipopolysaccharide injection. The study assessed the anti-inflammatory effects of SCTA in comparison to oral prednisone. Single eyes of 16 porcine models received either SC salt solution, 2.0 mg SCTA, or 0.1 or 1.0 mg/kg/d of prednisone every 24 h for a total of 3 days, with the other untreated eye acting as a control. The results demonstrated that SCTA (day 1) resulted in more rapid anti-inflammatory effects than oral prednisone (day 3). SCTA was found to be as effective as high-dose oral prednisone and superior to low-dose prednisone. On the first and second days of treatment, SCTA showed lower inflammation scores compared to controls. On the third day, both high-dose prednisone and SCTA had lower inflammation scores than controls. These findings highlighted the advantages of local drug administration with SCTA over systemic prednisone, which has the potential to lead to side effects such as hyperglycemia, immunosuppression, osteoporosis, and adrenal suppression with long-term use [172].

In another study by Gilger and colleagues (2013), the difference between IVTA and SCTA was investigated for the treatment of acute posterior uveitis in a similar porcine model. The researchers compared the efficacy and safety of different doses and administration routes of TA (0.2 mg or 2.0 mg TA using SC or IV injection). The results suggest that 0.2 mg and 2.0 mg of SCTA were equally effective as 2.0 mg IVTA in reducing inflammation and were similar in terms of IOP and OCT measurements. Eyes in the high-dose SCTA group had mean histologic inflammatory scores in the ocular posterior segment that were significantly lower than eyes treated with IVTA, as seen in Figure 7. Additionally, the mean vitreous humor cell count and protein concentration were lower in the high-dose SCTA group when compared to low-dose SCTA and IVTA groups. There were no significant differences in mean aqueous humor protein concentration among the groups, and there were AEs reported within 3 days of treatment [173].

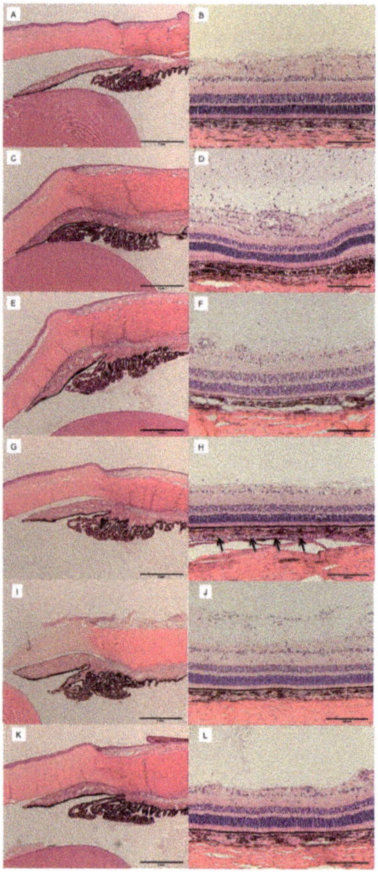

Figure 7. Ocular histopathology of eyes 3 days after IVT injection of balanced salt solution (BSS) or 100 ng of lipopolysaccharide (LPS) and 72 h after SCS or IVT injection of vehicle, 0.2 mg TA (low-dose TA), or 2.0 mg of TA (high-dose TA). Hematoxylin and eosin stain. (**A**) Anterior segment of eyes injected with BSS IVT and vehicle in SCS (group 1). (**B**) Posterior segment of eyes injected with BSS IVT and vehicle in SCS (group 1). (**C**) Anterior segment of eyes injected with LPS IVT and vehicle in SCS (group 2). (**D**) Posterior segment of eyes injected with LPS IVT and vehicle in SCS (group 2). (**E**) Anterior segment of eyes injected with LPS IVT and low-dose TA in SCS (group 3). (**F**) Posterior segment of eyes injected with LPS IVT and low-dose TA in SCS (group 3). (**G**) Anterior segment of eyes injected with LPS IVT and high-dose TA in SCS (group 4). (**H**) Posterior segment of eyes injected with LPS IVT and high-dose TA in SCS (group 4). Arrows indicate presence of TA in SCS. (**I**) Anterior segment of eyes injected with LPS IVT and low-dose TA IVT (group 5). (**J**) Posterior segment of eyes injected with LPS IVT and low-dose TA IVT (group 5). (**K**) Anterior segment of eyes injected with LPS IVT and high-dose TA IVT (group 6). (**L**) Posterior segment of eyes injected with LPS IVT and high-dose TA IVT (group 6). Reproduced with permission [173].

Similarly, Patel and collaborators (2013) conducted a study using a subretinal endotoxin-induced model of panuveitis in rabbits and found that 4.0 mg SCTA was equally effective as IVTA in reducing ocular inflammation. The study lasted for 22 days, and no AEs, including

IOP changes, were reported. After 24 h, eyes treated with SCTA showed less panuveitis than IVTA and control eyes. Both SCTA and IVTA resulted in significantly reduced viritis, aqueous flare, cellularity, and histopathological inflammation compared to controls [174].

In 2015, Chen and collaborators used a rabbit model of uveitis induced by lipopolysaccharide to compare the effects of 50 μL (2.0 mg) SCTA and subtenon injection of 20 mg TA. They found that SCTA was well tolerated and provided better therapeutic effects than subtenon 20 mg. Following SCTA, there was an acute elevation in IOP, with higher volumes of SCTA leading to higher IOP. The peak concentration of TA (<1.0 ng/mL) was detected in the retina and posterior vitreous, with nondetectable in the aqueous and 11.6 ng/mL in the plasma. SCTA demonstrated better efficacy with significantly lower aqueous humor cells, lower vitreous opacity scores, and reduced vitreous inflammation on histology when compared to subtenon TA [67].

Porcine models, with similarities in terms of anatomy, size, and retinal vascular pattern to the human eye, have offered valuable insights into the study of SC injection. While animal models are of critical importance, it should be noted that these animal models represent only acute disease and do not fully capture the chronic nature of uveitis, highlighting the need for human clinical trials. Following the improvement in BCVA that was observed in the study by Goldstein and colleagues, further exploration of the use of SCTA for treating ME due to uveitis was conducted by PEACHTREE, as seen previously. However, there still remains a need for these large, long-term, and masked controlled studies to evaluate the efficacy and safety of SCTA for treating the different types of uveitis without ME affecting different parts of the eye.

7.6. Suprachoroidal Injection for Glaucoma

Pharmacological treatments for lowering IOP in glaucoma patients often have low bioavailability when administered topically. This results in the need for multiple daily eye drops, leading to poor treatment adherence and systemic side effects [175–178]. SC injection, which offers higher drug bioavailability at the ciliary body, has gained interest in glaucoma research. Kim and collaborators (2014) found significant dose-sparing of anti-glaucoma medications, Sulprostone (a prostaglandin analog) and Brimonidine (an a2-adrenergic agonist), when injected into the supraciliary zone of the SCS of rabbits compared to topical administration. SC injection of both medications reduced IOP maximally by 3 mmHg in a dose-dependent manner for 9 h [179]. Chiang and colleagues (2016) were able to sustain levels of Brimonidine in the SCS using Brimonidine-loaded poly (lactic acid) microspheres for the treatment of glaucoma for 1 month. In rabbits, these microspheres were found to reduce IOP by 6 mmHg initially and then, by progressively lower amounts for over 1 month. AEs included mild conjunctival redness treated with antibiotic or steroid ointment, difficulty healing at the injection site, and a histological foreign body response to the microspheres with no serious AEs [180].

By employing a direct injection approach into the anterior portion of the SC space, Kim et al. effectively demonstrated therapeutic IOP reduction with lower doses compared to topical treatment in animals. This injection site, termed the supraciliary zone of the SCS, closely neighbors the site of action of many anti-glaucoma drugs, namely the ciliary body. However, prior to initiating human trials to assess the safety and efficacy of the SCS for targeting glaucoma treatment, it is imperative to conduct more extensive safety studies involving more animal models and comparative investigations against current standard treatments. Interestingly, Chiang's study was able to demonstrate that therapeutic loaded microspheres can also lengthen the time of therapy for up to 1 month. While further refinement of microspheres is needed for optimal results, their study demonstrated that sustained levels of medications in the SCS can be achieved for the treatment of glaucoma for up to 1 month. Notably, high-viscosity formulations injected into this space ensure minimal diffusion toward posterior eye structures, thus enhancing therapeutic effects. These studies collectively underscore the need for additional research aimed at optimizing anti-glaucoma treatment in the supraciliary zone for a longer duration of action using varying drug formulations, viscosities, particle suspensions, particle size, and osmotic and ionic characteristics.

Furthermore, the potential space between the sclera and choroid can temporarily be expanded without long-term AEs and has been well tolerated in animals and humans [66,173,181]. To find a medication and surgery-free method to treat glaucoma, Chae and collaborators (2020) found that SCS expansion using an in situ-forming hydrogel, as seen in Figure 8, reduced IOP in rabbit models for 1 and 4 months, respectively. Their hypothesis was that SCS expansion increases the drainage of aqueous humor from the eye through the uveovortex pathway [182]. No AEs were reported, but minor hemorrhage and fibrosis were observed at the injection site.

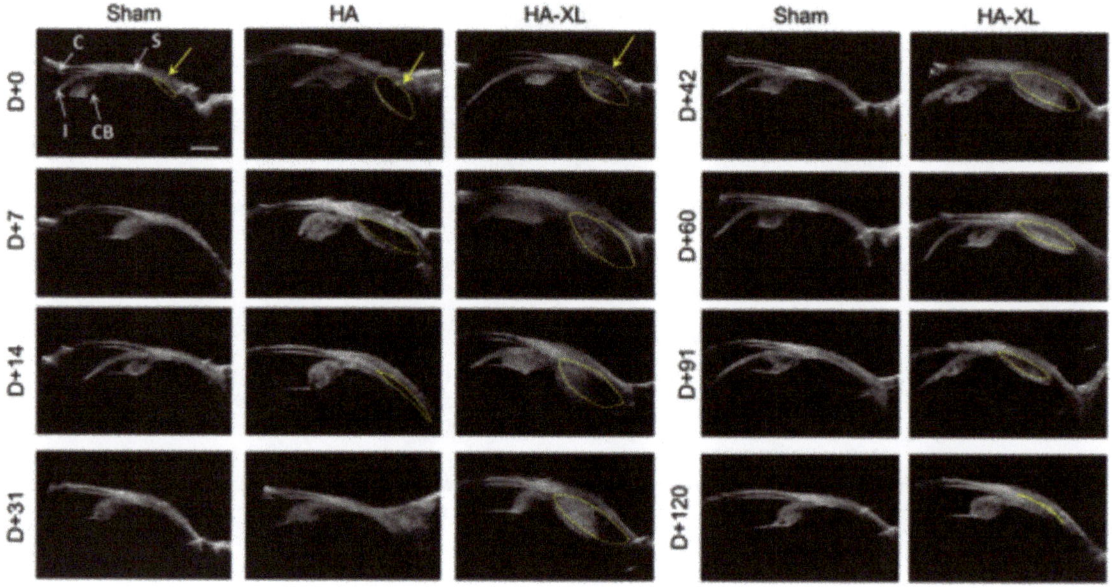

Figure 8. Ultrasound biomicroscopy imaging of hydrogel-injected eyes. Rabbit eyes were injected with Hanks' Balanced Salt Solution (Sham), commercial hyaluronic acid hydrogel (HA), or in situ-forming hyaluronic acid hydrogel group (HA-XL) and imaged over time. The yellow arrow indicates the approximate injection site, and the yellow dashed line roughly outlines the expanded suprachoroidal space. Images are representative of seven eyes per group (HA-XL group), two eyes per group (Sham), or the only eye available from the HA group. Abbreviations—C: Cornea; CB: Ciliary Body; I: Iris; S: Sclera. D + 0 refers to day zero after injection; D + 7 to 7 days after, etc. Scale bar: 2 mm. Reproduced with permission [182].

Hao and colleagues (2022) confirmed these findings by assessing the effect of an in situ-forming polyzwitterion polycarboxybetaine hydrogel, which decreased IOP for 6 weeks. The treatment was well tolerated with no serious AEs, minimal inflammatory reaction, and histopathological evidence that the SCS became expanded post hydrogel injection [183]. The use of a non-pharmacological approach through SC injection shows promising results in terms of IOP reduction with minor AEs in animal models, such as inflammatory reactions at the injection site. These results pave the way for clinical trials assessing the safety and efficacy of SC expansion to manage glaucoma in humans; however, none have been initiated at present. If shown to be safe and efficacious in human studies, the combination of SC expansion and SC anti-glaucoma medications could stand to lower the incidence of blindness from glaucoma.

7.7. Suprachoroidal Injection for Uveal Melanoma

AU-011, also known as Belzupacap Sarotalocan, is a promising treatment for ocular melanoma. This compound triggers cellular necrosis through an immune-mediated response when light is activated. Savinainen and collaborators (2020) found that AU-011 was well distributed in the choroid and resulted in effective anticancer activity due to its long duration of action in rabbit models of choroidal melanoma. Notably, a 100 μL dose of AU-011 remained in the choroid for several days, with distribution across 75% of the posterior globe. Tumor regression and cancer cell necrosis were observed histologically [74]. In 2021, the same researchers determined that SC AU-011 outperformed IV injection in terms of tumor distribution and bioavailability and decreased unintended exposure in a similar rabbit model of choroidal melanoma. Staining showed SC injection resulted in AU-011 tumor penetration at levels five times higher than IV injection, which remained up to 48 h post-injection. In contrast, IV injection resulted in AU-011 staying primarily on the tumor surface. After SC administration, negligible levels of AU-011 were present in the vitreous, and high exposure levels were present in the tumor and choroid–retina [184]. While these two studies focused on AU-011 as a therapeutic in the treatment of choroidal melanoma, Kang and colleagues (2011) found that suprachoroidally injected resin beads and fluorescent microspheres were successfully delivered using a microcatheter to the site of intraocular melanoma. They found no inflammatory reaction associated with the injection [185].

AU-011 stands at the forefront of choroidal melanoma research as an alternative to radiotherapy in preventing vision loss. The interim results of an ongoing multi-center trial for primary choroidal melanoma by IV AU-011 injection have shown the treatment to be well tolerated and produce adequate tumor control, in addition to maintaining vision [186]. Following these results, Demirci and collaborators (2022) demonstrated that SC injection of AU-011 was also safe in the dose escalation phase of the trial. In this phase, 17 subjects with primary indeterminate lesions and small choroidal melanoma received up to three cycles of 3 weekly SC AU-011 injections (max dose of 80 μg) with two rounds of laser. In terms of AEs, 24% experienced anterior chamber inflammation, 12% experienced conjunctival hyperemia, 21% had eye pain, and 12% reported punctate keratitis with no serious AEs related to treatment [187].

While brachytherapy is currently the standard of treatment for uveal melanoma, it is associated with extraocular muscle trauma, radiation toxicity in the form of radiation retinopathy and maculopathy, and ocular conditions such as strabismus, cataracts, and glaucoma [188]. Animal studies have shown that SC injection allows for adequate drug delivery directly to the tumor with a quick onset of action at lower doses. This targeted delivery can increase the range of tumor sizes that can be treated and enable direct penetration while reducing the risk of AEs. The efficacy results of the clinical trial by Demirci and collaborators, to be released later this year, stand to revolutionize the treatment of choroidal melanoma [189]. As ocular AEs can still occur using this method of injection, including changes to BCVA, larger multicenter studies with longer follow-ups are required to assess its safety and to determine long-term remission rates. Future RCTs between patients undergoing radiotherapy, IV AU-011, and SC AU-011 could determine the treatment with the best efficacy and safety profile for patients with uveal melanoma.

7.8. Suprachoroidal Injection for Myopia

Currently, there is a lack of animal and clinical studies investigating the use of SC injection for the treatment of myopia. However, Venkatesh and Takkar (2017) proposed that injecting biological cement into the SCS could halt the pathological elongation of the eyeball associated with this condition [190]. In pathological myopia, the sagittal axial length of the eye is longer than expected, which can lead to complications, such as RD [14,191]. However, at present, there is a need for preclinical animal studies to assess safety prior to initiating human trials. While the injection of cement is currently used in a variety of orthopedic conditions, its therapeutic potential in the eye may be limited by the eye's aqueous environment. Elevating pressure in this area to induce beneficial alterations in elongation mechanics could potentially lead to ocular complications, including trauma. Given the availability of non-invasive, affordable, and effective treatments for myopia, such as glasses and atropine, there might be limited motivation to explore the utilization of SC injection for myopia treatment.

7.9. Suprachoroidal Injection for Ocular Inflammatory Diseases

Ketorolac, a short-acting nonsteroidal inflammatory drug, is commonly used topically to relieve ocular inflammation and the resulting pain. However, its topical administration results in suboptimal therapeutic drug levels or AEs with increasing drug dosages. Side effects can include burning and stinging, as well as delayed corneal healing and conjunctival hyperemia [192]. IV injection carries the risk of vitreous opacity and various retinal pathologies [193]. In an animal study involving 54 rabbits, Wang and collaborators (2012) found that IV injection of 250 μg/0.05 mL Ketorolac Tromethamine resulted in higher intraocular concentrations for a longer duration in comparison to SC and IC groups. Mean maximum concentrations of Ketorolac in the vitreous and retina-choroid were highest for IV, followed by the SC and IC injections. In the retina-choroid, there was a statistically significant larger amount of Ketorolac with IV injection compared to SC injection. The half-life of Ketorolac was also longer with IV injection, with plasma concentrations below 0.4 μg/mL in all three groups. Ketorolac remained detectable in the retina-choroid for 24 and 8 h after the IV and SC injection, respectively [194]. Liu and colleagues found unilateral SC injections of 3.0 mg and 6.0 mg Ketorolac Tromethamine in rabbits to be safe as compared to controls in a 2012 animal study. Electroretinography showed no abnormal changes at 1 to 4 weeks post-injection, and the histomorphology of retinal cells was preserved at 4 weeks when compared to the control group [195].

At present, there is limited research on the use of SC Ketorolac in the treatment of ocular inflammatory diseases. Current evidence indicates that up to 6.0 mg of SC Ketorolac was safe from functional and anatomical perspectives on the rabbit retina, warranting larger animal studies to demonstrate efficacy and further safety. Wang and collaborators observed an increase in the maximum mean concentrations of Ketorolac in the vitreous and retina–choroid and an increased half-life for IV as opposed to SC injection. This finding aligns with other CNV animal models showing faster Bevacizumab and Pazopanib clearance with SC injection due to factors that can affect the duration of therapeutic action, such as the drug formulation, volume, viscosity, particle size, in addition to osmotic and ionic characteristics [152,153]. Thus, further studies are required to assess the optimization of Ketorolac drug formulations to obtain a longer duration of action in the SCS. The efficacy and safety of SC injection of Ketorolac should also be compared with other methods of delivery to the eye, including IV injection, retrobulbar injection, and topical administration, to determine the most efficacious approach for patients with a variety of inflammatory diseases, including scleritis, uveitis, keratitis, and conjunctivitis in future larger, multicenter human trials. Interestingly, there have been studies assessing the use of IV injection of Ketorolac, including nonsteroidal anti-inflammatory drugs, as opposed to corticosteroids, in the treatment of CME, DME, CNV, uveitis, and AMD [196–199]. Due to the low AE profile of nonsteroidal anti-inflammatory drugs compared to corticosteroids, particularly in relation to cataract progression and IOP elevation, further research on its administration using SC injection is warranted.

8. Conclusions

Throughout this review, we have endeavored to shed light on the potential of SC injection as an innovative and effective technique for targeted drug delivery to the posterior segment of the eye. Our comprehensive review of the most recent literature has provided compelling evidence of the utility of this minimally invasive method in addressing the challenges associated with traditional treatment approaches. SC injections present a significant advancement over conventional administration routes, such as eye drops and

IV injections, offering increased drug bioavailability, extended duration of action, and a marked reduction in off-target adverse effects.

While suprachoroidal injection offers a promising and innovative approach to targeted drug delivery for various ocular conditions, its widespread use is hindered by several current challenges:

1. Biomechanical Considerations: Optimizing the chemical and physical properties of the injectate (such as size and viscosity) is crucial for different indications and diseases, depending on the anatomical location. This requires the refinement of current techniques, including injection speed and approach (single quadrant vs. multiple quadrant), to ensure the precise delivery of the correct amount of drug to the appropriate anatomical site for the desired duration of action;
2. Need for Further Clinical Studies: More phase 3 clinical trials will be essential for broader clinical adoption. As it stands, most studies of indications other than macular edema are either preclinical or early-stage clinical trials. Comprehensive late-stage clinical research is paramount to assess the efficacy, safety, and applicability of suprachoroidal injections across various ocular and retinal conditions;
3. Clinical Translation Challenges: Factors such as drug storage, cost-effectiveness, and efficiency compared to IV injection (the current go-to administration route for posterior segment diseases due to its efficacy) must be carefully considered. Reimbursement considerations also play a vital role in the practical implementation of this technique;
4. Transition Challenges: The shift away from IV to SC injections will not be instantaneous. Strong evidence and concerted efforts will be required for clinicians to be willing to adapt to and learn this new technique and to overcome logistical issues such as in-office procedures.

Despite these challenges, the potential of SC injection is undeniable. Looking forward, it is encouraging to envision a future in which SC injection can be used in conjunction with biotech products, genes, and cell-based therapies to initiate a new era of personalized treatments. This could revolutionize the field of ophthalmology, enhance patient care, and improve outcomes in ocular disease management.

While there is certainly more work to be performed, the path is clear for the continuation of rigorous research into this technique. The potential of SC injection in reshaping the landscape of ocular drug delivery provides a compelling call to action for researchers, clinicians, and stakeholders in the field of ophthalmology. Guided by the powerful intersection of interdisciplinary collaboration, we aim to illuminate a future where devastating vision loss from diseases such as retinitis pigmentosa, severe diabetic retinopathy, and advanced age-related macular degeneration is no longer a life sentence. Together, we strive to restore not only sight but hope, dignity, and quality of life for those grappling with the darkness of these ocular diseases.

Author Contributions: Conceptualization, K.Y.W.; writing—original draft preparation, K.Y.W., J.K.F., and T.G.; writing—review and editing, K.Y.W., J.K.F., T.G., M.Z., and S.D.T.; supervision, M.Z. and S.D.T. All authors have read and agreed to the published version of the manuscript.

Funding: This research received no external funding.

Institutional Review Board Statement: Not applicable.

Informed Consent Statement: Not applicable.

Data Availability Statement: Data sharing is not applicable.

Acknowledgments: Lysa Houadj contributed to Section 6; Tasnim Tabassum contributed to Section 5; Sophie Valence, referencing and formatting; Roselyn Luo and Ashley Jong, figures.

Conflicts of Interest: The authors declare no conflict of interest.

Appendix A

Table A1. Suprachoroidal injection in ocular diseases.

No	Disease	Drug	Treatment	Key Findings	Study Design	Phase	Study Title
Macular edema secondary to non-infectious uveitis							
1	Macular edema secondary to non-infectious uveitis	TA	Single unilateral SC injection of TA, 4 mg (0.1 mL of 40 mg/mL) at day 0 and week 12 vs. SC sham injection at day 0 and week 12	At week 24: -BCVA gain > 15 ETDRS letters: 46.9% (intervention) vs. 15.6% (control) ($p < 0.0001$) -Early improvement: noticed by week 4 -CST reduction: −153 μm (intervention) vs. −18 μm (control) ($p < 0.001$) -ME resolution (CST < 300 μm): 53% (intervention) vs. 2% (control) ($p < 0.001$) -Need for rescue therapy: 13.5% (intervention) vs. 72% (control) -Time to rescue therapy: 89 days (intervention) vs. 36 days (control) -AEs, including IOP elevation: less in intervention group -Cataract AE rates: comparable in both groups -No serious AEs	Randomized, controlled, double-masked, multi-center	Clinical trial (phase III)	Efficacy and safety of suprachoroidal CLS-TA for macular edema secondary to noninfectious uveitis (PEACHTREE) [94]
2	Macular edema secondary to non-infectious uveitis	TA	Single unilateral SC injection of TA, 4 mg (0.1 mL of 40 mg/mL) vs. SC sham injection In patients ≤50 years and >50 years of age	At week 24: -BCVA gain: similar between age groups; greater improvements in intervention group at all visits -CST reduction: change from baseline greater in intervention than sham group in all age groups at all visits -Need for rescue therapy: lower in intervention than sham groups across age groups -Incidences of increased IOP and cataract AEs: similar between intervention and sham groups in all age groups (no statistical analysis)	Randomized, controlled, double-masked, multi-center	Post-hoc analysis of phase III clinical trial	Suprachoroidal triamcinolone acetonide injectable suspension for macular edema associated with uveitis: visual and anatomic outcomes by age [95]

Table A1. *Cont.*

No	Disease	Drug	Treatment	Key Findings	Study Design	Phase	Study Title
3	Macular edema secondary to non-infectious uveitis	TA	Single unilateral SC injection of TA, 4 mg (0.1 mL of 40 mg/mL) vs. SC sham injection In patients with concurrent use of systemic corticosteroid or steroid-sparing therapy vs. no use	Among UME patients receiving no steroid-sparing therapy, at week 24: -ETDRS letter change: +15.6 (intervention) vs. +4.9 (control) ($p < 0.001$) -CST change: −169.8 µm (intervention) vs. −10.3 µm (control) ($p < 0.001$) -Need for rescue therapy: 14.7% (SCTA) vs. 69.4% (control) Among patients receiving steroid therapy, at week 24: -ETDRS letter change: +9.4 (intervention) vs. −3.2 (control) ($p = 0.019$) -CST change: −108.3 µm (intervention) vs. −43.5 µm (control) ($p = 0.190$) -Need for rescue therapy: 10.7% (intervention) vs. 80% (control) -AEs: no serious AEs in either group	Randomized, controlled, double-masked, multi-center	Post-hoc analysis of phase III clinical trial	Suprachoroidal CLS-TA with and without systemic corticosteroid and/or steroid sparing therapy: a post-hoc analysis of the phase 3 PEACHTREE clinical trial [96]
4	Macular edema secondary to non-infectious uveitis	TA	SC injection of TA, 4 mg (0.1 mL of 40 mg/mL) at baseline and week 12 vs. SC injection of sham at baseline and week 12	Over 48 weeks: -Need for rescue therapy: 39.3% (intervention) vs. 60% (control) -Medium time to rescue therapy: 257 days (intervention) vs. 55.5 days (control) -At least 1 ocular AE: 64.3% (intervention) vs. 60% (control); most common being subcapsular cataract -At least 1 elevated IOP reading (>10 mm Hg): 14.3% (intervention) vs. 0% (control)	Observational extension study of PEACHTREE trial	Parent study was clinical trial (phase III)	Extension study of the safety and efficacy of CLS-TA for treatment of macular oedema associated with non-infectious uveitis (MAGNOLIA) [97]
5	Macular edema secondary to non-infectious uveitis	TA	Single unilateral SC injection of TA 4 mg (0.1 mL of 40 mg/m) at day 0 and week 12	At 24 weeks: -BCVA improvement: 68.9 to 75.0 at week 8 and 75.9 at week 24 -CST improvement: 335.9 µm to 284.0 µm at week 24 -IOP elevation > 10 mmHg, >30 mmHg: 15.8%, 5.3% of participants with 87.5% treated with IOP lowering drops -Cataract AEs: 10.5% of participants, only 1 was treatment-related -Treatment related AEs: 18.4% of participants -Serious AEs related to treatment: None	Nonrandomized, single arm, multi-center	Clinical trial (phase III)	Suprachoroidal CLS-TA for non-infectious uveitis: an open-label, safety trial (AZALEA) [93]

Table A1. *Cont.*

No	Disease	Drug	Treatment	Key Findings	Study Design	Phase	Study Title
6	Macular edema secondary to non-infectious uveitis	TA	Single unilateral, SC injection TA, 40 mg/mL (4 mg in 100 μL) vs. Single unilateral, SC injection TA, 8 mg/mL (0.8 mg in 100 μL)	-CST reduction: −135 μm at month 1 ($p = 0.0056$), −164 μm at month 2 ($p = 0.0017$) (4 mg group); −78 μm at month 2 (0.8 mg group) -ETDRS letter change: +7.7 at month 1 ($p = 0.0001$), +9.2 at month 2 ($p = 0.0004$); 65% had improvement of >5 ETDRS letters (4 mg group) -Anterior cell grade: 60% resolution (change to score of 0 for those >0 at baseline) (4 mg group) -Vitreous haze score: 80% improvement (for those >0 at baseline) (4 mg group) -At least 1 AE: 47% (4 mg group) vs. 100% (0.8 mg group), none requiring treatment -Serious AEs related to treatment or increase in IOP: none	Dose randomized, controlled, masked, multi-center	Clinical trial (phase II)	Suprachoroidal injection of triamcinolone acetonide, CLS-TA, for macular edema due to noninfectious uveitis (DOGWOOD) [98]
7	Macular edema secondary to non-infectious uveitis	TA	Single unilateral SC injection of TA, 4 mg (0.1 mL of 40 mg/mL)	-CMT reduction: >50% reduction at 1 month ($p < 0.001$) with a further reduction of 22% by month 3 ($p < 0.001$) -Resolution of ME: 100% of patients -BCVA gain: significant improvement from baseline at month 1 and month 3 ($p < 0.001$) -AE: lenticular changes in 5 -No significant difference in IOP by 3 months	Prospective, nonrandomized, interventional study, uni-center	Clinical trial (phase I/II)	Safety and efficacy of suprachoroidal injection of triamcinolone in treating macular edema secondary to noninfectious uveitis [99]
8	Macular edema secondary to uveitis, vascular disorders and diabetes	TA	SC injection of TA, 4 mg (0.1 mL of 40 mg/mL)	-BCVA gain: significant improvement observed -Early improvement at 1 week -IOP: highest at 6 months in 11–15 mmHg cases and highest at 1 month in 16–20 mmHg cases	Prospective interventional study, uni-center	Clinical trial (phase I/II)	Visual outcome after suprachoroidal injection of triamcinolone acetate in cystoid macular edema of different pathology [100]

Table A1. *Cont.*

No	Disease	Drug	Treatment	Key Findings	Study Design	Phase	Study Title
Diabetic macular edema							
9	Diabetic macular edema	Aflibercept in combination with TA	Single unilateral IV injection of Aflibercept, 2 mg (0.05 mL) followed by single unilateral SC injection of TA, 4 mg (0.1 mL) in same eye of treatment-naïve participants vs. Single unilateral SC injection of TA, 4 mg (0.1 mL) alone in previously treated participants	-Average number of SCTA injections: 3.3 (monotherapy) vs. 2.6 (combination) At 6 months: -Mean CST reduction: −128 μm (monotherapy) vs. −91 μm (combination) -Mean ETDRS letter change: +1.1 (monotherapy) vs. +8.5 (combination) -AEs: elevated IOP (2 patients), cataracts (3 patients), pain during the procedure (1 patient)	Nonrandomized, open-label, parallel-design, multi-center	Clinical trial (phase I/II)	Suprachoroidal triamcinolone acetonide for diabetic macular edema: the HULK trial [102]
10	Diabetic macular edema	Aflibercept in combination with TA	Single unilateral IV injection of Aflibercept, 2 mg (0.05 mL) followed by single unilateral SC injection of TA, 4 mg (0.1 mL) in same eye of treatment-naïve participants vs. Single unilateral SC injection of TA, 4 mg (0.1 mL) alone in previously treated participants	-Mean time from last SCTA delivery to final AS-OCT: 4.8 (range: 1.0–9.9) months -Mean SCS width at final AS-OCT: 8.4 μm (combination) vs. 8.1 μm (monotherapy) ($p = 0.698$) -Mean SCS width: 9.9 μm to 75.1 μm ($p < 0.001$) immediately before to 30 min after SC injection; normalized to 14.9 μm 1 month after final injection ($p = 0.221$) -Anatomical differences from baseline: none in both groups	Nonrandomized, controlled	Clinical trial (phase I/II)	Suprachoroidal space alterations following delivery of triamcinolone acetonide: post-hoc analysis of the phase 1/2 HULK study of patients with diabetic macular edema [4]
11	Diabetic macular edema	Aflibercept in combination with TA	IV injection of Aflibercept, 2 mg (0.05 mL) followed by SC injection of TA, 4 mg (0.1 mL) at months 0 and 3 vs. Monthly IV injection of Aflibercept, 2 mg (0.05 mL) followed by SC injection of sham for 3 months	By week 24: -Mean ETDRS letter change: +11.4 (combination) vs. +13.8 (monotherapy) ($p = 0.228$) -Mean CST reduction: −212.1 μm (combination) vs. −178.6 μm (monotherapy) ($p = 0.089$) -Number of treatments required: 2.6 (combination) vs. 4.6 (monotherapy) -AEs: no serious AEs related to treatment in either group	Randomized, controlled, double-masked, parallel design, multi-center	Clinical trial (phase II)	Suprachoroidal CLS-TA plus intravitreal aflibercept for diabetic macular edema: a randomized, double-masked, parallel-design, controlled study (The TYBEE trial) [103]

Table A1. *Cont.*

No	Disease	Drug	Treatment	Key Findings	Study Design	Phase	Study Title
12	Diabetic macular edema	TA in combination with IVB	SC injection of TA, 0.1 mL of 40 mg/mL + IVB, 1.25 mg of 0.05 mL; another injection of IVB (same dose) at 1 month and 2 months vs. SC sham injection of TA + IVB, 1.25 mg of 0.05 mL; another injection of IVB (same dose) at 1 month and 2 months	-Mean BCVA change (log MAR): -0.37 ± 0.24 ($p < 0.001$) (combination) vs. -0.20 ± 0.20 (monotherapy) ($p = 0.004$) at 12 weeks [between-group analysis ($p = 0.014$)]; combination group showed improvements from baseline at week 4 ($p = 0.046$) and 24 weeks later ($p < 0.001$) -Mean CST reduction: higher in combination group vs. monotherapy group ($p = 0.019$) -AEs: no serious AEs related to treatment in either group	Randomized, double-masked, parallel design, uni-center	Clinical trial (Phase II/III)	Suprachoroidal injection of triamcinolone acetonide plus intravitreal bevacizumab in diabetic macular edema: a randomized pilot trial [104]
13	Diabetic macular edema	TA	SC injection of TA, 4 mg (0.1 mL of 40 mg/mL) vs. IVB, 2.5 mg/0.01 mL	-Mean ETDRS letter change: +5 after 3 months; higher in the SCTA vs. IVB group ($p = 0.002$) -Mean CST reduction: at least 10% from baseline after 1 and 3 months; higher in SCTA vs. IVB group ($p = 0.01$ and $p = 0.04$, respectively) -Efficacy: 37.5% (SCTA) vs. 29.5% (IVB) ($p = 0.03$)	Prospective observational study, uni-center	Clinical trial (Phase I/II)	Comparison of suprachoroidal injection of triamcinolone acetonide versus intravitreal bevacizumab in primary diabetic macular odema [106]
14	Diabetic macular edema	TA	SC injection of TA, 4 mg (0.1 mL of 40 mg/mL) vs. IV of TA, 4 mg (0.1 mL of 40 mg/mL) vs. SC injection of TA, 2 mg (0.1 mL of 20 mg/mL)	-Mean BCVA gain: significant improvements in all 3 groups at 1 and 3 months; greatest improvement in 4 mg SCTA group by 1 month, BVCA returned to near baseline values at 6 months, except the 4 mg SCTA group -Mean CMT reduction: significantly decreased in all groups at 1 and 3 months; highest reduction in 4 mg SCTA group; CMT increased again after 3 months and returned to near baseline values at 6 months, except 4 mg SCTA group which maintained a mean reduction of 60.18 μm -AEs: no signs of infection, acute rise of IOP on injection day, nor serious AEs in any group	Prospective, interventional, randomized, uni-center	Clinical trial (Phase II)	Suprachoroidal versus intravitreal triamcinolone acetonide for the treatment of diabetic macular edema [107]
15	Diabetic macular edema	TA in combination with IVB	Single IVB 1.25 mg + single SC injection of TA, 2 mg vs. Single IVB 1.25 mg only	At 1 month: -Mean CMT reduction: $-113 + 10$ μm (combination) vs. $-81 + 10$ μm (monotherapy) ($p < 0.001$) -AEs: <33% reported mild to moderate pain	Randomized, uni-center	Clinical trial (Phase II)	Comparison of suprachoroidal triamcinolone injection with intravitreal bevacizumab vs. intravitreal bevacizumab only in treatment of refractory diabetic macular edema [105]

Table A1. *Cont.*

No	Disease	Drug	Treatment	Key Findings	Study Design	Phase	Study Title
16	Diabetic macular edema (refractory)	TA	Single IV injection of TA, 4 mg (0.1 mL of 40 mg/mL) vs. Single SC injection of TA, 4 mg (0.1 mL of 40 mg/mL)	-Mean BVCA gain: improved compared to baseline in both groups at 6 weeks; no difference between groups at 1 month -Mean CMT reduction: reduced in both groups at 6 weeks; comparable between groups at 1 month -Elevated IOP: higher in the IVTA vs. SCTA group at months 3 and 6 ($p < 0.003$); -Cataract progression: slower in SCTA vs. IVTA group -Serious AEs: none in either group	Randomized, parallel arm, uni-center	Clinical trial (Phase II)	Comparison between suprachoroidal triamcinolone and intravitreal triamcinolone acetonide in patients of resistant diabetic macular edema [108]
17	Diabetic macular edema post pars plana vitrectomy (PPV)	TA	SC injection of TA, 4 mg (0.1 mL of 40 mg/mL) post PPV	-Mean BVCA gain (log MAR): 0.75 ± 0.40 μm at baseline to 0.40 ± 0.33 μm at 8 weeks ($p = 0.003$) -Mean CMT reduction: 35% reduction by week 1 ($p = 0.003$); 43.9% by week 4 ($p = 0.003$), 45.74% reduction by 8 weeks ($p = 0.003$) -Retreatment: none required -AEs: no statistically significant change in IOP, no serious AEs	Retrospective, single arm case series	Not applicable	Suprachoroidal injection of triamcinolone acetonide using a custom-made needle to treat diabetic macular edema post pars plana vitrectomy: a case series [109]
18	Diabetic macular edema (refractory)	TA	Single SC injection of TA, 4 mg (0.1 mL of 40 mg/mL)	-Mean BCVA improvement (logMAR): from 1.193 ± 0.2 at baseline to 0.76 ± 0.3 at 12 months (p-value < 0.001); eyes with more baseline CMT and worse baseline BCVA achieved worse final BCVA at 12 months -Mean CMT reduction: 478.7 ± 170.2μm at baseline to 230.2 ± 47.4 μm at 12 months ($p < 0.001$) -AEs: mean IOP increased significantly 1 month post injection but returned to baseline levels at month 3	Prospective, nonrandomized, single arm, uni-center	Clinical trial (Phase I/II)	Effectiveness of suprachoroidal injection of triamcinolone acetonide in resistant diabetic macular edema using a modified microneedle [110]
19	Diabetic macular edema (refractory)	TA	Single SC injection of TA, 4 mg (0.1 mL of 40 mg/mL)	At 3 months: -Mean CMT reduction: from 776.21.0 ± 19.17 to 251.14 ± 6.27 μm ($p < 0.001$) -Mean BCVA improvement: 0.10 ± 0.005 to 0.37 ± 0.01 ($p < 0.001$) -Mean IOP: reduced from 13.01 ± 0.10 to 13.26 ± 0.10 mmHg ($p < 0.001$) -AEs: no serious AEs related to treatment	Nonrandomized, single arm, uni-center	Clinical trial (Phase I/II)	Suprachoroidal injection of triamcinolone acetonide for management of resistant diabetic macular oedema [111]
20	Diabetic macular edema (refractory)	TA	SC injection of TA, 4 mg (0.1 mL of 40 mg/mL)	-Mean CST reduction: from 612.89 ± 195.58 μm (baseline) to 308.59 ± 56.75 μm at 1 month and 304.89 ± 54.29 μm at 3 months ($p < 0.00001$) -Mean BCVA improvement: reduced at 3 months ($p < 0.05$) -Mean IOP: no statistically significant change at 1 or 3 months	Case series, uni-center	Not applicable	To determine the efficacy of suprachoroidal triamcinolone injection for the treatment of refractory diabetic macular edema [112]

Table A1. *Cont.*

No	Disease	Drug	Treatment	Key Findings	Study Design	Phase	Study Title
21	Diabetic macular edema (refractory)	TA	Single, unilateral SC injection of TA, 4 mg (0.1 mL of 40 mg/mL)	-Mean CST reduction: from 636.5 ± 200.11 µm (baseline) to 304.54 ± 67.43 (at 1 month, $p < 0.00001$) and to 302.66 ± 66.93 µm (at 3 months, $p < 0.00001$) -Mean BCVA gain: improved from 0.8 ± 0.24 ETDRS letters to 0.47 ± 0.3 (at 1 month, $p < 0.05$) and to 0.45 + 0.27 (at 3 months, $p < 0.05$) -Mean IOP: no difference from baseline at 1 and 3 months	Prospective, nonrandomized interventional, uni-center	Clinical trial (Phase I/II)	Efficacy and safety of suprachoroidal triamcinolone acetonide in cases of resistant diabetic macular edema [113]
22	Diabetic macular edema (refractory)	TA	SC injections of TA, 4 mg (0.1 mL of 40 mg/mL)	-Number of prior injections received: 6.2 (maximum 12, minimum 4) -Mean CST reduction: 612.8 ± 198.3 µm (baseline) to 308.6 ± 62.6 µm (at 1 month) to 302.72 ± 58.64 µm (at 3 months) -Mean BCVA improvement: from 0.8 ± 0.19 (baseline) to 0.49 ± 0.29 (at 1 month) and 0.39 ± 0.20 (at 3 months) -Mean IOP: from 12.32 mmHg (baseline) to 14.82 mmHg (at 1 month) and to 14.48 mmHg (at 3 months)	Retrospective, nonrandomized, single arm, uni-center, case series	Not applicable	Efficacy and safety of suprachoroidal triamcinolone acetonide in cases of resistant diabetic macular edema [114]
23	Diabetic macular edema (refractory)	TA	Single SC injection of TA, 4 mg (0.1 mL of 40 mg/mL) at baseline and administered every 3 months during the follow-up period (12 months) if intraretinal cysts, intraretinal or subretinal fluid persisted and CMT remained >250 µm	-Number of injections needed: 37.6% eyes required 2 injections; 23.5% of eyes required 3 injections -Mean CMT reduction: significant after 12-months ($p < 0.001$); positive correlation between final CMT and frequency of injection ($p < 0.001$) -Mean BVCA improvement: from 1.194 ± 0.1 (baseline) to 0.75 ± 0.2 (at 12 months, $p < 0.001$) -Mean IOP: reached a maximum value at 1 month; then, gradually declined using topical beta blockers; glaucoma surgery not required in any patients -IS/OS disruption and NSD: associated with worse final BVCA ($p < 0.001$) -AEs: no systemic or serious AEs related to treatment	Prospective, nonrandomized, single arm, uni-center	Clinical trial (Phase I/II)	Efficacy of suprachoroidal triamcinolone acetonide injection in the treatment of resistant diabetic macular edema [115]
24	Diabetic macular edema	TA	Posterior subtendon injection of TA (40 mg) in combination with VISCOAT (20 mg sodium chondroitin sulfate + 15 mg sodium hyaluronate) vs. Posterior subtendon injection of TA (40 mg) alone vs. SC injection of TA, 4 mg (0.1 mL of 40 mg/mL)	-Mean BCVA improvement: highest in SCTA group with VISCOAT -Mean CMT reduction: lowest in SCTA group with VISCOAT; reduction from baseline at all follow-up periods in all groups ($p < 0.0001$), significant reduction at 1, 3 and 6 months in SCTA group formulated with VISCOAT ($p < 0.001$); no difference in CMT between 1 month, 3 months, and 6 months in SCTA group -Retreatment: lowest frequency in SCTA group with VISCOAT	Prospective, nonrandomized, uni-center	Clinical trial (Phase II)	Suprachoroidal triamcinolone versus posterior subtenon triamcinolone alone or formulated in the management of diabetic macular edema [116]

Table A1. *Cont.*

No	Disease	Drug	Treatment	Key Findings	Study Design	Phase	Study Title
25	Diabetic macular edema	AAV8 vector	Comparison of 3 different doses of RGX-314 (AAV8) administered suprachoroidally, one of which will be infused with topical steroid	-Recruitment ongoing Preliminary results (3-month data of 15 patients): -Diabetic retinopathy improvement: 33% in treatment arm had a ≥2 improvement in diabetic retinopathy severity score vs. 0% in in control arm -AEs: no intraocular inflammation observed; common observed AEs not considered treatment-related	Randomized, dose-escalation study	Clinical trial (Phase II)	RGX-314 gene therapy administered in the suprachoroidal space for participants with diabetic retinopathy (DR) without center involved-diabetic macular edema (CI-DME) (ALTITUDE) [117]
Macular edema secondary to retinal vein occlusion							
26	Macular edema secondary to RVO	TA in combination with IV Aflibercept	SC injection of TA, 0.1 mL of 40 mg/mL + 2 mg IV of Aflibercept vs. SC sham injection + 2 mg IV injection of Aflibercept	-Number of retreatments: 23 (combination) vs. 9 (monotherapy) (−61%; $p = 0.013$), % of participants requiring no re-treatments was increased (78% vs. 30%; $p = 0.003$) -Mean BCVA imporvement: higher in combination arm vs. monotherapy arm at month 1 ($p = 0.20$) and month 2 ($p = 0.04$) -Mean CST reduction: reduced to normal values at month 1 and remained there at months 2 and 3 in combination arm, decreased at month 1 and increased at months 2 and 3 in monotherapy arm -Frequency of CST resolution (CST ≤ 310 µm): higher in combination arm at months 1, 2, and 3 vs. monotherapy arm	Randomized, triple masked, multi-center	Clinical trial (Phase II)	Suprachoroidal triamcinolone acetonide for retinal vein occlusion: results of the TANZANITE study [119]
27	Macular edema secondary to RVO	TA in combination with IV injection of Aflibercept	Single unilateral, SC injection of TA, 40 mg/mL (4 mg in 100 µL) following a 2 mg IV injection of Aflibercept vs. Single unilateral, SC sham procedure following a 2 mg IV injection of Aflibercept	-Retreatment: not required in 74% (17/23 patients) in combination arm vs. only 17% (4/23 patients) in monotherapy arm -Mean BCVA improvement: higher improvements observed as early as month 1 and maintained through month 3 in combination arm	Extension of TANZANITE trial (randomized, parallel design, triple masked, multi-center)	Clinical trial (Phase II)	TANZANITE extension study in patients with macular edema associated with retinal vein occlusion [120]
28	Macular edema secondary to RVO	TA in combination with IV of Aflibercept	IV Aflibercept (2 mg/0.05 mL) + SC TA (4 mg/100 µL) injections vs. IV Aflibercept (2 mg/0.05 mL) + sham SC procedure	-Mean BCVA gain: ~50.0% of patients in both groups reported a ≥15 ETDRS letters improvement at 8 week; results comparable between groups -No additional benefit of the combination therapy was observed leading to study discontinuation	Randomized, triple masked, controlled, parallel group, multi-center	Clinical trial (Phase III)	Suprachoroidal injection of triamcinolone acetonide with IVT aflibercept in subjects with macular edema following RVO (SAPPHIRE) [121]

Table A1. *Cont.*

No	Disease	Drug	Treatment	Key Findings	Study Design	Phase	Study Title
29	Macular edema secondary to RVO	TA in combination with IV injection of Ranibizumab	IV Ranibizumab (0.5 mg/0.05 mL) + SCTA (4 mg/0.10 mL) vs. IVB (1.25 mg/0.05 mL) + SCTA (4 mg/0.10 mL) vs. IV Ranibizumab (0.5 mg/0.05 mL) + sham SC injection or IVB (1.25 mg/0.05 mL) + sham SC injection	-Early discontinuation due to the SAPPHIRE study outcomes	Randomized, masked, controlled, parallel group, multi-center	Clinical trial (Phase III)	Suprachoroidal injection of triamcinolone acetonide with IVT anti-VEGF in subjects with macular edema following RVO (TOPAZ) [122]
30	Macular edema secondary to BRVO	TA in combination with IV Ranibizumab	IV injection of 0.05 mL (0.5 mg) of Ranibizumab + SCTA (Group 1) vs. IV injection of 0.05 mL (0.5 mg) of Ranibizumab only (Group 2) Both groups received monthly Ranibizumab injection PRN for 1 year	-Number of injections: 2.47 ± 1.2 (group 2) vs. 4.4 ± 1.5 (group 1) -Mean CMT reduction: significant reduction in both groups at 12 months ($p < 0.001$); group 2 showed greater reduction than group 1 at 1 month ($p = 0.008$); after 12 months, CMT was similar in both groups -Recurrent ME: higher in group 1 compared to group 2 -Predictors of final BCVA: baseline CMT and number of injections in group 1; baseline BCVA only predictor in group 2	Prospective, randomized interventional study, uni-center	Clinical trial (Phase II)	Modified microneedle for suprachoroidal injection of triamcinolone acetonide combined with intravitreal injection of ranibizumab in branch retinal vein occlusion patients [123]
31	Macular edema secondary to RVO	TA	Single SCinjection of TA, 4 mg (0.1 mL of 40 mg/mL)	-Mean BCVA gain: >15 letter increase in 68.7% participants at week 1, 62.5% at month 1, 50% at month 2 and 50% at month 3 ->70 ETDRS letter score: 81.25% at week 1 75% at month 1, 75% at month 2, 75% at month 3 -Mean CST reduction: associated with improvements in BCVA -Mean IOP: no significant changes, with an increase ranging from 0.75 mmHg at week 1 ($p = 0.09$) and 0.5 mmHg at 3 months ($p = 0.72$)	Nonrandomized, open-label, single arm, uni-center	Clinical trial (Phase I/II)	Suprachoroidal triamcinolone acetonide for the treatment of macular edema associated with retinal vein occlusion: a pilot study [124]
32	Macular edema secondary to RVO	TA	SC injection of TA, 4 mg (0.1 mL of 40 mg/mL)	-Mean BCVA gain: significant improvement from baseline at 3 months ($p = 0.003$) -Mean central retinal thickness reduction: significantly decreased from 342.2 ± 40.2 µm to 289 ± 47.5 µm at 3 months ($p = 0.002$)	Uni-center, case series	Not applicable	Effect of supra-choroidal triamcinolone injection on best-corrected visual acuity and central retinal thickness in patients with macular edema secondary to retinal vein occlusion [125]

Table A1. *Cont.*

No	Disease	Drug	Treatment	Key Findings	Study Design	Phase	Study Title
33	Macular edema secondary to RVO	TA, Aflibercept	Single unilateral, SCinjection of 40 mg/mL (4 mg in 100 μL) TA following a 2 mg IV injection of Aflibercept vs. Single unilateral, SC sham procedure following a 2 mg IV injection of Aflibercept	-Mean vascular choroidal thickness (VCT), stromal choroidal thickness (SCT) and total choroidal thickness (TCT): slight trend toward choroidal thinning in both groups at 3 months, but none reached significance (p = 0.231–0.342) -SCS thickening: 13.4 μm (combination) vs. 5.3 μm (monotherapy) at 3 months (p = 0.130) -SCS expansion: 39.5% eyes demonstrated visible SCS at baseline; significant expansion after SCTA injection (16.2 μm to 27.8 μm at 3 months; p = 0.033)	Randomized, masked, parallel design, multi-center	Clinical trial (Phase II)	Choroidal changes after suprachoroidal injection of triamcinolone in eyes with macular edema secondary to retinal vein occlusion [200]
34	Macular edema with subfoveal hard exudates (SHE) secondary to central or branch RVO or diffuse DME	TA in combination with IVB	Single injection or IVB (1.25 mg/0.05 mL) + SCTA (4.0 mg/0.1 mL)	-Mean ETDRS letter change: ≥2 lines in 4/6 eyes; remained unchanged in 2 eyes -Mean OCT macular thickness: decreased from 603.5 ± 348.5 μm (baseline) to 276.3 ± 40.7 μm (at 12 months) -Mean OCT macular volume: decreased from 9.44 ± 2.16 μm (baseline) to 7.62 ± 0.55 μm (at 12 months) -SHE resolution: mostly resolved at 1 month and 2 months in all eyes and ME was significantly reduced -AEs: no serious AEs observerd	Prospective, nonrandomized, case series	Not applicable	Suprachoroidal drug infusion for the treatment of severe subfoveal hard exudates [126]
35	RVO, DME, Vogt Koyanaji Harada Disease	TA	SC injection of TA, 4 mg (0.1 mL of 40 mg/mL	-Results pending study completion	Randomized, parallel assignment, interventional	NA	One year results for suprachoroidal triamcinolone acetonide injection in various retinal diseases [127]
Post-operative/pseudophakic cystoid macular edema							
36	Diabetic macular edema (refractory)	TA	Single SCTA 4 mg (0.1 mL of 40 mg/mL) vs. Single IVTA, 4 mg (0.1 mL of 40 mg/mL)	-Mean BCVA gain (logMAR): improved from baseline in both groups; comparable between groups at 1 month (p = 0.605) and 3 months (p = 0.313) -Mean CFT reduction: statistically significant difference in CFT at 3 months, with less reduction in the IVTA group than the SCTA group (p = 0.028) -AEs: mean IOP significantly higher in the IVTA group compared to the SCTA group at 1 month (p = 0.01) and 3 months (p = 0.028) -DME recurrence rate at 1 month: 50% (IVTA group) vs. 0% (SCTA group) -DME recurrence rate at 3 months: 70% (IVTA group) vs. 30.8% (SCTA group)	Randomized, multi-center	Clinical trial (Phase II)	A randomized trial comparing suprachoroidal and intravitreal injection of triamcinolone acetonide in refractory diabetic macular edema due to epiretinal membrane [128]

Table A1. *Cont.*

No	Disease	Drug	Treatment	Key Findings	Study Design	Phase	Study Title
37	Pseudophakic cystoid macular edema/cystoid macular edema	TA	SCTA 4 mg (0.1 mL of 40 mg/mL) at day 0	At 3 months: -Mean CST reduction: from 535.0 ± 157.24 (baseline) to 319.55 ± 127.30 µm ($p < 0.001$) -Mean BCVA gain: from 1.05 ± 0.41 (baseline) to 0.73 ± 0.41 logMAR ($p < 0.001$) -Mean IOP: from 15.05 ± 2.54 (baseline) to 15.85 ± 3.60 mm Hg ($p = 0.185$) -AEs: no serious AEs	Retrospective, non-comparative case-series	Not applicable	A simple technique for suprachoroidal space injection of triamcinolone acetonide in treatment of macular edema [129]
38	Pseudophakic cystoid macular edema	TA	SCTA 4 mg (0.1 mL of 40 mg/mL)	-Mean BCVA gain (logMAR): 0.3 at week 4; improvements maintained to 6 months -Mean CMT reduction: 473.5 µm (baseline) to 287 µm -Mean IOP: remained within normal limits -AEs: none related to uveitis or glaucoma	Retrospective, single arm case series	Not applicable	Modified inexpensive needle for suprachoroidal triamcinolone acetonide injections in pseudophakic cystoid macular edema [130]
39	Pseudophakic cystoid macular edema	TA	SCTA of 0.1 mL TA	-Case summary: 52 year old female received SC injection of TA due to inability to afford monthly IV anti-VEGF and IV dexamethasone -Mean IOP: reduced from 19 mmHg to 15 mmHg; persisted without raised spikes until week 24 -BCVA recovery: from 20/80 to 20/50 at week 1, 20/40 at 8 weeks and 20/30 at 24 weeks -OCT findings: significant thickness decrease within 24 h (348 µm); after 8 weeks, improvement in retinal thickness to normal (265 µm), complete anatomical resolution at 24 weeks -AEs: none	Case report	Not applicable	A manually made needle for treating pseudophakic cystoid macular edema by injecting triamcinolone acetonide in the suprachoroidal space: a case report [131]
40	Central serous chorioretinopathy, Irvine-gass syndrome, pars planitis, cystoid macular edema	TA	SCTA in patients diagnosed with central serous chorioretinopathy and Irving-Gass Syndrome	-Results pending study completion	Randomized, parallel assignment, interventional	Clinical trial (Phase II/III)	Suprachoroidal triamcinolone acetonide injection in two chorioretinal diseases: one year results [132]
Photoreceptor loss							
41	Gene therapy	AAV5 vector	Single SC injection of 100 µL of sc-AAV5-smCBA-hGFP vector at a concentration of 4.5 × 1013 vector genomes/mL in rabbits	-Efficacy of transfection: comparable among all treated eyes by microscopic examination -GFP expression: occurred at the level of the choroid, RPE, photoreceptors and retinal ganglion cells in whole mounts of treated eyes (no direct staining performed); absence of GFP In controls -Inflammatory response: no evidence of inflammation or tissue destruction	Animal experimental study	Preclinical (animal study)	Ab-externo AAV-mediated gene delivery to the suprachoroidal space using a 250 micron flexible microcatheter [65]

Table A1. *Cont.*

No	Disease	Drug	Treatment	Key Findings	Study Design	Phase	Study Title
42	Gene therapy	AAV2, AAV5 or AAV2 (triple) containing 3 tyrosine-phenylalanine mutations on its capsid surface	SC or vitreal/subretinal injections of AAV2, AAV5, or AAV2 (triple) vector containing 3 tyrosine-phenylalanine mutations on its capsid surface; vector doses were either 1×10^{12} and 4×10^{12}, or 1×10^{12} and 9×10^{12} particles/mL). vs. SC delivery of basic saline solution (BSS)	- GFP expression: found in eyes that received both vitrectomy/subretinal and SC injections; strong expression in AAV2(triple) treatment, intermediate expression in AAV2 treatment, minimal expression in AAV5 treatment, no GFP expression in BSS-injected eyes -Transduction profiles: not significantly influenced by vector concentration	Animal experimental study	Preclinical (animal study)	Comparison of suprachoroidal delivery via an Ab-externo approach with the iTrack microcatheter versus vitrectomy and subretinal delivery for 3 different AAV serotypes for gene transfer to the retina [133]
43	Gene therapy	AAV2 vector	AAV2 administration in mice using intrastromal, intracameral, IV, subretinal, or SC injections	-Transduction: of stroma, ciliary body, retinal ganglion cells, outer retina, and RPE, irrespective of delivery route; transduction of multiple retinal layers without causing retinal detachment	Animal experimental study	Preclinical (animal study)	Comparison of AAV Serotype2 transduction by various delivery routes to the mouse eye [134]
44	Gene therapy	AAV8, AAV9, AAV2, RGX-314 vectors	SC injections of 2.85×10^{10} gene copies (GCs) of AAV8.GFP, 2.85×10^{10} GCs of AAV9.GFP, 2.0×10^{10} GCs of AAV2.GFP in rats SC or subretinal injection of 1.2×10^{8} GCs of RGX-314 in rats SC injection of 50 µL containing 4.75×10^{11} GCs of AAV8.GFP in nonhuman primates and pigs	-GFP expression: widespread throughout the RPE and photoreceptors in rats, nonhuman primates, and pigs; SC and subretinal injection of same vector dose resulted in comparable expression which could be increased by multiple SC vector injections -Transduction of the RPE and photoreceptors: strong after SC injection of AAV9.GFP, similar to AAV8.GFP, but poor after SC injection of AAV2.GFP -Suppression of VEGF-induced vasodilation and vascular leakage: suppression by SC injection of RGX-314 comparable to subretinal injection in rats	Animal experimental study	Preclinical (animal study)	AAV8-vectored suprachoroidal gene transfer produces widespread ocular transgene expression [135]

Table A1. *Cont.*

No	Disease	Drug	Treatment	Key Findings	Study Design	Phase	Study Title
45	Gene therapy	AAV2, AAV5 vectors	SC injections of 7.8×10^9 GC of AAV2tYF-CBA-hGFP, 7.8×10^9 GC of AAV2tYF-GRK1-hGFP, 7.8×10^9 GC of AAV5-GRK1-hGFP, or 6.87×10^9 GC of AAV2-CBA-hGFP in Norway Brown rats	-Duration of GFP expression: peak expression observed within 2 weeks, except for AAV2tYF-GRK1-hGFP, which showed further increase between 2 and 4 weeks -Strength of GFP expression: highest and more extensive for AAV2tYF-GRK1-hGFP; AAV2-CBA-hGFP; expression extended approximately 1/4 circumference in the RPE and all layers of the retina; injection of AAV5-GRK1-hGFP resulted in lowest GFP expression at 2 and 4 weeks -Areas of GFP expression: for AAV2tYF-GRK1-GFP and AAV5tYF-GRK1-GFP expression limited to photoreceptors, including inner segments, outer segments, and some cell bodies; extent of GFP expression was around 1/4 and 1/6 eye circumference, respectively	Animal experimental study	Preclinical (animal study)	Transgene expression in RPE and retina after suprachoroidal delivery of AAV vectors [136]
46	Gene therapy	AAV8 vector	SC, subretinal and IVT injections of AAV8.GFP in primates (7×10^{11} or 7×10^{12} vector genomes per eye using a 700-µm-long 30-gauge microneedle)	-Transduction: diffuse, peripheral transduction of mostly the RPE (SC delivery) vs. robust focal transduction near injection site with some transduction of retinal ganglion neurons (subretinal delivery) vs. only scant peripapillary expression mostly nasal to the optic disc (IV delivery) -Duration of GFP expression: transient, reaching maximal expression at 1 month but decreased by months 2 and 3 for SC AAV8 -Inflammatory response: more local infiltration of retinal microglia, choroidal macrophages, leukocytes and T-cells for SC; subretinal injection showed minimal microglial activation, fewer leukocytes and T-cells compared to SC; IV injection showed minimal microglial activation and almost no leukocytes or T-cells; higher systemic humoral response after IV delivery -Tolerance of injection: comparable between groups	Animal experimental study	Preclinical (animal study)	Suprachoroidal and subretinal injections of AAV using transscleral microneedles for retinal gene delivery in nonhuman primates [24]
47	Gene therapy	AAV8 vector	SC, subretinal, and IV injections (100 µL) of AAV8 (7×10^{12} or 10^{12} vector genes per eye) and TA (40 mg) in primates	-Humoral response: minimal antibody response by SC injection with greater responses to GFP; IV injection induced an early and higher robust humoral response to the viral capsid -Cell-mediated immune response: no appreciable T-cell responses to AAV8 capsid after SC injection with some T cell responses to GFP beginning as early as 1 month -Systemic distribution: higher genome copies of vector in spleen and liver for IV injection compared to SC injection or subretinal injection	Animal experimental study	Preclinical (animal study)	Host immune responses after suprachoroidal delivery of AAV8 in nonhuman primate eyes [138]

Table A1. *Cont.*

No	Disease	Drug	Treatment	Key Findings	Study Design	Phase	Study Title
48	Gene therapy	AAV serotypes	SC injections of 1.0 µL fluorescein sodium (1.0×10^{-6}%) or 1 of 3 AAV serotypes via injection of scAAVs-CBA-EGFP solution in mice	-Transduction: occurred in outer retina and the RPE in all 3 AAV serotypes; 3 AAVs displayed varied efficiency and cell specificity; widespread distribution across different layers of the mouse retina -Inflammatory response activation of inflammatory cells depending on the dosage used -AEs: retinal detachment was avoided	Animal experimental study	Preclinical (animal study)	Suprachoroidal injections of AAV for retinal gene delivery in mouse [201]
49	Gene therapy	AAV1, AAV2, AAV6, AAV8, and AAV9 vectors	SC, subretinal, and IV delivery of AAV1, AAV2, AAV6, AAV8, and AAV9 with GFP in rats vs. Buffer-injected controls for each route of delivery	-Inflammatory response: response induced by AAV2 and AAV6 vectors for all routes of delivery with AAV6 inducing the highest levels when delivered suprachoroidally; AAV1-induced inflammation was highest when delivered suprachoroidally, whereas minimal inflammation was seen with IV delivery; AAV8 and AAV9 induced least amount of inflammation across all delivery routes -Cell-mediated immune response: AAV1, AAV2, and AAV6 each induced adaptive immune cells into neural retina	Animal experimental study	Preclinical (animal study)	The degree of adeno-associated virus-induced retinal inflammation varies based on serotype and route of delivery: intravitreal, subretinal, or suprachoroidal [202]
50	Gene therapy	AAV2 serotypes (AAV2/1, AAV2/2, AAV2/6, AAV2/8, and AAV2/9) vectors	SC, subretinal, and IV injections of AAV2-viral particles; >3 injections per serotype per route of delivery (5×10^{12} vector genes/mL for a total dose of 5×10^{10} vector genes) in rats	-Transduction: successful in the RPE and outer nuclear layer (ONL) for all serotypes with AAV2/1 subretinal delivery showing the highest transduction efficiency and minimal inner subretinal delivery; SC tropism comparable to subretinal delivery, but wider distribution and greater average ONL transduction efficiency for all serotypes; retinal transduction primarily in inner retina for IV delivery with AAV2/6 showing the highest transduction	Animal experimental study	Preclinical (animal study)	Retinal tropism and transduction of adeno-associated virus varies by serotype and route of delivery (intravitreal, subretinal, or suprachoroidal) in rats [203]
51	Gene therapy	DNA nanoparticles (DNPs)	Single bilateral SC injection (0.1 mL) of ellipsoid-shaped DNPs, rod-shaped DNPs or saline in non-human primates and rabbits	-Tolerance: well-tolerated in both animal models -Luciferase activity in non-human primates: ellipsoid-shaped DNPs had persistent luciferase activity up to day 22; rod-shaped DNPs showed a significant decrease in choroid and the RPE - Luciferase activity in rabbits: both rod and ellipsoid-shaped DNPs injected in SCS alongside rod-shaped DNPs injected subretinally, exhibited similar luciferase activity after week 1	Animal experimental study	Preclinical (animal study)	Suprachoroidally delivered DNA nanoparticles transfect chorioretinal cells in non-human primates and rabbits [137]
52	Gene therapy	DNA nanoparticles (DNPs)	Unilateral SC injection (0.1 mL) of ellipsoid-shaped DNPs, rod-shaped DNPs, or saline in rabbits Unilateral subretinal injection (0.05 mL) of rod-shaped DNPs in rabbits	-Tolerance: well-tolerated, resulted in reversible opening of the SCS -Luciferase activity: high activity in the retina and the RPE; mean luciferase activity comparable between treatment groups -Drug distribution: greater surface area coverage after SC administration	Animal experimental study	Preclinical (animal study)	Suprachoroidally delivered DNA nanoparticles transfect retina and retinal pigment epithelium/choroid in rabbits [139]

Table A1. *Cont.*

No	Disease	Drug	Treatment	Key Findings	Study Design	Phase	Study Title
53	Gene therapy	Poly (β-amino ester)s nanoparticles (PBAE NPs)	SC injections of PBAE NPs containing 1 µg of pEGFP-N1 (an expression plasmid in which a cytomegalovirus promoter drives expression of GFP (CMV-GFP)) SC injections of PBAE NPs containing 1 µg of pVEGF SC injections of PBAE NPs containing 1 µg of p3sFlt1Fc or 1 µg of a CMV-Luciferase expression plasmid (pCMV-Luc) (control) followed by intravitreous injection of 100 ng of recombinant VEGF165 2 weeks later All injections occurred in Brown Norway rats	-GFP expression after SC injection of PBAE NPs containing pEGFP-NP: expression in anterior retina around the entire eye circumference; less expression in the RPE and photoreceptors compared to SC injection of 2.85×10^{10} GC of AAV8.GFP, fluorescence not strong enough to be visualized on flat mounts; multiple injections markedly increase expression; expression maintained without substantial decline at least through 8 months -Neovascularization after SC injection of NPs containing VEGF expression plasmid: severe subretinal neovascularization starting in the periphery near injection site and extended posteriorly progressing to subretinal fibrosis -Suppression of VEGF-induced retinal vascular leakage and neovascularization: resulted after SC injection of p3sFlt1Fc NPs	Animal experimental study	Preclinical (animal study)	Suprachoroidal gene transfer with nonviral nanoparticles [140]
54	Dry age-related macular degeneration (AMD) and Stargardt's macular dystrophy (SMD)	Adipose tissue-derived mesenchymal stem cell (ADMSC) implantation	SC implantation of adipose tissue-derived mesenchymal stem cell (ADMSC) implantation	-Beneficial outcomes: improvements in visual acuity, visual field, and electroretinogram recordings -AEs: no complications in the 6-month follow-up period -Choroidal thickening: observed on OCT scans, indicating increased choroidal perfusion	Prospective, single arm, uni-center	Clinical trial (Phase I/II)	First Year Results of Suprachoroidal Adipose Tissue Derived Mesenchymal Stem Cell Implantation in Degenerative Macular Diseases [204]

Table A1. *Cont.*

No	Disease	Drug	Treatment	Key Findings	Study Design	Phase	Study Title
55	Retinitis pigmentosa patients	Umbilical cord derived mesenchymal stem cell (UCMSC) implantation	SC umbilical cord derived mesenchymal stem cell (UCMSC) implantation	-Mean BCVA and visual field scores: both improved after treatment during the 12-month study period ($p < 0.05$); negative correlation between BCVA improvement and disease scores and grades -Mean score and mean grade of disease: improved after treatment ($p < 0.05$)	Prospective, uin-center	Clinical trial (Phase I/II)	Does stem cell implantation have an effect on severity of retinitis pigmentosa: evaluation with a classification system? [143]
56	Retinitis pigmentosa patients	Umbilical cord derived mesenchymal stem cell (UCMSC) implantation	SC umbilical cord derived mesenchymal stem cell (UCMSC) implantation in patients ≤18 years old	-Mean BCVA gain: improved from baseline ($p < 0.05$); declined in 56% of 46 eyes during 1st year; no improvement in untreated eyes -Mean visual field: improvement after treatment ($p < 0.05$); 65% of 46 eyes had improvement at 1 year -Mean CMT reduction: not significant from baseline ($p > 0.05$) -Mean mfERG: improvement after treatment ($p < 0.05$) -AEs: none	Prospective, uni-center	Clinical trial (Phase I/II)	Suprachoroidal umbilical cord derived mesenchymal stem cell implantation for the treatment of retinitis pigmentosa in pediatric patients [144]
57	Photoreceptor loss due to neovascular age-related macular degeneration, DME, RVO	BD311 integration-deficient lentiviral vector (IDLV) expressing VEGFA antibody	Single SC injection of IDLV expressing VEGFA antibody, 500 uL	-Recruiting participants, results pending study completion	Prospective, interventional, single arm	Clinical trial (Phase I)	VEGFA-targeting gene therapy to treat retinal and choroidal neovascularization diseases [164]
58	Retinitis pigmentosa patients	Umbilical cord derived mesenchymal stem cell (UCMSC) implantation	SC mesenchymal stem cell implanted vs. SC mesenchymal spheroidal stem cell implantation	-Study results pending	Prospective, clinical case series	Not applicable	Spheroidal mesenchymal stem cells in retinitis pigmentosa [145]

Table A1. *Cont.*

No	Disease	Drug	Treatment	Key Findings	Study Design	Phase	Study Title
59	Solar retinopathy	TA	SC injection of 0.1 mL TA with a custom-made needle	-Case summary: 17-year-old female with decreased vision due to solar retinopathy received single SCTA injection without any surgical complications -Mean BCVA gain: 0.7 at 1 week, 0.8 as 12 weeks; full recovery by week 4 -AEs: no serious AEs as of 12 weeks -Mean IOP: increased to 28 mmHg in week 7, controlled by topical eye drops (timolol) to 15 mmHg	Case report	Not applicable	Managing solar retinopathy with suprachoroidal triamcinolone acetonide injection in a young girl: a case report [146]
Choroidal neovascularization (CNV)							
60	Choroidal neovascularizaiton	Pazopanib, Bevacizumab, Fusion protein hI-con1	IVB injection, 2.5 mg vs. IV Pazopanib injection, 1 mg vs. IV 300 μg hI-con1 vs. SC Pazopanib injection, 1 mg vs. 10 vehicle controls (SC+ IV)	-CNV height: smaller in IV pazopanib (90 ± 20 μm) vs. control (180 ± 20 μm; $p = 0.009$); smaller maximum height in IV Pazopanib (173 ± 43 μm) vs. SC Pazopanib (478 ± 105 μm; $p = 0.018$); small decrease with IV Bevacizumab vs. controls -CNV surface area: no difference between the 3 treatment groups; with hI-con1 lesions were thinner than controls -Lesion size: smaller for all vs. controls	Animal experimental study	Preclinical trial (animal study)	A pharmacodynamic analysis of choroidal neovascularization in a porcine model using three targeted drugs [151]
61	Choroidal neovascularizaiton	Bevacizumab	1250 μg/50 μL SC Bevacizumab	-% bevacizumab recovered: 88.4 ± 0.9% at 15 min, 4.6 ± 0.5% at 1 day, and 0.2 ± 0.1% at 2 days after injection -Drug distribution (at 15 min): 76% in choroid, 13% in sclera and 2.9% in retina, 1.0% in vitreous, 0.5% in aqueous humor, 0.9% in anterior chamber, 0.6% in lens and 0.1% in optic nerve -Drug distribution (at day 1): 34% in choroid, 27% in sclera and 23% in retina, 11% in vitreous, 0.7% in aqueous humor, 1.6% in anterior chamber, 3.8% in lens and 0.3% in optic nerve -Drug distribution (At day 2): 0.5% in choroid, 3.3% in sclera, 0.5% in retina, 55% in vitreous, 3% in aqueous humor, 36% in anterior chamber, 1.1% in lens and 0.6% in optic nerve	Animal experimental study	Preclinical trial (animal study)	Pharmacokinetics and biodistribution of Bevacizumab following suprachoroidal injection into the rabbit eye using a microneedle [152]
62	Choroidal neovascularizaiton	Bevacizumab	SC injection of Bevacizumab cross-linked with polycaprolactone dimethacrylate and hydroxyethyl methacrylate	-Drug release: sustained manner > 4 months -Bevacizumab's mechanism of action: not affected in animal models	Animal experimental study	Preclinical trial (animal study)	Light activated, in-situ forming gel for sustained suprachoroidal delivery of Bevacizumab [66]

Table A1. *Cont.*

No	Disease	Drug	Treatment	Key Findings	Study Design	Phase	Study Title
63	Choroidal neovascularizaiton	Bevacizumab	SC injection of an in-situ forming hydrogel comprised Bevacizumab and hyaluronic acid (HA)	-Duration of drug release: >6 months -Tolerance: well tolerated by clinical exam, fundus imaging, histological analysis, and IOP measurement	Animal experimental study	Preclinical trial (animal study)	Six-month sustained delivery of anti-VEGF from in-situ forming hydrogel in the suprachoroidal space [80]
64	Choroidal neovascularizaiton	Acriflavine	Intraocular injection of 100 ng Acriflavine vs. SC injection of 300 ng Acriflavine vs. Topical administration of Acriflavine	-Inner retina fluorescence: SC injection caused fluorescence in quadrant of injection at 1 h with entire retinal and choroid spread by day 1 (detectable for 5 days), strong suppression of CNV at Bruch's membrane rupture sites at day 7 vs. topical administration caused fluorescence in retina and the RPE within 5 min, detectable for 6–12 h -CNV reduction: dramatic at 14 days after rupture of Bruch's membrane (SC); also reduced (topical)	Animal experimental study	Preclinical trial (animal study)	The HIF-1 antagonist Acriflavine: visualization in retina and suppression of ocular neovascularization [154]
65	Choroidal neovascularizaiton	Acriflavine	SC injection of Acriflavine poly lactic-co-glycolic acid formulated micro particle	-CNV suppression: suppressed for at least 9 weeks (IV injection) in mice vs. 18 weeks (SC injection) in rats -Full-field electroretinogram function: modest reduction in IV, no reduction in SC injection; normal electroretinogram scotopic a- and b- wave amplitudes at 28 days with SC injection -Other outcomes: normal retinas, retinal histology, and IOP at 28 days with SC injection; active component of Acriflavine had steady-state levels in the low nM range in RPE/choroid/retina for at least 16 weeks	Animal experimental study	Preclinical trial (animal study)	Sustained delivery of Acriflavine from suprachoroidal space provides long term suppression of choroidal neovascularization [84]
66	Choroidal neovascularizaiton	VEGFR-1 (sFlt-1)-encoding plasmid	SC injection of soluble VEGFR-1 (sFlt-1)-encoding plasmid into the with an electrical field	-Transduction: at least 1 month of the RPE -AEs: none -Inhibition of CNV: significant levels achieved 15 days after transfection	Animal experimental study	Pre-clinical study (animal study)	Suprachoroidal electrotransfer: a novel gene delivery method to transfect the choroid and the retnia without detaching the retina [88]

Table A1. *Cont.*

No	Disease	Drug	Treatment	Key Findings	Study Design	Phase	Study Title
Neovascular age related macular degeneration							
67	Neovascular age related macular degeneration	RGX-314	Cohort 1: SC 2.5 × 10^{11} RGX genomic copies/eye vs. monthly 0.5 mg SC Ranibizumab Cohort 2: SC 5 × 10^{11} RGX genomic copies/eye vs. monthly 0.5 mg SC Ranibizumab Cohort 3: SC 5 × 10^{11} RGX genomic copies/eye vs. SC 5 × 10^{11} RGX genomic copies/eye in patients who are neutralizing antibody positive	-Tolerance: well tolerated in cohorts 1–3 with no serious AEs -AEs: mild AEs related to treatment occurred in cohorts 1 and 2 through 6 months; 23% mild intraocular inflammation (similar incidence across dose levels), all cases resolved within days to weeks on topical corticosteroid -BCVA and CRT: stable at 6 months in patients dosed with RGX-314 in cohorts 1 and 2 -Anti-VEGF reduction: >70% in cohorts 1 and 2 -Retreatment: 29% (cohort 1) and 40% (cohort 2) received no anti-VEGF injections for over 6 months following RGX-314 injection	Randomized, interventional, open-label	Clinical trial (phase II)	Suprachoroidal delivery of RGX-314 gene therapy for neovascular age related macular degeneration: The phase II AAVIATE study [157]

Table A1. *Cont.*

No	Disease	Drug	Treatment	Key Findings	Study Design	Phase	Study Title
68	Neovascular age related macular degeneration	RGX-314	Cohort 1: SC 2.5 × 10^{11} RGX genomic copies/eye vs. Monthly 0.5 mg SC Ranibizumab Cohort 2: SC 5 × 10^{11} RGX genomic copies/eye vs. Monthly 0.5 mg SC Ranibizumab Cohort 3: SC 5 × 10^{11} RGX genomic copies/eye vs. SC 5 × 10^{11} RGX genomic copies/eye in patients who are neutralizing antibody positive	-Pending full study results	Randomized, interventional, open-label	Clinical trial (phase II)	RGX-314 gene therapy administered in the suprachoroidal space for participants with neovascular age-related macular degeneration (nAMD) (AAVIATE) [156]
69	Neovascular age related macular degeneration	Bevacizumab Triamci-nolone	SC Bevacizumab and TA	-AEs: no serious AEs related to treatment -IOP elevation: 4.76% of eyes at 3 months, medically controlled -Nuclear sclerotic cataracts: increase in 10.5% of eyes	Nonrandomized, single arm, interventional, uni-center	Clinical trial (phase I)	Safety of submacular suprachoroidal drug administration via a microcatheter: retrospective analysis of European treatment results [158]
70	Neovascular age related macular degeneration	Bevacizumab	SC injection of 100 µL Bevacizumab	-AEs: moderate pain only, no serious AEs -IOP: no serious elevation -Rescue therapy: none required for two months	Single-center, open-label	Clinical trial (phase I)	Suprachoroidal microinjection of Bevacizumab is well tolerated in human patients [159]
71	Neovascular age related macular degeneration	Aflibercept	4 mg SC Aflibercept vs. SC saline	-Neovascularization reduction: ~4862 ± 192 $pixels^2$ on fluorescein angiography (control) vs. ~3318 ± 353 $pixels^2$ (intervention) based on evaluation of neovascular leak area at week 3 ($p < 0.001$)	Animal experimental study	Preclinical trial (animal study)	Efficacy of suprachoroidal Aflibercept in a laser induced choroidal neovascularization model [160]

Table A1. *Cont.*

No	Disease	Drug	Treatment	Key Findings	Study Design	Phase	Study Title
72	Neovascular age related macular degeneration	CLS011A	4 mg (100 µL) SC CLS011A	-Tolerance: well-tolerated till day 91 with no signs of toxicity -Drug distribution: not detected at quantifiable levels in plasma or aqueous humor; quantifiable at all times in vitreous humor, retina, and sclera/choroid-RPE -Drug concentration gradient: sclera/choroid-RPE > retina > vitreous humor -Drug elimination: half-life of 102 days, >60% remaining at 3 months	Animal experimental study	Preclinical trial (animal study)	Pharmacokinetics including ocular distribution characteristics of suprachoroidally administered CLS011A in rabbits could be beneficial for wet AMD therapeutic candidate [161]
73	Neovascular age related macular degeneration	Axitinib	SC 0.03, 0.10, 0.50, and 1.0 mg of Axitinib following IV 2 mg Aflibercept	-Preliminary safety data: no treatment related serious AEs -Final safety data to be released	Interventional, prospective, non-randomized, sequential assignment	Clinical trial (phase I/II)	Safety and tolerability study of suprachoroidal injection of CLS-AX following anti-VEGF therapy in neovascular AMD (OASIS) [162]
74	Neovascular age-related macular degeneration	Axitinib	Subjects who received SC 0.1 mg, 0.5 mg, and 1.0 mg Axitinib in the parent study will be followed for an additional 12 weeks	-Study ongoing	Observational, prospective cohort	Parent study was a phase II clinical trial	Extension study to evaluate the long-term outcomes of subjects in the CLS-AX CLS1002-101 study [163]

Table A1. *Cont.*

No	Disease	Drug	Treatment	Key Findings	Study Design	Phase	Study Title
75	Neovascular age related macular degeneration	Axitinib	100 µL SC Axitinib 0.03 mg/eye of vs. 100 µL SC Axitinib 0.1 mg/eye Once weekly for two weeks SC 0.2 mg/5 µLs/eye Axitinib in rabbit with laser induced choroidal neovascularization vs. SC saline in rabbit with laser induced choroidal neovascularization 4 mg SC Axitinib in pig with laser induced choroidal neovascularization vs. SC saline in pig with laser induced choroidal neovascularization	-Tolerance: well tolerated -Drug concentration: no Axitinib detected in plasma or aqueous humor; sustained, high exposure through 10-week study, highest in the sclera/choroid/RPE, retina, vitreous -Drug levels in choroid–retina: >1000× higher in humans vs. in-vitro value through 6 months -Drug efficacy: reduced CNV by Axitibin in 40% eyes with clinically important lesions (scores of 3 or 4); general improvement (scores of 0 to 2) by day 21 vs. control group -Fluorescein leakage: reduced at weeks 1 and 2 ($p < 0.009$ for both) by SC Axitinib vs. control	Animal experimental study	Preclinical trial (animal study)	Suprachoroidal CLS-AX (Axitinib injectable suspension), as a potential long-acting therapy for neovascular age-related macular degeneration (nAMD) [92]
76	Neovascular age related macular degeneration	Axitinib	100 µL SC Axitinib 0.03 mg/eye (Group 1) vs. 100 µL SC Axitinib 0.01 (Group 2)	-Tolerance: well tolerated -Drug distribution: sustained and high exposure of Axitinib the RPE-choroid–sclera throughout 10-week study -Drug concentration: 138 ng/g at week 10, 4400 ng/g for Groups 1 and 2 (1153× and 36,667× higher than in-vitro value, respectively); Axitinib not detected in either aqueous humor or plasma -Mean retina drug levels: maximum of 4480 ng/g (Group 1) and 6260 ng/g (Group 2) at 24 h -Mean vitreous drug levels: 4 to 5 orders of magnitude lower than in retina -Estimation of human drug levels: SC 0.1 mg/eye may provide Axitinib levels in choroid–retina > 1000× higher than in-vitro value until 6 months	Animal experimental study	Preclinical trial (animal study)	Pharmacokinetics and ocular tolerability of suprachoroidal CLS-AX (Axitinib injectable suspension) in rabbits [205]

Table A1. *Cont.*

No	Disease	Drug	Treatment	Key Findings	Study Design	Phase	Study Title
78	Serous pigment epithelium detachment due to neovascular age related macular degeneration	Bevacizumab	2 SC injections, 1 month apart, of 0.1 mL Bevacizumab	-BCVA change (logMAR): reduced from 0.604 (baseline) to 0.146667 at 8 weeks ($p < 0.05$) -Size and height of pigment epithelium detachment on OCT: reduced from 676.8 ± 156.4 μm (baseline) to 108.6 ± 52.4 μm ($p < 0.05$) at 8 weeks -IOP: rise immediately after injection, normalized with 500 mg oral acetazolamide -AEs: pain -IOP: no change	Prospective, interventional, single group	Clinical trial (phase I)	Role of suprachoroidal anti-VEGF injections in recalcitrant serous pigment epithelium detachment [165]
Retinal detachment							
79	Retinal detachment due to Vogt–Koyanagi Harada Disease	TA	4 mg SCTA and systemic steroids vs. Systemic steroids only	-BCVA gain: higher in SCTA eyes at 1 month and 3 months (p-value = 0.026) - CFT reduction: CFT higher in control eyes at 1 month and 3 months (p-value 0.028) -Mean IOP: comparable between groups	Prospective, parallel group	Clinical trial (phase II)	Suprachoroidal Triamcinolone Acetonide injection: a novel therapy for serous retinal detachment due to Vogt–Koyanagi Harada Disease [167]
80	Serous choroidal detachment due to rhegmatogenous retinal detachment	TA	4 mg SC TA before vitrectomy or scleral buckle surgery	-Fluid reduction: >50% reduction in %50 eyes by day 3 and %20 eyes by day 5 -Treatment response: failed in 30% requiring surgical drainage before proceeding with vitrectomy -AEs: none during procedure -Elevated IOP: transient rise (30 mmHg) in %10 following vitrectomy managed with therapy	Prospective, noncomparative, interventional pilot study	Clinical trial (phase I)	Safety and efficacy of suprachoroidal Triamcinolone Acetonide for the management of serous choroidal detachment prior to rhegmatogenous retinal detachment surgery: a pilot study [166]
81	Rhegmatogenous retinal detachment	Sodium hyaluronate	Sodium hyaluronate injected into the SCS before retinal hole scleral freezing and laser photocoagulation	-Reattachment: required in 50%; 33% partly anatomically reattached with subretinal fluid; 16.67% failed reattachment and received vitrectomy with silicone oil tamponade or sclera buckling surgery -AEs: no severe AEs related to treatment	Prospective, interventional, single group	Clinical trial (phase I)	Suprachoroidal injection of sodium hyaluronate in the treatment of 12 patients with rhegmatogenous retinal detachment [168]
82	Retinal detachment	Sodium hyaluronate	Fractions of sodium hyaluronate injected into the SCS	-Buckling effect: short-lived between 12 and 72 h -Drug distribution: sodium hyaluronate present in SCS for >10–14 days -Dosage effect: no significant differences between buckles by sodium hyaluronate (1 and 2%), or by cross-linked sodium hyaluronate	Animal experimental study	Preclinical trial (animal study)	Suprachoroidal injection of sodium hyaluronate as an 'internal' buckling procedure [169]

Table A1. *Cont.*

No	Disease	Drug	Treatment	Key Findings	Study Design	Phase	Study Title
83	Retinal detachment	Air	1.5 mL air injected into SCS	-Treatment response: 5 cases responded satisfactorily -AEs: 1 case of vitreous hemorrhage -Relapse: in 2 cases -Further treatment: in 1 case	Case series	Not applicable	Suprachoroidal air injection for detached retina [170]
Other diseases							
84	Non-infectious intermediate, posterior, or pan-uveitis	TA	SC injection of 4 mg TA in 100 μL	-AEs: 38 reported, 89% mild or moderate in severity: uveitis progression (18%), cataract progression (3%) requiring surgery, ocular pain (16%); all systemic AEs unrelated to treatment; no treatment-related increases in IOP -BCVA: improvement in all eyes, >2-line improvement in 4 patients (who did not need additional therapy) through week 26	Open-label, clinical study	Clinical trial (phase I/II)	Suprachoroidal corticosteroid administration: a novel route for local treatment of non-infectious uveitis [171]
85	Acute posterior uveitis	TA, Prednisone	Group 1:50 μL injection of balanced salt solution vs. Group 2:1 mg/kg/d oral prednisone for 3 days vs. Group 3:2 mg SC TA injection vs. Group 4:0.1 mg/kg/day oral prednisone for 3 days vs. control eye	-Inflammatory score: on day 1 and 2 only, group 3 had mean cumulative inflammation scores significantly lower than group 1 ($p \leq 0.04$); by day 3, group 2 and 3 had lower mean cumulative inflammation scores than group 1 ($p < 0.034$); group 4 had mean cumulative inflammation scores not significantly different than BSS treated eyes at any time ($p > 0.05$) -Mean histologic inflammation scores of the anterior and posterior segment: significantly lower in group 3 than eyes in group 1	Animal experimental study	Preclinical trial (animal study)	Evaluation of suprachoroidal CLS-TA and oral Prednisone in a porcine model of uveitis [172]
86	Acute posterior uveitis	TA	SC injection of 0.2 mg or 2.0 mg TA vs. IV injection of 0.2 mg or 2.0 mg of TA	-Drug efficacy: comparable reduction in inflammation in posterior segment of both SCTA (0.2 mg and 2 mg) and high-dose IVTA (2.0 mg); low-dose SCTA (0.2 mg) also effective in reducing inflammation but low-dose IVTA (0.2 mg) was not - Vitreous humor cell count and protein concentration: lower in high dose SCTA vs. low dose SCTA and IVTA groups - Aqueous humor protein concentration: no differences between the groups -AEs: none for SCTA group within 3 days -IOP and OCT measurements: similar between SCTA and 2.0 mg IVTA groups	Animal experimental study	Preclinical trial (animal study)	Treatment of acute posterior uveitis in a porcine model by injection of Triamcinolone Acetonide into the suprachoroidal space using microneedles [173]

Table A1. *Cont.*

No	Disease	Drug	Treatment	Key Findings	Study Design	Phase	Study Title
87	Panuveitis	TA	4 mg SCTA vs. 4 mg IVTA vs. SC Injection of vehicle as control	-AEs: none, including rise in IOP -Drug efficacy: higher panuveitis in control and IVTA treated eyes after 24 h; vitritis, aqueous flare, and cellularity less severe in both SCTA and IVTA treated eyes vs. control -Iris vessel dilation and tortuosity: greater reduction in SC group than IVTA group -Inflammatory response: significant reduction in SCTA group; histology showed marked reduction in SCTA and IVTA vs. control	Animal experimental study	Preclinical trial (animal study)	Evaluation of suprachoroidal microinjection of Triamcinolone Acetonide in a model of panuveitis in albino rabbits [174]
88	Experimental uveitis	TA	50 µL (2 mg) SCTA vs. Subtenon injection of 20 mg TA	- IOP: acute rise post-injection; higher rise with higher volume ($p < 0.0001$); equivalent volume of indocyanine green solution led to smaller rise than SCTA -Drug concentration: SCTA group, 1912 ng/mL in posterior vitreous and 400,369 ng/mL in retina; maximum in plasma was 11.6 ng/mL; exposure to posterior retina was 523,910 times greater than that to aqueous and 29,516 times more than systemic TA exposure -Efficacy for lipopolysaccharide-induced uveitis: less aqueous humor cells and lower vitreous opacity scores in 2 mg SCTA group compared to 20 mg subtenon group ($p < 0.05$) -Inflammatory response: less vitreous inflammation in SCTA group compared to subtenon group ($p < 0.0001$) -Tolerance: SCTA well tolerated -Drug distribution: excellent penetration into posterior retina in SCTA group vs. subtenon group	Animal experimental study	Preclinical trial (animal study)	Safety and pharmacodynamics of suprachoroidal injection of Triamcinolone Acetonide as a controlled ocular drug release model [67]
89	Glaucoma	Sulprostone, Brimoni-dine	Supraciliary injection of 10 µL Sulprostone or 10 µL Brimonidine vs. Topical administration of 0.05 mg/mL Sulprostone, 1 drop or 1.5 mg/mL Brimonidine, 1 drop	-IOP: SC Sulprostone and Brimonidine reduced IOP by 3 mmHg in a dose-dependent mannber over 9 h -Dose sparing: ~100-fold dose sparing vs. topical administration -Safety study: comparable kinetics of IOP elevation immediately after supraciliary and IV injection of placebo formulations	Animal experimental study	Preclinical trial (animal study)	Targeted delivery of antiglaucoma drugs to the supraciliary space using microneedles [179]
90	Glaucoma	Brimonidine	SC Brimonidine-loaded microspheres using poly (lactic acid) microspheres	-IOP: reduce initially by 6 mmHg; then, by progressively smaller amounts for >1 month -Tolerance: overall well, mild conjunctival redness and injection site healing delays -Histological examination: foreign-body reaction to the microspheres	Animal experimental study	Preclinical trial (animal study)	Sustained reduction in intraocular pressure by supraciliary delivery of Brimonidine-loaded poly (lactic acid) microspheres for the treatment of glaucoma [180]

Table A1. *Cont.*

No	Disease	Drug	Treatment	Key Findings	Study Design	Phase	Study Title
91	Glaucoma	NA	Hyaluronic acid in situ-forming hydrogel	-IOP: reduced for >1 month, observed for 4 months -AEs: none other than minor hemorrhage and fibrosis at injection site	Animal experimental study	Preclinical trial (animal study)	Drug-free, nonsurgical reduction in intraocular pressure for four months after suprachoroidal injection of hyaluronic acid hydrogel [182]
92	Glaucoma	NA	In situ-forming polyzwitterion polycarboxybetaine hydrogel	-Tolerance: well-tolerated with minimal inflammatory reaction -Histopathology assessment: SCS expansion with hydrogel -IOP: decreased for 6 weeks, correlated with SCS expansion	Animal experimental study	Preclinical trial (animal study)	Suprachoroidal injection of polyzwitterion hydrogel for treating glaucoma [183]
93	Uveal melanoma	AU-011	SC injection of AU-011 followed by photoactivation 1/week for 3 consecutive weeks	-Drug distribution: volume-dependent fashion in the choroid within 30 min. 100 μL distributed to ~75% of posterior globe -Drug clearance: not cleared from choroid for several days -Tumor regression: seen in all rabbits after SC 100 μL AU-011 -Histological evaluation: evidence of tumor responses	Animal experimental study	Preclinical trial (animal study)	Ocular distribution and efficacy after suprachoroidal injection of AU-011 for treatment of ocular melanoma [74]
94	Uveal melanoma	AU-011	SC AU-011 injection vs. IV AU-011 injection	-Drug distribution: negligible levels in vitreous, high exposure levels in tumor (up to 48 h) and choroid/retina for SC injection; high exposure in tumor for IV injection (up to 48 h) -Drug concentration: exposure of AU-011 in tumor ~5× higher for SC injection; mean AU-011 concentrations were 12,459 ± 5190 and 1996 ± 421 ng/mL for SC and IV injection, respectively, for 48 h -Positive IHC staining: AU-011 was present in tumor after both SC and IV injection; AU-011 staining observed penetrating throughout tumor for SC injection vs. localizing on the apex or vitreal surface of tumor for IV injection	Animal experimental study	Preclinical trial (animal study)	Ocular distribution and exposure of AU-011 after suprachoroidal or intravitreal administration in an orthotropic rabbit model of human uveal melanoma [184]
95	Uveal melanoma	Fluorescent parti-cles, Resin beads	SC injection of 10 μm fluorescent particles vs. SC injection of resin beads	-Fundus examination: yellow-tinted area (fluorescent particles) around tumor in posterior pole -Histological examination: polystyrene microspheres or resin beads located in SCS -Inflammatory response: not associated with microspheres -Drug distribution: microbeads present in SCS	Animal experimental study	Preclinical trial (animal study)	Suprachoroidal injection of microspheres with microcatheter in a rabbit model of uveal melanoma [185]

Table A1. *Cont.*

No	Disease	Drug	Treatment	Key Findings	Study Design	Phase	Study Title
96	Uveal melanoma	AU-011	3 cycles of 3 weekly AU-011 treatments via SC administration with a maximum dose of 80 µg with 2 laser applications	-AE related to treatment: anterior chamber inflammation (24%), conjunctival hyperemia (12%), eye pain (12%), punctate keratitis (12%) -No dose-limiting toxicities, treatment-related serious or grade 3/4 AEs, vitritis or vision loss; 2 subjects had 5 serious AEs unrelated to treatment	Randomized, multi-center	Clinical trial (phase II)	A phase II trial of AU-011, an investigational, virus-like drug conjugate (VDC) for the treatment of primary indeterminate lesions and small choroidal melanoma (IL/CM) using suprachoroidal administration [187]
97	Myopia	Biologic agents	NA	NA	NA	NA	Suprachoroidal injection of biological agents may have a potential role in the prevention of progression and complications in high myopia [190]
98	Ocular inflammatory diseases	Ketorolac	Intracameral injection of Ketorolac 250 µg/0.05 mL (Group A) vs. IV Ketorolac 250 µg/0.05 mL (Group B) vs. SC Ketorolac 250 µg/0.05 mL (Group C)	-Maximum drug concentration in vitreous: 0.378 ± 0.19 µg/mL at 0.5 h (Group A) vs. 156.2 ± 20.74 µg/mL at 0.5 h (Group B) vs. 0.873 ± 0.34 µg/mL at 0.5 h (Group C) -Maximum drug concentration in retina-choroid: 3.15 ± 0.49 µg/g at 0.5 h (Group A); 208.0 ± 21.67 µg/g at 1 h (Group B); 56.71 ± 22.64 µg/g at 0.5 h (Group C)-Drug concentration: <2 µg/g in retina-choroid in group C; plasma concentration < 0.4 µg/mL in all 3 group-Area under the curve: 866.1 ± 52.67 µg/g·h in retina-choroid in group B vs. 77.10 ± 25.90 µg/g·h in group C ($p < 0.01$) -Drug elimination: half-life was 3.09 h (Group B) vs. 1.19 h (Group C) ($p< 0.01$); Ketorolac in retina-choroid until 24 h (Group B) and 8 h (Group C)	Animal experimental study	Preclinical trial (animal study)	Pharmacokinetic comparison of Ketorolac after intracameral, intravitreal, and suprachoroidal administration in rabbits [194]
99	Ocular inflammatory diseases	Ketorolac	SC 3 mg Ketorolac vs. SC 6 mg Ketorolac vs. Control (left eye)	-Electroretinography results: no abnormal changes in rod cell response, maximum rod cell or cone cell mixing reaction, oscillation potential, cone cell response, waveform, amplitude, and potential of 30 Hz scintillation response at 1, 2, and 4 weeks, comparable with control eye -Light microscopy: normal histology in each retinal layer at 4 weeks	Animal experimental study	Preclinical trial (animal study)	Suprachoroidal injection of Ketorolac Tromethamine does not cause retinal damage [195]

References

1. Wu, K.Y.; Joly-Chevrier, M.; Akbar, D.; Tran, S.D. Overcoming Treatment Challenges in Posterior Segment Diseases with Biodegradable Nano-Based Drug Delivery Systems. *Pharmaceutics* **2023**, *15*, 1094. [CrossRef]
2. Ghate, D.; Edelhauser, H.F. Ocular Drug Delivery. *Expert Opin. Drug Deliv.* **2006**, *3*, 275–287. [CrossRef] [PubMed]
3. Patel, S.R.; Lin, A.S.P.; Edelhauser, H.F.; Prausnitz, M.R. Suprachoroidal Drug Delivery to the Back of the Eye Using Hollow Microneedles. *Pharm. Res.* **2011**, *28*, 166–176. [CrossRef] [PubMed]
4. Lampen, S.I.R.; Khurana, R.N.; Noronha, G.; Brown, D.M.; Wykoff, C.C. Suprachoroidal Space Alterations Following Delivery of Triamcinolone Acetonide: Post-Hoc Analysis of the Phase 1/2 HULK Study of Patients with Diabetic Macular Edema. *Ophthalmic Surg. Lasers Imaging Retina* **2018**, *49*, 692–697. [CrossRef]
5. Bhattacharyya, S.; Hariprasad, S.M.; Albini, T.A.; Dutta, S.K.; John, D.; Padula, W.V.; Harrison, D.; Joseph, G. Suprachoroidal Injection of Triamcinolone Acetonide Injectable Suspension for the Treatment of Macular Edema Associated with Uveitis in the United States: A Cost-Effectiveness Analysis. *Value Health* **2022**, *25*, 1705–1716. [CrossRef]
6. Dubashynskaya, N.; Poshina, D.; Raik, S.; Urtti, A.; Skorik, Y.A. Polysaccharides in Ocular Drug Delivery. *Pharmaceutics* **2019**, *12*, 22. [CrossRef]
7. Naftali Ben Haim, L.; Moisseiev, E. Drug Delivery via the Suprachoroidal Space for the Treatment of Retinal Diseases. *Pharmaceutics* **2021**, *13*, 967. [CrossRef]
8. Margolis, R.; Spaide, R.F. A Pilot Study of Enhanced Depth Imaging Optical Coherence Tomography of the Choroid in Normal Eyes. *Am. J. Ophthalmol.* **2009**, *147*, 811–815. [CrossRef]
9. Mahabadi, N.; Al Khalili, Y. Neuroanatomy, Retina. In *StatPearls*; StatPearls Publishing: Treasure Island, FL, USA, 2023.
10. Kaplan, H.J. Anatomy and Function of the Eye. In *Chemical Immunology and Allergy*; Niederkorn, J.Y., Kaplan, H.J., Eds.; KARGER: Basel, Switzerland, 2007; pp. 4–10. ISBN 978-3-8055-8187-5.
11. Vurgese, S.; Panda-Jonas, S.; Jonas, J.B. Scleral Thickness in Human Eyes. *PLoS ONE* **2012**, *7*, e29692. [CrossRef] [PubMed]
12. Patel, S.R.; Berezovsky, D.E.; McCarey, B.E.; Zarnitsyn, V.; Edelhauser, H.F.; Prausnitz, M.R. Targeted Administration into the Suprachoroidal Space Using a Microneedle for Drug Delivery to the Posterior Segment of the Eye. *Investig. Ophthalmol. Vis. Sci.* **2012**, *53*, 4433–4441. [CrossRef]
13. Ciulla, T.; Yeh, S. Microinjection via the Suprachoroidal Space: A Review of a Novel Mode of Administration. *Am. J. Manag. Care* **2022**, *28*, S243–S252. [CrossRef] [PubMed]
14. Meng, W.; Butterworth, J.; Malecaze, F.; Calvas, P. Axial Length of Myopia: A Review of Current Research. *Ophthalmologica* **2011**, *225*, 127–134. [CrossRef] [PubMed]
15. Del Amo, E.M.; Rimpelä, A.-K.; Heikkinen, E.; Kari, O.K.; Ramsay, E.; Lajunen, T.; Schmitt, M.; Pelkonen, L.; Bhattacharya, M.; Richardson, D.; et al. Pharmacokinetic Aspects of Retinal Drug Delivery. *Prog. Retin. Eye Res.* **2017**, *57*, 134–185. [CrossRef] [PubMed]
16. Emi, K.; Pederson, J.E.; Toris, C.B. Hydrostatic Pressure of the Suprachoroidal Space. *Investig. Ophthalmol. Vis. Sci.* **1989**, *30*, 233–238.
17. Krohn, J.; Bertelsen, T. Light Microscopy of Uveoscleral Drainage Routes after Gelatine Injections into the Suprachoroidal Space. *Acta Ophthalmol. Scand.* **1998**, *76*, 521–527. [CrossRef]
18. Krohn, J.; Bertelsen, T. Corrosion Casts of the Suprachoroidal Space and Uveoscleral Drainage Routes in the Human Eye. *Acta Ophthalmol. Scand.* **1997**, *75*, 32–35. [CrossRef]
19. Chiang, B.; Kim, Y.C.; Edelhauser, H.F.; Prausnitz, M.R. Circumferential Flow of Particles in the Suprachoroidal Space Is Impeded by the Posterior Ciliary Arteries. *Exp. Eye Res.* **2016**, *145*, 424–431. [CrossRef]
20. Urtti, A. Challenges and Obstacles of Ocular Pharmacokinetics and Drug Delivery. *Adv. Drug Deliv. Rev.* **2006**, *58*, 1131–1135. [CrossRef]
21. Wu, K.Y.; Ashkar, S.; Jain, S.; Marchand, M.; Tran, S.D. Breaking Barriers in Eye Treatment: Polymeric Nano-Based Drug-Delivery System for Anterior Segment Diseases and Glaucoma. *Polymers* **2023**, *15*, 1373. [CrossRef]
22. Carnahan, M.C.; Goldstein, D.A. Ocular Complications of Topical, Peri-Ocular, and Systemic Corticosteroids. *Curr. Opin. Ophthalmol.* **2000**, *11*, 478–483. [CrossRef]
23. Tyagi, P.; Kadam, R.S.; Kompella, U.B. Comparison of Suprachoroidal Drug Delivery with Subconjunctival and Intravitreal Routes Using Noninvasive Fluorophotometry. *PLoS ONE* **2012**, *7*, e48188. [CrossRef] [PubMed]
24. Yiu, G.; Chung, S.H.; Mollhoff, I.N.; Nguyen, U.T.; Thomasy, S.M.; Yoo, J.; Taraborelli, D.; Noronha, G. Suprachoroidal and Subretinal Injections of AAV Using Transscleral Microneedles for Retinal Gene Delivery in Nonhuman Primates. *Mol. Ther. Methods Clin. Dev.* **2020**, *16*, 179–191. [CrossRef] [PubMed]
25. Agrahari, V.; Mandal, A.; Agrahari, V.; Trinh, H.M.; Joseph, M.; Ray, A.; Hadji, H.; Mitra, R.; Pal, D.; Mitra, A.K. A Comprehensive insight on ocular pharmacokinetics. *Drug Deliv. Transl. Res.* **2016**, *6*, 735–754. [CrossRef] [PubMed]
26. Loftsson, T.; Stefánsson, E. Aqueous Eye Drops Containing Drug/Cyclodextrin Nanoparticles Deliver Therapeutic Drug Concentrations to Both Anterior and Posterior Segment. *Acta Ophthalmol.* **2022**, *100*, 7–25. [CrossRef] [PubMed]
27. Uchino, M.; Yokoi, N.; Shimazaki, J.; Hori, Y.; Tsubota, K.; on behalf of the Japan Dry Eye Society. Adherence to Eye Drops Usage in Dry Eye Patients and Reasons for Non-Compliance: A Web-Based Survey. *J. Clin. Med.* **2022**, *11*, 367. [CrossRef]

28. Foley, L.; Larkin, J.; Lombard-Vance, R.; Murphy, A.W.; Hynes, L.; Galvin, E.; Molloy, G.J. Prevalence and Predictors of Medication Non-Adherence among People Living with Multimorbidity: A Systematic Review and Meta-Analysis. *BMJ Open* **2021**, *11*, e044987. [CrossRef]
29. Holló, G. The Side Effects of the Prostaglandin Analogues. *Expert Opin. Drug Saf.* **2007**, *6*, 45–52. [CrossRef]
30. Santulli, R.J.; Kinney, W.A.; Ghosh, S.; Decorte, B.L.; Liu, L.; Tuman, R.W.A.; Zhou, Z.; Huebert, N.; Bursell, S.E.; Clermont, A.C.; et al. Studies with an Orally Bioavailable Alpha V Integrin Antagonist in Animal Models of Ocular Vasculopathy: Retinal Neovascularization in Mice and Retinal Vascular Permeability in Diabetic Rats. *J. Pharmacol. Exp. Ther.* **2008**, *324*, 894–901. [CrossRef]
31. Shirasaki, Y.; Miyashita, H.; Yamaguchi, M. Exploration of Orally Available Calpain Inhibitors. Part 3: Dipeptidyl Alpha-Ketoamide Derivatives Containing Pyridine Moiety. *Bioorg. Med. Chem.* **2006**, *14*, 5691–5698. [CrossRef]
32. Kampougeris, G.; Antoniadou, A.; Kavouklis, E.; Chryssouli, Z.; Giamarellou, H. Penetration of Moxifloxacin into the Human Aqueous Humour after Oral Administration. *Br. J. Ophthalmol.* **2005**, *89*, 628–631. [CrossRef]
33. Sakamoto, H.; Sakamoto, M.; Hata, Y.; Kubota, T.; Ishibashi, T. Aqueous and Vitreous Penetration of Levofloxacin after Topical and/or Oral Administration. *Eur. J. Ophthalmol.* **2007**, *17*, 372–376. [CrossRef] [PubMed]
34. Shirasaki, Y. Molecular Design for Enhancement of Ocular Penetration. *J. Pharm. Sci.* **2008**, *97*, 2462–2496. [CrossRef] [PubMed]
35. Kaur, I.P.; Smitha, R.; Aggarwal, D.; Kapil, M. Acetazolamide: Future Perspective in Topical Glaucoma Therapeutics. *Int. J. Pharm.* **2002**, *248*, 1–14. [CrossRef] [PubMed]
36. Gipson, I.K.; Argüeso, P. Role of Mucins in the Function of the Corneal and Conjunctival Epithelia. *Int. Rev. Cytol.* **2003**, *231*, 1–49. [CrossRef]
37. Geroski, D.H.; Edelhauser, H.F. Transscleral Drug Delivery for Posterior Segment Disease. *Adv. Drug Deliv. Rev.* **2001**, *52*, 37–48. [CrossRef]
38. Hosseini, K.; Matsushima, D.; Johnson, J.; Widera, G.; Nyam, K.; Kim, L.; Xu, Y.; Yao, Y.; Cormier, M. Pharmacokinetic Study of Dexamethasone Disodium Phosphate Using Intravitreal, Subconjunctival, and Intravenous Delivery Routes in Rabbits. *J. Ocul. Pharmacol. Ther.* **2008**, *24*, 301–308. [CrossRef]
39. Weijtens, O.; Feron, E.J.; Schoemaker, R.C.; Cohen, A.F.; Lentjes, E.G.; Romijn, F.P.; van Meurs, J.C. High Concentration of Dexamethasone in Aqueous and Vitreous after Subconjunctival Injection. *Am. J. Ophthalmol.* **1999**, *128*, 192–197. [CrossRef]
40. Kim, S.H.; Csaky, K.G.; Wang, N.S.; Lutz, R.J. Drug Elimination Kinetics Following Subconjunctival Injection Using Dynamic Contrast-Enhanced Magnetic Resonance Imaging. *Pharm. Res.* **2008**, *25*, 512–520. [CrossRef]
41. Prausnitz, M.R.; Noonan, J.S. Permeability of Cornea, Sclera, and Conjunctiva: A Literature Analysis for Drug Delivery to the Eye. *J. Pharm. Sci.* **1998**, *87*, 1479–1488. [CrossRef]
42. Modi, Y.S.; Tanchon, C.; Ehlers, J.P. Comparative Safety and Tolerability of Anti-VEGF Therapy in Age-Related Macular Degeneration. *Drug Saf.* **2015**, *38*, 279–293. [CrossRef]
43. Massa, H.; Nagar, A.M.; Vergados, A.; Dadoukis, P.; Patra, S.; Panos, G.D. Intravitreal Fluocinolone Acetonide Implant (ILUVIEN®) for Diabetic Macular Oedema: A Literature Review. *J. Int. Med. Res.* **2019**, *47*, 31–43. [CrossRef] [PubMed]
44. Adelman, R.A.; Parnes, A.J.; Bopp, S.; Saad Othman, I.; Ducournau, D. Strategy for the Management of Macular Edema in Retinal Vein Occlusion: The European VitreoRetinal Society Macular Edema Study. *BioMed Res. Int.* **2015**, *2015*, 870987. [CrossRef] [PubMed]
45. Gao, L.; Zhao, X.; Jiao, L.; Tang, L. Intravitreal Corticosteroids for Diabetic Macular Edema: A Network Meta-Analysis of Randomized Controlled Trials. *Eye Vis.* **2021**, *8*, 35. [CrossRef] [PubMed]
46. Hussain, R.M.; Hariprasad, S.M.; Ciulla, T.A. Treatment Burden in Neovascular AMD:Visual Acuity Outcomes Are Associated with Anti-VEGF Injection Frequency. *Ophthalmic Surg. Lasers Imaging Retina* **2017**, *48*, 780–784. [CrossRef] [PubMed]
47. Ciulla, T.A.; Bracha, P.; Pollack, J.; Williams, D.F. Real-World Outcomes of Anti-Vascular Endothelial Growth Factor Therapy in Diabetic Macular Edema in the United States. *Ophthalmol. Retina* **2018**, *2*, 1179–1187. [CrossRef] [PubMed]
48. Ciulla, T.; Pollack, J.S.; Williams, D.F. Visual Acuity Outcomes and Anti-VEGF Therapy Intensity in Macular Oedema Due to Retinal Vein Occlusion: A Real-World Analysis of 15 613 Patient Eyes. *Br. J. Ophthalmol.* **2021**, *105*, 1696–1704. [CrossRef]
49. Chin, H.-S.; Park, T.-S.; Moon, Y.-S.; Oh, J.-H. Difference in clearance of intravitreal triamcinolone acetonide between vitrectomized and nonvitrectomized eyes. *Retina* **2005**, *25*, 556–560. [CrossRef]
50. Multicenter Uveitis Steroid Treatment Trial Research Group. The Multicenter Uveitis Steroid Treatment (MUST) Trial: Rationale, Design and Baseline Characteristics. *Am. J. Ophthalmol.* **2010**, *149*, 550–561.e10. [CrossRef]
51. Writing Committee for the Multicenter Uveitis Steroid Treatment (MUST) Trial and Follow-up Study Research Group. Association between Long-Lasting Intravitreous Fluocinolone Acetonide Implant vs. Systemic Anti-Inflammatory Therapy and Visual Acuity at 7 Years Among Patients with Intermediate, Posterior, or Panuveitis. *JAMA* **2017**, *317*, 1993–2005. [CrossRef]
52. Holekamp, N.M.; Campochiaro, P.A.; Chang, M.A.; Miller, D.; Pieramici, D.; Adamis, A.P.; Brittain, C.; Evans, E.; Kaufman, D.; Maass, K.F.; et al. Archway Randomized Phase 3 Trial of the Port Delivery System with Ranibizumab for Neovascular Age-Related Macular Degeneration. *Ophthalmology* **2022**, *129*, 295–307. [CrossRef]
53. Heier, J.S.; Khanani, A.M.; Quezada Ruiz, C.; Basu, K.; Ferrone, P.J.; Brittain, C.; Figueroa, M.S.; Lin, H.; Holz, F.G.; Patel, V.; et al. Efficacy, Durability, and Safety of Intravitreal Faricimab up to Every 16 Weeks for Neovascular Age-Related Macular Degeneration (TENAYA and LUCERNE): Two Randomised, Double-Masked, Phase 3, Non-Inferiority Trials. *Lancet* **2022**, *399*, 729–740. [CrossRef] [PubMed]

54. Genentech: Press Releases | Friday, 28 January 2022. Available online: https://www.gene.com/media/press-releases/14943/2022-01-28/fda-approves-genentechs-vabysmo-the-firs (accessed on 6 July 2023).
55. Genentech: Press Releases | Friday, 22 October 2021. Available online: https://www.gene.com/media/press-releases/14935/2021-10-22/fda-approves-genentechs-susvimo-a-first- (accessed on 6 July 2023).
56. Pitkänen, L.; Ruponen, M.; Nieminen, J.; Urtti, A. Vitreous Is a Barrier in Nonviral Gene Transfer by Cationic Lipids and Polymers. *Pharm. Res.* **2003**, *20*, 576–583. [CrossRef] [PubMed]
57. Peeters, L.; Sanders, N.N.; Braeckmans, K.; Boussery, K.; Van de Voorde, J.; De Smedt, S.C.; Demeester, J. Vitreous: A Barrier to Nonviral Ocular Gene Therapy. *Investig. Ophthalmol. Vis. Sci.* **2005**, *46*, 3553–3561. [CrossRef] [PubMed]
58. Dalkara, D.; Kolstad, K.D.; Caporale, N.; Visel, M.; Klimczak, R.R.; Schaffer, D.V.; Flannery, J.G. Inner Limiting Membrane Barriers to AAV-Mediated Retinal Transduction from the Vitreous. *Mol. Ther. J. Am. Soc. Gene Ther.* **2009**, *17*, 2096–2102. [CrossRef]
59. Kansara, V.; Muya, L.; Wan, C.-R.; Ciulla, T.A. Suprachoroidal Delivery of Viral and Nonviral Gene Therapy for Retinal Diseases. *J. Ocul. Pharmacol. Ther.* **2020**, *36*, 384–392. [CrossRef]
60. Russell, S.; Bennett, J.; Wellman, J.A.; Chung, D.C.; Yu, Z.-F.; Tillman, A.; Wittes, J.; Pappas, J.; Elci, O.; McCague, S.; et al. Efficacy and Safety of Voretigene Neparvovec (AAV2-HRPE65v2) in Patients with RPE65-Mediated Inherited Retinal Dystrophy: A Randomised, Controlled, Open-Label, Phase 3 Trial. *Lancet* **2017**, *390*, 849–860. [CrossRef]
61. Maguire, A.M.; Russell, S.; Chung, D.C.; Yu, Z.-F.; Tillman, A.; Drack, A.V.; Simonelli, F.; Leroy, B.P.; Reape, K.Z.; High, K.A.; et al. Durability of Voretigene Neparvovec for Biallelic RPE65-Mediated Inherited Retinal Disease: Phase 3 Results at 3 and 4 Years. *Ophthalmology* **2021**, *128*, 1460–1468. [CrossRef]
62. REGENXBIO Announces Additional Positive Interim Phase I/IIa and Long-Term Follow-Up Data of RGX-314 for the Treatment of Wet AMD | Regenxbio Inc. Available online: https://ir.regenxbio.com/news-releases/news-release-details/regenxbio-announces-additional-positive-interim-phase-iiia-and/ (accessed on 6 July 2023).
63. Jung, J.H.; Chae, J.J.; Prausnitz, M.R. Targeting Drug Delivery within the Suprachoroidal Space. *Drug Discov. Today* **2019**, *24*, 1654–1659. [CrossRef]
64. Hancock, S.E.; Wan, C.-R.; Fisher, N.E.; Andino, R.V.; Ciulla, T.A. Biomechanics of Suprachoroidal Drug Delivery: From Benchtop to Clinical Investigation in Ocular Therapies. *Expert Opin. Drug Deliv.* **2021**, *18*, 777–788. [CrossRef]
65. Peden, M.C.; Min, J.; Meyers, C.; Lukowski, Z.; Li, Q.; Boye, S.L.; Levine, M.; Hauswirth, W.W.; Ratnakaram, R.; Dawson, W.; et al. Ab-Externo AAV-Mediated Gene Delivery to the Suprachoroidal Space Using a 250 Micron Flexible Microcatheter. *PLoS ONE* **2011**, *6*, e17140. [CrossRef]
66. Tyagi, P.; Barros, M.; Stansbury, J.W.; Kompella, U.B. Light Activated, In Situ Forming Gel for Sustained Suprachoroidal Delivery of Bevacizumab. *Mol. Pharm.* **2013**, *10*, 2858–2867. [CrossRef]
67. Chen, M.; Li, X.; Liu, J.; Han, Y.; Cheng, L. Safety and Pharmacodynamics of Suprachoroidal Injection of Triamcinolone Acetonide as a Controlled Ocular Drug Release Model. *J. Control. Release* **2015**, *203*, 109–117. [CrossRef]
68. Kansara, V.S.; Hancock, S.E.; Muya, L.W.; Ciulla, T.A. Suprachoroidal Delivery Enables Targeting, Localization and Durability of Small Molecule Suspensions. *J. Control. Release* **2022**, *349*, 1045–1051. [CrossRef] [PubMed]
69. Yeh, S.; Ciulla, T. Suprachoroidal Triamcinolone Acetonide Injectable Suspension for Macular Edema Associated with Noninfectious Uveitis: An In-Depth Look at Efficacy and Safety. *Am. J. Manag. Care* **2023**, *29*, S19–S28. [PubMed]
70. Fisher, N.; Yoo, J.; Hancock, S.E.; Andino, R.V. *A Novel Technique to Characterize Key Fluid Mechanic Properties of the SC Injection Procedure in an In Vivo Model*; Clear Association for Research in Vision and Ophthalmology Annual Meeting: Atlanta, GA, USA, 2018.
71. Fisher, N.; Wan, C. Suprachoroidal Delivery with the SCS Microinjector™: Characterization of Operational Forces. *Investig. Ophthalmol. Vis. Sci.* **2020**, *61*, 24.
72. Moisseiev, E.; Loewenstein, A.; Yiu, G. The Suprachoroidal Space: From Potential Space to a Space with Potential. *Clin. Ophthalmol.* **2016**, *10*, 173–178. [CrossRef] [PubMed]
73. Gu, B.; Liu, J.; Li, X.; Ma, Q.; Shen, M.; Cheng, L. Real-Time Monitoring of Suprachoroidal Space (SCS) Following SCS Injection Using Ultra-High Resolution Optical Coherence Tomography in Guinea Pig Eyes. *Investig. Ophthalmol. Vis. Sci.* **2015**, *56*, 3623–3634. [CrossRef]
74. Savinainen, A.; Grossniklaus, H.; Kang, S.; Rasmussen, C.; Bentley, E.; Krakova, Y.; Struble, C.B.; Rich, C. Ocular Distribution and Efficacy after Suprachoroidal Injection of AU-011 for Treatment of Ocular Melanoma. *Investig. Ophthalmol. Vis. Sci.* **2020**, *61*, 3615.
75. Chiang, B.; Venugopal, N.; Grossniklaus, H.E.; Jung, J.H.; Edelhauser, H.F.; Prausnitz, M.R. Thickness and Closure Kinetics of the Suprachoroidal Space Following Microneedle Injection of Liquid Formulations. *Investig. Ophthalmol. Vis. Sci.* **2017**, *58*, 555–564. [CrossRef]
76. Jung, J.H.; Park, S.; Chae, J.J.; Prausnitz, M.R. Collagenase Injection into the Suprachoroidal Space of the Eye to Expand Drug Delivery Coverage and Increase Posterior Drug Targeting. *Exp. Eye Res.* **2019**, *189*, 107824. [CrossRef]
77. Nork, T.M.; Katz, A.W.; Kim, C.B.Y.; Rasmussen, C.A.; Wabers, H.D.; Bentley, E.; Struble, C.B.; Savinainen, A. Distribution of Aqueous Solutions Injected Suprachoroidally (SC) in Rabbits. *Investig. Ophthalmol. Vis. Sci.* **2020**, *61*, 320.
78. Oshika, T.; Bissen-Miyajima, H.; Fujita, Y.; Hayashi, K.; Mano, T.; Miyata, K.; Sugita, T.; Taira, Y. Prospective Randomized Comparison of DisCoVisc and Healon5 in Phacoemulsification and Intraocular Lens Implantation. *Eye* **2010**, *24*, 1376–1381. [CrossRef] [PubMed]

79. Kim, Y.C.; Oh, K.H.; Edelhauser, H.F.; Prausnitz, M.R. Formulation to Target Delivery to the Ciliary Body and Choroid via the Suprachoroidal Space of the Eye Using Microneedles. *Eur. J. Pharm. Biopharm.* **2015**, *95*, 398–406. [CrossRef] [PubMed]
80. Jung, J.H.; Kim, S.S.; Chung, H.; Hejri, A.; Prausnitz, M.R. Six-Month Sustained Delivery of Anti-VEGF from in-Situ Forming Hydrogel in the Suprachoroidal Space. *J. Control. Release* **2022**, *352*, 472–484. [CrossRef] [PubMed]
81. Chiang, B.; Wang, K.; Ethier, C.R.; Prausnitz, M.R. Clearance Kinetics and Clearance Routes of Molecules From the Suprachoroidal Space After Microneedle Injection. *Investig. Ophthalmol. Vis. Sci.* **2017**, *58*, 545–554. [CrossRef]
82. Mustafa, M.B.; Tipton, D.L.; Barkley, M.D.; Russo, P.S.; Blum, F.D. Dye Diffusion in Isotropic and Liquid-Crystalline Aqueous (Hydroxypropyl)Cellulose. *Macromolecules* **1993**, *26*, 370–378. [CrossRef]
83. FITC-Dextran Fluorescein Isothiocyanate Dextran. 2011. Available online: https://www.semanticscholar.org/paper/FITC-Dextran-Fluorescein-isothiocyanate-dextran/01c8e9539524bc604f6b45a6bbb06dd03507d82f (accessed on 30 May 2023).
84. Hackett, S.F.; Fu, J.; Kim, Y.C.; Tsujinaka, H.; Shen, J.; Lima E Silva, R.; Khan, M.; Hafiz, Z.; Wang, T.; Shin, M.; et al. Sustained Delivery of Acriflavine from the Suprachoroidal Space Provides Long Term Suppression of Choroidal Neovascularization. *Biomaterials* **2020**, *243*, 119935. [CrossRef]
85. Edwards, A.; Prausnitz, M.R. Fiber Matrix Model of Sclera and Corneal Stroma for Drug Delivery to the Eye. *AIChE J.* **1998**, *44*, 214–225. [CrossRef]
86. Jung, J.H.; Desit, P.; Prausnitz, M.R. Targeted Drug Delivery in the Suprachoroidal Space by Swollen Hydrogel Pushing. *Investig. Ophthalmol. Vis. Sci.* **2018**, *59*, 2069–2079. [CrossRef]
87. Jung, J.H.; Chiang, B.; Grossniklaus, H.E.; Prausnitz, M.R. Ocular Drug Delivery Targeted by Iontophoresis in the Suprachoroidal Space Using a Microneedle. *J. Control. Release* **2018**, *277*, 14–22. [CrossRef]
88. Touchard, E.; Berdugo, M.; Bigey, P.; El Sanharawi, M.; Savoldelli, M.; Naud, M.-C.; Jeanny, J.-C.; Behar-Cohen, F. Suprachoroidal Electrotransfer: A Nonviral Gene Delivery Method to Transfect the Choroid and the Retina without Detaching the Retina. *Mol. Ther. J. Am. Soc. Gene Ther.* **2012**, *20*, 1559–1570. [CrossRef] [PubMed]
89. Edelhauser, H.F.; Verhoeven, R.S.; Burke, B.; Struble, C.B.; Patel, S.R. Intraocular Distribution and Targeting of Triamcinolone Acetonide Suspension Administered Into the Suprachoroidal Space. *Investig. Ophthalmol. Vis. Sci.* **2014**, *55*, 5259.
90. Muya, L.; Kansara, V.; Cavet, M.E.; Ciulla, T. Suprachoroidal Injection of Triamcinolone Acetonide Suspension: Ocular Pharmacokinetics and Distribution in Rabbits Demonstrates High and Durable Levels in the Chorioretina. *J. Ocul. Pharmacol. Ther.* **2022**, *38*, 459–467. [CrossRef] [PubMed]
91. Hancock, S.E.; Phadke, A.; Kansara, V.; Boyer, D.; Rivera, J.; Marlor, C.; Podos, S.; Wiles, J.; McElheny, R.; Ciulla, T.A.; et al. Ocular Pharmacokinetics and Safety of Suprachoroidal A01017, Small Molecule Complement Inhibitor, Injectable Suspension in Rabbits. *Investig. Ophthalmol. Vis. Sci.* **2020**, *61*, 3694.
92. Kaiser, P.K.; Ciulla, T.; Kansara, V. Suprachoroidal CLS-AX (Axitinib Injectable Suspension), as a Potential Long-Acting Therapy for Neovascular Age-Related Macular Degeneration (NAMD). *Investig. Ophthalmol. Vis. Sci.* **2020**, *61*, 3977.
93. Henry, C.R.; Shah, M.; Barakat, M.R.; Dayani, P.; Wang, R.C.; Khurana, R.N.; Rifkin, L.; Yeh, S.; Hall, C.; Ciulla, T. Suprachoroidal CLS-TA for Non-Infectious Uveitis: An Open-Label, Safety Trial (AZALEA). *Br. J. Ophthalmol.* **2022**, *106*, 802–806. [CrossRef]
94. Yeh, S.; Khurana, R.N.; Shah, M.; Henry, C.R.; Wang, R.C.; Kissner, J.M.; Ciulla, T.A.; Noronha, G. Efficacy and Safety of Suprachoroidal CLS-TA for Macular Edema Secondary to Noninfectious Uveitis: Phase 3 Randomized Trial. *Ophthalmology* **2020**, *127*, 948–955. [CrossRef]
95. Henry, C.R.; Kapik, B.; Ciulla, T.A. Suprachoroidal Triamcinolone Acetonide Injectable Suspension for Macular Edema Associated with Uveitis: Visual and Anatomic Outcomes by Age. *Investig. Ophthalmol. Vis. Sci.* **2022**, *63*, 3206-A0432.
96. Merrill, P.T.; Henry, C.R.; Nguyen, Q.D.; Reddy, A.; Kapik, B.; Ciulla, T.A. Suprachoroidal CLS-TA with and without Systemic Corticosteroid and/or Steroid-Sparing Therapy: A Post-Hoc Analysis of the Phase 3 PEACHTREE Clinical Trial. *Ocul. Immunol. Inflamm.* **2021**, 1–8. [CrossRef]
97. Khurana, R.N.; Merrill, P.; Yeh, S.; Suhler, E.; Barakat, M.R.; Uchiyama, E.; Henry, C.R.; Shah, M.; Wang, R.C.; Kapik, B.; et al. Extension Study of the Safety and Efficacy of CLS-TA for Treatment of Macular Oedema Associated with Non-Infectious Uveitis (MAGNOLIA). *Br. J. Ophthalmol.* **2022**, *106*, 1139–1144. [CrossRef]
98. Yeh, S.; Kurup, S.K.; Wang, R.C.; Foster, C.S.; Noronha, G.; Nguyen, Q.D.; Do, D.V.; DOGWOOD Study Team. Suprachoroidal injection of triamcinolone acetonide, CLS-TA, for macular edema due to noninfectious uveitis: A Randomized, Phase 2 Study (DOGWOOD). *Retina* **2019**, *39*, 1880–1888. [CrossRef] [PubMed]
99. Hanif, J.; Iqbal, K.; Perveen, F.; Arif, A.; Iqbal, R.N.; Jameel, F.; Hanif, K.; Seemab, A.; Khan, A.Y.; Ahmed, M. Safety and Efficacy of Suprachoroidal Injection of Triamcinolone in Treating Macular Edema Secondary to Noninfectious Uveitis. *Cureus* **2021**, *13*, e20038. [CrossRef] [PubMed]
100. Munir, M.S.; Rehman, R.; Nazir, S.; Sharif, N.; Chaudhari, M.Z.; Saleem, S. Visual Outcome after Suprachoroidal Injection of Triamcinolone Acetate in Cystoid Macular Edema of Different Pathology. *Pak. J. Med. Health Sci.* **2022**, *16*, 164. [CrossRef]
101. Chen, J.; Wang, H.; Qiu, W. Intravitreal Anti-Vascular Endothelial Growth Factor, Laser Photocoagulation, or Combined Therapy for Diabetic Macular Edema: A Systematic Review and Network Meta-Analysis. *Front. Endocrinol.* **2023**, *14*, 1096105. [CrossRef]
102. Wykoff, C.C.; Khurana, R.N.; Lampen, S.I.R.; Noronha, G.; Brown, D.M.; Ou, W.C.; Sadda, S.R.; HULK Study Group. Suprachoroidal Triamcinolone Acetonide for Diabetic Macular Edema: The HULK Trial. *Ophthalmol. Retina* **2018**, *2*, 874–877. [CrossRef] [PubMed]

103. Barakat, M.R.; Wykoff, C.C.; Gonzalez, V.; Hu, A.; Marcus, D.; Zavaleta, E.; Ciulla, T.A. Suprachoroidal CLS-TA plus Intravitreal Aflibercept for Diabetic Macular Edema: A Randomized, Double-Masked, Parallel-Design, Controlled Study. *Ophthalmol. Retina* **2021**, *5*, 60–70. [CrossRef]
104. Fazel, F.; Malekahmadi, M.; Feizi, A.; Oliya, B.; Tavakoli, M.; Fazel, M. Suprachoroidal Injection of Triamcinolone Acetonide plus Intravitreal Bevacizumab in Diabetic Macular Edema: A Randomized Pilot Trial. *BMC Ophthalmol.* **2023**, *23*, 40. [CrossRef]
105. Shahid, M.H.; Rashid, F.; Tauqeer, S.; Ali, R.; Farooq, M.T.; Aleem, N. Comparison of Suprachoroidal Triamcinolone Injection with Intravitreal Bevacizumab Vs Intravitreal Bevacizumab Only in Treatment of Refractory Diabetic Macular Edema. *Pak. J. Med. Health Sci.* **2022**, *16*, 301. [CrossRef]
106. Anwar, F.; Khan, A.A.; Majhu, T.M.; Javaid, R.M.M.; Ghaffar, M.T.; Bokhari, M.H. Comparison of Suprachoroidal Injection of Triamcinolone Acetonide Versus Intravitreal Bevacizumab in Primary Diabetic Macular Odema. *Pak. J. Med. Health Sci.* **2022**, *16*, 304. [CrossRef]
107. Zakaria, Y.G.; Salman, A.G.; Said, A.M.A.; Abdelatif, M.K. Suprachoroidal versus Intravitreal Triamcinolone Acetonide for the Treatment of Diabetic Macular Edema. *Clin. Ophthalmol.* **2022**, *16*, 733–746. [CrossRef]
108. Shaikh, K.; Ahmed, N.; Kazi, U.; Zia, A.; Aziz, M.Z. Comparison between Suprachoroidal Triamcinolone and Intravitreal Triamcinolone Acetonide in Patients of Resistant Diabetic Macular Edema. *Pak. J. Ophthalmol.* **2023**, *39*. [CrossRef]
109. Marashi, A.; Zazo, A. Suprachoroidal Injection of Triamcinolone Acetonide Using a Custom-Made Needle to Treat Diabetic Macular Edema Post Pars Plana Vitrectomy: A Case Series. *J. Int. Med. Res.* **2022**, *50*, 03000605221089807. [CrossRef] [PubMed]
110. Nawar, A.E. Effectiveness of Suprachoroidal Injection of Triamcinolone Acetonide in Resistant Diabetic Macular Edema Using a Modified Microneedle. *Clin. Ophthalmol.* **2022**, *16*, 3821–3831. [CrossRef] [PubMed]
111. Ateeq, A.; Majid, S.; Memon, N.A.; Hayat, N.; Somroo, A.Q.; Fattah, A. Suprachoroidal Injection of Triamcinolone Acetonide for Management of Resistant Diabetic Macular Oedema. *JPMA J. Pak. Med. Assoc.* **2023**, *73*, 239–244. [CrossRef] [PubMed]
112. Chandni, A.; Bhatti, S.R.; Khawer, F.; Ijaz, M.; Rafique, D.; Choudhry, T.A. To Determine the Efficacy of Suprachoroidal Triamcinolone Injection for the Treatment of Refractory Diabetic Macular Edema. *Pak. J. Med. Health Sci.* **2022**, *16*, 400. [CrossRef]
113. Tayyab, H.; Ahmed, C.N.; Sadiq, M.A.A. Efficacy and Safety of Suprachoroidal Triamcinolone Acetonide in Cases of Resistant Diabetic Macular Edema. *Pak. J. Med. Sci.* **2020**, *36*, 42–47. [CrossRef]
114. Ahmad, Y.; Memon, S.U.H.; Bhatti, S.A.; Nawaz, F.; Ahmad, W.; Saleem, M. Efficacy and Safety of Suprachoroidal Triamcinolone Acetonide in Cases of Resistant Diabetic Macular Edema. *Pak. J. Med. Health Sci.* **2023**, *17*, 324. [CrossRef]
115. Butt, S.; Iqbal, R.; Siddiq, S.; Waheed, K.; Javed, T. Efficacy of Suprachoroidal Triamcinolone Acetonide Injection in the Treatment of Resistant Diabetic Macular Edema. *Biol. Clin. Sci. Res. J.* **2023**, *2023*, 202. [CrossRef]
116. Tharwat, E.; Ahmed, R.E.H.; Eltantawy, B.; Ezzeldin, E.R.; Elgazzar, A.F. Suprachoroidal Triamcinolone versus Posterior Subtenon Triamcinolone Either Alone or Formulated in the Management of Diabetic Macular Edema. *Int. Ophthalmol.* **2022**. [CrossRef]
117. Dhoot, D.S. Suprachoroidal Delivery of RGX-314 for Diabetic Retinopathy: The Phase II ALTITUDE™ Study. *Investig. Ophthalmol. Vis. Sci.* **2022**, *63*, 1152.
118. Veiga Reis, F.; Dalgalarrondo, P.; da Silva Tavares Neto, J.E.; Wendeborn Rodrigues, M.; Scott, I.U.; Jorge, R. Combined Intravitreal Dexamethasone and Bevacizumab Injection for the Treatment of Persistent Diabetic Macular Edema (DexaBe Study): A Phase I Clinical Study. *Int. J. Retina Vitr.* **2023**, *9*, 13. [CrossRef]
119. Campochiaro, P.A.; Wykoff, C.C.; Brown, D.M.; Boyer, D.S.; Barakat, M.; Taraborelli, D.; Noronha, G.; Tanzanite Study Group. Suprachoroidal Triamcinolone Acetonide for Retinal Vein Occlusion: Results of the Tanzanite Study. *Ophthalmol. Retina* **2018**, *2*, 320–328. [CrossRef] [PubMed]
120. Clearside Biomedical's TANZANITE Extension Study in Patients with Macular Edema Associated with Retinal Vein Occlusion Presented at the 40th Annual Macula Society Meeting | Clearside Biomedical, Inc.-IR Site. Available online: https://ir.clearsidebio.com/news-releases/news-release-details/clearside-biomedicals-tanzanite-extension-study-patients-macular (accessed on 15 July 2023).
121. Clearside Biomedical, Inc. *SAPPHIRE: A Randomized, Masked, Controlled Trial to Study the Safety and Efficacy of Suprachoroidal CLS-TA in Conjunction with Intravitreal Aflibercept in Subjects with Retinal Vein Occlusion*; Clearside Biomedical, Inc.: Alpharetta, GA, USA, 2021.
122. Clearside Biomedical, Inc. *A Randomized, Masked, Controlled Trial to Study the Safety and Efficacy of Suprachoroidal CLS-TA in Combination with an Intravitreal Anti-VEGF Agent in Subjects with Retinal Vein Occlusion*; Clearside Biomedical, Inc.: Alpharetta, GA, USA, 2021.
123. Nawar, A.E. Modified Microneedle for Suprachoroidal Injection of Triamcinolone Acetonide Combined with Intravitreal Injection of Ranibizumab in Branch Retinal Vein Occlusion Patients. *Clin. Ophthalmol.* **2022**, *16*, 1139–1151. [CrossRef] [PubMed]
124. Ali, B.M.; Azmeh, A.M.; Alhalabi, N.M. Suprachoroidal Triamcinolone Acetonide for the Treatment of Macular Edema Associated with Retinal Vein Occlusion: A Pilot Study. *BMC Ophthalmol.* **2023**, *23*, 60. [CrossRef] [PubMed]
125. Muslim, I.; Chaudhry, N.; Javed, R.M.M. Effect of Supra-Choroidal Triamcinolone Injection on Best-Corrected Visual Acuity and Central Retinal Thickness in Patients with Macular Edema Secondary to Retinal Vein Occlusion. *Pak. J. Ophthalmol.* **2022**, *38*. [CrossRef]
126. Rizzo, S.; Ebert, F.G.; Bartolo, E.D.; Barca, F.; Cresti, F.; Augustin, C.; Augustin, A. Suprachoroidal drug Infusion for the Treatment of Severe Subfoveal Hard Exudates. *Retina* **2012**, *32*, 776. [CrossRef]

127. Abdelshafy, A. *One Year Results for Suprachoroidal Triamcinolone Acetonide Injection in Various Retinal Diseases*; Benha University: Benha, Egypt, 2022.
128. Abdelshafy Tabl, A.; Tawfik Soliman, T.; Anany Elsayed, M.; Abdelshafy Tabl, M. A Randomized Trial Comparing Suprachoroidal and Intravitreal Injection of Triamcinolone Acetonide in Refractory Diabetic Macular Edema Due to Epiretinal Membrane. *J. Ophthalmol.* **2022**, *2022*, 7947710. [CrossRef] [PubMed]
129. Zhang, D.-D.; Che, D.-Y.; Zhu, D.-Q. A Simple Technique for Suprachoroidal Space Injection of Triamcinolone Acetonide in Treatment of Macular Edema. *Int. J. Ophthalmol.* **2022**, *15*, 2017–2021. [CrossRef]
130. Oli, A.; Waikar, S. Modified Inexpensive Needle for Suprachoroidal Triamcinolone Acetonide Injections in Pseudophakic Cystoid Macular Edema. *Indian J. Ophthalmol.* **2021**, *69*, 765–767. [CrossRef]
131. Marashi, A.; Zazo, A. A Manually Made Needle for Treating Pseudophakic Cystoid Macular Edema by Injecting Triamcinolone Acetonide in the Suprachoroidal Space: A Case Report. *Am. J. Ophthalmol. Case Rep.* **2022**, *25*, 101254. [CrossRef]
132. Abdelshafy, A. *Suprachoroidal Triamcinolone Acetonide Injection in Two Chorioretinal Diseases: One Year Results*; Benha University: Benha, Egypt, 2022.
133. Martorana, G.; Levine, M.; Peden, M.; Boye, S.; Lukowski, Z.; Min, J.; Meyers, C.; Boye, S.; Sherwood, M. Comparison of Suprachoroidal Delivery via an Ab-Externo Approach with the ITrack Microcatheter versus Vitrectomy and Subretinal Delivery for 3 Different AAV Serotypes for Gene Transfer to the Retina. *Investig. Ophthalmol. Vis. Sci.* **2012**, *53*, 1931.
134. Woodard, K.T.; Vance, M.; Gilger, B.; Samulski, R.J.; Hirsch, M. 544. Comparison of AAV Serotype2 Transduction by Various Delivery Routes to the Mouse Eye. *Mol. Ther.* **2016**, *24*, S217–S218. [CrossRef]
135. Ding, K.; Shen, J.; Hafiz, Z.; Hackett, S.F.; Silva, R.L.E.; Khan, M.; Lorenc, V.E.; Chen, D.; Chadha, R.; Zhang, M.; et al. AAV8-Vectored Suprachoroidal Gene Transfer Produces Widespread Ocular Transgene Expression. *J. Clin. Investig.* **2019**, *129*, 4901–4911. [CrossRef] [PubMed]
136. Ding, K.; Shen, J.; Hackett, S.; Campochiaro, P.A. Transgene Expression in RPE and Retina after Suprachoroidal Delivery of AAV Vectors. *Investig. Ophthalmol. Vis. Sci.* **2020**, *61*, 4490.
137. Kansara, V.; Yoo, J.; Cooper, M.J.; Laird, O.S.; Taraborelli, D.; Moen, R.; Noronha, G. Suprachoroidally Delivered Non-Viral DNA Nanoparticles Transfect Chorioretinal Cells in Non-Human Primates and Rabbits. *Investig. Ophthalmol. Vis. Sci.* **2019**, *60*, 2909.
138. Chung, S.H.; Mollhoff, I.N.; Mishra, A.; Sin, T.-N.; Ngo, T.; Ciulla, T.; Sieving, P.; Thomasy, S.M.; Yiu, G. Host Immune Responses after Suprachoroidal Delivery of AAV8 in Nonhuman Primate Eyes. *Hum. Gene Ther.* **2021**, *32*, 682–693. [CrossRef]
139. Kansara, V.S.; Cooper, M.; Sesenoglu-Laird, O.; Muya, L.; Moen, R.; Ciulla, T.A. Suprachoroidally Delivered DNA Nanoparticles Transfect Retina and Retinal Pigment Epithelium/Choroid in Rabbits. *Transl. Vis. Sci. Technol.* **2020**, *9*, 21. [CrossRef]
140. Shen, J.; Kim, J.; Tzeng, S.Y.; Ding, K.; Hafiz, Z.; Long, D.; Wang, J.; Green, J.J.; Campochiaro, P.A. Suprachoroidal Gene Transfer with Nonviral Nanoparticles. *Sci. Adv.* **2020**, *6*, eaba1606. [CrossRef]
141. Lin, Y.; Ren, X.; Chen, Y.; Chen, D. Interaction Between Mesenchymal Stem Cells and Retinal Degenerative Microenvironment. *Front. Neurosci.* **2021**, *14*, 617377. [CrossRef]
142. Habot-Wilner, Z.; Noronha, G.; Wykoff, C.C. Suprachoroidally Injected Pharmacological Agents for the Treatment of Chorio-Retinal Diseases: A Targeted Approach. *Acta Ophthalmol.* **2019**, *97*, 460–472. [CrossRef]
143. Öner, A.; Kahraman, N.S. Does Stem Cell Implantation Have an Effect on Severity of Retinitis Pigmentosa: Evaluation with a Classification System? *Open J. Ophthalmol.* **2021**, *11*, 36–48. [CrossRef]
144. Oner, A.; Kahraman, N.S. Suprachoroidal Umbilical Cord Derived Mesenchymal Stem Cell Implantation for the Treatment of Retinitis Pigmentosa in Pediatric Patients. *Am. J. Stem Cell Res.* **2023**, *5*, 1–7.
145. Özkan, B. Suprachoroidal Spheroidal Mesenchymal Stem Cell Implantation in Retinitis Pigmentosa: Clinical Results of 6 Months Follow-Up. 2023. Available online: clinicaltrials.gov (accessed on 6 July 2023).
146. Marashi, A.; Baba, M.; Zazo, A. Managing Solar Retinopathy with Suprachoroidal Triamcinolone Acetonide Injection in a Young Girl: A Case Report. *J. Med. Case Rep.* **2021**, *15*, 577. [CrossRef] [PubMed]
147. Gohil, R.; Crosby-Nwaobi, R.; Forbes, A.; Burton, B.; Hykin, P.; Sivaprasad, S. Caregiver Burden in Patients Receiving Ranibizumab Therapy for Neovascular Age Related Macular Degeneration. *PLoS ONE* **2015**, *10*, e0129361. [CrossRef] [PubMed]
148. Saxena, N.; George, P.P.; Hoon, H.B.; Han, L.T.; Onn, Y.S. Burden of Wet Age-Related Macular Degeneration and Its Economic Implications in Singapore in the Year 2030. *Ophthalmic Epidemiol.* **2016**, *23*, 232–237. [CrossRef]
149. Sampat, K.M.; Garg, S.J. Complications of Intravitreal Injections. *Curr. Opin. Ophthalmol.* **2010**, *21*, 178–183. [CrossRef]
150. Fallico, M.; Maugeri, A.; Lotery, A.; Longo, A.; Bonfiglio, V.; Russo, A.; Avitabile, T.; Pulvirenti, A.; Furino, C.; Cennamo, G.; et al. Intravitreal Anti-Vascular Endothelial Growth Factors, Panretinal Photocoagulation and Combined Treatment for Proliferative Diabetic Retinopathy: A Systematic Review and Network Meta-Analysis. *Acta Ophthalmol.* **2021**, *99*, e795–e805. [CrossRef]
151. Tran, J.; Craven, C.; Wabner, K.; Schmit, J.; Matter, B.; Kompella, U.; Grossniklaus, H.E.; Olsen, T.W. A Pharmacodynamic Analysis of Choroidal Neovascularization in a Porcine Model Using Three Targeted Drugs. *Investig. Ophthalmol. Vis. Sci.* **2017**, *58*, 3732–3740. [CrossRef]
152. Mansoor, S.; Patel, S.R.; Tas, C.; Pacha-Ravi, R.; Kompella, U.B.; Edelhauser, H.F.; Prausnitz, M.R. Pharmacokinetics and Biodistribution of Bevacizumab Following Suprachoroidal Injection into the Rabbit Eye Using a Microneedle. *Investig. Ophthalmol. Vis. Sci.* **2012**, *53*, 498.

153. Olsen, T.W.; Feng, X.; Wabner, K.; Csaky, K.; Pambuccian, S.; Cameron, J.D. Pharmacokinetics of Pars Plana Intravitreal Injections versus Microcannula Suprachoroidal Injections of Bevacizumab in a Porcine Model. *Investig. Ophthalmol. Vis. Sci.* **2011**, *52*, 4749–4756. [CrossRef]
154. Zeng, M.; Shen, J.; Liu, Y.; Lu, L.Y.; Ding, K.; Fortmann, S.D.; Khan, M.; Wang, J.; Hackett, S.F.; Semenza, G.L.; et al. The HIF-1 Antagonist Acriflavine: Visualization in Retina and Suppression of Ocular Neovascularization. *J. Mol. Med.* **2017**, *95*, 417–429. [CrossRef] [PubMed]
155. Olsen, T.W.; Sanderson, S.; Feng, X.; Hubbard, W.C. Porcine Sclera: Thickness and Surface Area. *Investig. Ophthalmol. Vis. Sci.* **2002**, *43*, 2529–2532.
156. AbbVie. *A Phase 2, Randomized, Dose-Escalation, Ranibizumab-Controlled Study to Evaluate the Efficacy, Safety, and Tolerability of RGX-314 Gene Therapy Delivered Via One or Two Suprachoroidal Space (SCS) Injections in Participants with Neovascular Age-Related Macular Degeneration (NAMD) (AAVIATE)*; AbbVie: Wellington, New Zealand, 2023.
157. Khanani, A.M. Suprachoroidal Delivery of RGX-314 Gene Therapy for Neovascular AMD: The Phase II AAVIATE™ Study. *Investig. Ophthalmol. Vis. Sci.* **2022**, *63*, 1497.
158. Tetz, M.; Rizzo, S.; Augustin, A.J. Safety of Submacular Suprachoroidal Drug Administration via a Microcatheter: Retrospective Analysis of European Treatment Results. *Ophthalmologica* **2012**, *227*, 183–189. [CrossRef]
159. Morales-Canton, V.; Fromow-Guerra, J.; Salinas Longoria, S.; Romero Vera, R.; Widmann, M.; Patel, S.; Yerxa, B. Suprachoroidal Microinjection of Bevacizumab Is Well Tolerated in Human Patients. *Investig. Ophthalmol. Vis. Sci.* **2013**, *54*, 3299.
160. Patel, S.R.; Kissner, J.; Farjo, R.; Zarnitsyn, V.; Noronha, G. Efficacy of Suprachoroidal Aflibercept in a Laser Induced Choroidal Neovascularization Model. *Investig. Ophthalmol. Vis. Sci.* **2016**, *57*, 286.
161. Kissner, J.; Patel, S.R.; Prusakiewicz, J.J.; Alton, D.; Bikzhanova, G.; Geisler, L.; Burke, B.; Noronha, G. *Pharmacokinetics including Ocular Distribution Characteristics of Suprachoroidally Administered CLS011A in Rabbits Could Be Beneficial for a Wet AMD Therapeutic Candidate*; ASSOC Research Vision Ophthalmology Inc.: Seattle, WA, USA, 2016.
162. Clearside Biomedical, Inc. *OASIS: Open-Label, Dose-Escalation, Phase 1/2a Study of the Safety and Tolerability of Suprachoroidally Administered CLS-AX Following Intravitreal Anti-VEGF Therapy in Subjects with Neovascular Age-Related Macular Degeneration*; Clearside Biomedical, Inc.: Alpharetta, GA, USA, 2022.
163. Clearside Biomedical, Inc. *Extension Study to Evaluate the Long-Term Outcomes of Subjects Following CLS-AX Administration for Age-Related Macular Degeneration in the CLS-AX CLS1002-101 Study*; Clearside Biomedical, Inc.: Alpharetta, GA, USA, 2023.
164. Shanghai BDgene Co., Ltd. *A Safety and Efficacy Study of VEGFA-Targeting Gene Therapy to Treat Refractory Retinal and Choroidal Neovascularization Diseases*; Shanghai BDgene Co., Ltd.: Shanghai, China, 2022.
165. Datta, D.; Khan, P.; Khan, L.; Singh, A. Role of Suprachoroidal Anti-VEGF Injections in Recalcitrant Serous Pigment Epithelium Detachment. *Ophthalmol. Res. Int. J.* **2023**, *18*, 1–10. [CrossRef]
166. Kohli, G.M.; Shenoy, P.; Halim, D.; Nigam, S.; Shetty, S.; Talwar, D.; Sen, A. Safety and Efficacy of Suprachoroidal Triamcinolone Acetonide for the Management of Serous Choroidal Detachment Prior to Rhegmatogenous Retinal Detachment Surgery: A Pilot Study. *Indian J. Ophthalmol.* **2022**, *70*, 1302–1306. [CrossRef]
167. Tabl, A.A.; Elsayed, M.A.; Tabl, M.A. Suprachoroidal Triamcinolone Acetonide Injection: A Novel Therapy for Serous Retinal Detachment Due to Vogt-Koyanagi Harada Disease. *Eur. J. Ophthalmol.* **2022**, *32*, 3482–3488. [CrossRef]
168. Gao, Y.; An, J.; Zeng, Z.; Lou, H.; Wu, G.; Lu, F. Suprachoroidal injection of sodium hyaluronate in the treatment of 12 patients with rhegmatogenous retinal detachment. *Chin. J. Ocul. Fundus Dis.* **2019**, *6*, 274–278.
169. Mittl, R.N.; Tiwari, R. Suprachoroidal Injection of Sodium Hyaluronate as an "internal" Buckling Procedure. *Ophthalmic Res.* **1987**, *19*, 255–260. [CrossRef] [PubMed]
170. Smith, R. Suprachoroidal Air Injection for Detached Retina. *Br. J. Ophthalmol.* **1952**, *36*, 385–388. [CrossRef] [PubMed]
171. Goldstein, D.A.; Do, D.; Noronha, G.; Kissner, J.M.; Srivastava, S.K.; Nguyen, Q.D. Suprachoroidal Corticosteroid Administration: A Novel Route for Local Treatment of Noninfectious Uveitis. *Transl. Vis. Sci. Technol.* **2016**, *5*, 14. [CrossRef]
172. Noronha, G.; Blackwell, K.; Gilger, B.C.; Kissner, J.; Patel, S.R.; Walsh, K.T. Evaluation of Suprachoroidal CLS-TA and Oral Prednisone in a Porcine Model of Uveitis. *Investig. Ophthalmol. Vis. Sci.* **2015**, *56*, 3110.
173. Gilger, B.C.; Abarca, E.M.; Salmon, J.H.; Patel, S. Treatment of Acute Posterior Uveitis in a Porcine Model by Injection of Triamcinolone Acetonide into the Suprachoroidal Space Using Microneedles. *Investig. Ophthalmol. Vis. Sci.* **2013**, *54*, 2483–2492. [CrossRef] [PubMed]
174. Patel, S.; Carvalho, R.; Mundwiler, K.; Meschter, C.; Verhoeven, R. Evaluation of Suprachoroidal Microinjection of Triamcinolone Acetonide in a Model of Panuveitis in Albino Rabbits. *Investig. Ophthalmol. Vis. Sci.* **2013**, *54*, 2927.
175. Ghate, D.; Edelhauser, H.F. Barriers to Glaucoma Drug Delivery. *J. Glaucoma* **2008**, *17*, 147–156. [CrossRef]
176. Konstas, A.G.; Stewart, W.C.; Topouzis, F.; Tersis, I.; Holmes, K.T.; Stangos, N.T. Brimonidine 0.2% given Two or Three Times Daily versus Timolol Maleate 0.5% in Primary Open-Angle Glaucoma. *Am. J. Ophthalmol.* **2001**, *131*, 729–733. [CrossRef]
177. Robin, A.L.; Novack, G.D.; Covert, D.W.; Crockett, R.S.; Marcic, T.S. Adherence in Glaucoma: Objective Measurements of Once-Daily and Adjunctive Medication Use. *Am. J. Ophthalmol.* **2007**, *144*, 533–540. [CrossRef]
178. Gurwitz, J.H.; Glynn, R.J.; Monane, M.; Everitt, D.E.; Gilden, D.; Smith, N.; Avorn, J. Treatment for Glaucoma: Adherence by the Elderly. *Am. J. Public Health* **1993**, *83*, 711–716. [CrossRef]
179. Kim, Y.C.; Edelhauser, H.F.; Prausnitz, M.R. Targeted Delivery of Antiglaucoma Drugs to the Supraciliary Space Using Microneedles. *Investig. Ophthalmol. Vis. Sci.* **2014**, *55*, 7387–7397. [CrossRef] [PubMed]

180. Chiang, B.; Kim, Y.C.; Doty, A.C.; Grossniklaus, H.E.; Schwendeman, S.P.; Prausnitz, M.R. Sustained Reduction of Intraocular Pressure by Supraciliary Delivery of Brimonidine-Loaded Poly(Lactic Acid) Microspheres for the Treatment of Glaucoma. *J. Control. Release* **2016**, *228*, 48–57. [CrossRef] [PubMed]
181. Einmahl, S.; Savoldelli, M.; D'Hermies, F.; Tabatabay, C.; Gurny, R.; Behar-Cohen, F. Evaluation of a Novel Biomaterial in the Suprachoroidal Space of the Rabbit Eye. *Investig. Ophthalmol. Vis. Sci.* **2002**, *43*, 1533–1539.
182. Chae, J.J.; Jung, J.H.; Zhu, W.; Gerberich, B.G.; Bahrani Fard, M.R.; Grossniklaus, H.E.; Ethier, C.R.; Prausnitz, M.R. Drug-Free, Nonsurgical Reduction of Intraocular Pressure for Four Months after Suprachoroidal Injection of Hyaluronic Acid Hydrogel. *Adv. Sci.* **2021**, *8*, 2001908. [CrossRef] [PubMed]
183. Hao, H.; He, B.; Yu, B.; Yang, J.; Xing, X.; Liu, W. Suprachoroidal Injection of Polyzwitterion Hydrogel for Treating Glaucoma. *Biomater. Adv.* **2022**, *142*, 213162. [CrossRef]
184. Savinainen, A.; Grossniklaus, H.E.; King, S.; Wicks, J.; Rich, C.C. Ocular Distribution and Exposure of AU-011 after Suprachoroidal or Intravitreal Administration in an Orthotopic Rabbit Model of Human Uveal Melanoma. *Investig. Ophthalmol. Vis. Sci.* **2021**, *62*, 2861.
185. Kang, S.J.; Patel, S.R.; Berezovsky, D.E.; Zhang, Q.; Yang, H.; Grossniklaus, H.E. Suprachoroidal Injection of Microspheres with Microcatheter in a Rabbit Model of Uveal Melanoma. *Investig. Ophthalmol. Vis. Sci.* **2011**, *52*, 1459.
186. Mruthyunjaya, P.; Schefler, A.C.; Kim, I.K.; Bergstrom, C.; Demirci, H.; Tsai, T.; Bhavsar, A.R.; Capone, A.; Marr, B.; McCannel, T.A.; et al. A Phase 1b/2 Open-Label Clinical Trial to Evaluate the Safety and Efficacy of AU-011 for the Treatment of Choroidal Melanoma. *Investig. Ophthalmol. Vis. Sci.* **2020**, *61*, 4025.
187. Demirci, H.; Narvekar, A.; Murray, C.; Rich, C. 842P A Phase II Trial of AU-011, an Investigational, Virus-like Drug Conjugate (VDC) for the Treatment of Primary Indeterminate Lesions and Small Choroidal Melanoma (IL/CM) Using Suprachoroidal Administration. *Ann. Oncol.* **2022**, *33*, S934. [CrossRef]
188. Peddada, K.V.; Sangani, R.; Menon, H.; Verma, V. Complications and Adverse Events of Plaque Brachytherapy for Ocular Melanoma. *J. Contemp. Brachyther.* **2019**, *11*, 392–397. [CrossRef]
189. Aura Biosciences. *A Phase 2 Open-Label, Ascending Single and Repeat Dose Escalation Trial of Belzupacap Sarotalocan (AU-011) via Suprachoroidal Administration in Subjects with Primary Indeterminate Lesions and Small Choroidal Melanoma*; Aura Biosciences: Boston, MA, USA, 2023.
190. Venkatesh, P.; Takkar, B. Suprachoroidal Injection of Biological Agents May Have a Potential Role in the Prevention of Progression and Complications in High Myopia. *Med. Hypotheses* **2017**, *107*, 90–91. [CrossRef] [PubMed]
191. Morgan, I.G.; Ohno-Matsui, K.; Saw, S.-M. Myopia. *Lancet* **2012**, *379*, 1739–1748. [CrossRef] [PubMed]
192. Gaynes, B.I.; Fiscella, R. Topical Nonsteroidal Anti-Inflammatory Drugs for Ophthalmic Use: A Safety Review. *Drug Saf.* **2002**, *25*, 233–250. [CrossRef] [PubMed]
193. Kompella, U.B.; Kadam, R.S.; Lee, V.H.L. Recent Advances in Ophthalmic Drug Delivery. *Ther. Deliv.* **2010**, *1*, 435–456. [CrossRef]
194. Wang, M.; Liu, W.; Lu, Q.; Zeng, H.; Liu, S.; Yue, Y.; Cheng, H.; Liu, Y.; Xue, M. Pharmacokinetic Comparison of Ketorolac after Intracameral, Intravitreal, and Suprachoroidal Administration in Rabbits. *Retina* **2012**, *32*, 2158–2164. [CrossRef]
195. Liu, S.; Liu, W.; Ma, Y.; Liu, K.; Wang, M. Suprachoroidal Injection of Ketorolac Tromethamine Does Not Cause Retinal Damage. *Neural Regen. Res.* **2012**, *7*, 2770–2777. [CrossRef]
196. Maldonado, R.M.; Vianna, R.N.G.; Cardoso, G.P.; de Magalhães, A.V.; Burnier, M.N. Intravitreal Injection of Commercially Available Ketorolac Tromethamine in Eyes with Diabetic Macular Edema Refractory to Laser Photocoagulation. *Curr. Eye Res.* **2011**, *36*, 768–773. [CrossRef]
197. Giannantonio, C.; Papacci, P.; Purcaro, V.; Cota, F.; Tesfagabir, M.G.; Molle, F.; Lepore, D.; Baldascino, A.; Romagnoli, C. Effectiveness of Ketorolac Tromethamine in Prevention of Severe Retinopathy of Prematurity. *J. Pediatr. Ophthalmol. Strabismus* **2011**, *48*, 247–251. [CrossRef]
198. Margalit, E.; Boysen, J.L.; Zastrocky, J.P.; Katz, A. Use of Intraocular Ketorolac Tromethamine for the Treatment of Chronic Cystoid Macular Edema. *Can. J. Ophthalmol. J. Can. Ophtalmol.* **2010**, *45*, 409–410. [CrossRef]
199. Kim, S.J.; Toma, H.S. Inhibition of Choroidal Neovascularization by Intravitreal Ketorolac. *Arch. Ophthalmol.* **2010**, *128*, 596–600. [CrossRef]
200. Willoughby, A.S.; Vuong, V.S.; Cunefare, D.; Farsiu, S.; Noronha, G.; Danis, R.P.; Yiu, G. Choroidal Changes after Suprachoroidal Injection of Triamcinolone in Eyes with Macular Edema Secondary to Retinal Vein Occlusion. *Am. J. Ophthalmol.* **2018**, *186*, 144–151. [CrossRef]
201. Tian, B.; Xie, J.; Su, W.; Sun, S.; Su, Q.; Gao, G.; Lin, H. Suprachoroidal Injections of AAV for Retinal Gene Delivery in Mouse. *Investig. Ophthalmol. Vis. Sci.* **2021**, *62*, 1177.
202. Wiley, L.A.; Boyce, T.M.; Meyering, E.E.; Ochoa, D.; Sheehan, K.M.; Stone, E.M.; Mullins, R.F.; Tucker, B.A.; Han, I.C. The Degree of Adeno-Associated Virus-Induced Retinal Inflammation Varies Based on Serotype and Route of Delivery: Intravitreal, Subretinal, or Suprachoroidal. *Hum. Gene Ther.* **2023**, *34*, 530–539. [CrossRef] [PubMed]
203. Han, I.C.; Cheng, J.L.; Burnight, E.R.; Ralston, C.L.; Fick, J.L.; Thomsen, G.J.; Tovar, E.F.; Russell, S.R.; Sohn, E.H.; Mullins, R.F.; et al. Retinal Tropism and Transduction of Adeno-Associated Virus Varies by Serotype and Route of Delivery (Intravitreal, Subretinal, or Suprachoroidal) in Rats. *Hum. Gene Ther.* **2020**, *31*, 1288–1299. [CrossRef] [PubMed]

204. Kahraman, N.S.; Gonen, Z.B.; Sevim, D.G.; Oner, A. First Year Results of Suprachoroidal Adipose Tissue Derived Mesenchymal Stem Cell Implantation in Degenerative Macular Diseases. *Int. J. Stem Cells* **2021**, *14*, 47–57. [CrossRef] [PubMed]
205. Muya, L.; Kansara, V.; Ciulla, T. Pharmacokinetics and Ocular Tolerability of Suprachoroidal CLS-AX (Axitinib Injectable Suspension) in Rabbits. *Investig. Ophthalmol. Vis. Sci.* **2020**, *61*, 4925.

pharmaceutics

MDPI

Review

Innovative Strategies for Drug Delivery to the Ocular Posterior Segment

Andrea Gabai [1], Marco Zeppieri [1,*], Lucia Finocchio [1,2] and Carlo Salati [1]

[1] Department of Ophthalmology, University Hospital of Udine, 33100 Udine, Italy
[2] Department of Ophthalmology, Nuovo Ospedale Santo Stefano, 59100 Prato, Italy
* Correspondence: markzeppieri@hotmail.com; Tel.: +39-0432-552743

Abstract: Innovative and new drug delivery systems (DDSs) have recently been developed to vehicle treatments and drugs to the ocular posterior segment and the retina. New formulations and technological developments, such as nanotechnology, novel matrices, and non-traditional treatment strategies, open new perspectives in this field. The aim of this mini-review is to highlight promising strategies reported in the current literature based on innovative routes to overcome the anatomical and physiological barriers of the vitreoretinal structures. The paper also describes the challenges in finding appropriate and pertinent treatments that provide safety and efficacy and the problems related to patient compliance, acceptability, effectiveness, and sustained drug delivery. The clinical application of these experimental approaches can help pave the way for standardizing the use of DDSs in developing enhanced treatment strategies and personalized therapeutic options for ocular pathologies.

Keywords: drug delivery systems (DDSs); nanotechnology; matrices; ocular posterior segment; vitreoretinal

1. Introduction

New drug delivery methods to target specific ocular tissues and treat debilitating ocular diseases have been proposed in the past decade. Of all ocular diseases, 55% originate from the posterior segment [1]. Retinal diseases, such as age-related macular degeneration (AMD), diabetic retinopathy (DR), diabetic macular edema (DME), endophthalmitis, viral retinitis, proliferative vitreoretinopathy (PVR), posterior uveitis, retinal vascular occlusions, retinitis pigmentosa (RP), and inherited retinal diseases (IRDs), represent the leading cause of vision impairment [2,3].

The presence of static barriers (different layers of the cornea, sclera, retina, blood–aqueous (BAB) and (BRB) blood–retinal barriers) (Figure 1) and dynamic barriers (conjunctival and choroidal blood flow, tear turnover, and lymphatic clearance) represent an obstacle to the delivery of a drug to a particular ocular tissue and to treating these retinal diseases [4]. The research field based on ocular "drug delivery", which refers to numerous innovative techniques to target retinal tissue and overcome ocular barriers, has witnessed huge growth in recent years.

Depending on disease type, drug property, and target site, drugs can be administered through different routes, including topical, intravitreal, periocular, and systemic. Several types of ophthalmic drug delivery systems (DDSs) are currently available on the market, and range from eyedrops, eye ointments, gels, and ocular inserts, such as eye dosage formulations that are created to increase the holding time of drugs in the eye. Topical drug instillation on the ocular surface is a common and non-invasive application method for the treatment modalities of eye disorders. This route, however, offers suboptimal ocular bioavailability. Studies have shown that 90% of eyedrops available on the market only provide 5% of drug bioavailability, while the rest of the drug gets washed away through different elimination routes, such as tear fluid, nasolacrimal secretion, protein binding, enzymatic degradation, or metabolism by protease and esterase enzyme [5]. Despite the

Citation: Gabai, A.; Zeppieri, M.; Finocchio, L.; Salati, C. Innovative Strategies for Drug Delivery to the Ocular Posterior Segment. *Pharmaceutics* **2023**, *15*, 1862. https://doi.org/10.3390/pharmaceutics15071862

Academic Editors: Rosario Pignatello, Montse Mitjans Arnal, Hugo Almeida, Carmelo Puglia and Debora Santonocito

Received: 18 May 2023
Revised: 19 June 2023
Accepted: 29 June 2023
Published: 1 July 2023

limits of topical treatments, current studies have reported promising results for substances delivered to the retina, which suggests that topical treatment of retinal diseases might be possible in the future [6,7].

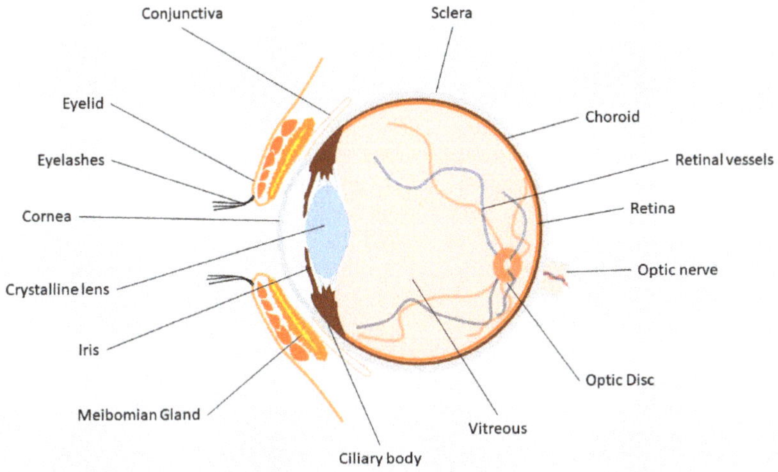

Figure 1. Ocular anatomy.

Injection into the globe is very often recommended for drug delivery into the posterior region, but it is painful, causes patient non-compliance, has risks of infection, and is associated with various side effects. Over the past decade, thanks to advances in nanotechnology and the development of many drug delivery systems, such as implants, in situ gel, contact lenses, microneedles, liposomes, nanomicelles, dendrimers, and other nanoparticles (NPs), numerous drug-delivery solutions have been proposed. The polymeric nature of these various technologies includes the distinction between microparticles, which are polymeric systems larger than 1 μm, and nanoparticles that have a smaller diameter. Structurally, these particles can be broadly described as micro/nanospheres, when the loaded drug is integrated in the matrix and nano/microcapsules, when the drug is enclosed in a polymeric shell. Although most of the studies in this field are still in the preclinical stages, micro/nanotechnology-based DDSs possess great potential to solve the shortcomings of currently available drug delivery systems. These new strategies can potentially allow safe and effective drug administration to the ocular posterior segment and retina [8–11].

In this mini-review, we attempt to focus on and highlight promising strategies reported in the current literature based on innovative routes to overcome the anatomical and physiological barriers of the vitreoretinal structures. We also describe the challenges in finding appropriate and pertinent treatments for delivering therapeutic agents to retinal tissues in a safe and effective manner.

2. Ocular Barriers

Pharmaceutical formulations via the anterior segment, mostly liquid solutions, or suspensions, are the most common treatment used in ophthalmology. These locally administered drops include a broad range of molecules, such as antibiotics, anti-inflammatory agents, anti-glaucomatous drops, lubricants, and diagnostic agents. Topical formulations tend to be used for the ocular surface and do not allow topical drugs to reach therapeutic concentrations in the posterior ocular segment (vitreous, retina, choroid) due to several anatomical and functional barriers.

2.1. Lacrimal Wash-Out and Mucosal Capillary Circulation

The first and most important factor that decreases topic drop efficacy in the posterior segment is the continuous lacrimal wash-out of the ocular surface. This shortens the contact between eyedrops and the ocular surface so that an instilled volume of topical drug is usually drained via the nasolacrimal duct in approximately 2 min [12]. Capillary vessels, both in the nasal mucosa and conjunctiva, also prevent a portion of the active drug from reaching therapeutic concentration within the eye by dispersing molecules in the systemic blood flow [13].

2.2. Cornea

The epithelium of the cornea is the principal barrier of this multilayered bio-membrane. Epithelial cells are lipophilic, tightly interconnected, organized in a 3 to 6 layer structure, and continuously replaced with newer cells migrating from the limbus to the corneal apex. The intercellular tight junctions limit the paracellular passage of hydrophilic molecules and ions, making the cornea much more permeable to lipophilic drugs, and capable of transcellular passage. The corneal stroma, which is rich in collagen fibrils and glycosaminoglycan, is hydrophilic, thus limiting the absorption rate of lipophilic molecules crossing the epithelium. The endothelium, with its monolayer structure, seems to offer little resistance to lipophilic substances. For these reasons, corneal permeation is currently the preferred way to deliver lipophilic drugs with a small molecular weight in the anterior chamber [14,15].

2.3. Conjunctiva

Studies have reported that the conjunctiva is approximately 20 times more permeable than the cornea, and that allows for the absorption of more hydrophilic and larger molecules, thus offering a potential route of administration for new therapeutic proteins and peptides [16–18].

2.4. Sclera

The sclera is composed of collagen fibers embedded in mucopolysaccharides, thus making it more permeable to drugs than the cornea and less than the conjunctiva. It is important to remember that the conjunctiva is the most vascularized and porous structure of the ocular surface [19]. Scleral permeation mostly occurs through passive diffusion, with a permeability coefficient inversely related to the molecular weight of the permeating substances [16,20].

2.5. BAB and BRB

Systemic drug administration provides low ocular bioavailability (<5%) due to the limited fraction of the entire blood reaching the eye and the presence of the BAB and BRB, which render systemic administration effective only for drugs with high therapeutic index, and for treatments given in high doses, such as antibiotics and antiviral agents [13,21].

Non-pigmented ciliary cells and endothelial cells of the irideal vessels are the main elements of the BAB. The tight intersections of this structure render the wall of the capillaries impermeable to the plasma albumin, thus avoiding access to the aqueous humor and limiting the passage of hydrophilic drugs from the systemic circulation to the anterior chamber. The disruption of BAB in inflammatory conditions can allow systemic drugs to freely distribute to the anterior chamber [13].

The blood flow through the choroidal vasculature passively contributes to the clearance of systemic drugs, preventing penetration into the eye. The choroidal vessel walls, however, are rather permeable, so blood and drugs can easily leak through. A more active barrier to penetration is represented by the retinal pigment epithelium (RPE) and Bruch's membrane, which constitute the outer part of the BRB. Retinal vessel endothelium and intertwining connections also block drug passage from systemic circulation to the retina and vitreous, constituting the inner part of the BRB [13,22,23]. The metabolic, molecular, and pharmacokinetic characteristics of blood–ocular barriers are not completely known;

future histological and molecular pathologic studies are needed to better understand the underlying mechanisms involved in these structures.

3. Methods

We conducted a search of the literature published between 1 January 2002 and 28 February 2023 using MEDLINE (PubMed). The database was first searched using the key words "drug delivery system, ocular posterior segment, AND vitreoretinal, AND nanotechnologies AND matrices". We considered only studies in English and those with an abstract. The reference lists of all retrieved articles were assessed to identify additional relevant studies. The research of articles was performed using PubMed (https://pubmed.ncbi.nlm.nih.gov, accessed on 28 February 2023).

Only articles with an abstract were considered. Studies in which small case series were described and those that assessed surgical techniques were analyzed. Each study was independently assessed by at least two reviewers (A.G., L.F., and M.Z.), and rating decisions were based on the consensus of the reviewing authors. A total of 233 references were included in the review. This search strategy was limiting in the midst of the vast literature, which could have thus potentially and unintentionally excluded opinion leaders in this field of research.

4. Innovative Drug Delivery Systems

4.1. Nanomedicine

Systems and devices developed for scientific purposes, with a size scale of cellular and molecular structures ranging from 1 to 1000 nanometer (1 nanometer = 10^{-9} m), are commonly defined as nanotechnology. Nanoparticles (NPs) possess ideal characteristics for ocular drug delivery due to their nanometric and controllable size, and their ability to protect the carried active molecule from degradation, allowing it to be released in a targeted manner and at a controlled rate [24]. In addition, the NP surface area is highly specific and mucoadhesive in comparison to larger bulk polymers due to its high interface availability for hydrogen and ionic bonding, or hydrophobic interaction with mucous surfaces [25]. Drug-loaded NPs with sizes between 50 and 500 nm are the most adapted for ocular delivery, overcoming physiological barriers and mucin mesh [26–28]. NPs larger than 1000 nm, however, are unfit to pass through mucous channels, poorly adhere to mucus surfaces, and are easily cleared from them. Nanomaterials studied for retinal diseases consist of amphiphilic molecules, such as liposomes and micelles, polymers, such as dendrimers, and organic and non-organic nanoparticles. The properties of these NPs play a crucial role in their effectiveness in ocular drug delivery. The high surface-to-volume ratio makes them ideal vehicles for therapeutic and targeting agents. Their size must be large enough to avoid drug leakage and dispersion into the blood vessels, and small enough to permit its penetration across the ocular barriers and/or allow for intraocular injection and permanence, when needed.

4.1.1. Liposomes

Liposomes are spherical vesicular structures comprised of amphiphilic molecules, such as phospholipids and sterols, organized to form a lipidic bilayer membrane enclosing an inner aqueous space. Smaller unilamellar liposomes are composed of a bilayer membrane, typically up to 100 nm. Larger versions can have a diameter > 100 nm. Multilamellar liposomimial vesicles, composed of several bilayers, tend to be larger than 500 nm. This architecture, resembling a cellular membrane, provides good biocompatibility and the capability of liposomes to carry considerable quantities of both hydrophobic and hydrophilic drugs and to present variable surface polymers to target different cells and tissues [29].

Liposome-based drug delivery has been studied since 1960 and was the first medical nanotechnology to receive Food and Drugs Administration (FDA) approval in 1995. Verteporfin (Visudyne, Bausch, and Lomb), used to treat choroidal neovascularization (CNV) secondary to AMD, was one of the first commercially available products to adopt liposomes. Choroidal neovascularization was also experimentally treated with liposomes via intravitreal injection, embedding polyethilen glycol (PEG) in the liposomial wall, and via intravenous injection of cationic liposomes loaded with paclitaxel [30–32]. Liposomes loaded with the immunosuppressant tacrolimus have been injected into the vitreous to treat autoimmune uveoretinitis. Topical instillation of eyedrops containing TA-loaded liposomes has been shown to improve refractory macular edema both anatomically and functionally [33].

In a study conducted by Gu et al., dexamethasone was successfully delivered in the posterior ocular segment using liposomes. The authors obtained a therapeutic concentration of this drug in the choroid and retina within 2 h from instillation of eyedrops containing dexamethasone salt-loaded liposomes [34]. Despite these promising results, liposome-based ocular therapies present critical drawbacks. NPs cause allergic and hypersensitivity reactions in animal models [35]. Cationic liposomes, in particular, seem more at risk of triggering inflammatory responses [36]. Moreover, liposome aggregation can occur as a consequence of their instability during storage and transportation, resulting in blurred vision with poor functional outcomes, and the need for excipients to stabilize and preserve them limits their therapeutic employment [37,38].

4.1.2. Nanomicelles

Nanomicelles are spherical nanostructures with a hydrophobic stiff core, ideal to encapsulate hydrophobic drugs, and an hydrophilic outer surface facing the aqueous medium. They are usually formulated of a small size (5–30 nm), which makes them ideal for delivering their pharmaceutical content to subcellular targets. Micelles are structurally stable but susceptible to environmental changes (pH, temperature, ionic strength) that can easily precipitate their content (i.e., during storage). Standard, reverse, or unimolecular micelles can be created depending on the amphiphilic molecule and solvent we choose. Furthermore, these NPs have a prolonged circulation time, since they are not recognized by hepatic macrophages, and present a low tendency to aggregate [39,40].

Anti-viral prodrugs were successfully carried to the retina in vivo, using micelles of polyoxyethylene hydroigenated castor oil, across the ocular barriers, after topical administration [41]. Nanomicelles resulting from the polymerization of octoxynol, vitamin E, and tocopherol-PEG-succinate have been used topically to deliver rapamycin to the choroid and retina in vivo, avoiding undesirable concentrations of this antiblastic in the vitreous and with limited cytotoxicity in vitro [42].

Among the hydrophobic drugs that can be vehiculated inside nanomicelles to treat posterior ocular pathologies, we found cyclosporine-A, cyclosporine, and curcumin [43–45]. Conjunctival/scleral injection seems a better way to deliver drugs than intraocular injection. Following the conjunctival/scleral route, micelles diffuse through the scleral water channels and then reach the retina without retinal damage after multiple injections [46,47]. Micellar core cross-linking using functional groups and lowering the critical solution temperature have been shown to improve the duration and solubility of nanomicellar preparations [48]. Intravenous administration of nanomicelles was also investigated by Ideta et al. Polyion nanomicelles, encapsulating fluorescein istiocyanate-labeled poly-L-lysine, accumulated around CNV in a rat model of exudative AMD for as long as 168 h after intravenous injection. However, signs of toxicity were detected, demanding further studies on nanomicelle characteristics and administration pathways [49].

Nanotubes can be considered a particular type of nanomicelle. Panda et al. reported the successful intraocular delivery of pazopanib using dipeptidic phenylalanine-alpha and beta-hydroxyphenilalalnine nanotubes as carriers. The preparation was administered via intravitreal injection, obtaining sustained pazopanib concentration in the vitreous, retina, RPE, and choroid for 15 days [50].

4.1.3. Nanospheres and Solid Lipids

Nanospheres are particles encapsulated in polymeric delivery systems. They self-assemble with a uniform distribution of their content, which reduces damage and inflammation in their target tissues. This differentiates them from nanocapsules, which are similar but less uniform polymeric structures [35]. Nanospheres with diameters varying from 50 to 200 nm have been successfully tested in rabbits [51].

Solid lipids are another nanotechnology used to deliver drugs and genes to the retina. As suggested by their name, these particles consist of a solid lipid core stabilized with surfactants. This simple structure makes them resistant, long-standing, and even resistant to autoclave sterilization, but biodegradable and economical to produce, not requiring solvents. Solid lipids have been employed to deliver non-viral gene vectors to RPE cells and photoreceptors in a murine model of X-linked juvenile retinoschisis (XLRS) [52].

4.1.4. Dendrimers

Dendrimers are ramified polymers characterized by a symmetrical core and the presence of functional groups on each branch, with neutral, negative, or positive activity [53,54]. The size usually ranges from 1 to 100 nm, depending on their complexity. PAMAM dendrimers have been used to deliver DEX in vivo, both with topical and subconjunctival administration, in diabetic retinopathy (DR) model rats [55]. Intravitreal and intravenous administration in vivo also showed anti-inflammatory action in murine models by targeting retinal microglia and macrophages, offering interesting perspectives for the treatment of retinopathies where inflammation is dysregulated, such as AMD, DR, and retinal vein occlusion [56]. Neuroinflammation was reduced and photoreceptor loss was halted for 4 weeks in retinal degeneration mice using intravitreal PAMAM dendrimers carrying steroids [57].

Dendrimer clearance was seen to be slowed in target tissues, where it is more needed, than in non-target organs, such as the healthy eye, and interestingly, in comparison to the half-life of other drugs, such as bevacizumab [58].

Dendrimers loaded with brimonidine-tartrate were demonstrated to be more effective than the ordinary topical formulation of this drug in glaucomatous model rats [59]. Similarly, IOP reduction was observed with acetazolamide-loaded dendrimers in albino rabbits [60]. Mouse models of retinoblastoma responded well to PAMAM dendrimers loaded with carboplatin, which, after subconjunctival injection and scleral penetration, reached the tumor, suppressing its vasculature for 22 days [61].

Considerable concerns remain about dendrimers' safety due to their cytotoxicity. Since the main mechanism for their toxic effect seems to be the disruptive interaction between the positive charge on the dendrimer and the negatively charged biological membranes, several strategies to impede this interaction have been studied, such as acetylation, PEGylation, and peptide conjugation [62].

4.1.5. Organic Nanopolymers

Several types of biodegradable polymers have been developed to deliver ocular drugs in a safe, effective, and sustained way. Among these chemical compounds, we found polyvinylpyrrolidone (PVP), polylactic acid (PLA), polyglycolide (PGA), and their copolymers poly(lactic-co-glycolic acid) (PLGA), poly(n-butyl cyanoacrylate) (PBCA), and polycaprolactone (PCL) [22].

PVP can be injected in hydrogel form, presenting stable retention at the injection site, lasting several weeks. Polymers of PVP have been tested as artificial vitreous substances (cross-linked PVP), lens regeneration scaffolds, and slow-release implants for anti-glaucomatous drugs, acting for 300 days [63–66]. Small fluorescent hydrophobic molecules conjugated to PVP were effectively delivered to retinal cells after intravenous administration in rats by Tawfik et al. [67]. These results indicate that PVP nanoparticles are promising carriers for hydrophobic drugs in the retina. Nevertheless, other studies have shown possible side effects of this compound, such as corneal and vitreous opacification and inflammation, suggesting that further investigations are required to ameliorate this delivery strategy [68].

PLGA, a well-established and FDA-approved polymer used for the preparation of drug-delivering nanoparticles due to its biodegradability, is the most used drug delivery polymer in ophthalmology. Innovative uses of PLGA to treat retinal disorders have been reported by several authors. PLGA NPs loaded with dexamethasone and injected into the vitreous were able to sustain 50% of the drug level for one month, as compared to the 7 days obtained injecting a simple dexamethasone solution [69]. Light-responsive implants containing PLGA NPs were injected in situ to deliver peptides to the posterior segment [70]. Fragments of plasminogen with anti-angiogenic effect (K5) were delivered to the retina, per intravitreal injection, loaded in PLGA-chitosan nanoparticles. Expressed K5 was detectable in the murine model retina more than 2 weeks after the injection, whereas inflammation resolved in 3 days [71]. Transferrin conjugation to PLGA NPs allowed precise delivery via intravenous injection of a plasmid expressing an anti-VEGF receptor to endothelial cells and the RPE of choroidal neovascular lesions in rats [72]. PLGA NPs loaded with brinzolamide effectively reduced IOP in rabbits, releasing the anti-glaucomatous drug up to 10 days after their subconjunctival injection [73]. Overall, the use of PLGA as a drug-vehicle presents some drawbacks, including weak protein stability, suboptimal loading efficiency, and abrupt drug release.

Bourges et al. tested the intravitreal injection of PLA NPs loaded with fluorochromes in rats. They observed a sustained presence of fluorochromes in the mice's retinal cells for 1 month, with detectable levels in the ganglion cells for up to 4 months [74]. Dexamethasone loaded on PLA NPs and administered intravenously to uveoretinitis model rats was demonstrated to be effective in controlling inflammation [75].

PCL, a polyester derived from polymerization of caprolactone, can also be loaded with dexamethasone. This implant provided a therapeutic concentration of dexamethasone for one year in rabbit eyes [76]. Immunosuppression with cyclosporine loaded in PCL NPs was studied by Yenice et al. They reported a drug bioavailability 10 to 15-fold higher with this formulation than with its solution in castor oil [77].

PCL copolymerization with PEG, forming PEG-PCL-PEG polymers, resulted in a biocompatible triblock nanocarrier that was potentially effective in retinal drug delivery, whereas combinations of PCL with PLA or PGA were seen to induce permeability and crystallinity alterations [78].

The first NPs for ocular drug delivery were polymers of PBCA, following their broad use as drug delivery carriers [79]. PBCA NPs present favorable characteristics for this function, including stability, biocompatibility, biodegradability, targetability, and the capability to cross the blood–brain barrier when coated with polysorbate 80 [80–85]. In vivo confocal neuroimaging (ICON) allowed some authors to be the first to record in real time the NP crossing of BRB [86–88]. The effects of the nanoparticles' size and zeta potential on their capability to trespass the biological barriers were also studied, showing that larger PBCA NPs (272 versus 172 nm) with intermediate z potential (5 V versus 0 V and 15 V) were more likely to concentrate in the retina. Their accumulation in RGCs, together with their well-documented safety profile in humans, makes this polymer a viable option for delivering retinal therapies [89,90].

4.1.6. Chitosan and Chitosan-Based Nanotechnologies

Chitosan (CS), a highly diffused polysaccharide (the second most abundant in nature), represents an important structural component of the exoskeleton of several insects, crustaceans, and fungi. This substance has been used as a penetration enhancer in pharmaceutical research and industry for decades [91]. The favorable properties of CS include the absence of cytotoxicity, high biocompatibility and biodegradability, and a polycationic and mucoadhesive nature. For these reasons, the addition of CS to ocular topical drugs represents a safe and effective strategy for prolonging the drug presence in the precorneal area and making the active drug more bioavailable. Several studies have been conducted on the use of CS and its derivatives for drug-loaded NPs, liposomes, and solid lipid matrixes to improve their adhesion and penetration across ocular tissues.

Chitosan Nanoparticles

The encapsulation of ophthalmic drugs in CS-coated NPs and their administration in solution have been shown to prolong their residence time in the precorneal area [92–94]. NPs for ocular formulations generally do not exceed 10 μm to avoid foreign body sensation and ocular irritation. CS NPs are generally spherical and smooth, therefore possessing an optimal surface area-to-volume ratio that also enhances their reactive surface and therapeutic potential. Several methods have been proposed to prepare different types of CS NPs, such as ionotropic gelation, spray drying, water-in-oil emulsion crosslinking, reverse micelle formation, emulsion droplet coalescence, nanoprecipitation, or self-assembly, with the first usually preferred due to its relative simplicity and convenience. Several drugs have been loaded in CS NPs to treat different diseases in the posterior segment of the eye, including implants containing bevacizumab-loaded CS NPs [95] and PLGA microparticles entrapping ranibizumab-loaded C NPs [96] for the treatment of choroidal neovascularization (vide infra), CS NPs for delivery of daptomycin in bacterial endophthalmitis, although showing lower antimicrobial susceptibility as compared to the antibiotic in its free form [97].

Carboxymethyl chitosan (CMCS) was used by Wang et al. to coat nanocomposite carriers used to deliver dexamethasone (DEX) to the posterior pole. Topical eyedrops containing coated nanocomposites, non-coated nanocomposites, and commercially available DEX were instilled in albino rabbits. Retina-choroid homogenates were then analyzed using high-performance liquid chromatography (HPLC), showing higher concentration and longer permanence of DEX when delivered by CMCS-coated nanocomposites than by non-coated composites or commercial DEX eyedrops. The nanocomposite absorption was seen to occur mainly via the conjunctival-scleral pathway using in vivo fluorescence imaging. The cellular uptake was studied in vitro on human conjunctival cells, and appeared to be energy dependent, consisting of clathrin-mediated endocytosis, as demonstrated by a 54% reduction in cellular uptake in the presence of specific inhibitors of this clathrin-mediated mechanism [98].

Polymeric nanocarriers made of CS-grafted poly(ethylene glycol) methacrylate (CS-g-PEGMA) were loaded with bevacizumab in a study by Savin et al. The authors crosslinked the polymer using either sodium tripolyphosphate (TPP) or Na_2SO_4, forming 200–900 nm or 1000–1500 nm NPs due to lower and higher molecular crosslinking density, respectively, and obtained a prolonged and sustained drug release with a small burst effect [99].

Chitosan Micelles

CS has been tested as a component of polymeric micelles to facilitate the ocular release of several ocular drugs. Xu et al. synthesized a CS derivative (CS oligosaccharide-valyvaline-stearic acid) to prepare dexamethasone-loaded nanomicelles (30 nm) for the topical treatment of macula edema [100].

The presence of the oligosaccharide was a key factor in reaching the posterior ocular pole via the conjunctival route, and the positive electric potential on the naonomicelle surface (+30 mV) favored their adhesion to the anionic ocular surface. In vitro analysis demonstrated sustained drug release without bursts and no toxic effects.

Chitosan Lipid Nanoparticles and Liposomes

As a polysaccharide, CS can be used to prepare lipid NPs (LNPs) and liposomes. LNPs consist of a lipidic core stabilized by a surfactant on the surface that stabilizes the particle in an aqueous environment. These characteristics make LNPs potential vehicles for lipophilic molecules by all administration routes, although their drug-loading efficacy is relatively poor. As for micelles, their content can be expulsed rather easily during storage.

Different from LNPs, liposomes consist of a double surfactant layer, structurally resembling a living cell, that can include both lipophilic and hydrophilic compounds and makes these particles highly biocompatible and biodegradable with low inner toxicity. Li et al. tested the ocular penetration enhancement effects of a CS coating on liposomes containing triamcinolone acetonide (TA), an intermediate-acting corticosteroid employed to treat ocular inflammatory and angiogenic conditions. After topical administration to mice, the presence of TA in the posterior segment was tested using optical coherence tomography (OCT). The OCT scans showed a stronger signal from the retinal surface of mice treated with CS-coated liposomes than in controls receiving non-coated liposomes, although the difference in signal strength was not significant. The TA effect on the signal was detectable 10 min after instillation, peaked at 6 h, and lasted up to 12 and 10 h in subjects receiving coated and non-coated preparation, respectively, thus indicative of a chitosan effect on the TA permanence time [101]. The effectiveness of these CS-coated liposomes was further studied by Cheng et al., showing their efficiency in relieving laser-induced retinal edema without toxic effects [102].

Similar results were observed by Khalil et al., who prepared CS-coated liposomes encapsulating TA, and administered as topical treatment to rat models. After 15 days, the drug was detectable in the ocular posterior chamber in vivo [103].

Chitosan in Combined Drug Delivery Systems

The drug targeting and release modulation of CS-containing nanocarriers can be further ameliorated by combining them with other delivery vehicles, such as polymeric coatings, larger molecules, gels, lenses, and inserts. PLGA has been experimentally associated with CS for retinal drug delivery. Elsaid and his collaborators formulated a system-within-system matrix consisting of PLGA microparticles containing CS-based nanoparticles to deliver ranibizumab to the vitreous. The authors showed that the presence of CS enhanced ranibizumab loading and release thanks to the bonds between the drug and the nanoparticles [96].

NPs loaded with the anti-VEGF molecule bevacizumab were inserted by Badiee et al. into a hyaluronic acid (HA)/zinc implant. The system presented a homogeneous NP distribution and offered sustained drug release over two months in vitro [95].

A CS-based injectable hydrogel for the delivery of retinal progenitor stem cells was fabricated by Jiang et al. for the treatment of retinal degeneration. Oxidized dextran (Odex) was bonded with the CS amine groups to form the hydrogel. The proliferation of retinal progenitor cells and their differentiation toward neurons was favored by the CS/Odex hydrogel [104].

A modified CS-based hydrogel was synthesized by Moreno et al. for the administration of ranibizumab and adflibercept, two for neovascular AMD and corneal neovessels. The investigators created a thiolated, more densely cross-linked hydrogel capable of retaining the drug-load molecules for a more prolonged time, preventing burst release in vitro [105].

Abe et al. created a silicone-made refillable reservoir for transscleral drug delivery containing 1% CS and 3% gelatin matrix for the treatment of retinal diseases. The gel itself resulted in a 5-day drug release, with an initial burst, whereas its insertion in the reservoir extended it by 2–5 times. In vitro, and up to 12 weeks in vivo [106].

4.1.7. Metallic and Other Inorganic Nanomaterials

Gold, silver, and platinum NPs have shown important therapeutic properties. The ability to permeate the BRP seems to be size dependent. Gold NPs of a 20 nm size can cross this barrier, even after intravenous administration, differently from 100 nm NPs [107]. Silver NPs demonstrated anti-angiogenic effects in AMD models. Vascular permeability is also impaired by these nanoparticles, interfering with pathologic endothelial mechanisms occurring in retinal diseases, such as retinopathy of prematurity (ROP), RP, and DR [108,109]. Similarly, gold NPs were seen to contrast angiogenesis and inflammation in retinal pathologies [110]. Intravitreal injections of magnetic nanoparticles (MNPs) delivered neuronal growth factors (NGF) to the retina for neuroprotection in Xenopus embryos. In detail, injecting MNPS-GNF complexes prevented retinal ganglion cell apoptosis, whereas injection of free GNF did not [111].

Cerium NPs, also called nanoceria, delivered by intravitreal injection, protected retinal cells from oxidation, caspase-induced apoptosis, and retinal degeneration in AMD model mice [112,113]. A decrease in rod cell apoptosis and an augment of retinal lipid peroxidation were obtained in RP model rats treated with nanoceria, proving their important antioxidant properties and potential application in other types of retinal degeneration [114,115]. Nanoceria were detectable for more than 1 year after its intravitreal injection in murine models, without development of inflammatory or other pathological side effects, indicating a sustained and safe action of this type of NP [116].

Silicate antiangiogenic properties emerged from studies on intravitreal silicate-based NPs in mice with oxygen-induced retinopathy [117]. A helical vector containing a silica scaffold and a magnetic element of iron or nickel was experimented with to deliver therapeutic substances to the retina. The vector was precisely moved through the vitreous applying a magnetic field ab externo coated in perfluorocarbon liquid to reduce attrition, and its position was monitored in real time by OCT imaging [118].

Relevant potential risks in using inorganic materials in vivo derive from their poor or absent biodegradation or clearance [119]. Metal nanoparticles 20 to 80 nm in diameter showed toxic effects on photoreceptors in vitro and damage to the blood–retinal barrier derived from intravitreal injection of NPs containing titanium [120,121]. Therefore, further studies are required to assess and optimize the safety of therapeutic delivery systems based on these materials.

4.1.8. Encapsulated Cell Technology

A new technology using encapsulated human RPE cells has been developed by Neurothec Pharmaceuticals. NT-501 (Renexus®) consists of an implantable polymeric scaffold, encapsulating cells that are genetically modified to secrete ciliary neurotrophic factor (CNTF). This capsule-containing cells is composed of a semipermeable membrane surrounding a scaffold made of polyethylene terephthalate strands, which protects the cells from the immune system while allowing the passage of nutrients and therapeutic molecules. A titanium loop is attached to the extremity of this capsule, allowing anchorage to the scleral wall after surgical implantation via the pars plana. Initially developed to treat RP and dry AMD, this device has also been considered in the management of patients with glaucoma and type 2 macular teleangectasia. Studies have reported that NT-501 slowed retinal degeneration and stabilized patients' reading speed [122–124].

4.2. Other Topical Absorption Enhancers

Technologies to enhance the absorption of topical drugs have recently emerged as a promising solution to increase bioavailability. Ocular penetration enhancers (PEs) are chemical or biological agents that are associated with topical drugs, such as excipients or additives, and are used to increase the ability of the active drug to overcome ocular barriers and penetrate the eye. Several types of PEs have been reported in the literature, and most of them limit the drug delivery action to the anterior chamber. Benzalkonium chloride (BAC) and different types of cell-penetrating peptides, however, have shown significant results in internalizing drugs across cellular membranes to the posterior segment [125–128]. These peptides have been initially studied to carry drugs across skin, respiratory tract mucosae, blood–brain barrier (BBB), and, more recently, into the ocular tissues.

4.2.1. Cell-Penetrating Peptides (CPPs)

CPPs are short-chain peptides, usually composed of 30 or less amino acid residues, capable of trespassing membranes with no need for chiral interactions with surface receptors. The transactivator of transcription (TAT), a protein transduction domain (PTD) and one of the most studied CPPs, was investigated by Wang et al. to deliver growth factors to retinal tissue in vivo. The group performed studies in which TAT was conjugated with acidic fibroblast growth factor (aFGF) and topically administered by eyedrops to rats with retinal ischemia reperfusion. Immunohistochemical (IHC) studies documented the presence of TAT-aFGF in retinal tissue 30 min after instillation. The major concentration was observed in the ganglion cell layer (GCL), suggesting a cell-specific uptake mechanism of TAT, with a peak between 30 and 60 min after administration and detectable presence for up to 8 h. The histological and electrophysiological analysis of the treated eyes also identified a reduction in GCL apoptosis and a faster functional recovery compared to non-treated and aFGF-only treated eyes. The absence of TAT-aFGF in the deeper corneal stroma and endothelium indicated to the authors the involvement of a non-corneal absorption route [129].

Zhang et al. also reported that TAT is an effective carrier for treating retinal diseases in animal models. They conjugated TAT to endostatin (Es), an inhibitor of choroidal neovascularization (CNV), and topically administered TAT-Es to experimental mice. IHC exams revealed a good retinal distribution of TAT-Es in treated subjects, and a significant reduction in their CNV areas in comparison to controls and to mice treated with unconjugated Es. Furthermore, the CNV area reduction obtained with topical TAT-Es was comparable to that induced in controls receiving intravitreal bevacizumab and intravitreal TAT-Es. Endocytosis, majorly micropinocytosis, was suggested as the principal uptake mechanism in this study, with clathrin- and caveolae-mediated endocytosis and energy-independent direct translocation serving as secondary mechanisms [130].

TAT conjugated with Es or with Es and an arginine-glycine-aspartic tripeptide (RGD) was tested by Li et al. on experimental mice with oxygen-induced retinopathy. The investigators aimed at verifying the inhibitory properties of this fusion protein on angiogenesis and neo-vessels formation. The retinal concentration at 1 h from topical instillation was seen to be 14-fold higher than Es alone by ELISA testing, with TAT-Es-RGD slightly more concentrated than TAT-Es, due to the specific RGD binding properties with the integrins on the angiogenic endothelial cell surface. Histologically, the investigators observed the significant angio-inhibitory effects of topical TAT-Es and TAT-Es-RGD, as a reduction of vessel tufts and avascular areas on fluorescein microscopy, and as a reduction in endothelial cell nuclei breaking through the inner limiting membrane on microscopy. No difference was observed between the groups of mice treated with non-conjugated Es and Es-RGD and the control group of untreated mice. Moreover, vascular endothelial growth factor (VEGF) levels detected by IHC similarly dropped in response to topical TAT-Es-RGD and intravitreal anti-VEGF [131].

In a study by Chu et al., dual TAT-RGD peptides were bound to PEG-PLGA nanoparticles (NP) to enhance the penetration in murine eyes affected by laser-induced CNV. Confocal microscopy of choroid-and-retina samples from the CNV areas revealed the highest NP presence, expressed as fluorescence intensity, in mice treated with eyedrops containing TAT-RGD-NPs, when compared to mice receiving topical NP alone (11-fold higher), with TAT-NP and RGD-NP preparations resulting in intermediate fluorescence intensities. RGD was confirmed in this study to concentrate specifically in the CNV area due to its affinity with the endothelial integrin α-V β-3 [132].

Retinal protection was obtained in rats by Atlasz et al. by topical administration of TAT bound to two peptides: vasoactive intestinal peptide (VIP) and pituitary adenylate cyclase-activating polypeptide (PACAP), with considerable retinoprotective and anti-inflammatory activity, respectively. Similar to other studies, conjugation with TAT allowed these therapeutic molecules to target retinal cells more efficiently. This was demonstrated by fluorescence microscopy, which showed a much higher fluorescence per retinal unit area in rats receiving PACAP-TAT/ VIP-TAT eyedrops in comparison with rats receiving PACAP/VIP. The authors also calculated the efficiency for traversing the eye to the retina, finding it 3-fold higher in PACAP-TAT/ VIP-TAT than in PACAP/VIP [133].

Penetratin, another CPP derived from *Drosophila melanogaster*, has been reported to act as a drug PE in several studies. Liu et al. were the first to report the penetration efficiency and biodistribution of topically administered penetratin in both anterior and posterior ocular structures. Fluorescence microscopy showed internalization of this agent within 10 min of the eyedrop instillation, with maximum uptake in the photoreceptors and RPE layers. Accumulation was detectable for up to 6 h, with a peak around 30 min after administration. Penetratin also showed low conjunctival cytotoxicity in vitro, with an IC50 value of 2.5 mM, which was lower than TAT IC50 (2 mM), and 100% of cellular viability even at concentrations as high as 30 mM. Penetration into the posterior segments tends to be favored by its cationic and amphipathic nature, in addition to the helicoidal structure (polyproline type 2) of this agent [134].

Further studies by Liu et al. demonstrated the penetration and retinal localization of a topical preparation of penetratin conjugated with polyamidoamine (PAMAM) dendrimers delivering red fluorescent protein plasmid (pRFP) in retinal cells. Fluorescence microscopy detected penetratin-PAMAM-pRFP in the posterior segment after 10 min, with an accumulation peak at 1 to 2 h and persistence for up to 8 h. The molecular complex was mostly observed in photoreceptors and the RPE, in which the fluorescence was more intense. Similarly, the transfected gene expression was evident in photoreceptors, inner plexiform, and outer plexiform layers and absent in control subjects treated with non-conjugated plasmid [135].

Penetratin hydrophobic derivates were seen to perform even better by Jiang et al., who compared them with wild-type penetratin and penetratin hydrophilic derivates. All three types of peptides, administered in vivo by eyedrops, showed penetration in the anterior and posterior ocular segments after 10 min, peaking at 1 h. Hydrophobic derivates reached the highest retinal concentration among them, resulting in the most intense fluorescence on microscopy. Hydrophilic derivates, however, resulted in a weaker fluorescence compared to the wild-type penetratin. As a possible explanation for these findings, the authors suggested a higher presence of a helix structure in the hydrophobic peptides that could facilitate the interaction with biological membranes and permeation across them. In vitro toxicity assays on human corneal and conjunctival cells, using MTT, and ex vivo biocompatibility testing on excised rabbit corneas and sclera also showed good results [136].

Yang et al. conjugated penetratin and RGD peptide with PEG-PAMAM dendrimers nanocarriers (NCs) and demonstrated that these 2 peptides enhanced ocular permeation and posterior segment localization after topical ocular administration in mice. Conjugation of NCs with penetratin or RGD-penetratin resulted in higher peptide retinal concentration, evident as a 3 times more intense retinal fluorescence, and a prolonged permanence in the retinal tissue, expressed as a longer fluorescence emission (24 h vs. 12 h), in comparison to mice receiving non-conjugated NCs. No cytotoxicity emerged in vitro by testing these NCs on human corneal epithelial cells and umbilical vein endothelial cells. PEG conjugation seemed to reduce PAMAM cytotoxicity, preventing direct contact between cells and amines [137].

A specific peptide for ocular delivery (POD) was investigated by Johnson et al. to vehicle drugs to the posterior segment in vivo. They instilled this carrier-drug complex in mice as topical eyedrops, and by using microscopical studies, the authors revealed localization of this agent in the sclera, choroid, and the optic nerve dura after 45 min, being eliminated at 24 h. No localization was observed in the controls treated with the non-conjugated drug. The uptake seemed to be temperature dependent, whereas inhibitors of endocytosis in vitro did not stop internalization, excluding endocytosis as a key element [138].

A novel CPP based on poly-arginine was tested by de Cogan et al. to deliver anti-VEGF in animal models. Topical treatment was administered to Sprague-Dawley rats and wild-type mice populations to study the pharmacokinetic and angio-inhibitory aspects of the CPP-drug complex, respectively. ELISA testing revealed a 10–11 times higher drug concentration in the target tissue when the anti-VEGF was conjugated with CPP. The angio-inhibitory effect CPP drug was recorded as a reduction of the CNV and scarring area using fluorescein angiography (FA), IHC, and infrared imaging on choroid/RPE samples. A similar response was achieved with intravitreal anti-VEGF, whereas non-treated mice and those receiving the non-conjugated anti-VEGF eyedrops showed no response. No cytotoxicity emerged when this compound was tested on murine retinal cells, human ARPE-19 cells, and human corneal fibroblasts in vitro [139].

4.2.2. Cyclodextrins

Cyclodextrins (CDs) are a group of oligosaccharides composed of six (α-CD), seven (β-CD) or eight (γ-CD) glucose molecules. They possess a truncated cone shape, with a more lipophilic central cavity and a more hydrophilic outer surface. This configuration provides protection from degradation and potential environmental detrimental factors (e.g., reactive molecules). The solubility in water of CDs in their natural forms is relatively poor but can be artificially enhanced to derive molecules such as 2-hydroxyoropyl-β-CD (HPβCD), sulphobutyl ether-CD (SBEβCD), methylated-β CD (MβCD) and 2-hydroxypropyl- γCD (HPγCD), which can be used to augment the topical absorption of hydrophobic drugs. The concentration of dexamethasone in the anterior and posterior ocular segment has been studied by Sigurdsson et al. The study reported that two hours after topical ocular administration of 0.5% dexamethasone/MβCD aggregates in albino rabbits, the drug retinal concentration were 33 ± 7 ng/g in the study eye vs. 14 ± 3 ng/g in the control eye, indicating that 19 ng/g (58%) was derived from topical absorption and 14 ng/g (42%) from systemic absorption. In the vitreous and optic nerves, the portions of dexamethasone topically absorbed were 55% and 17%, respectively [140]. Loftsson et al. compared the ocular absorption in albino rabbits of 1.5% dexamethasone either aggregated with MβCD (solution) or γCD (suspension). The dexamethasone 1.5%/γCD aggregated suspension resulted in 49% of retinal dexamethasone derived from topical administration vs. 14% using the dexamethasone 1.5%/MβCD aggregates solution, whereas in the vitreous humor, the portions of drug coming from the topical instillation were 86% and 73%, respectively, for these two preparations. In the study, the authors observed that suspensions containing dexamethasone/γCD aggregates effectively targeted the ocular posterior segment, especially the retina, and that γCD limits the systemic absorption of the drug by 80% [141].

Clinical studies involving CDs in the topical treatment of diabetic macula edema have been conducted by Tanito et al. The investigators administered 1.5% dexamethasone/γCD eyedrops 3 times per day in 19 patients affected by diabetic macular edema, obtaining a significant central macular thickness (CMT) reduction at week 4 from 512 ± 164 μm to 399 ± 154 μm (p = 0.0016), with a ≥ 10% reduction in 12 out of 19 patients and a mean reduction of −20.3% (range −65.4% to + 9.8%), significantly higher in vitrectomized (−47%) than in un-vitrectomized (−15%) eyes (p = 0.009). LogMAR VA also significantly improved from baseline (mean ± SD) 0.52 ± 0.41) to week 4 (0.37 ± 0.40) (p = 0.0025) with 14 of 19 eyes (74%) improving by more than 0.1. Intraocular pressure slightly increased from (mean ± SD) 15.2 ± 3.1 mmHg at baseline to 17.4 ± 4.2 mmHg (p = 0.0015) at week 4, then returning to pretreatment values at week 8 (15.8 ± 4.0) [142].

In a randomized controlled trial, Ohira et al. compared the effects of topical 1.5% dexamethasone/γCD (12 eyes) tapered every 4 weeks from 3 to 2 and finally to 1 time per day, and, as a control, the results of one subtenon injection of 20 mg of triamcinolone acetonide (10 eyes) in patients with diabetic macular edema. Both LogMAR VA and CMT significantly improved in both groups from baseline to 4 weeks (treatment group: from Log MAR 0.41 ± 0.3 to 0.09 ± 0.15, $p < 0.05$; from 483 ± 141 μm to 99 ± 169 μm, $p < 0.05$; control group: from Log MAR 0.42 ± 0.28 to 0.1 ± 0.14, $p < 0.01$; from 494 ± 94 μm to 106 ± 88 μm, $p < 0.001$) and to 8 weeks (treatment group: Log MAR 0.11 ± 0.13, $p < 0.05$; 141 ± 211 μm, $p < 0.01$; control group: Log MAR 0.08 ± 0.16, not significant; 106 ± 92 μm, $p < 0.001$). CMT was reduced ≥ 20% in one-half of the topically treated patients and 60% of the controls. VA improved by 2 or more lines in 42% of the topically treated patients vs. 20% of the control group. A modest IOP elevation was detected in the treatment group only at 4, 8, and 12 weeks, whereas both groups showed a transient lowering in cortisol and adrenocorticotropic hormone (ACTH), indicating systemic absorption, and lasting, in the topical therapy group, up to 4 weeks after the treatment suspension. No significant glycemic alterations were observed. This study confirmed the anatomical and functional improvements of topical 1.5% dexamethasone/γCD aggregated suspensions, which were comparable to those obtained with a sub-tenon injection of triamcinolone acetonide [143].

Studies have reported noninfectious posterior uveitis treated with 1.5% dexamethasone/γCD aggregated suspension. Shulman et al. administered this preparation in 5 uveitic patients (1 female and 4 males, age range 45–65 years) affected by vitritis (3 eyes) and macular edema (5 eyes), starting with 4 instillations per day and tapering the drug by 1 drop per day every 10 days. The study was open-label and non-comparative. Macular edema completely resolved in 4 eyes, relapsed at week 12 after initial response in one case. VA improved in 3 eyes, remained stable in 3 eyes, and decreased in the other 2 eyes, also because of cataract in one of them, with median VA significantly improved at week 4, but returning to baseline values at 12 weeks. Vitritis completely resolved in 2 eyes, but improved in the third. One patient, who was known to be a steroid-responder prior to the study, actually presented with IOP elevation after the treatment [144].

Uveitis and macular edema were also treated with eyedrops containing 1.5% dexamethasone/γCD particles in studies by Krag & Hassellund. They administered the topical preparation in 3 cases. The posology was 4 times daily for one month in the affected eye in one case, obtaining macular edema reabsorption, therefore switched to conventional topical dexamethasone, with edema recurrence after one month. The second case was bilateral: one eye was treated with 2 drops of preparation, instilled 4 times per day for three weeks, then tapered to 1 drop 3 times per day, whereas the other eye underwent an intravitreal implant of Ozurdex. Both eyes responded well, showing edema resolution. The third patient also presented with bilateral uveitic macular edema, which had recurred in both eyes 3 months after intravitreal Ozurdex. The recurrence was treated in one eye with topical 1.5% dexamethasone/γCD 6 times daily for one week, then 4 times daily for another week, but without success. The CME augment required a second Ozurdex implant [145].

4.2.3. BAC

BAC is a widely used preservative in ocular topical formulations. It acts as a PE by damaging the anatomical barriers of the ocular surface and facilitating the penetration of solutes and solvents through the external ocular epithelia. Studies on nanoparticles administered via eyedrops in association with BAC were performed on mice by Mahaling and Katti. The enhancement power of BAC was not as strong as expected on fluorescence biomicroscopy, although increased bioavailability of BAC-coated nanoparticles was recorded in the retina, choroid, and sclera compared with non-coated nanoparticles [146].

4.2.4. Iontophoresis

Iontophoresis can also be used to transport drugs across ocular membranes with a non-invasive mechanism. This technique uses a low-amplitude electrical current delivered in a continuous or pulsatile way without damaging the ocular tissues. Iontophoretic treatment for the posterior segment forces the passage of dedicated topical drug formulations through the transscleral pathway to avoid anterior anatomical barriers.

Several preclinical studies have shown interesting results in delivering corticosteroids to the inner ocular structures, including the vitreous, choroid, and retina. Hemisuccinate methylprednisolone (HMP) was administered to rabbits using transscleral iontophoresis, reaching higher and more sustained concentrations than with intravenous administration, and with minimal systemic absorption and ocular complications [147].

Cathodal transscleral iontophoresis, experimented on rabbits, allowed us to obtain intraocular concentrations of topical DEX higher than those obtained via passive diffusion of the same preparation. The concentration measured in the vitreous was well above the concentration needed to suppress inflammation [148].

Preliminary encouraging results on the transscleral iontophoretic administration of dexamethasone phosphate and its favorable molecular characteristics (high water solubility, 2 negative charges at physiologic Ph) led to the development of dedicated patented devices, such as the EyeGate II delivery system (EGDS; EyeGate Pharmaceuticals, Inc, Encintas, CA,

USA.). The device contains an electrode housed in an annular ocular applicator, which produces ions that push the drug, a dedicated dexamethasone phosphate formulation, through the conjunctiva and sclera by electrochemical repulsion [149].

A phase-1 clinical trial has recently started to deliver bevacizumab and ranibizumab using an iontophoretic device called Visulex-1; however, concerns about skin exposure to prolonged electric currents have been reported [150–152].

4.3. Sustained Drug-Release Systems

4.3.1. Ocular Inserts

Ocular inserts (Ois) are sterile, non-implantable, thin, multilayered routes of administration with a solid or semisolid consistency developed to achieve better ocular bioavailability and sustained drug action over a prolonged period [153,154]. They have been designed to overcome eyedrop limitations and increase the contact time between the preparation and the conjunctival tissue to ensure a sustained and accurate release suited for topical or systemic treatments [155]. They are placed in the fornix of the conjunctival sac of the lower eyelid and, less frequently, in the upper fornix or on the cornea, offering an alternative approach to the difficult problem of limited pre-corneal drug residence time [156]. Such systems can achieve prolonged therapeutic drug concentrations in ocular target tissues while limiting systemic exposure and side effects and improving patient adherence to therapy [157]. Based upon solubility, they can be classified as insoluble (osmotic, diffusion, contact lens); soluble (based on natural polymers, e.g., collagen, or based on synthetic or semi-synthetic polymers, e.g., cellulose derivatives, such as HPMC, HPC, MC, etc.); and bioerodible [158].

Ois have been used to treat conditions, such as glaucoma, Ocusert ®(pilocarpine-alginate), NODS ®, New Ophthalmic Delivery System (pilocarpine) dry eye, and allergy [159–162]. In addition, Ois has been utilized for the treatment of common ocular infections, such as bacterial keratitis [163–165]. Ois loaded with cyclosporine (Cys) has been reported by Grimaudo et al. [166]. Ois based on sodium hyaluronate (HA) nanofibers loaded with the antioxidant compound ferulic acid (FA) and the antimicrobial peptide ε-polylysine (ε-PL) have shown high antibacterial activity against Pseudomonas aeruginosa and Staphylococcus aureus [163–167]. Other Ois have been developed and loaded with Ketorolac Tromethamine (KT) Eudragit ®, Atorvastatin Cakcium (ATC) to treat ocular inflammatory conditions [168–171]. Moreover, Ois offers the possibility of targeting internal ocular tissues through non-corneal conjunctival-scleral penetration routes to reach the ocular posterior segment. A new technique used to develop new synthetic Ois is electrospinning, which is a method that obtains nanofibers that have the property to encapsulate and control the release profile of multiple drugs [172]. Nanofibers, due to their unique structural features, show great promise for drug delivery to the retinal segment following topical application. Preclinical results have shown that preservative-free polycaprolactone (PCL) electrospun nanofibers can be considered a primary drug carrier for the delivery of fluocinolone acetonide into the posterior eye segment, particularly for retinal epithelium [173]. The melt-cast method has been used to fabricate topical Ois for the delivery of indomethacin, prednisolone sodium phosphate, and ciprofloxacin hydrochloride commonly employed in the treatment of ocular inflammation and infections. Studies have shown that these devices generated significantly higher drug levels in all ocular tissues, including the retina-choroid, when compared to their control formulations, demonstrating that the melt-cast/melt-extruded films could shift the paradigm for drug delivery to the posterior segment of the eye [174]. More recently, the effects of Ois for the administration of progesterone (PG), a sexual hormone characterized by neuroprotection activity and used for the treatment of posterior degenerative ocular diseases associated with oxidative stress, have been evaluated using permeation enhancer technology. Due to the fact that the PG is a hydrophobic drug, it was incorporated in β-cyclodextrins in order to solubilize it. A controlled diffusion of PG was obtained by in vitro grafting of 59% polyvinyl alcohol (PVA), 39% polyvinylpyrrolidone K30 (PVP-K30), and 2% propylene glycol (PGL). Ex vivo analyses assessed trans-corneal and trans-scleral diffusion of PG and allowed the authors to conclude that the PG-loaded Ois can be suitable for the treatment of various posterior eye diseases such as DR, AMD, cataracts, glaucoma, and retinitis [175]. Ois are placed in the conjunctival fornix or on the cornea and increase the contact time between the drug and the conjunctival/corneal tissue in order to ensure a long-lasting, controlled, and precise release of the preparation. In this way, they overcome the problem of limited pre-corneal drug residence time, leading to increased bioavailability. By avoiding the use of preservatives, they decrease the likelihood of sensitivity reactions and minimize systemic side effects. Other advantages include precision dosing with controlled release and minimal systemic absorption, reduced administration frequency, and improved patient compliance. Electrospinning allows nanofibers to be obtained that encapsulate and control the release profile of numerous drugs to the posterior eye segment [172]. Moreover, the melt-cast method allows the generation of higher drug levels in ocular tissues, including the retina and choroid [174]. Despite these advantages, the major disadvantages of Ois reside in patient non-compliance with frequent feelings, such as the entry of a foreign body into the eye, difficulty in self-insertion or removal, potential accidental loss and movement around the eye that could interfere with vision. Ois can be specifically formulated to address the unique characteristics of retinal diseases, such as the need for long-term treatment and the delicate nature of the retina. Research and development in this area is ongoing, with a focus on optimizing the design, drug release, and biocompatibility of ocular inserts for the treatment of retinal diseases. These advancements hold great promise in improving the outcomes and quality of life of patients with retinal conditions.

4.3.2. Ocular Implants

Intraocular/intravitreal implants are relatively new routes of administration designed to be inserted into the eye to achieve a sustained release mechanism of the drug in the vitreous and to provide a long-term therapeutic effect in a controlled and prolonged way. They can bypass the BRB, avoid burst release, provide a reduction in the dose, and deliver therapeutics at a constant rate directly at the ocular site, with no need to perform repeated injections intravitreally. These implants have an increased half-life, reduced peak plasma levels, and improved patient compliance [176,177]. The mechanism of drug release from implants showed three phases, which include an early burst, a middle diffusive phase, and a final burst. There are two major categories of materials used in the development of these implants: non-biodegradables and biodegradables.

Non-biodegradable implants (NBI), such as scleral, intra-scleral (disc), and intravitreal implants (encapsulated cell), do not experience changes in structure and require two surgical procedures, which entails one for implantation and a second one for removal or replacement. They are larger in size, thus requiring a larger incision for implantation. They are made up of ethylene vinyl acetate (EVA), polyvinyl alcohol (PVA), or polysulfone capillary fiber (PCF).

Biodegradables implants (BI), such as injectable microparticles, intravitreal implant (injectable rod), intra-scleral, and epi-scleral implant (disc, scleral implant (plug), degrade and disintegrate over time. All the components from the implant are eliminated autonomously; thus, only a single surgical procedure is needed for insertion [176]. They are made of polylactic acid (PLA), polyglycolic acid (PGA), PLGA, or polycaprolactones.

With regards to the currently available NBIs, the first insert was developed and approved in 1996 Vitrasert® (Bausch and Lomb, Rochester, NY, USA) was designed for the treatment of cytomegalovirus retinitis with ganciclovir. It has been demonstrated to control inflammation, reduce recurrences in patients with viral retinitis, and improve visual acuity [40,178]. Retisert (Bausch & Lomb, Rochester, NY, USA) is an intravitreal NBI of a corticosteroid, fluocinolone acetonide, which the FDA approved in 2005 for treating chronic non-infectious uveitis [179]. The main indications for this insert include chronic non-infectious posterior uveitis (NIPU), but it has also been shown to be effective in DME and macular edema (ME) secondary to central retinal vein occlusion (RVO) [180,181]. Iluvien

(Alimera Sciences Inc., Alpharetta, GA, USA) is the smallest NBI of FA. It is cylindrically shaped and has a composition similar to Retisert. This insert is used to treat DME but is also currently being evaluated in phase 2 trials for dry AMD, retinal vein occlusion, and non-infectious uveitis [182,183].

Yutiq (EyePoint Pharmaceuticals, Inc., MA, USA) is similar to Iluvien and is another intravitreal NBI of FA that received FDA approval in 2018 for the treatment of chronic NIPU [184]. I-vation (SurModics, Eden Prairie, MN, USA) is an NBI that releases triamcinolone acetonide (TA) and is used to treat DME [185,186]. The Ranibizumab Port Delivery System (PDS) is a new intraocular DDS for continuously delivering an anti-vascular endothelial growth factor (VEGF) antibody, ranibizumab, for the treatment of neovascular AMD (nAMD). It is made up of an ocular implant and four ancillary devices that are utilized for initially filling ranibizumab, surgical implantation, refilling exchange, and explantation [187].

The DEX implant (Ozurdex, Allergan Inc., Irvine, CA, USA) is a dexamethasone intravitreal implant composed of poly lactic-co-glycolic acid (PLGA), a synthetic aliphatic polyester predominantly biodegraded via non-enzymatic hydrolysis of the ester linkages under physiological conditions. It contains 0.7 mg dexamethasone, which is released sustainably in the vitreous for up to 6 months. This device received FDA approval in June 2009 for treating retinal vein occlusion-associated macular edema and in 2010 for treating non-infectious posterior uveitis. The main indications include RVO (central and branch) associated with ME, DME, and NIPU. It also has off-label use in Irvine Gass syndrome, nAMD, vasoproliferative retinal tumors, retinal telangiectasia, Coats' disease, radiation maculopathy, retinitis pigmentosa, and macular edema secondary to scleral buckle and pars plana vitrectomy [188]. The DEX implant offers prolonged and targeted drug delivery and is placed directly into the vitreous to maximize its therapeutic effect while minimizing systemic side effects. By delivering a consistent and controlled amount of dexamethasone, it can maintain therapeutic drug levels over an extended period. Moreover, patients may experience a reduced treatment burden compared to other forms of medication, thus improving their convenience and compliance. On the other half, potential disadvantages may consist of invasiveness, limited indications and reversibility, and side effects, such as increased intraocular pressure, cataract formation, and infection. Verisome (Ramscor, Inc., Menlo Park, CA, USA) is a long-acting intravitreal injectable drug delivery system for different drugs, and it is with TA to treat chronic cystoid macular edema (CME) due to RVO and with ranibizumab to treat nAMD [186–189].

Ocular implants can provide a sustained and controlled mechanism of drug release over an extended period. They are designed to release medications slowly and maintain therapeutic levels in the eye for a longer duration. This allows for a more consistent therapeutic effect and reduces the need for frequent administration of eyedrops or injections, enhancing patient compliance and convenience. These types of DDSs can enhance drug bioavailability by increasing the residence time of the drug in the eye and in a direct manner at the site of action, ensuring efficient delivery and reducing systemic absorption and consequent potential side effects. They can overcome the challenges associated with short drug half-lives and rapid clearance and can shield drugs from degradation by tear fluid and enzymes, enhancing their stability and prolonging their shelf life. While ocular implants offer several advantages, they also have potential disadvantages. Biodegradable implants generally require a single surgical procedure, while non-biodegradable implants require two surgical procedures under local or general anesthesia, increasing some inherent risks, including infections, bleeding, and damage to surrounding tissues. Additionally, the need for surgery may not be suitable for all patients, especially those who are not surgical candidates or have contraindications. Another disadvantage is irreversibility because some ocular implants, such as sustained-release devices, are designed to remain in the eye for an extended period of time; therefore, they cannot be easily removed or adjusted once implanted. While this may be advantageous for long-term treatment, it can pose challenges if there are complications, adverse reactions, or the need to change the treatment plan.

Another limitation is the lack of flexibility due to the fact that, once implanted, it may not be possible to modify the drug or change the medication regimen easily. Like any foreign body, ocular implants carry a risk of complications, including infection, inflammation, implant migration, erosion, or extrusion, which can compromise the effectiveness of the treatment and may require further medical or surgical intervention. In retinal disease, ocular implants have shown promising results in improving visual function, restoring vision, and providing targeted drug delivery to the retina. It is important to note that these routes of administration are still evolving, and their effectiveness may vary depending on the specific retinal condition, patient characteristics, and implant design.

4.3.3. Hydrogels

Hydrogels are well-defined structures composed of a wide variety of hydrophilic monomers connected with crosslinked bonds, which are capable of swelling when placed in water or an aqueous environment [190]. They are highly soft and elastic in nature, have physicochemical similarities with ocular fluids, and are adequate for intraocular use [176]. Hydrogels have been developed to deliver proteins, peptides, and antibodies, as the formation of the hydrogel can occur at ambient temperature conditions. These components are currently used in clinical research utilizing soft contact lenses and foldable intraocular lenses to deliver drugs to the anterior segment and to the posterior segment of the eye and have been considered in the treatment of diabetic retinopathy, age-related macular degeneration, or rhegmatogenous retinal detachment [177,191–193].

Several in situ hydrogel systems are prepared with hyaluronic acid, chitosan, poloxamer, hydroxypropyl methylcellulose (HPMC), and polycaprolactone. These components have demonstrated safe use as depot systems in the ocular environment. They can be injected into the vitreous cavity through a small gauge needle, as "in situ", which then transforms into gel in response to internal and/or external stimuli mediated by pH, temperature, ions, or enzymes [194]. The sol-gel phase transition occurs within seconds to minutes, entrapping, and stabilizing the therapeutic proteins in an aqueous polymeric network [195]. After injection, the hydrogel forms a reservoir, allowing for the continuous release of loaded protein molecules over time [196,197]. Drug release occurs via diffusion-controlled and degradation-controlled processes from the reservoir [198,199].

Hydrogels can play a vital role in the development of nanotechnologies for the delivery of drugs to the eye. Regarding posterior segment delivery, polymeric natural-based hydrogels and synthetic hydrogels are characterized by easy injectability and long residence times, thus potentially promising candidates for ideal vitreous substitutes [200]. It has been demonstrated that polysaccharide crosslinked hydrogels showed sustained release of bevacizumab for three days with a low initial burst, while thermosensitive hydrogels exhibited sustained release of bevacizumab for 18 days [201]. In a recent study, the hyaluronic acid-bearing furan with 4 arm-PEG10K-maleimide (4APM-HAFU) (ratio 1:5) hydrogel formulation was easily injected into the vitreous cavity using a small needle (29G) and showed sustained release of bevacizumab >400 days by a combination of diffusion, swelling, and degradation. A bioassay showed that the released bevacizumab remained bioactive [202].

This hydrogel platform offers high potential for the sustained release of therapeutic antibodies to treat ocular diseases, such as age-related macular degeneration. An injectable antibody-loaded supramolecular nanofiber hydrogel has been created by simply mixing betamethasone phosphate (BetP), a clinical anti-inflammatory drug, anti-VEGF, the gold-standard anti-VEGF drug for AMD treatment, with $CaCl_2$. Upon intravitreal injection, such BetP-based hydrogel (BetP-Gel), while enabling a long-term sustained release of anti-VEG, can also scavenge reactive oxygen species to reduce local inflammation and prolong the effective treatment time of conventional anti-VEGF therapy [203]. Overall, various pre-clinical studies on rabbit eye models have shown good biocompatibility of anti-VEGF-loaded hydrogel after intravitreal injection, exhibiting sustained release properties [195,204,205]. These agents may be readily translated into clinical use for AMD treatment with the potential to replace current anti-VEGF therapy.

In vivo investigation with fibrin hydrogels revealed high short-term subretinal biocompatibility of this type of DDS, which is a suitable scaffold for human Embryonic Stem Cell- Derived Retinal Pigment Epithelial Cells (hESC-RPE) transplantation, which could be a new grafting material for tissue engineering RPE cells [206]. A small series of rhegmatogenous retinal detachment models with short-term follow-up provide preliminary evidence to support the favorable biocompatibility and efficacy of the hyaluronic acid (HA) hydrogel as a promising retinal patch for sealing retinal breaks in retinal detachment repair [207]. Moreover, gene delivery using an injectable hydrogel has also been studied as a treatment for retinitis pigmentosa [208,209].

Hydrogels can be combined with microparticles/nanoparticles (NPs) in order to form a hybrid "combined-DDS" for the controlled delivery of therapeutics, especially for localized applications, which can be useful to increase therapeutic efficacy and to limit particle movement in the eye. An injectable hydrogel loaded with retinal-targeted, biodegradable hybrid NPs with a hyaluronic acid coating has been developed to improve in vivo distribution throughout the vitreous and delivery to retinal cells. It has been shown to greatly improve the administration of sensitive therapeutic molecules to the retina by exploiting both the targeting ability and protective effect of NPs while prolonging their release [210]. The use of anti-VEGF-loaded microspheres suspended within an injectable, egener-responsive hydrogel has shown controlled, extended, and bioactive release for approximately 200 days of ranibizumab and aflibercept in vitro. [211]. In a laser-induced CNV model in nonhuman primate models, Kim et al. demonstrated that an aflibercept-loaded microsphere and hydrogel combination system was an effective treatment for up to 6 months post-injection, without adverse events [212]. Recently, a biodegradable microparticle- and nanoparticle-hydrogel DDS was developed to obtain the simultaneous release of aflibercept and dexamethasone. The Combo-DDS has proven to be an effective method for simultaneously releasing dexamethasone and aflibercept for up to six months. This may eliminate the need for separate dosing regimens of anti-VEGF and corticosteroids for patients with wet AMD [213]. The key advantages of hydrogels include the fact that they can provide sustained and controlled release of drugs within intraocular tissues, such as the aqueous humor and vitreous cavity. The gel-like structure of hydrogels allows for the gradual release of drugs, ensuring a sustained therapeutic effect and reducing the frequency of drug administration. Furthermore, certain ocular drugs, particularly biologics, exhibit low stability and/or short half-life when present in the vitreous humor. By encapsulating these biologics within hydrogels, both drug stability and release duration can be improved. In some ocular conditions, such as retinal diseases, monotherapy may not be adequate to achieve optimal therapeutic efficacy, and hydrogels can integrate different drugs into a single platform, simplifying the treatment regimen and improving patient compliance. Therefore, combination therapy has emerged as a crucial strategy for enhancing clinical outcomes through synergistic effects. This class of DDSs can be designed to specifically target the ocular posterior segment and retina. By incorporating drugs into hydrogels, they can be delivered directly to the desired site of action, minimizing systemic exposure, and reducing potential side effects. This targeted drug delivery approach enhances therapeutic efficacy while minimizing off-target effects. Hydrogels can enhance drug penetration through ocular tissues, including the cornea and sclera, to reach the ocular posterior segment and retina because their gel-like nature can promote sustained contact with eye tissues, facilitating better drug permeation and bioavailability in these deep ocular layers. Disadvantages include the fact that hydrogels may have limitations in terms of their loading capacity for drugs. The gel matrix can accommodate a certain amount of drug molecules, and exceeding this limit may lead to reduced gel integrity or compromised release kinetics. This limitation can restrict the use of hydrogels for high-dose drug delivery or when large quantities of drugs need to be administered. Hydrogels, especially those with higher viscosity, may face challenges in effectively penetrating dense ocular tissues, such as the cornea. Their viscosity can impede diffusion and hinder the efficient delivery of drugs to the desired target sites. This limitation may require additional strategies or modifications to enhance the penetration capabilities of hydrogel-based DDSs. While hydrogels can provide sustained drug release, their long-term stability can be a concern because, over time, they may undergo physical or chemical changes, leading to alterations in their drug release profiles. Factors such as degradation, water evaporation, or interactions with ocular fluids can affect the stability and performance of hydrogel-based DDSs. Ensuring long-term stability is essential for maintaining consistent drug release over extended periods.

While hydrogels offer several advantages as DDSs to the ocular posterior segment, further research is still needed to optimize their performance, ensure long-term stability, and address the specific challenges associated with these targeted applications. Nonetheless, hydrogels hold great promise for delivering therapeutics to these critical ocular regions, potentially revolutionizing the treatment of posterior segment and retinal disorders.

4.3.4. Contact Lens

The use of contact lenses (CLs) as routes of administration has been increasingly evaluated in recent years [214]. The idea of using CLs as carriers of active ingredients is a relatively new strategy that is still being developed and improved. There are two main groups of contact lenses depending on the designed material: soft contact lenses made of hydrogel or silicone hydrogel polymers, and rigid gas-permeable contact lenses. Therapeutic contact lenses include polymeric carriers, such as drug-containing polymer nanoparticles and polymeric implants [215]. In recent years, studies have focused on ways to extend the drug residence time and improve the bioavailability of various lens-based DDSs. Surface modifying methods include dip-coating (soaking), diffusion barrier insertion (Vitamin E), incorporation of functional monomers, ligands, and a polymeric matrix, molecular imprinting, cyclodextrin vaccination, incorporation of colloidal, drug-loaded nanoparticles, or other colloidal nanostructured systems, and surface coating by multilayer film deposition of colloidal nanoparticles or ligands [215]. The advantages of using control-released drug systems in the form of contact lenses are the drug dosing regimen, bioavailability, and prolonged residence time of drugs in the eye [216,217]. The use of contact lenses as a reservoir of drugs is a promising treatment system for: chronic eye diseases (such as glaucoma); ocular allergies; controlled release of antimicrobial peptides on the ocular surface; and drug delivery with antiviral, antifungal, anti-inflammatory, and/or immunosuppressive agents [218–222].

A commercially approved silicon hydrogel CL named ACUVUE® OASYS®, has been modified to control the delivery of pirfenidone (PFD) to ameliorate corneal inflammation and fibrosis conditions [223]. The same authors used the ACUVUE® Oasys® and the 1-DAY ACUVUE® TruEyeTM lens soaked with vitamin E. These CL have been employed to evaluate the release profiles of ketorolac tromethamine (KT) and flurbiprofen sodium (FS), which have shown a better drug delivery dosage in the treatment of ocular inflammatory conditions [224]. CLs based on methacrylic acid (MAA) loaded with acyclovir (ACV) and valacyclovir (VACV) have been used to treat ocular keratitis caused by the herpes simplex virus (HSV) [221]. Moxifloxacin (MF) and dexamethasone (DM) were loaded on chitosan-, glycerol-, and polyethylene glycol (PEG)-based CLs, which were developed using the solvent casting approach. These CLs showed efficacy in delivering MF and DM in the treatment of postoperative conditions to prevent ocular infections [225]. Silicone hydrogel soft CLs loaded with brinzolamide or latanoprost have also been developed, allowing constant release of the drug and thus representing a good alternative to eyedrops for treating glaucoma [226,227].

Regarding drug delivery to the posterior segment of the eye, Alvarez-Rivera et al. developed CLs suitable for the local prevention/treatment of diabetes-related eye pathologies. The main idea was to incorporate functional groups into the polymer matrix that could reversibly interact with epalrestat, an aldose reductase inhibitor used for the treatment of diabetic neuropathy, promoting drug accumulation and diffusion through the cornea [228]. Moreover, it has been hypothesized that ocular drug flux to the retina can be improved by providing sustained drug delivery directly to the cornea, increasing drug concentrations at the ocular surface, increasing drug residence time at the ocular surface, and using mechanical forces as a permeation enhancer. In vitro and ex vivo experiments have been performed, and the results have shown that these drug-loaded hydrogels may be useful as ocular devices for regulating the posterior release of epalrestat, thus facilitating its accumulation and diffusion across the cornea [229]. Recently, soft hydrogel CLs have been employed to obtain a sustained release of naringenin (NAR), a flavonoid anti-inflammatory and antioxidant substance used for treating posterior eye segment disease, such as age-related macular degeneration [230,231].

A sustained drug-eluting contact lens positioned directly over the cornea has been developed for drug delivery to the eye, including the retina. This contact lens has shown sustained drug delivery to the retina at therapeutic levels using a dexamethasone delivery system (Dex-DS), which consists of a dexamethasone-polymer film encapsulated inside a contact lens. Rabbits wearing Dex-DS achieved retinal drug concentrations that were 200 times greater than those from intensive (hourly) dexamethasone drops. Conversely, Dex-DS demonstrated lower systemic dexamethasone concentrations. In an efficacy study in rabbits, Dex-DS successfully inhibited retinal vascular leakage induced by intravitreal injection of vascular endothelial growth factor (VEGF) [232]. Recently, a drug-loaded contact lens combined with electrodes placed on cadaver rabbit eyes and positioned diametrically opposite and beyond the limbus has been shown to potentially deliver ionic drugs directly to the vitreous. Incorporation of an electric field with multiple electrodes on a single lens can effectively deliver ionic drugs to the posterior region at levels comparable to current methods, with the benefits of being safer and less invasive [233]. CLs offer several advantages over traditional methods of drug administration, providing enhanced effectiveness and patient convenience. This type of route of administration allows the delivery of drugs directly to the ocular posterior segment and retina, enabling targeted drug delivery, minimizing systemic exposure, and reducing potential side effects. Contact lenses can be designed to release drugs continuously over an extended period, ensuring consistent therapeutic concentration at the target site and enhancing treatment efficacy while reducing the frequency of drug administration. This type of route of administration provides a larger surface area for drug absorption compared to traditional delivery methods, such as eyedrops, allowing for better drug penetration into the ocular tissues, enhancing bioavailability, and optimizing the therapeutic effect. Moreover, modern contact lenses are designed to provide excellent comfort and vision, and by incorporating drug delivery capabilities, patients can benefit from both vision correction and therapeutic drug administration simultaneously. This approach eliminates the need for multiple interventions, enhancing patient convenience and acceptance. This type of route of administration is a non-invasive method that reduces the associated risks and complications while offering a less intimidating option for patients. The ease of administration also makes contact lens-based drug delivery suitable for long-term treatment plans. The drug release rate, duration, and dosage can be adjusted based on the specific needs of each patient's condition. This level of customization allows for personalized treatment strategies and optimized therapeutic outcomes. Contact lenses can accommodate various types of drugs, including small molecules, biologics, nanoparticles, and gene therapies. Nevertheless, there are also some potential disadvantages and challenges that need to be considered. CLs have a limited capacity to carry drugs due to their small size and thickness. This can restrict the amount of drug that can be loaded into the lens, potentially limiting the duration of drug release or requiring frequent lens replacement. The release kinetics of drugs from CLs may vary depending on factors, such as lens material, drug characteristics, and environmental conditions. Achieving a consistent and controlled release profile can be challenging, potentially leading to unpredictable drug concentrations at the target site. Factors such as tear film composition, blinking patterns, and lens movement on the eye can influence drug release and bioavailability. Certain drugs, particularly larger molecules or those with specific formulation requirements, may not be suitable for contact lens-based delivery. This limitation may restrict the versatility of this route of administration in some cases. The compatibility of different drugs with contact lens materials and their ability to maintain stability during storage and wear can limit the range of drugs that can be delivered using this approach. It is important to note that research and technological advancements are continuously addressing these challenges to improve the feasibility and reliability of CLs for ocular posterior segment and retinal therapies. With further innovation and refinement, these disadvantages can potentially be overcome, leading to more effective and patient-friendly ocular drug delivery methods. While the contact lens-based route of administration for the ocular posterior segment and retinal therapies holds tremendous promise, further research and development are still required to overcome challenges related to drug loading, release kinetics, and biocompatibility.

4.3.5. Microneedles

In recent years, due to intense research and advancements in microtechnology, there has been remarkable interest in the development of microneedles (MNs)-based systems as an alternative, non-invasive form for administering drugs to the eye in order to minimize tissue damage, reduce the disruption of membrane continuity, eliminate the risk of pathogen infections, and improve overall safety.

Simultaneously with the development of single-microneedle technologies, research has focused on microneedle systems/patches for ocular drug delivery, recently, and successfully applied to the cornea or sclera [234]. Ocular microneedles are DDSs that show passive delivery of molecules via arrays of solid MNs coated with drug formulations that dissolve a few minutes after insertion. They provide passive diffusion of therapeutics, overcoming the transport barriers of epithelial tissues, eliminating clearance by conjunctival mechanisms, and minimizing retinal damage [79]. The most common microneedle classifications are based on geometry, the material applied to obtain the systems, the method of fabrication, the drug loading technique, and the mode of drug delivery [235].

Regarding the use of MNs as DDSs to the posterior segment of the eye, a lot of research has been conducted recently. Injection into the suprachoroidal space (SCS) represents an alternative method of ocular drug delivery to the posterior segment allowed by MN-based DDSs because it facilitates targeted distribution to affected chorioretinal tissues through the suprachoroidal pathway. This allows potential efficacy benefits, compartmentalization away from unaffected anterior segment tissues, and a high degree of bioavailability. The commercially approved SCS Microinjector® (Clearside Biomedical, Inc., Alpharetta, GA, USA) was specifically designed to provide non-surgical, reliable, and in-office access to the SCS. Indeed, the first and only FDA-approved SC therapy (CLS-TA) is administered via the SCS Microinjector. (Bausch+ Lomb and Clearside Biomedical 2021) Triamcinolone acetonide injectable suspension (Xipere®, Bausch + Lomb) was successfully used as a novel formulation optimized for use with the SCS Microinjector® [236]. This presents an opportunity for safe and effective drug delivery for the treatment of uveitic macular edema and, potentially, for broader use with other drugs to treat other ocular diseases that impact chorioretinal tissues, such as age-related macular degeneration, diabetic retinopathy, and choroidal melanoma [237,238].

Roy et al. presented two types of patches for the delivery of triamcinolone acetonide (TA): a microneedle scleral patch (MSP) and a microneedle corneal patch (MCP). Ex vivo experiments performed on porcine eye globe showed that, in comparison to MCP and TA nanosuspension, MSP obtained much greater TA concentrations in the vitreous humor and choroidoretinal complex after 5 min of application [239]. Amer and Chen fabricated PVA hydrogel-based microneedle arrays for the delivery of immunoglobin G1, a model protein resembling bevacizumab, applied in the treatment of age-related macular degeneration (AMD). The in vitro tests showed an extended release of the active compound compared to the rapid release after injection. The authors indicated that the MN-based arrays show a much more uniform drug release profile than the single injections [240]. Wu and co-workers developed nanoparticle-loaded bilayer dissolving microneedle arrays for the sustained delivery of proteins to the posterior ophthalmic segment. The MNs had adequate mechanical stability to puncture the sclera and degrade very quickly, releasing the nanoparticles (NPs) in less than 3 min. The slow disintegration of the NP-forming matrices resulted in the release of the active ingredient in a prolonged manner [241].

Some of the advantages of MNs as DDSs to the ocular posterior segment consist in the fact that they enable precise, controlled, and targeted delivery of drugs, thanks to their minimally invasive nature. MNs create micropores at the level of the sclera/suprachoroidal space which enhance bioavailability and ensure that a higher concentration of the drug reaches the desired site, increasing the therapeutic efficacy while minimizing the required dosage. Compared to traditional ocular DDSs, such as injections, microneedles provide a non-invasive and pain-free alternative method. They can be designed to deliver drugs in a sustained manner, allowing for prolonged therapeutic effects without the need for frequent administration and improving patient compliance with medication regimens. By avoiding the need for preservatives or exposure to harsh conditions, such as high temperatures or pH, microneedles minimize the risk of drug degradation and ensure that the therapeutic agent reaches the ocular posterior segment in its active form. MNs also have some potential disadvantages that should be considered. Their fabrication can be technically complex and challenging. Achieving the desired dimensions, needle strength, and sharpness while ensuring biocompatibility and reproducibility can be demanding. Developing scalable manufacturing processes for commercial production is an ongoing area of research. Although MNs are designed to be minimally invasive, there is still a risk of injury during the insertion process. Their small size restricts the amount of drugs that can be loaded onto or within them. This limitation may pose a challenge for drugs that require higher doses or those with low solubility. MNs are often made from materials that may have limited stability, especially in terms of long-term storage. Factors such as degradation, moisture absorption, or changes in mechanical properties over time can impact their performance and effectiveness. It is important to note that, while these disadvantages exist, ongoing research and development efforts are focused on addressing these challenges and improving the performance and safety of MN-based ocular DDSs.

Overall, MNs can be considered a minimally invasive compromise between topical formulations, which are acceptable but reveal poor effectiveness, and direct injections, which are more effective but invasive. With this novel approach, the drug can be delivered to the target site with good precision and minimized the risk of tissue damage, pain, and infection [234,242].

5. Conclusions and Future Perspectives

The development of innovative DDSs to increase the passage of therapeutic molecules across the ocular barriers to the posterior ocular segment, with minimally invasive, safe, and affordable technologies, is a rapidly growing research field. Figure 2 shows the different materials used in the current DDSs, while Table 1 lists the characteristics, pros, and cons of each. Various alternatives to ordinary intravitreal injection have been proposed to overcome the clinical and logistic burdens for the patient and for the healthcare providers that are intrinsic to this type of treatment and the chronic nature of most posterior segment disorders. Nanotechnologies, alternative drug penetration enhancers, and various types of in situ devices for sustained drug release have been extensively tested, many, for the moment, only on animal models, in vitro, or with limited numbers and indications on humans. They seem capable of delivering targeted retinal treatments with promising results, but more in vivo studies are required to confirm these experimental results. The addition of mucoadhesive polymers and aggregation with micro/nanomolecular carriers have been shown to enhance drug bioavailability and promote the prolonged release of therapeutic concentrations. Nanoparticles in general have the advantages of small size, considerable surface area, and high mucoadhesivity, whereas the particles' stability and loading capability is not always optimal. For these reasons, NPs have often been integrated with more complex polymeric structures, such as gel, to integrate the controlled delivery of the first with the higher stability and prolonged retention time of the second. Nevertheless, several aspects of the drug penetration mechanism are still to be clarified, as if it may trigger toxic reactions or harmful alterations to the ocular barriers [121].

Table 1. Strategies for drug delivery to the ocular posterior segment.

		Brief Description	Developmental Stage	Advantages	Disadvantages
Nanomedicine	Liposomes	Membrane-like vesicular structures carrying drugs across ocular barriers, e.g., Visudyne (Bausch&Lomb) to deliver verteporfin to the retina in nAMD Dexamethasone and tacrolimus also experimented with using liposomes to treat vitreoretinal inflammation and macular edema	Approved (Visudyne)	• Good biocompatibility and biodegradability • Low toxicity • Better drug-loading capacity compared to other lipidic nano vesicles • Effective protection of carried molecules	• Unstable preparation (aggregation during transportation and storage with loss of transparency) • Need for stabilizing excipients • Questionable physicochemical properties • Possibile inflammatory and hypersensitivity reactions
	Nanomicelles	Amphiphilic monolayered vesicles carrying drugs. Topical preparations able to vehicle drugs to the retina via the conjunctival-scleral route in a safe and non-invasive way. Intravitreal administration is more invasive but may be useful to obtain sustained drug release (e.g., intravitreal pazopanib-loaded nanotubes)	Pre-clinical	• Small size allows for sub-cellular targeting • Water-insoluble drug loading capacity • Simple and stable structure with spontaneous formation and low aggregation tendency • Long circulation time (by-pass hepatic macrophages)	• Considerably susceptible to environmental changes: easy content precipitation • Hydrophobic load only
	Nanospheres and nanocapsules	Self-assembling polymeric nanospheres and nanocapsules	Pre-clinical	• Easy formation: self-assembling • Uniform drug-load distribution: less inflammatory	• Low drug-loading efficacy • Need encapsulation in polymeric delivery systems
	Solid lipids	Solid lipid core stabilized by surfactants. Stable, extremely resistant (autoclave), and economic	Pre-clinical	• Resisting (autoclave) and long standing structure • Biodegradable • Inexpensive production	• Susceptible to content expulsion during storage • Hydrophobic load only
	Dendrimers	Ramified polymers consisting in a core with functional groups on its branches Intravitreal steroids, subconjunctival antiblastic, and topical antiglaucomatous molecules have been tested on animal models	Pre-clinical	• Good targeting capability • Versatile structure • Advantageous slow clearance in target tissues	• Potentially cytotoxic

Table 1. *Cont.*

		Brief Description	Developmental Stage	Advantages	Disadvantages
Nanomedicine	Organic nanopolymers	Chemical compounds acting as carrier for retinal drugs including dexamethasone and anti-VEGF, enhancing their bioavailability and targeting and prolonging their release	Pre-clinical	• Biocompatible, stable, biodegradable materials with well-documented safety profile in humans • Easily targetable compounds • Can be combined with different nanoparticles • Blood–retina barrier crossing documented in vivo	• Corneal and vitreous opacification and inflammation reported with PVP • PLGA presents weak protein stability, inefficient drug loading, abrupt release profile • Crystallinity alteration induced by copolymers.
	Chitosan	Highly diffuse polysaccharide used for decades in pharmaceutics. Versatile penetration enhancer employed as a coating or component of different drug-loaded particles and drug delivery systems.	Approved products containing chitosan	• Natural molecule with no cititoxicity • High biocompatibility and biodegradability • Mucoadhesive nature	
	Metals and other inorganic materials	Metallic nanoparticles with intrinsic therapeutic properties. Magnetism can be used to direct ab-externo metallic nanocarriers to target tissues (e.g., helical vectors containing iron and nickel)	Pre-clinical	• Antiangiogenic activity (silver, gold, silicate) • Inflammatory effects (gold) • Ability to reduce vascular permeability (silver) • Antiapoptotic and antioxidant action (nanoceria)	• Poor biodegradability and clearance • Potentially toxic and cell damage (photoreceptors) • Compromise BRB integrity
	Encapsulated cells	Implantable polymeric scaffold containing human RPE cells secreting growth factors	Pre-clinical	• Sustained secretion from living cells • Potentially applicable to multiple types of cells and diseases	• Invasive implantation • Metallic device, not biodegradable
Topical drugs penetration enhancers	Cell-penetrating peptides	Short chains of peptides trespassing membranes. Studied on animal models of choroidal neovascularization, retinal neovascularization and oxygen-induced retinopathy	Pre-clinical	• High targetability • No cytotoxicity • Non-corneal pathways involved	
	Cyclodextrins	Oligosaccharides with a truncated cone-shape, more lipophilic centrally and a more hydrophilic on the outer surface, which can be used to aggregate with and augment the topical absorption of hydrophobic drugs	P2	• Biodegradable molecules • Good protection and stabilization of the carried drug • Improved solubility, bioadhesion, and permeation of the treatment • Targeted and sustained drug delivery	• Poor hydrosolubility and affinity with hydrophobic drugs, requiring addition of moieties

Table 1. *Cont.*

		Brief Description	Developmental Stage	Advantages	Disadvantages
Topical drugs penetration enhancers	Benzalkonium chloride	Enhancing penetration by breaking down tight junction of corneal epithelia.	Pre-clinical as enhancer for posterior segment disease treatment	• Widely used and approved molecule	• Intrinsic damage to ocular barriers
	Iontophoresis	Application of low-amplitude electrical current to vehicle drugs across the conjunctival-scleral barrier	P1 (Visulex) Launched (EyeGate II)	• Anterior ocular surface sparing technique (transconjunctival-transscleral pathway)	• Expensive technology • Dedicated device and drug formulation required • Concerns about skin exposure to prolonged electric current
Sustained Drug-release Systems	Ocular inserts	Sterile, non-implantable, thin, multi-layered routes of administration with solid or semisolid consistency	Pre-clinical	• Increased contact time/bioavailability • Long-lasting, controlled, and precise release • Minimal systemic absorption • Reduced administration frequency	• Patient non-compliance with foreign body sensation • Difficulty in self-insertion or removal • Potential accidental loss • Potential obstacle to vision due to movement around the eye
	Non-biodegradable Ocular Implants	Scleral and intrascleral (disc) implants and intravitreal implants (encapsulated cells) which do not experience change in structure and are made up of ethylene vinyl acetate, polyvinyl alcohol, polysulfone capillary fiber	Approved	• Prolonged drug release • Improved drug bioavailability • Enhanced therapeutic efficacy • Reduced dosing frequency	• Surgical procedure • Non-biodegradable • Irreversibility • Limited drug flexibility • Implant-related complications
	Biodegradable Ocular Implants	Injectable microparticles, intravitreal implant (injectable rod), intra-scleral and epi-scleral implant (disc, plug) which degrade and disintegrate over time. They are made up of polylactic acid, polyglycolic acid, PLGA, or polycaprolactones	Approved		
	Hydrogels	Three-dimensional network structures of crosslinked hydrophilic monomers which can deliver drugs via multiple administration routes such as topical administration, intracameral injection and intravitreal injection	Pre-clinical	• Controlled and sustained drug release • Site-specific drug delivery • Enhanced drug stability and penetration • Possible combination therapy	• Limited drug-loading capacity • Difficulty penetrating dense ocular tissues • Lack of long-term stability

Table 1. *Cont.*

		Brief Description	Developmental Stage	Advantages	Disadvantages
Sustained Drug-release Systems	Contact lens	Contact lenses act as a drug-reservoir, incorporating functional monomers or nanoparticles in a polymeric matrix	Pre-clinical or approved	• Targeted delivery • Prolonged drug release • Improved bioavailability • Enhanced patient comfort • Non-invasive approach	• Limited drug capacity • Variable drug release • Individual variability • Limited drug selection
	Microneedles	Drug-loaded arrays of microneedles, inserted in sclera/suprachoroidal space	Pre-clinical or approved	• Enhanced targeted delivery • Improved drug bioavailability • Non-invasive method • Sustained release • Preservation of drug integrity	• Technical challenges • Possible risk of ocular damage and infection • Limited drug payload • Limited stability and shelf life

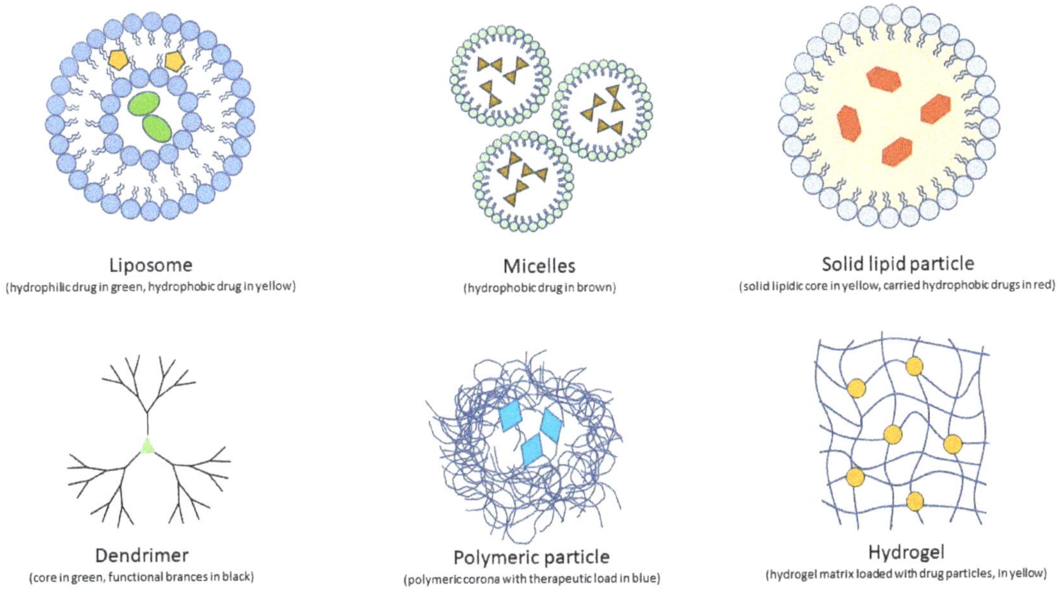

Figure 2. Material used in Drug Delivery Systems (DDSs).

Apart from nanotechnologies, other systems have been developed and studied to enhance drug delivery. CPPs, for example, are characterized by a general lack of cell and tissue specificity. Although TAT and penetrates were seen to somehow accumulate in the retina after topical administration, the use of specific CPPs to target different eye structures demands further investigation since the available data derive from studies using different in vivo models and conditions. In vivo experiments are generally conducted on rats or mice. This is often a necessary choice, and differences between murine and human eyes in relevant aspects, including ocular volumes and delivery path lengths, must be considered when interpreting the results of this type of study. Furthermore, evidence of ocular toxicity and uptake of CPPs is collected with experiments on isolated human conjunctival/corneal/RPE cell lines. Although these in vitro results are considered more replicable and less susceptible to effects derived from species-dependent differences, some drawbacks remain. The first difficulty derives from the differences in CPP behavior in different cell lines. For example, it is known that non-adherent cell lines show a higher permeability toward CPPs [243]. A second issue concerns the prediction of the results obtained in vitro when translated in vivo. In the latter set-up, not only pharmacokinetic factors, such as lacrimal wash-out and blood and lymphatic absorption, but also a different CPP interaction with cells integrated in an organized tissue and organism could make the difference. For instance, a reduction in the cellular uptake of peptides for ocular delivery was observed after incubation with proteoglycans, which are naturally present on the cellular surface and intercellular spaces in vivo [138].

Iontophoresis seems to offer a potential route to enhance the transscleral-transconjunctival absorption of topical drugs directed to the vitreous and retina. Again, preclinical studies have been conducted on animals, and some concerns have emerged regarding safety due to the exposure to prolonged electric current and feasibility in terms of logistic and technological costs, especially in comparison to other topical treatments [122].

Different types of implants and inserts have been proposed to grant the controlled and sustained release of ocular drugs, reducing the number of drug administrations, with benefits on the patient comfort and compliance, and reducing the number of necessary accesses to the health care providers for treatment and monitoring. These devices, however, have some limitations. The positioning and size of the implant must be considered to avoid vision obscuration. To this extent, injection of particles below 300 nm is recommended. Light scattering and other vision disturbances can occur because of the aggregation of particles after injection into the vitreous. Systems allowing the sustained release of drugs from nanoparticles may thus offer an advantage. Even with modern technology, it is still rather challenging to load a sufficient amount of drug into small particles, which need to be released for at least a few weeks after a single administration. This factor represents the true bottleneck in developing a successful intravitreal treatment of this kind. For these reasons, sustained efficacy of action in the posterior segment might be achieved by subconjunctival injection of products with slow choroidal clearance or by using a formulation that provides gradually releasing drugs in the suprachoroidal space. Overall, research in this sector only produced a few implants now available for clinical use, with some of the most promising solutions, such as nanotechnologies, not really translating the good results obtained in preclinical studies into clinical trials. Furthermore, according to some authors, this might also be due to the scarce investment of nanotechnologies in the development of neurological and ocular treatments, with more tangible efforts made to develop oncological and imaging agents [123].

Despite these considerations, the existence of different types of implants and polymeric materials, with many of them already approved for clinical use, and the continuous development of new drugs to treat diffuse pathologies, such as AMD and RD, makes efficiency in drug delivery a highly dynamic field with interesting and crucial applications. Therapeutic efficacy is certainly the primary objective of any DDS; however, a patient's comfort is also crucial since it considerably affects compliance with treatment, which is also a key factor, especially when it comes to ocular treatments. More trials on existing technologies and the development of new strategies will allow for advancements in therapeutic efficiency with reduced side effects and better compliance in treating pathologies of the posterior ocular segment.

Author Contributions: Conceptualization, A.G., M.Z. and L.F.; methodology, A.G., M.Z. and L.F.; validation, A.G., M.Z., L.F. and C.S.; formal analysis, A.G. and L.F.; investigation, A.G. and L.F.; resources, C.S.; writing—original draft preparation, A.G. and L.F.; writing—review and editing A.G., M.Z. and L.F.; visualization, A.G., M.Z., L.F. and C.S.; supervision, M.Z. and C.S.; project administration, M.Z. and C.S. All authors have read and agreed to the published version of the manuscript.

Funding: This research received no external funding.

Institutional Review Board Statement: Not applicable.

Informed Consent Statement: Not applicable.

Data Availability Statement: Not applicable.

Conflicts of Interest: The authors declare no conflict of interest.

References

1. Edelhauser, H.F.; Rowe-Rendleman, C.L.; Robinson, M.R.; Dawson, D.G.; Chader, G.J.; Grossniklaus, H.E.; Rittenhouse, K.D.; Wilson, C.G.; Weber, D.A.; Kuppermann, B.D.; et al. Ophthalmic Drug Delivery Systems for the Treatment of Retinal Diseases: Basic Research to Clinical Applications. *Investig. Opthalmology Vis. Sci.* **2010**, *51*, 5403–5420. [CrossRef] [PubMed]
2. Thrimawithana, T.R.; Young, S.; Bunt, C.R.; Green, C.; Alany, R.G. Drug delivery to the posterior segment of the eye. *Drug Discov. Today* **2011**, *16*, 270–277. [CrossRef] [PubMed]
3. Bansal, P.; Garg, S.; Sharma, Y.; Venkatesh, P. Posterior Segment Drug Delivery Devices: Current and Novel Therapies in Development. *J. Ocul. Pharmacol. Ther.* **2016**, *32*, 135–144. [CrossRef]
4. Awwad, S.; Ahmed, A.H.M.; Sharma, G.; Heng, J.S.; Khaw, P.T.; Brocchini, S.; Lockwood, A. Principles of pharmacology in the eye. *Br. J. Pharmacol.* **2017**, *174*, 4205–4223. [CrossRef]
5. Gholizadeh, S.; Wang, Z.; Chen, X.; Dana, R.; Annabi, N. Advanced nanodelivery platforms for topical ophthalmic drug delivery. *Drug Discov. Today* **2021**, *26*, 1437–1449. [CrossRef] [PubMed]
6. Löscher, M.; Seiz, C.; Hurst, J.; Schnichels, S. Topical Drug Delivery to the Posterior Segment of the Eye. *Pharmaceutics* **2022**, *14*, 134. [CrossRef] [PubMed]
7. Kang-Mieler, J.J.; Rudeen, K.M.; Liu, W.; Mieler, W.F. Advances in ocular drug delivery systems. *Eye* **2020**, *34*, 1371–1379. [CrossRef]

8. Yadav, D.; Varma, L.T.; Yadav, K. Drug delivery to posterior segment of the eye: Conventional delivery strategies their barriers and restrictions. In *Drug Delivery for the Retina and Posterior Segment Disease*; Patel, J.K., Sutariya, V., Kanwar, J.R., Pathak, Y.V., Eds.; Springer: Cham, Switzerland, 2018; pp. 51–67. [CrossRef]
9. Akhter, M.H.; Ahmad, I.; Alshahrani, M.Y.; Al-Harbi, A.I.; Khalilullah, H.; Afzal, O.; Altamimi, A.S.A.; Najib Ullah, S.N.M.; Ojha, A.; Karim, S. Drug Delivery Challenges and Current Progress in Nanocarrier-Based Ocular Therapeutic System. *Gels* **2022**, *8*, 82. [CrossRef]
10. Wang, R.; Gao, Y.; Liu, A.; Zhai, G. A review of nanocarrier-mediated drug delivery systems for posterior segment eye disease: Challenges analysis and recent advances. *J. Drug Target.* **2021**, *29*, 687–702. [CrossRef]
11. Joseph, R.R.; Venkatraman, S.S. Drug delivery to the eye: What benefits do nanocarriers offer? *Nanomedicine* **2017**, *12*, 683–702. [CrossRef]
12. Urtti, A.; Salminen, L. Minimizing systemic absorption of topically administered ophthalmic drugs. *Surv. Ophthalmol.* **1993**, *37*, 435–456. [CrossRef] [PubMed]
13. Urtti, A. Challenges and obstacles of ocular pharmacokinetics and drug delivery. *Adv. Drug Deliv. Rev.* **2006**, *58*, 1131–1135. [CrossRef] [PubMed]
14. Maurice, D.M.; Mishima, S. Ocular pharmacokinetics. In *Handbook of Experimental Pharmacology*; Sears, M.L., Ed.; Springer: Berlin/Heidelberg, Germany, 1984; Volume 69, pp. 16–119.
15. Hornof, M.; Toropainen, E.; Urtti, A. Cell culture models of the ocular barriers. *Eur. J. Pharm. Biopharm.* **2005**, *60*, 207–225. [CrossRef]
16. Prausnitz, M.R.; Noonan, J.S. Permeability of cornea, sclera, and conjunctiva: A literature analysis for drug delivery to the eye. *J. Pharm. Sci.* **1998**, *87*, 1479–1488. [CrossRef]
17. Hämäläinen, K.M.; Kontturi, K.; Murtomäki, L.; Auriola, S.; Urtti, A. Estimation of pore size and porosity of biomembranes from permeability measurements of polyethylene glycols using an effusion-like approach. *J. Control. Release* **1997**, *49*, 97–104. [CrossRef]
18. Geroski, D.H.; Edelhauser, H.F. Transscleral drug delivery for posterior segment disease. *Adv. Drug Deliv. Rev.* **2001**, *52*, 37–48. [CrossRef] [PubMed]
19. Hämäläinen, K.M.; Kananen, K.; Auriola, S.; Kontturi, K.; Urtti, A. Characterization of paracellular aqueous penetration routes in cornea conjunctiva sclera. *Investig. Ophthalmol. Vis. Sci.* **1997**, *38*, 627–634.
20. Raghava, S.; Hammond, M.; Kompella, U.B. Periocular routes for retinal drug delivery. *Exp. Opin. Drug Deliv.* **2004**, *1*, 99–114. [CrossRef]
21. Loftsson, T.; Sigurdsson, H.H.; Konrádsdóttir, F.; Gísladóttir, S.; Jansook, P.; Stefánsson, E. Topical drug delivery to the posterior segment of the eye: Anatomical and physiological considerations. *Pharmazie* **2008**, *63*, 171–179.
22. Tawfik, M.; Chen, F.; Goldberg, J.L.; Sabel, B.A. Nanomedicine and drug delivery to the retina: Current status and implications for gene therapy. *Naunyn-Schmiedeberg's Arch. Pharmacol.* **2022**, *395*, 1477–1507. [CrossRef]
23. Cunha-Vaz, J.G. The blood-retinal barriers. *Doc. Ophthalmol.* **1976**, *41*, 287–327. [CrossRef]
24. Das, S.; Suresh, P.K. Drug delivery to the eye: Special reference to nanoparticle. *Int. J. Drug Deliv.* **2010**, *2*, 12–21. [CrossRef]
25. Zamboulis, A.; Nanaki, S.; Michailidou, G.; Koumentakou, I.; Lazaridou, M.; Ainali, N.M.; Xanthopoulou, E.; Bikiaris, D.N. Chitosan and its Derivatives for Ocular Delivery Formulations: Recent Advances and Developments. *Polymers* **2020**, *12*, 1519. [CrossRef] [PubMed]
26. Almeida, H.; Amaral, M.H.; Lobão, P.; Silva, A.C.; Lobo, J.M.S. Applications of polymeric and lipid nanoparticles in ophthalmic pharmaceutical formulations: Present and future considerations. *J. Pharm. Sci.* **2014**, *17*, 278–293. [CrossRef] [PubMed]
27. Lai, S.K.; O'Hanlon, D.E.; Harrold, S.; Man, S.T.; Wang, Y.Y.; Cone, R.; Hanes, J. Rapid transport of large polymeric nanoparticles in fresh undiluted human mucus. *Proc. Natl. Acad. Sci. USA* **2007**, *104*, 1482–1487. [CrossRef] [PubMed]
28. Lai, S.K.; Wang, Y.Y.; Hida, K.; Cone, R.; Hanes, J. Nanoparticles reveal that human cervicovaginal mucus is riddled with pores larger than viruses. *Proc. Natl. Acad. Sci. USA* **2010**, *107*, 598–603. [CrossRef]
29. Kompella, U.B.; Amrite, A.C.; Pacha Ravi, R.; Durazo, S.A. Nanomedicines for back of the eye drug delivery, gene delivery, and imaging. *Prog. Retin. Eye Res.* **2013**, *36*, 172–198. [CrossRef]
30. Kaur, I.P.; Kakkar, S. Nanotherapy for posterior eye diseases. *J. Control. Release* **2014**, *193*, 100–112. [CrossRef]
31. Liu, H.-A.; Liu, Y.-L.; Ma, Z.-Z.; Wang, J.-C.; Zhang, Q. A Lipid Nanoparticle System Improves siRNA Efficacy in RPE Cells and a Laser-Induced Murine CNV Model. *Investig. Opthalmol. Vis. Sci.* **2011**, *52*, 4789–4794. [CrossRef]
32. Gross, N.; Ranjbar, M.; Evers, C.; Hua, J.; Schulze, B.; Michaelis, U.; Hansen, L.L.; Agostini, H.T. Choroidal neovascularization reduced by targeted drug delivery with cationic liposome-encapsulated paclitaxel or targeted photodynamic therapy with verteporfin encapsulated in cationic liposomes. *Mol. Vis.* **2013**, *19*, 54.
33. Crommelin, D.J.; van Hoogevest, P.; Storm, G. The role of liposomes in clinical nanomedicine development. What now? Now what? *J. Control. Release* **2020**, *318*, 256–263. [CrossRef]
34. Gu, Y.; Xu, C.; Wang, Y.; Zhou, X.; Fang, L.; Cao, F. Multifunctional nanocomposites based on liposomes layered double hydroxides conjugated with glycylsarcosine for efficient topical drug delivery to the posterior segment of the eye. *Mol. Pharm.* **2019**, *16*, 2845–2857. [CrossRef] [PubMed]
35. Kamaleddin, M.A. Nano-ophthalmology: Applications and considerations. *Nanomedicine* **2017**, *13*, 1459–1472. [CrossRef] [PubMed]

36. Lv, H.; Zhang, S.; Wang, B.; Cui, S.; Yan, J. Toxicity of cationic lipids and cationic polymers in gene delivery. *J. Control. Release* **2006**, *114*, 100–109. [CrossRef] [PubMed]
37. Bochot, A.; Fattal, E. Liposomes for intravitreal drug delivery: A state of the art. *J. Control. Release* **2012**, *161*, 628–634. [CrossRef]
38. Bachu, R.D.; Chowdhury, P.; Al-Saedi, Z.H.; Karla, P.K.; Boddu, S.H.S. Ocular drug delivery barriers—Role of nanocarriers in the treatment of anterior segment ocular diseases. *Pharmaceutics* **2018**, *10*, 28. [CrossRef]
39. Cholkar, K.; Patel, A.; Dutt Vadlapudi, A.K.; Mitra, A. Novel nanomicellar formulation approaches for anterior posterior segment ocular drug delivery. *Recent Pat. Nanomed.* **2012**, *2*, 82–95. [CrossRef]
40. Patel, A.; Cholkar, K.; Agrahari, V.; Mitra, A.K. Ocular drug delivery systems: An overview. *World J. Pharmacol.* **2013**, *2*, 47–64. [CrossRef]
41. Mandal, A.; Cholkar, K.; Khurana, V.; Shah, A.; Agrahari, V.; Bishit, R.; Pal, D.; Mitra, A.K. Topical formulation of self-assembled antiviral prodrug nanomicelles for targeted retinal delivery. *Mol. Pharm.* **2017**, *14*, 2056–2069. [CrossRef]
42. Cholkar, K.; Gunda, S.; Earla, R.; Pal, D.; Mitra, A.K. Nanomicellar Topical Aqueous Drop Formulation of Rapamycin for Back-of-the-Eye Delivery. *AAPS PharmSciTech* **2015**, *16*, 610–622. [CrossRef]
43. Velagaleti, P.R.; Anglade, E.; Khan, I.J.; Gilger, B.C. Topical delivery of hydrophobic drugs using a novel mixed nanomicellar technology to treat diseases of the anterior and posterior segments of the eye. *Drug Deliv. Technol.* **2010**, *10*, 42–47.
44. Alshamrani, M.; Sikder, S.; Coulibaly, F.; Mandal, A.; Pal, D.; Mitra, A.K. Self-assembling topical nanomicellar formulation to improve curcumin absorption across ocular tissues. *AAPS PharmSciTech* **2019**, *20*, 254. [CrossRef] [PubMed]
45. Mandal, A.; Gote, V.; Pal, D.; Ogundele, A.; Mitra, A.K. Ocular pharmacokinetics of a topical ophthalmic nanomicellar solution of cyclosporine Cequa®for dry eye disease. *Pharm. Res.* **2019**, *36*, 36. [CrossRef]
46. Vadlapudi, A.D.; Mitra, A.K. Nanomicelles: An emerging platform for drug delivery to the eye. *Ther. Deliv.* **2013**, *4*, 1–3. [CrossRef] [PubMed]
47. Vadlapudi, A.D.; Cholkar, K.; Vadlapatla, R.K.; Mitra, A.K. Aqueous nanomicellar formulation for topical delivery of biotinylated lipid prodrug of acyclovir: Formulation development and ocular biocompatibility. *J. Ocul. Pharmacol. Ther.* **2014**, *30*, 49–58. [CrossRef]
48. Trivedi, R.; Kompella, U.B. Nanomicellar formulations for sustained drug delivery: Strategies and underlying principles. *Nanomedicine* **2010**, *5*, 485–505. [CrossRef] [PubMed]
49. Ideta, R.; Yanagi, Y.; Tamaki, Y.; Tasaka, F.; Harada, A.; Kataoka, K. Effective accumulation of polyion complex micelle to experimental choroidal neovascularization in rats. *FEBS Lett.* **2004**, *557*, 21–25. [CrossRef]
50. Panda, J.J.; Yandrapu, S.; Kadam, R.S.; Chauhan, V.S.; Kompella, U.B. Self-assembled phenylalanine-α β-dehydrophenylalanine nanotubes for sustained intravitreal delivery of a multi-targeted tyrosine kinase inhibitor. *J. Control. Release* **2013**, *172*, 1151. [CrossRef]
51. Honda, M.; Asai, T.; Oku, N.; Araki, Y.; Tanaka, M.; Ebihara, N. Liposomes and nanotechnology in drug development: Focus on ocular targets. *Int. J. Nanomed.* **2013**, *8*, 495–504. [CrossRef]
52. Apaolaza, P.S.; Del Pozo-Rodriguez, A.; Solinis, M.A.; Rodriguez, J.M.; Friedrich, U.; Torrecilla, J.; Weber, B.H.F.; Rodríguez-Gascón, A. Structural recovery of the retina in a retinoschisin-deficient mouse after gene replacement therapy by solid lipid nanoparticles. *Biomaterials* **2016**, *90*, 40–49. [CrossRef]
53. Kalomiraki, M.; Thermos, K.; Chaniotakis, N.A. Dendrimers as tunable vectors of drug delivery systems and biomedical and ocular applications. *Int. J. Nanomed.* **2016**, *11*, 1.
54. Kokaz, S.F.; Deb, P.K.; Borah, P.; Bania, R.; Venugopala, K.N.; Nair, A.B.; Singh, V.; Al-Shar'I, N.A.; Hourani, W.; Tekade, R.K. Dendrimers: Properties and applications in biomedical field. *Nanoeng. Biomater.* **2022**, *2*, 215–243.
55. Yavuz, B.; Pehlivan, S.B.; Vural, I.; Ünlü, N. In Vitro/In Vivo Evaluation of Dexamethasone—PAMAM Dendrimer Complexes for Retinal Drug Delivery. *J. Pharm. Sci.* **2015**, *104*, 3814–3823. [CrossRef] [PubMed]
56. Whitcup, S.M.; Nussenblatt, R.B.; Lightman, S.L.; Hollander, D.A. Inflammation in Retinal Disease. *Int. J. Inflamm.* **2013**, *2013*, 724648. [CrossRef] [PubMed]
57. Iezzi, R.; Guru, B.R.; Glybina, I.V.; Mishra, M.K.; Kennedy, A.; Kannan, R.M. Dendrimer-based targeted intravitreal therapy for sustained attenuation of neuroinflammation in retinal degeneration. *Biomaterials* **2012**, *33*, 979–988. [CrossRef]
58. Kambhampati, S.P.; Clunies-Ross, A.J.M.; Bhutto, I.; Mishra, M.; Edwarda, M.; McLeod, D.S.; Kannan, R.M.; Lutty, G. Systemic and Intravitreal Delivery of Dendrimers to Activated Microglia/Macrophage in Ischemia/Reperfusion Mouse Retina. *Investig. Opthalmol. Vis. Sci.* **2015**, *56*, 4413–4424. [CrossRef]
59. Lancina, M.G., III; Singh, S.; Kompella, U.B.; Husain, S.; Yang, H. Fast dissolving dendrimer nanofiber mats as alternative to eye drops for more efficient antiglaucoma drug delivery. *ACS Biomater. Sci. Eng.* **2017**, *3*, 1861–1868. [CrossRef]
60. Mishra, V.; Jain, N.K. Acetazolamide encapsulated dendritic nano-architectures for effective glaucoma management in rabbits. *Int. J. Pharm.* **2014**, *461*, 380–390. [CrossRef]
61. Kang, S.J.; Durairaj, C.; Kompella, U.B.; O'Brien, J.M.; Grossniklaus, H.E. Subconjunctival nanoparticle carboplatin in the treatment of murine retinoblastoma. *Arch. Ophthalmol.* **2009**, *127*, 1043–1047. [CrossRef]
62. Albertazzi, L.; Gherardini, L.; Brondi, M.; Sato, S.S.; Bifone, A.; Pizzorusso, T.; Ratto, G.M.; Bardi, G. In vivo distribution and toxicity of PAMAM dendrimers in the central nervous system depend on their surface chemistry. *Mol. Pharm.* **2013**, *10*, 249–260. [CrossRef]

63. Robinson, B.V.; Sullivan, F.M.; Borzelleca, J.F.; Schwartz, S.L. *PVP: A Critical Review of the Kinetics and Toxicology of Polyvinylpyrrolidone Povidone*; CRC Press: Boca Raton, FL, USA, 2018.
64. Bruining, M.J.; Edelbroek-Hoogendoorn, P.S.; Blaauwgeers, H.G.; Mooyh, C.M.; Hendrikse, F.H.; Koole, L.H. New biodegradable networks of poly(N-vinylpyrrolidinone) designed for controlled nonburst degradation in the vitreous body. *J. Biomed. Mater. Res.* **1999**, *47*, 189–197. [CrossRef]
65. Hong, Y.; Chirila, T.V.; Vijayasekaran, S.; Dalton, P.D.; Tahija, S.G.; Cuypers, M.J.; Constable, I.J. Crosslinked poly-1-vinyl-2-pyrrolidinone as a vitreous substitute. *J. Biomed. Mater. Res.* **1996**, *30*, 441–448. [CrossRef]
66. Gupta, S.V. Physicochemical requirements for polymers and poly-mer-based nanomaterial for ophthalmic drug delivery. In *Nano-Biomaterials for Ophthalmic Drug Delivery*; Pathak, Y., Sutariya, V., Hirani, A.A., Eds.; Springer: Cham, Switzerland, 2016; pp. 131–146.
67. Tawfik, M.; Zhang, X.; Grigartzik, L.; Heiduschka, P.; Hintz, W.; Heinrich-Noack, P.; van Wachem, B.; Bernhard, A.S. Gene therapy with caspase-3 small interfering RNA-nanoparticles is neuroprotective after optic nerve damage. *Neural Regen. Res.* **2021**, *16*, 2534. [PubMed]
68. Colthurst, M.J.; Williams, R.L.; Hiscott, P.S.; Grierson, I. Biomaterials used in the posterior segment of the eye. *Biomaterials* **2000**, *21*, 649–665. [CrossRef]
69. Zhang, L.; Li, Y.; Zhang, C.; Wang, Y.; Song, C. Pharmacokinetics and tolerance study of intravitreal injection of dexamethasone-loaded nanoparticles in rabbits. *Int. J. Nanomed.* **2009**, *4*, 175. [CrossRef]
70. Bisht, R.; Jaiswal, J.K.; Rupenthal, I.D. Nanoparticle-loaded biodegradable light-responsive in situ forming injectable implants for effective peptide delivery to the posterior segment of the eye. *Med. Hypotheses* **2017**, *103*, 5–9. [CrossRef] [PubMed]
71. Park, K.; Chen, Y.; Hu, Y.; Maypo, A.S.; Kompella, U.B.; Longera, R.; Ma, J. Nanoparticle-mediated expression of an angiogenic inhibitor ameliorates ischemia-induced retinal neovascularization and diabetes-induced retinal vascular leakage. *Diabetes* **2009**, *58*, 1902–1913. [CrossRef]
72. Singh, S.R.; Grossniklaus, H.E.; Kang, S.J.; Edelhauser, H.F.; Ambati, B.K.; Kompella, U.B. Intravenous transferrin RGD peptide dual-targeted nanoparticles enhance anti-VEGF intraceptor gene delivery to laser-induced CNV. *Gene Ther.* **2009**, *16*, 645–659. [CrossRef]
73. Salama, H.A.; Ghorab, M.; Mahmoud, A.A.; Hady, M.A. PLGA nanoparticles as subconjunctival injection for management of glaucoma. *AAPS PharmSciTech* **2017**, *18*, 2517–2528. [CrossRef]
74. Bourges, J.L.; Gautier, S.E.; Delie, F.; Bejjani, R.A.; Jeanny, J.; Gurny, R.; Benezra, D.; Behar-Cohen, F.F. Ocular drug delivery targeting the retinal pigment epithelium using polylactide nanoparticles. *Investig. Ophthalmol. Vis. Sci.* **2003**, *44*, 3562–3569. [CrossRef] [PubMed]
75. Sakai, T.; Kohno, H.; Ishihara, T.; Higaki, M.; Saito, S.; Matsushima, M.; Kitahara, K. Treatment of experimental autoimmune uveoretinitis with poly lactic acid nanoparticles encapsulating betamethasone phosphate. *Exp. Eye Res.* **2006**, *82*, 657–663. [CrossRef] [PubMed]
76. Fialho, S.L.; Behar-Cohen, F.; Silva-Cunha, A. Dexamethasone-loaded poly ε-caprolactone intravitreal implants: A pilot study. *Eur. J. Pharm. Biopharm.* **2008**, *68*, 637–646. [CrossRef] [PubMed]
77. Yenice, İ.; Mocan, M.C.; Palaska, E.; Bochot, A.; Bilensoy, E.; Vural, I.; Irkeç, M.; Hincal, A.A. Hyaluronic acid coated poly-ε-caprolactone nanospheres deliver high concentrations of cyclosporine A into the cornea. *Exp. Eye Res.* **2008**, *87*, 162–167. [CrossRef] [PubMed]
78. Yin, H.; Gong, C.; Shi, S.; Liu, X.; Wei, Y.; Qian, Z. Toxicity evaluation of biodegradable thermosensitive PEG-PCL-PEG hydrogel as a potential in situ sustained ophthalmic drug delivery system. *J. Biomed. Mater. Res. B Appl. Biomater.* **2010**, *92*, 129–137. [CrossRef]
79. Li, V.H.; Wood, R.W.; Kreuter, J.; Harmia, T.; Robinson, J.R. Ocular drug delivery of progesterone using nanoparticles. *J. Microencapsul.* **1986**, *3*, 213–218. [CrossRef]
80. Vote, B.J.; Elder, M.J. Cyanoacrylate glue for corneal perforations: A description of a surgical technique a review of the literature. *Clin. Exp. Ophthalmol.* **2000**, *28*, 437–442. [CrossRef]
81. Ramge, P.; Unger, R.E.; Oltrogge, J.B.; Zenker, D.; Begley, D.; Kreuter, J.; Von Briesen, H. Polysorbate-80 coating enhances uptake of polybutylcyanoacrylate PBCA -nanoparticles by human and bovine primary brain capillary endothelial cells. *Eur. J. Neurosci.* **2000**, *12*, 1931–1940. [CrossRef]
82. Leggat, P.A.; Smith, D.R.; Kedjarune, U. Surgical applications of cyanoacrylate adhesives: A review of toxicity. *ANZ J. Surg.* **2007**, *77*, 209–213. [CrossRef]
83. Wilson, B. Brain targeting PBCA nanoparticles and the blood–brain barrier. *Nanomedicine* **2009**, *4*, 499–502. [CrossRef]
84. Voigt, N.; Henrich-Noack, P.; Kockentiedt, S.; Hintz, W.; Tomas, J.; Sabel, B.A. Surfactants not size or zeta-potential influence blood–brain barrier passage of polymeric nanoparticles. *Eur. J. Pharm. Biopharm.* **2014**, *87*, 19–29. [CrossRef]
85. Voigt, N.; Henrich-Noack, P.; Kockentiedt, S.; Hintz, W.; Tomas, J.; Sabel, B.A. Toxicity of polymeric nanoparticles in vivo and in vitro. *J. Nanopart. Res.* **2014**, *16*, 2379. [CrossRef] [PubMed]
86. Sabel, B.A.; Engelmann, R.; Humphrey, M.F. In vivo confocal neuroimaging ICON of CNS neurons. *Nat. Med.* **1997**, *3*, 244–247. [CrossRef] [PubMed]
87. Prilloff, S.; Fan, J.; Henrich-Noack, P.; Sabel, B.A. In vivo confocal neuroimaging ICON: Non-invasive functional imaging of the mammalian CNS with cellular resolution. *Eur. J. Neurosci.* **2010**, *31*, 521–528. [CrossRef]

88. Henrich-Noack, P.; Prilloff, S.; Voigt, N.; Jin, J.; Hintz, W.; Tomas, J.; Sabel, B.A. In vivo visualisation of nanoparticle entry into central nervous system tissue. *Arch. Toxicol.* **2012**, *86*, 1099–1105. [CrossRef] [PubMed]
89. You, Q.; Hopf, T.; Hintz, W.; Rannabauer, S.; Voigt, N.; van Wachem, B.; Henrich-Noack, P.; Sabel, B.A. Major effects on blood-retinabarrier passage by minor alterations in design of polybutylcyanoacrylate nanoparticles. *J. Drug Target.* **2019**, *27*, 338–346. [CrossRef] [PubMed]
90. You, Q.; Sokolov, M.; Grigartzik, L.; Hintz, W.; van Wachem, B.; Henrich-Noack, P.; Sabel, B.A. How nanoparticle physicochemical parameters affect drug delivery to cells in the retina via systemic interactions. *Mol. Pharm.* **2019**, *16*, 5068–5075. [CrossRef]
91. Caramella, C.; Ferrari, F.; Bonferoni, M.C.; Rossi, S.; Sandri, G. Chitosan and Its Derivatives as Drug Penetration Enhancers. *J. Drug Deliv. Sci. Technol.* **2010**, *20*, 5–13. [CrossRef]
92. De Campos, A.M.; Sánchez, A.; Alonso, M.J. Chitosan nanoparticles: A new vehicle for the improvement of the delivery of drugs to the ocular surface. Application to cyclosporin A. *Int. J. Pharm.* **2001**, *224*, 159–168. [CrossRef]
93. Felt, O.; Furrer, P.; Mayer, J.M.; Plazonnet, B.; Buri, P.; Gurny, R. Topical use of chitosan in ophthalmology:Tolerance assessment and evaluation of precorneal retention. *Int. J. Pharm.* **1999**, *180*, 185–193. [CrossRef]
94. Taghe, S.; Mirzaeei, S. Preparation and characterization of novel, mucoadhesive of ofloxacin nanoparticles for ocular drug delivery. *Braz. J. Pharm. Sci.* **2019**, *55*, 1–12. [CrossRef]
95. Badiee, P.; Varshochian, R.; Rafiee-Tehrani, M.; Abedin Dorkoosh, F.; Khoshayand, M.R.; Dinarvand, R. Ocular implant containing bevacizumab-loaded chitosan nanoparticles intended for choroidal neovascularization treatment. *J. Biomed. Mater. Res. Part A* **2018**, *106*, 2261–2271. [CrossRef] [PubMed]
96. Elsaid, N.; Jackson, T.L.; Elsaid, Z.; Alqathama, A.; Somavarapu, S. PLGA microparticles entrapping chitosan-based nanoparticles for the ocular delivery of ranibizumab. *Mol. Pharm.* **2016**, *13*, 2923–2940. [CrossRef] [PubMed]
97. Silva, N.C.; Silva, S.; Sarmento, B.; Pintado, M. Chitosan nanoparticles for daptomycin delivery in oculartreatment of bacterial endophthalmitis. *Drug. Deliv.* **2015**, *22*, 885–893. [CrossRef] [PubMed]
98. Wang, Y.; Zhou, L.; Fang, L.; Cao, F. Multifunctional Carboxymethyl Chitosan Derivatives-Layered Double Hydroxide Hybrid Nanocomposites for Efficient Drug Delivery to the Posterior Segment of the Eye. *Acta Biomater.* **2020**, *104*, 104–114. [CrossRef]
99. Savin, C.L.; Popa, M.; Delaite, C.; Costuleanu, M.; Costin, D.; Peptu, C.A. Chitosan grafted-poly(ethyleneglycol) methacrylate nanoparticles as carrier for controlled release of bevacizumab. *Mater. Sci. Eng. C* **2019**, *98*, 843–860. [CrossRef]
100. Xu, X.; Sun, L.; Zhou, L.; Cheng, Y.; Cao, F. Functional chitosan oligosaccharide nanomicelles for topical ocular drug delivery of dexamethasone. *Carbohydr. Polym.* **2020**, *227*, 115356. [CrossRef]
101. Li, J.; Cheng, T.; Tian, Q.; Cheng, Y.; Zhao, L.; Zhang, X.; Qu, Y. A More Efficient Ocular Delivery System of Triamcinolone Acetonide as Eye Drop to the Posterior Segment of the Eye. *Drug Deliv.* **2019**, *26*, 188–198. [CrossRef]
102. Cheng, T.; Li, J.; Cheng, Y.; Zhang, X.; Qu, Y. Triamcinolone acetonide-chitosan coated liposomes efficiently treated retinal edema as eye drops. *Exp. Eye Res.* **2019**, *188*, 107805. [CrossRef]
103. Khalil, M.; Hasmi, U.; Riaz, R.; Rukh Abbas, S. Chitosan coated liposomes (CCL) containing triamcinolone acetonide for sustained delivery: A potential topical treatment for posterior segment diseases. *Int. J. Biol. Macromol.* **2020**, *143*, 483–491. [CrossRef]
104. Jiang, F.; Tang, Z.; Zhang, Y.; Ju, Y.; Gao, H.; Sun, N.; Liu, F.; Gu, P.; Zhang, W. Enhanced proliferation and differentiation of retinal progenitor cells through a self-healing injectable hydrogel. *Biomater. Sci.* **2019**, *7*, 2335–2347. [CrossRef]
105. Moreno, M.; Pow, P.Y.; Tabitha, T.S.T.; Nirmal, S.; Larsson, A.; Radhakrishnan, K.; Nirmal, J.; Quah, S.T.; Geifman Shochat, S.; Agrawal, R.; et al. Modulating release of ranibizumab and aflibercept from thiolated chitosan-based hydrogels for potential treatment of ocular neovascularization. *Expert Opin. Drug Deliv.* **2017**, *14*, 913–925. [CrossRef]
106. Nagai, N.; Saijo, S.; Song, Y.; Kaji, H.; Abe, T. A drug refillable device for transscleral sustained drug delivery to the retina. *Eur. J. Pharm. Biopharm.* **2019**, *136*, 184–191. [CrossRef]
107. Kim, J.H.; Kim, J.H.; Kim, K.W.; Kim, K.; Kim, M.H.; Yu, Y.S. Intravenously administered gold nanoparticles pass through the blood–retinal barrier depending on the particle size, and induce no retinal toxicity. *Nanotechnology* **2009**, *20*, 505101. [CrossRef] [PubMed]
108. Kalishwaralal, K.; Barathmanikanth, S.; Pandian, S.R.K.; Deepak, V.; Gurunathan, S. Silver nano—A trove for retinal therapies. *J. Control. Release* **2010**, *145*, 76–90. [CrossRef] [PubMed]
109. Sheikpranbabu, S.; Kalishwaralal, K.; Lee, K.J.; Vaidyanathan, R.; Eom, S.H.; Gurunathan, S. The inhibition of advanced glycation end-products-induced retinal vascular permeability by silver nanoparticles. *Biomaterials* **2010**, *31*, 2260–2271. [CrossRef] [PubMed]
110. Masse, F.; Ouellette, M.; Lamoureux, G.; Boisselier, E. Gold nanoparticles in ophthalmology. *Med. Res. Rev.* **2018**, *39*, 302–327. [CrossRef]
111. Giannaccini, M.; Pedicini, L.; De Matienzo, G.; Chiellini, F.; Dente, L.; Raffa, V. Magnetic nanoparticles: A strategy to target the choroidal layer in the posterior segment of the eye. *Sci. Rep.* **2017**, *7*, 43092. [CrossRef] [PubMed]
112. Kong, L.; Cai, X.; Zhou, X.; Wong, L.; Karakoti, A.S.; Seal, S.; McGinnis, J.F. Nanoceria extend photoreceptor cell lifespan in tubby mice by modulation of apoptosis/survival signaling pathways. *Neurobiol. Dis.* **2011**, *42*, 514–523. [CrossRef]
113. Kyosseva, S.V.; McGinnis, J.F. Cerium oxide nanoparticles as promising ophthalmic therapeutics for the treatment of retinal diseases. *World J. Ophthalmol.* **2015**, *5*, 23–30. [CrossRef]
114. Maccarone, R.; Tisi, A.; Passacantando, M.; Ciancaglini, M. Ophthalmic Applications of Cerium Oxide Nanoparticles. *J. Ocul. Pharmacol. Ther.* **2020**, *36*, 376–383. [CrossRef]
115. Wong, L.L.; Pye, Q.N.; Chen, L.; Seal, S.; McGinnis, J.F. Defining the Catalytic Activity of Nanoceria in the P23H-1 Rat, a Photoreceptor Degeneration Model. *PLoS ONE* **2015**, *10*, e0121977. [CrossRef] [PubMed]

116. Cai, X.; Seal, S.; McGinnis, J.F. Non-toxic retention of nanoceria in murine eyes. *Mol. Vis.* **2016**, *22*, 1176–1187. [PubMed]
117. Jo, D.H.; Kim, J.H.; Yu, Y.S.; Lee, T.G.; Kim, J.H. Antiangiogenic effect of silicate nanoparticle on retinal neovascularization induced by vascular endothelial growth factor. *Nanomedicine* **2012**, *8*, 784–791. [CrossRef] [PubMed]
118. Wu, Z.; Troll, J.; Jeong, H.H.; Wei, Q.; Stang, M.; Ziemssen, F.; Wang, Z.; Mingdong, D.; Schnichels, S.; Qui, T.; et al. A swarm of slippery micropropellers penetrates the vitreous body of the eye. *Sci. Adv.* **2018**, *4*, eaat4388. [CrossRef]
119. Jo, D.H.; Lee, T.G.; Kim, J.H. Nanotechnology and nanotoxicology in retinopathy. *Int. J. Mol. Sci.* **2011**, *12*, 8288–8301. [CrossRef]
120. Soderstjerna, E.; Bauer, P.; Cedervall, T.; Abdshill, H.; Johansson, F.; Englund Johansson, U. Silver and gold nanoparticles exposure to in vitro cultured retina—Studies on nanoparticle internalization, apoptosis, oxidative stress, glial- and microglial activity. *PLoS ONE* **2014**, *9*, e105359. [CrossRef]
121. Chan, Y.J.; Liao, P.L.; Tsai, C.H.; Cheng, Y.; Lin, F.; Ho, J.; Chen, C.; Li, C. Titanium dioxide nanoparticles impair the inner blood-retinal barrier and retinal electrophysiology through rapid ADAM17 activation claudin-5 degradation. *Part. Fibre Toxicol.* **2021**, *18*, 4. [CrossRef]
122. Zhang, K.; Hopkins, J.J.; Heier, J.S.; Birch, D.G.; Halperin, L.S.; Albini, T.A.; Brown, D.M.; Jaffe, G.J.; Tao, W.; Williams, G.A. Ciliary neurotrophic factor delivered by encapsulated cell intraocular implants for treatment of geographic atrophy in age-related macular degeneration. *Proc. Natl. Acad. Sci. USA* **2011**, *108*, 6241–6245. [CrossRef]
123. Zhang, K.; Zhang, L.; Weinreb, R.N. Ophthalmic drug discovery: Novel targets mechanisms for retinal diseases and glaucoma. *Nat. Rev. Drug Discov.* **2012**, *11*, 541–559. [CrossRef]
124. Wong, F.S.; Tsang, K.K.; Lo, A.C. Delivery of therapeutics to posterior eye segment: Cell-encapsulating systems. *Neural Regen. Res.* **2017**, *12*, 576–577.
125. Moiseev, R.V.; Morrison, P.W.J.; Steele, F.; Khutoryanskiy, V.V. Penetration Enhancers in Ocular Drug Delivery. *Pharmaceutics* **2019**, *11*, 321. [CrossRef] [PubMed]
126. Kaur, I.P.; Smitha, R. Penetration Enhancers and Ocular Bioadhesives: Two New Avenues for Ophthalmic Drug Delivery. *Drug Dev. Ind. Pharm.* **2002**, *28*, 353–369. [CrossRef] [PubMed]
127. Zambito, Y.; Di Colo, G. Chitosan and Its Derivatives as Intraocular Penetration Enhancers. *J. Drug Deliv. Sci. Technol.* **2010**, *20*, 45–52. [CrossRef]
128. Bechara, C.; Sagan, S. Cell-Penetrating Peptides: 20 Years Later, Where Do We Stand? *FEBS Lett.* **2013**, *587*, 1693–1702. [CrossRef] [PubMed]
129. Wang, Y.; Lin, H.; Lin, S.; Qu, J.; Xiao, J.; Huang, Y.; Xiao, Y.; Fu, X.; Yang, Y.; Li, X. Cell-Penetrating Peptide TAT-Mediated Delivery of Acidic FGF to Retina and Protection against Ischemia-Reperfusion Injury in Rats. *J. Cell. Mol. Med.* **2010**, *14*, 1998–2005. [CrossRef] [PubMed]
130. Zhang, X.; Li, Y.; Cheng, Y.; Tan, H.; Li, Z.; Qu, Y.; Mu, G.; Wang, F. Tat PTD-Endostatin: A Novel Anti-Angiogenesis Protein with Ocular Barrier Permeability via Eye-Drops. *Biochim. Biophys. Acta Gen. Subj.* **2015**, *1850*, 1140–1149. [CrossRef]
131. Li, Y.; Li, L.; Li, Z.; Sheng, J.; Zhang, X.; Feng, D.; Zhang, X.; Yin, F.; Wang, A.; Wang, F. Tat PTD-Endostatin-RGD: A Novel Protein with Anti-Angiogenesis Effect in Retina via Eye Drops. *Biochim. Biophys. Acta Gen. Subj.* **2016**, *1860*, 2137–2147. [CrossRef]
132. Chu, Y.; Chen, N.; Yu, H.; Mu, H.; He, B.; Hua, H.; Wang, A.; Sun, K. Topical Ocular Delivery to Laser-Induced Choroidal Neovascularization by Dual Internalizing RGD and TAT Peptide-Modified Nanoparticles. *Int. J. Nanomed.* **2017**, *12*, 1353–1368. [CrossRef]
133. Atlasz, T.; Werling, D.; Song, S.; Szabo, E.; Vaczy, A.; Kovari, P.; Tamas, A.; Reglodi, D.; Yu, R. Retinoprotective Effects of TAT-Bound Vasoactive Intestinal Peptide and Pituitary Adenylate Cyclase Activating Polypeptide. *J. Mol. Neurosci.* **2019**, *68*, 397–407. [CrossRef]
134. Liu, C.; Tai, L.; Zhang, W.; Wei, G.; Pan, W.; Lu, W. Penetratin, a Potentially Powerful Absorption Enhancer for Noninvasive Intraocular Drug Delivery. *Mol. Pharm.* **2014**, *11*, 1218–1227. [CrossRef]
135. Liu, C.; Jiang, K.; Tai, L.; Liu, Y.; Wei, G.; Lu, W.; Pan, W. Facile Noninvasive Retinal Gene Delivery Enabled by Penetratin. *ACS Appl. Mater. Interfaces* **2016**, *8*, 19256–19267. [CrossRef]
136. Jiang, K.; Gao, X.; Shen, Q.; Zhan, C.; Zhang, Y.; Xie, C.; Wei, G.; Lu, W. Discerning the Composition of Penetratin for Safe Penetration from Cornea to Retina. *Acta Biomater.* **2017**, *63*, 123–134. [CrossRef] [PubMed]
137. Yang, X.; Wang, L.; Li, L.; Han, M.; Tang, S.; Wang, T.; Han, J.; He, X.; He, X.; Wang, A.; et al. A Novel Dendrimer-Based Complex Co-Modified with Cyclic RGD Hexapeptide and Penetratin for Noninvasive Targeting and Penetration of the Ocular Posterior Segment. *Drug Deliv.* **2019**, *26*, 989–1001. [CrossRef] [PubMed]
138. Johnson, L.N.; Cashman, S.M.; Kumar-Singh, R. Cell-Penetrating Peptide for Enhanced Delivery of Nucleic Acids and Drugs to Ocular Tissues Including Retina and Cornea. *Mol. Ther.* **2008**, *16*, 107–114. [CrossRef] [PubMed]
139. De Cogan, F.; Hill, L.J.; Lynch, A.; Morgan-Warren, P.J.; Lechner, J.; Berwick, M.R.; Peacock, A.F.A.; Chen, M.; Scott, R.A.H.; Xu, H.; et al. Topical Delivery of Anti-VEGF Drugs to the Ocular Posterior Segment Using Cell-Penetrating Peptides. *Investig. Ophthalmol. Vis. Sci.* **2017**, *58*, 2578–2590. [CrossRef] [PubMed]
140. Sigurdsson, H.H.; Konradsdottir, F.; Loftsson, T.; Stefansson, E. Topical and systemic absorption in delivery of dexamethasone to the anterior and posterior segments of the eye. *Acta Ophthalmol. Scand.* **2007**, *85*, 598–602. [CrossRef]
141. Loftsson, T.; Hreinsdottir, D.; Stefansson, E. Cyclodextrin microparticles for drug delivery to the posterior segment of the eye: Aqueous dexamethasone eye drops. *J. Pharm. Pharmacol.* **2007**, *59*, 629–635. [CrossRef]

142. Tanito, M.; Hara, K.; Takai, Y.; Matsuoka, Y.; Nishimura, N.; Jansook, P.; Loftsson, T.; Stéfansson, E.; Ohira, A. Topical Dexamethasone-Cyclodextrin Microparticle Eye Drops for Diabetic Macular Edema. *Investig. Opthalmol. Vis. Sci.* **2011**, *52*, 7944–7948.
143. Ohira, A.; Hara, K.; Jóhannesson, G.; Tanito, M.; Ásgrímsdóttir, G.M.; Lund, S.H.; Loftsson, T.; Stéfansson, E. Topical dexamethasone γ-cyclodextrin nanoparticle eye drops increase visual acuity and decrease macular thickness in diabetic macular oedema. *Acta Ophthalmol.* **2015**, *93*, 610–615. [CrossRef]
144. Shulman, S.; Jóhannesson, G.; Stefánsson, E.; Loewenstein, A.; Rosenblatt, A.; Habot-Wilner, Z. Topical dexamethasone-cyclodextrin nanoparticle eye drops for non-infectious uveitic macular oedema and vitritis—A pilot study. *Acta Ophthalmol.* **2015**, *93*, 411–415. [CrossRef]
145. Krag, S.; Hessellund, A. Topical dexamethasone-cyclodextrin microparticle eye drops for uveitic macular oedema. *Acta Ophthalmol.* **2014**, *92*, e689–e690. [CrossRef]
146. Mahaling, B.; Katti, D.S. Understanding the Influence of Surface Properties of Nanoparticles and Penetration Enhancers for Improving Bioavailability in Eye Tissues In Vivo. *Int. J. Pharm.* **2016**, *501*, 1–9. [CrossRef]
147. Behar-Cohen, F.F.; El Aouni, A.; Gautier, S.; David, G.; Davis, J.; Chapon, P.; Parel, J.M. Transscleral Coulomb-controlled Iontophoresis of Methylprednisolone into the Rabbit Eye: Influence of Duration of Treatment, Current Intensity and Drug Concentration on Ocular Tissue and Fluid Levels. *Exp. Eye Res.* **2002**, *74*, 51–59. [CrossRef] [PubMed]
148. Güngör, S.; Delgado-Charro, M.B.; Ruiz-Perez, B.; Schubert, W.; Isom, P.; Moslemy, P.; Patane, M.A.; Guy, R.H. Trans-scleral iontophoretic delivery of low molecular weight therapeutics. *J. Control. Release* **2010**, *147*, 225–231. [CrossRef] [PubMed]
149. Cohen, A.E.; Assang, C.; Patane, M.A.; From, S.; Korenfeld, M.; Avion Study Investigators. Evaluation of dexamethasone phosphate delivered by ocular iontophoresis for treating noninfectious anterior uveitis. *Ophthalmology* **2012**, *119*, 66–73. [CrossRef] [PubMed]
150. Chopra, P.; Hao, J.; Li, S.K. Sustained release micellar carrier systems for iontophoretic transport of dexamethasone across human sclera. *J. Control. Release* **2012**, *160*, 96–104. [CrossRef] [PubMed]
151. Molokhia, S.A.; Jeong, E.K.; Higuchi, W.I.; Li, S.K. Examination of penetration routes distribution of ionic permeants during after transscleral iontophoresis with magnetic resonance imaging. *Int. J. Pharm.* **2007**, *335*, 46–53. [CrossRef]
152. Souza, J.G.; Dias, K.; Pereira, T.A.; Spuri Bernardi, D.; Lopez, R.F.V. Topical delivery of ocular therapeutics: Carrier systems physical methods. *J. Pharm. Pharmacol.* **2014**, *66*, 507–530. [CrossRef]
153. Dabral, K.; Uniyal, Y. Ocular inserts: Novel approach for drug delivery into eyes. *GSC Biol. Pharm. Sci.* **2019**, *7*, 001–007. [CrossRef]
154. Kumari, A.; Sharma, P.K.; Garg, V.K.; Garg, G. Ocular inserts—Advancement in therapy of eye diseases. *J. Adv. Pharm. Technol. Res.* **2010**, *1*, 291–296. [CrossRef] [PubMed]
155. Thakur, R.; Swami, G. Promising implication of ocuserts in ocular disease. *J. Drug Deliv. Ther.* **2012**, *2*, 2. [CrossRef]
156. Kearns, V.R.; Williams, R.L. Drug delivery systems for the eye. *Expert Rev. Med. Devices* **2009**, *6*, 277–290. [CrossRef]
157. Lee, S.S.; Hughes, P.; Ross, A.D.; Robinson, M.R. Biodegradable Implants for Sustained Drug Release in the Eye. *Pharm. Res.* **2010**, *27*, 2043–2053. [CrossRef]
158. Pelusi, L.; Mandatori, D.; Mastropasqua, L.; Agnifili, L.; Allegretti, M.; Nubile, M.; Pandolfi, A. Innovation in the Development of Synthetic and Natural Ocular Drug Delivery Systems for Eye Diseases Treatment: Focusing on Drug-Loaded Ocular Inserts, Contacts, and Intraocular Lenses. *Pharmaceutics* **2023**, *15*, 625. [CrossRef] [PubMed]
159. Brandt, J.D.; Sall, K.; DuBiner, H.; Benza, R.; Alster, Y.; Walker, G.; Semba, C.P. Six-month intraocular pressure reduction with a topical bimatoprost ocular insert: Results of a phase II randomized controlled study. *Ophthalmology* **2016**, *123*, 1685–1694. [CrossRef]
160. Manickavasagam, D.; Wehrung, D.; Chamsaz, E.A.; Sanders, M.; Bouhenni, R.; Crish, S.D.; Joy, A.; Oyewumi, M.O. Assessment of alkoxylphenacyl-based polycarbonates as a potential platform for controlled delivery of a model anti-glaucoma drug. *Eur. J. Pharm. Biopharm.* **2016**, *107*, 56–66. [CrossRef] [PubMed]
161. Franca, J.R.; Foureaux, G.; Fuscaldi, L.L.; Ribeiro, T.G.; Castilho, R.O.; Yoshida, I.M.; Cardoso, V.N.; Fernandes, S.O.A.; Cronemberg, S.; Nogueira, J.C.; et al. Chitosan/hydroxyethyl cellulose inserts for sustained-release of dorzolamide for glaucoma treatment: In vitro and in vivo evaluation. *Int. J. Pharm.* **2019**, *570*, 118662. [CrossRef] [PubMed]
162. Wang, L.; Jiang, Y.-Y.; Lin, N. Promise of latanoprost and timolol loaded combinatorial nanosheet for therapeutic applications in glaucoma. *J. King Saud Univ. Sci.* **2020**, *32*, 1042–1047. [CrossRef]
163. Dubald, M.; Bourgeois, S.; Andrieu, V.; Fessi, H. Ophthalmic Drug Delivery Systems for Antibiotherapy—A Review. *Pharmaceutics* **2018**, *10*, 10. [CrossRef]
164. Terreni, E.; Burgalassi, S.; Chetoni, P.; Tampucci, S.; Zucchetti, E.; Fais, R.; Ghelardi, E.; Lupetti, A.; Monti, D. Development and Characterization of a Novel Peptide-Loaded Antimicrobial Ocular Insert. *Biomolecules* **2020**, *10*, 664. [CrossRef]
165. Sadeghi, A.M.; Farjadian, F.; Alipour, S. Sustained release of linezolid in ocular insert based on lipophilic modified structure of sodium alginate. *Iran. J. Basic Med. Sci.* **2021**, *24*, 331–340.
166. Grimaudo, M.A.; Nicoli, A.; Santi, P.; Concheiro, A.; Alvarez-Lorenzo, C. Cyclosporine-loaded cross-linked inserts of sodium hyaluronan and hydroxypropyl-beta-cyclodextrin for ocular administration. *Carbohydr. Polym.* **2018**, *201*, 308–316. [CrossRef] [PubMed]
167. Grimaudo, M.A.; Concheiro, A.; Alvarez-Lorenzo, C. Crosslinked Hyaluronan Electrospun Nanofibers for Ferulic Acid Ocular Delivery. *Pharmaceutics* **2020**, *12*, 274. [CrossRef] [PubMed]

168. Mohammadi, G.; Mirzaeei, S.; Taghe, S.; Mohammadi, P. Preparation and Evaluation of EudragitI L100 Nanoparticles Loaded Impregnated with KT Tromethamine Loaded PVA -HEC Insertions for Ophthalmic Drug Delivery. *Adv. Pharm. Bull.* **2019**, *9*, 593–600. [CrossRef]
169. Girgis, G.N.S. Formulation and Evaluation of Atorvastatin Calcium-Poly-epsilon-Caprolactone Nanoparticles Loaded Ocular Inserts for Sustained Release and Antiinflammatory Efficacy. *Curr. Pharm. Biotechnol.* **2020**, *21*, 1688–1698. [CrossRef] [PubMed]
170. Bertens, C.J.; Martino, C.; van Osch, M.C.; Lataster, A.; Dias, A.J.; Biggelaar, F.J.V.D.; Tuinier, R.; Nuijts, R.M.; Gijs, M. Design of the ocular coil, a new device for non-invasive drug delivery. *Eur. J. Pharm. Biopharm.* **2020**, *150*, 120–130. [CrossRef]
171. Bertens, C.J.F.; Gijs, M.; Dias, A.A.J.; Biggelaar, F.J.H.M.V.D.; Ghosh, A.; Sethu, S.; Nuijts, R.M.M.A. Pharmacokinetics and efficacy of a ketorolac-loaded ocular coil in New Zealand white rabbits. *Drug Deliv.* **2021**, *28*, 400–407. [CrossRef]
172. Thakkar, S.; Misra, M. Electrospun polymeric nanofibers: New horizons in drug delivery. *Eur. J. Pharm. Sci.* **2017**, *107*, 148–167. [CrossRef]
173. Singla, J.; Bajaj, T.; Goyal, A.K.; Rath, G. Development of Nanofibrous Ocular Insert for Retinal Delivery of Fluocinolone Acetonide. *Curr. Eye Res.* **2019**, *44*, 541–550. [CrossRef]
174. Balguri, S.P.; Adelli, G.R.; Tatke, A.; Janga, K.Y.; Bhagav, P.; Majumdar, S. Melt-Cast Noninvasive Ocular Inserts for Posterior Segment Drug Delivery. *J. Pharm. Sci.* **2017**, *106*, 3515–3523. [CrossRef]
175. Alambiaga-Caravaca, A.M.; Domenech-Monsell, I.M.; Sebastián-Morelló, M.; Calatayud-Pascual, M.A.; Merino, V.; Rodilla, V.; López-Castellano, A. Development, characterization, and ex vivo evaluation of an insert for the ocular administration of progesterone. *Int. J. Pharm.* **2021**, *606*, 120921. [CrossRef]
176. Shastri, D.H.; Silva, A.C.; Almeida, H. Ocular Delivery of Therapeutic Proteins: A Review. *Pharmaceutics* **2023**, *15*, 205. [CrossRef] [PubMed]
177. Ben-Arzi, A.; Ehrlich, R.; Neumann, R. Retinal Diseases: The Next Frontier in Pharmacodelivery. *Pharmaceutics* **2022**, *14*, 904. [CrossRef] [PubMed]
178. Martin, D.F.; Parks, D.J.; Mellow, S.D.; Ferris, F.L.; Walton, R.C.; Remaley, N.A.; Chew, E.Y.; Ashton, P.; Davis, M.D.; Nussenblatt, R.B. Treatment of cytomegalovirus retinitis with an intraocular sustained-release ganciclovir implant. A randomized controlled clinical trial. *Arch. Ophthalmol.* **1994**, *112*, 1531–1539. [CrossRef]
179. Jaffe, G.J.; Martin, D.; Callanan, D.; Pearson, P.A.; Levy, B.; Comstock, T. Fluocinolone Acetonide Implant (Retisert) for Non-infectious Posterior Uveitis: Thirty-Four–Week Results of a Multicenter Randomized Clinical Study. *Ophthalmology* **2006**, *113*, 1020–1027. [CrossRef] [PubMed]
180. Jain, N.; Stinnett, S.S.; Jaffe, G.J. Prospective study of a fluocinolone acetonide implant for chronic macular edema from central retinal vein occlusion: Thirty-six-month results. *Ophthalmology* **2012**, *119*, 132–137. [CrossRef]
181. Pearson, P.A.; Comstock, T.L.; Ip, M.; Callanan, D.; Morse, L.S.; Ashton, P.; Levy, B.; Mann, E.S.; Eliott, D. Fluocinolone Acetonide Intravitreal Implant for Diabetic Macular Edema: A 3-Year Multicenter, Randomized, Controlled Clinical Trial. *Ophthalmology* **2011**, *118*, 1580–1587. [CrossRef]
182. Campochiaro, P.A.; Brown, D.M.; Pearson, A.; Chen, S.; Boyer, D.; Ruiz-Moreno, J.; Garretson, B.; Gupta, A.; Hariprasad, S.M.; Bailey, C.; et al. Sustained Delivery Fluocinolone Acetonide Vitreous Inserts Provide Benefit for at Least 3 Years in Patients with Diabetic Macular Edema. *Ophthalmology* **2012**, *119*, 2125–2132. [CrossRef]
183. Pearce, W.; Hsu, J.; Yeh, S. Advances in drug delivery to the posterior segment. *Curr. Opin. Ophthalmol.* **2015**, *26*, 233–239. [CrossRef]
184. Testi, I.; Pavesio, C. Preliminary evaluation of YUTIQ™ (fluocinolone acetonide intravitreal implant 0.18 mg) in posterior uveitis. *Ther. Deliv.* **2019**, *10*, 621–625. [CrossRef]
185. Christoforidis, J.B.; Chang, S.; Jiang, A.; Wang, J.; Cebulla, C.M. Intravitreal devices for the treatment of vitreous inflammation. *Mediat. Inflamm.* **2012**, *2012*, 126463. [CrossRef]
186. Wang, J.; Jiang, A.; Joshi, M.; Christoforidis, J. Drug delivery implants in the treatment of vitreous inflammation. *Mediat. Inflamm.* **2013**, *2013*, 780634. [CrossRef] [PubMed]
187. Ranade, S.V.; Wieland, M.R.; Tam, T.; Rea, J.C.; Horvath, J.; Hieb, A.R.; Jia, W.; Grace, L.; Barteselli, G.; Stewart, J.M. The Port Delivery System with ranibizumab: A new paradigm for long-acting retinal drug delivery. *Drug Deliv.* **2022**, *29*, 1326–1334. [CrossRef] [PubMed]
188. Iovino, C.; Mastropasqua, R.; Lupidi, M.; Bacherini, D.; Pellegrini, M.; Bernabei, F.; Borrelli, E.; Sacconi, R.; Carnevali, A.; D'aloisio, R.; et al. Intravitreal Dexamethasone Implant as a Sustained Release Drug Delivery Device for the Treatment of Ocular Diseases: A Comprehensive Review of the Literature. *Pharmaceutics* **2020**, *12*, 703. [CrossRef] [PubMed]
189. Mohan, S.; Ratra, D. Intravitreal Implants. In *StatPearls [Internet]*; StatPearls Publishing: Treasure Island, FL, USA, 2022.
190. Gholamali, I.; Yadollahi, M. Doxorubicin-loaded carboxymethyl cellulose/Starch/ZnO nanocomposite hydrogel beads as an anticancer drug carrier agent. *Int. J. Biol. Macromol.* **2020**, *160*, 724–7355. [CrossRef]
191. Sadasivam, R.; Packirisamy, G.; Goswami, M. Biocompatible soft hydrogel lens as topical implants for diabetic retinopathy. *Mater. Lett.* **2023**, *318*, 132174. [CrossRef]
192. Tan, C.S.; Ngo, W.K.; Chay, I.W.; Ting, D.S.; Sadda, S.R. Neovascular Age-Related Macular Degeneration (nAMD): A Review of Emerging Treatment Options. *Clin. Ophthalmol.* **2022**, *16*, 917–933. [CrossRef]

193. Zheng, C.; Xi, H.; Wen, D.; Ke, Y.; Zhang, X.; Ren, X.; Li, X. Biocompatibility and Efficacy of a Linearly Cross-Linked Sodium Hyaluronic Acid Hydrogel as a Retinal Patch in Rhegmatogenous Retinal Detachment Repairment. *Front. Bioeng. Biotechnol.* **2022**, *10*, 914675. [CrossRef]
194. Vermonden, T.; Censi, R.; Hennink, W.E. Hydrogels for protein delivery. *Chem. Rev.* **2012**, *112*, 2853–2888. [CrossRef]
195. Yu, Y.; Lau, L.C.; Lo, A.C.; Chau, Y. Injectable chemically crosslinked hydrogel for the controlled release of bevacizumab in vitreous: A 6-month in vivo study. *Transl. Vis. Sci. Technol.* **2015**, *4*, 5. [CrossRef]
196. Buwalda, S.J.; Vermonden, T.; Hennink, W.E. Hydrogels for therapeutic delivery: Current developments and future directions. *Biomacromolecules* **2017**, *18*, 316–330. [CrossRef]
197. Buwalda, S.J.; Bethry, A.; Hunger, S.; Kandoussi, S.; Coudane, J.; Nottelet, B. Ultrafast in situ forming poly(ethylene glycol)-poly(amido amine) hydrogels with tunable drug release properties via controllable degradation rates. *Eur. J. Pharm. Biopharm.* **2019**, *139*, 232–239. [CrossRef] [PubMed]
198. Bae, K.H.; Wang, L.S.; Kurisawa, M. Injectable biodegradable hydrogels: Progress and challenges. *J. Mater. Chem. B* **2013**, *1*, 5371. [CrossRef] [PubMed]
199. Franssen, O.; Vandervennet, L.; Roders, P.; Hennink, W.E. Degradable dextran hydrogels: Controlled release of a model protein from cylinders and microspheres. *J. Control. Release* **1999**, *60*, 211–221. [CrossRef] [PubMed]
200. Wang, T.; Ran, R.; Ma, Y.; Zhang, M. Polymeric hydrogel as a vitreous substitute: Current research, challenges, and future directions. *Biomed. Mater.* **2021**, *16*, 042012. [CrossRef]
201. Censi, R.; Vermonden, T.; Van, M.J. Photopolymerized thermosensitive hydrogels for tailorable diffusion-controlled protein delivery. *J. Control. Release* **2009**, *140*, 230–236. [CrossRef]
202. Ilochonwu, B.C.; Mihajlovic, M.; Maas-Bakker, R.F.; Rousou, C.; Tang, M.; Chen, M.; Hennink, W.E.; Vermonden, T. Hyaluronic Acid-PEG-Based Diels–Alder In Situ Forming Hydrogels for Sustained Intraocular Delivery of Bevacizumab. *Biomacromolecules* **2022**, *23*, 2914–2929. [CrossRef] [PubMed]
203. Gao, H.; Chen, M.; Liu, Y.; Zhang, D.; Shen, J.; Ni, N.; Tang, Z.; Ju, Y.; Dai, X.; Zhuang, A.; et al. Injectable Anti-Inflammatory Supramolecular Nanofiber Hydrogel to Promote Anti-VEGF Therapy in Age-Related Macular Degeneration Treatment. *Adv. Mater.* **2023**, *35*, e2204994. [CrossRef]
204. Janet, T.; Stuart, W.; Kevin, H.; Gary, O.; Gabe, F.; Nicole, M.; Tomas, N.; Benjamin, M.; Benjamin, Y. In-vitro release of Bevacizumab from hydrogel-based drug delivery systems. *Investig. Ophthalmol. Vis. Sci.* **2015**, *56*, 222.
205. Ilochonwu, B.C.; Urtti, A.; Hennink, W.E.; Vermonden, T. Intravitreal hydrogels for sustained release of therapeutic proteins. *J. Control. Release* **2020**, *326*, 419–441. [CrossRef]
206. Wei, Y.; Alexandre, U.; Ma, X. Hydrogels to Support Transplantation of Human Embryonic Stem Cell-Derived Retinal Pigment Epithelial Cells. *Brain Sci.* **2022**, *12*, 1620. [CrossRef]
207. Zheng, C.; Wen, D.; Xu, K.; Zhang, X.; Ren, X.; Li, X. Advances in biomaterials as a retinal patch for the repair of rhegmatogenous retinal detachment. *Front. Bioeng. Biotechnol.* **2022**, *10*, 997243. [CrossRef] [PubMed]
208. Han, Z.; Banworth, M.J.; Makkia, R.; Conley, S.M.; Al-Ubaidi, M.R.; Cooper, M.J.; Naash, M.I. Genomic DNA nanoparticles rescue rhodopsin-associated retinitis pigmentosa phenotype. *FASEB J.* **2015**, *29*, 2535–2544. [PubMed]
209. Zheng, M.; Mitra, R.N.; Filonov, N.A.; Han, Z. Nanoparticle-mediated rhodopsin cDNA but not intron-containing DNA delivery causes transgene silencing in a rhodopsin knockout model. *FASEB J.* **2016**, *30*, 1076–1086. [CrossRef] [PubMed]
210. Ottonelli, I.; Bighinati, A.; Adani, E.; Loll, F.; Caraffi, R.; Vandelli, M.A.; Boury, F.; Tosi, G.; Duskey, J.T.; Marigo, V.; et al. Optimization of an Injectable Hydrogel Depot System for the Controlled Release of Retinal-Targeted Hybrid Nanoparticles. *Pharmaceutics* **2023**, *15*, 25. [CrossRef] [PubMed]
211. Osswald, C.R.; Kang-Mieler, J.J. Controlled and extended in vitro release of bioactive anti-vascular endothelial growth factors from a microsphere-hydrogel drug delivery system. *Curr. Eye Res.* **2016**, *41*, 1216–1222. [CrossRef]
212. Kim, S.; Kang-Mieler, J.J.; Liu, W.; Wang, Z.; Yiu, G.; Teixeira, L.B.C.; Mieler, W.F.; Thomasy, S.M. Safety and Biocompatibility of Aflibercept-Loaded Microsphere Thermo-Responsive Hydrogel Drug Delivery System in a Nonhuman Primate Model. *Transl. Vis. Sci. Technol.* **2020**, *9*, 30. [CrossRef]
213. Rudeen, K.M.; Liu, W.; Mieler, W.F.; Kang-Mieler, J.J. Simultaneous Release of Aflibercept and Dexamethasone from an Ocular Drug Delivery System. *Curr. Eye Res.* **2022**, *47*, 1034–1042. [CrossRef]
214. Holgado, M.A.; Anguiano-Domínguez, A.; Martín-Banderas, L. Contact lenses as drug-delivery systems: A promising therapeutic tool. Lentes de contacto para vehiculizar principios activos: Una prometedora herramienta terapéutica. *Arch. Soc. Española Oftalmol. (Engl. Ed.)* **2020**, *95*, 24–33. [CrossRef]
215. Peral, A.; Martinez-Aguila, A.; Pastrana, C.; Huete-Toral, F.; Carpena-Torres, C.; Carracedo, G. Contact lenses as a drug delivery system for glaucoma: A Review. *Appl. Sci.* **2020**, *10*, 151. [CrossRef]
216. Stiler-Wyszyńska, S.; Golba, S.; Jurek-Suliga, J.; Kuczkowski, S. Review of the latest solutions in the use of contact lenses as controlled release systems for ophthalmic drugs. *Polym Med.* 2023; *ahead of print*. [CrossRef]
217. Franco, P.; De Marco, I. Contact Lenses as Ophthalmic Drug Delivery Systems: A Review. *Polymers* **2021**, *13*, 1102. [CrossRef] [PubMed]
218. Carvalho, I.M.; Marques, C.S.; Oliveira, R.S.; Coelho, P.B.; Costa, P.C.; Ferreira, D.C. Sustained drug release by contact lenses for glaucoma treatment—A review. *J. Control. Release* **2015**, *202*, 76–82. [CrossRef] [PubMed]

219. González-Chomón, C.; Silva, M.; Concheiro, A.; Alvarez-Lorenzo, C. Biomimetic contact lenses eluting olopatadine for allergic conjunctivitis. *Acta Biomater.* **2016**, *41*, 302–311. [CrossRef] [PubMed]
220. Malakooti, N.; Alexander, C.; Alvarez-Lorenzo, C. Imprinted contact lenses for sustained release of polymyxin B and related antimicrobial peptides. *J. Pharm. Sci.* **2015**, *104*, 3386–3394. [CrossRef] [PubMed]
221. Varela-Garcia, A.; Gomez-Amoza, J.L.; Concheiro, A.; Alvarez-Lorenzo, C. Imprinted Contact Lenses for Ocular Administration of Antiviral Drugs. *Polymers* **2020**, *12*, 2026. [CrossRef]
222. Phan, C.M.; Subbaraman, L.; Jones, L. Contact lenses for antifungal ocular drug delivery: A review. *Expert Opin. Drug Deliv.* **2014**, *11*, 537–546. [CrossRef] [PubMed]
223. Dixon, P.; Ghosh, T.; Mondal, K.; Konar, A.; Chauhan, A.; Hazra, S. Controlled delivery of pirfenidone through vitamin E-loaded contact lens ameliorates corneal inflammation. *Drug Deliv. Transl. Res.* **2018**, *8*, 1114–1126. [CrossRef]
224. Torres-Luna, C.; Hu, N.; Tammareddy, T.; Domszy, R.; Yang, J.; Wang, N.S.; Yang, A. Extended delivery of non-steroidal anti-inflammatory drugs through contact lenses loaded with Vitamin E and cationic surfactants. *Contact Lens Anterior Eye* **2019**, *42*, 546–552. [CrossRef]
225. Gade, S.K.; Nirmal, J.; Garg, P.; Venuganti, V.V.K. Corneal delivery of moxifloxacin and dexamethasone combination using drug-eluting mucoadhesive contact lens to treat ocular infections. *Int. J. Pharm.* **2020**, *591*, 120023. [CrossRef]
226. De Guzman, L.M.C.; De Guzman, G.Q.; Borromeo, E.C. Brinzolamide-loaded soft contact lens for ophthalmic delivery. *Ther. Deliv.* **2022**, *13*, 233–247. [CrossRef]
227. Dang, H.; Dong, C.; Zhang, L. Sustained latanoprost release from PEGylated solid lipid nanoparticle-laden soft contact lens to treat glaucoma. *Pharm. Dev. Technol.* **2022**, *27*, 127–133. [CrossRef] [PubMed]
228. Alvarez-Rivera, F.; Fernández-Villanueva, D.; Concheiro, A.; Alvarez-Lorenzo, C. α-Lipoic Acid in Soluplus(®) Polymeric Nanomicelles for Ocular Treatment of Diabetes-Associated Corneal Diseases. *J. Pharm. Sci.* **2016**, *105*, 2855–2863. [CrossRef] [PubMed]
229. Alvarez-Rivera, F.; Concheiro, A.; Alvarez-Lorenzo, C. Epalrestat-loaded silicone hydrogels as contact lenses to address diabetic eye complications. *Eur. J. Pharm. Biopharm.* **2018**, *122*, 126–136. [CrossRef]
230. Zaidun, N.H.; Thent, Z.C.; Latiff, A.A. Combating oxidative stress disorders with citrus flavonoid: Naringenin. *Life Sci.* **2018**, *208*, 111–122. [CrossRef] [PubMed]
231. Nguyen, D.; Dowling, J.; Ryan, R.; McLoughlin, P.; Fitzhenry, L. Controlled release of naringenin from soft hydrogel contact lens: An investigation into lens critical properties and in vitro release. *Int. J. Pharm.* **2022**, *621*, 121793. [CrossRef] [PubMed]
232. Ross, A.E.; Bengani, L.C.; Tulsan, R.; Maidana, D.E.; Salvador-Culla, B.; Kobashi, H.; Kolovou, P.E.; Zhai, H.; Taghizadeh, K.; Kuang, L.; et al. Topical sustained drug delivery to the retina with a drug-eluting contact lens. *Biomaterials* **2019**, *217*, 119285. [CrossRef]
233. Keith, C.; Anuj, C. Contact Lens Based Drug Delivery to the Posterior Segment via Iontophoresis in Cadaver Rabbit Eyes. *Pharm. Res.* **2019**, *36*, 87.
234. Moffatt, K.; Wang, Y.; Singh, T.R.R.; Donnelly, R.F. Microneedles for enhanced transdermal and intraocular drug delivery. *Curr. Opin. Pharmacol.* **2017**, *36*, 14–21. [CrossRef]
235. Gadziński, P.; Froelich, A.; Wojtyłko, M.; Białek, A.; Krysztofiak, J.; Osmałek, T. Microneedle-based ocular drug delivery systems—Recent advances and challenges. *Beilstein J. Nanotechnol.* **2022**, *13*, 1167–1184. [CrossRef]
236. [Press Release] Bausch + Lomb and Clearside Biomedical Announce FDA Approval of XIPERE™ (Triamcinolone Acetonide Injectable Suspension) for Suprachoroidal Use for the Treatment of Macular Edema Associated with Uveitis. 2021. Available online: https://ir.clearsidebio.com/news-relea (accessed on 12 March 2023).
237. Ciulla, T.; Yeh, S. Microinjection via the suprachoroidal space: A review of a novel mode of administration. *Am. J. Manag. Care* **2022**, *28* (Suppl. 13), S243–S252. [CrossRef]
238. Kansara, V.S.; Hancock, S.E.; Muya, L.W.; Ciulla, T.A. Suprachoroidal delivery enables targeting, localization and durability of small molecule suspensions. *J. Control. Release* **2022**, *349*, 1045–1051. [CrossRef] [PubMed]
239. Roy, G.; Garg, P.; Venuganti, V.V.K. Microneedle scleral patch for minimally invasive delivery of triamcinolone to the posterior segment of eye. *Int. J. Pharm.* **2022**, *612*, 121305. [CrossRef] [PubMed]
240. Amer, M.; Chen, R.K. Hydrogel-Forming Microneedle Arrays for Sustained and Controlled Ocular Drug Delivery. *ASME J. Med. Diagn.* **2020**, *3*, 041003. [CrossRef]
241. Wu, Y.; Vora, L.K.; Wang, Y.; Adrianto, M.F.; Tekko, I.A.; Waite, D.; Donnelly, R.F.; Thakur, R.R.S. Long-acting nanoparticle-loaded bilayer microneedles for protein delivery to the posterior segment of the eye. *Eur. J. Pharm. Biopharm.* **2021**, *165*, 306–318. [CrossRef]
242. Singh, R.R.T.; Tekko, I.; McAvoy, K.; McMillan, H.; Jones, D.; Donnelly, R.F. Minimally invasive microneedles for ocular drug delivery. *Expert Opin. Drug Deliv.* **2017**, *14*, 525–537. [CrossRef]
243. Jones, A.T.; Sayers, E.J. Cell entry of cell penetrating peptides: Tales of tails wagging dogs. *J. Control. Release* **2012**, *161*, 582–591. [CrossRef]

pharmaceuticals

Review

Honey-Related Treatment Strategies in Dry Eye Disease

Julia Prinz [1], Nicola Maffulli [2,3,4], Matthias Fuest [1], Peter Walter [1], Frank Hildebrand [1] and Filippo Migliorini [1,5,*]

[1] RWTH University Hospital of Aachen, 52074 Aachen, Germany
[2] Department of Medicine, Surgery and Dentistry, University of Salerno, 84081 Salerno, Italy
[3] Barts and The London School of Medicine and Dentistry, Mile End Hospital, Queen Mary University of London, 275 Bancroft Road, London E1 4DG, UK
[4] School of Pharmacy and Bioengineering, Keele University Faculty of Medicine, Thornburrow Drive, Stoke on Trent ST4 7QB, UK
[5] Department of Orthopaedics and Trauma Surgery, Academic Hospital of Bolzano (SABES-ASDAA), 39100 Bolzano, Italy
* Correspondence: migliorini.md@gmail.com; Tel.: +49-0241-80-35529

Abstract: This systematic review and meta-analysis investigated whether honey-related treatment strategies improve the signs and symptoms of patients with dry eye disease (DED). In March 2023, the following databases were accessed for clinical trials investigating the efficacy of honey-related treatment strategies in DED: PubMed, Web of Science, Google Scholar, and EMBASE. The following data were extracted at baseline and at the last follow-up: Ocular Surface Disease Index, tear breakup time, Schirmer I test, and corneal staining. Data from 323 patients were retrieved (53.3% female, mean age 40.6 ± 18.1 years). The mean follow-up was 7.0 ± 4.2 weeks. All the endpoints of interest significantly improved from baseline to the last follow-up: tear breakup time ($p = 0.01$), Ocular Surface Disease Index ($p < 0.0001$), Schirmer I test ($p = 0.0001$), and corneal staining ($p < 0.0001$). No difference was found in tear breakup time ($p = 0.3$), Ocular Surface Disease Index ($p = 0.4$), Schirmer I test ($p = 0.3$), and corneal staining ($p = 0.3$) between the honey-related treatment strategies and the control groups. According to our main results, honey-related treatment strategies are effective and feasible to improve symptoms and signs of DED.

Keywords: dry eye disease; xerophthalmus; keratoconjunctivitis sicca; honey; Manuka; Royal Jelly

Citation: Prinz, J.; Maffulli, N.; Fuest, M.; Walter, P.; Hildebrand, F.; Migliorini, F. Honey-Related Treatment Strategies in Dry Eye Disease. *Pharmaceuticals* **2023**, *16*, 762. https://doi.org/10.3390/ph16050762

Academic Editors: Réjean Couture, Rosario Pignatello, Hugo Almeida, Debora Santonocito and Carmelo Puglia

Received: 25 April 2023
Revised: 11 May 2023
Accepted: 12 May 2023
Published: 18 May 2023

1. Introduction

Dry eye disease (DED) is a common ocular condition with a prevalence rate of up to 74% [1–5]. The aetiology of DED is multifactorial [2]. Inflammatory or environmental conditions, such as allergens, contact lens wear, cigarette smoke, previous eye surgery, neurotrophic deficiency, exposure to pollutants, ultraviolet radiation, hormonal imbalance—especially in perimenopausal women—and oxidative stress are implicated in DED [6–8]. Additionally, tear film hyperosmolarity plays an important role in the pathogenesis of DED: damage of the corneal epithelium leads to cell death by apoptosis, followed by a loss of goblet cells and mucin expression, increasing the presence of inflammatory mediators, such as tumour necrosis factor α, interleukin 6, and matrix metallopeptidase 9 [9,10]. Symptoms associated with DED include foreign body sensation, blurred vision, pain, and photophobia [6,11]. Aqueous-deficient and evaporative DED can be distinguished, while numerous patients show signs of both subtypes [1]. Current treatment options mainly comprise artificial tears, lifestyle changes, topical steroids or cyclosporine, lacrimal punctal occlusion, and oral omega-3 fatty acids [12–16]. Though improving both symptoms and clinical findings, artificial tears do not treat the inflammation processes underlying DED [17]. Topical steroids have anti-inflammatory properties, and their efficacy in improving the signs and symptoms of DED have been demonstrated before [16,18]. However, their long-term use is not recommended, as ocular side effects such as the development of cataract or secondary glaucoma might occur [19,20]. Further anti-inflammatory treatment strategies for patients with DED include cyclosporine and lifitegrast [21]. Recently, the efficacy of naturally occurring anti-inflammatory agents as treatment strategies for patients with DED has been investigated [21]. Altogether, the interest in alternative treatment approaches for DED is growing [21].

Honey has been used in the management of ophthalmic diseases for thousands of years [22]. It mainly consists of carbohydrates, water, organic acids, proteins, amino acids, minerals, vitamins, enzymes, flavonoids, and antimicrobial components, such as hydrogen peroxide, sugar, and antimicrobial peptides [23,24]. The flavonoids, including pinocembrin, quercetin, chrysin, and phenolic acids might be accountable for the anti-bacterial, anti-oxidant, anti-inflammatory, immunomodulatory and analgesic properties of honey [25]. Additionally, the anti-bacterial, anti-oxidant, and anti-fungal effects of honey have been attributed to the anti-microbial effects of glucose oxidase, and a high osmolarity which might inhibit bacterial growth [22,24,26]. More than 300 varieties of honey exist, depending on the heterogeneity of plants and environmental conditions [23]. Manuka honey contains a proprietary mix of honey from the Australian and New Zealand *Leptospermum* species (known as Manuka) [27]. Its anti-bacterial efficacy includes activity against methicillin-resistant *Staphylococcus aureus* and *Pseudomonas aeruginosa* [28]. Royal Jelly is mainly secreted by the worker honeybees (*Apis mellifera*) and is required for the nutrition of the queen honeybee [29]. It is secreted from the hypopharyngeal and mandibular glands of the worker bees [29]. In general, medical-grade honey is free of toxic contaminants after sterilisation by gamma irradiation, according to standard medical regulations [30]. The efficacy of honey in the treatment of ophthalmic diseases such as chemical and thermal burns, corneal bacterial ulcers, postoperative corneal oedema, bullous keratopathy, neurotrophic keratitis, vernal keratoconjunctivitis, and catarrhal keratoconjunctivitis has been demonstrated by previous studies [22,31–34]. It has been attributed to the capacity of honey to stimulate immune cells and promote reepithelialisation, as well as angiogenesis [35].

The present study investigated whether honey supplementation improves the clinical signs and symptoms in patients with DED at the last follow-up compared to baseline. Moreover, a meta-analysis comparing honey-derived therapies vs. placebo or artificial tears was conducted.

2. Results

2.1. Study Selection

The eligibility criteria are described in detail in paragraph 4.1. The literature search resulted in 124 randomized clinical trials which evaluated the efficacy of topical or systemic honey application in patients with DED. Of them, 63 were excluded because of duplication. Another 46 articles were excluded because they did not match the eligibility criteria. Ten further studies did not report quantitative data under the endpoints of interest and were therefore excluded from further analysis. Finally, five randomized clinical trials were eligible for the final analysis. The flow chart of the literature search is shown in Figure 1.

2.2. Study Risk of Bias Assessment

Given the randomized design of the patient allocation in all included studies, the risk of selection bias was low. A moderate risk of detection bias was evidenced. Additionally, the performance bias was considered low. The risk of attrition bias was low, and the risk of reporting and other biases was moderate. Overall, the risk of bias graph evidenced a low risk of publication bias in the included studies. The results of the methodological quality assessment for the selection bias, performance bias, detection bias, attrition bias, reporting bias, and other biases for the included studies are shown in Figure 2.

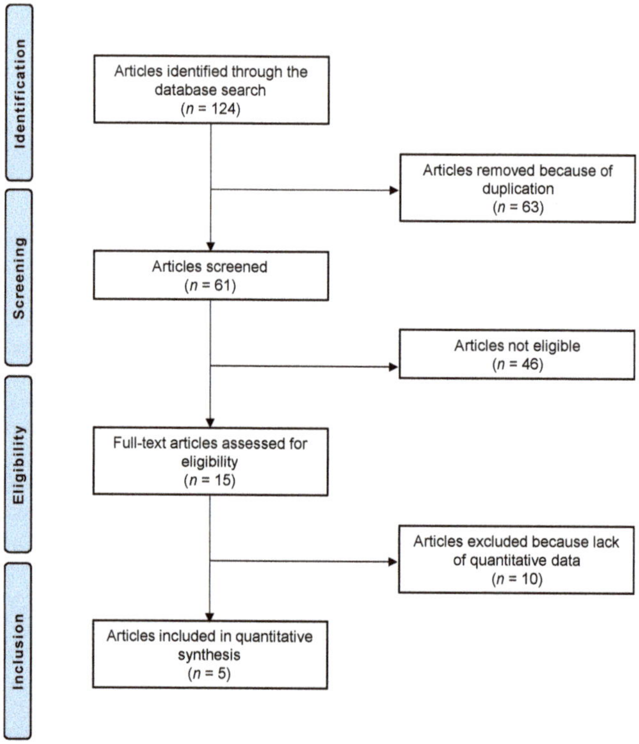

Figure 1. PRISMA flow chart of the literature search.

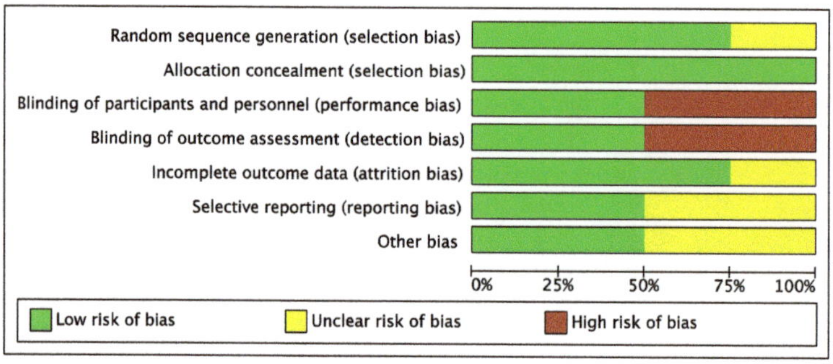

Figure 2. Methodological quality assessment.

2.3. Risk of Publication Bias

The funnel plot was performed to evaluate the risk of publication bias of the present study. All the effects were located within the shape of acceptability, and they demonstrated a symmetrical disposition. These features of the plot indicate a low risk of publication bias (Figure 3).

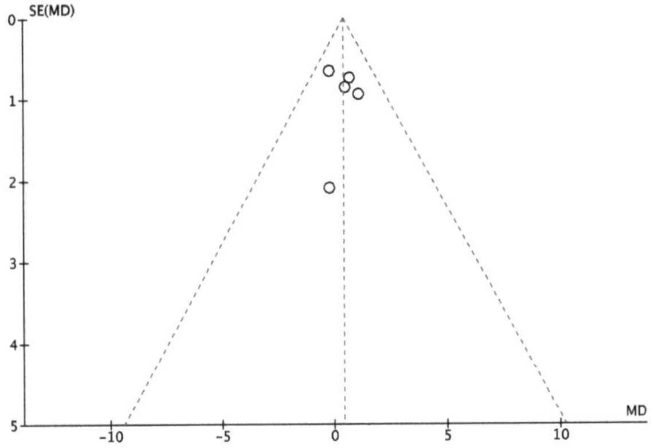

Figure 3. Funnel plot to evaluate the risk of publication bias.

2.4. Study Characteristics and Results of Individual Studies

Data from 323 patients were retrieved from the included studies. The study generalities and patient characteristics of the included studies are shown in greater detail in Table 1.

Table 1. Generalities and patients baseline of the included study.

Author, Year	Journal	Follow-Up (Weeks)	Treatment	Patients (*n*)	Mean Age	Women (%)
Albietz et al., 2017 [36]	Clin. Exp. Optom.	8	Honey (Optimel Manuka gel) plus conventional therapy	37	58.9	42.9
			Honey (Optimel Manuka drops) plus conventional therapy	37	62.2	42.4
			Conventional therapy	40	61.4	41.2
Craig et al., 2020 [37]	Ocul. Surf.	13	Honey (Manuka microemulsion)	53	60.0	60.0
			No treatment	53	60.0	60.0
Inoue et al., 2017 [29]	PLoS ONE	8	Honey (Royal Jelly)	22	29.6	28.6
			Placebo	19	37.0	54.5
Tan et al., 2020 [38]	Br. J. Ophthalmol.	4	Honey (Optimel Manuka+ honey eye drops)	21	22.2	57.1
			Artificial tears	21	20.6	76.2
Wong et al., 2017 [27]	Cont. Lens Anterior Eye	2	Honey (Optimel Manuka drops)	10	25.7	55.0
			Artificial tears	10	25.7	55.0

2.5. Efficacy of Honey-Related Treatment Strategies

All the endpoints of interest significantly changed from baseline to the last follow-up: At the last follow-up, the tear breakup time was significantly increased (+1.1 s; $p = 0.01$), the Ocular Surface Disease Index score was significantly reduced (−12.8 points; $p < 0.0001$), the Schirmer I test was significantly increased (+1.8 mm; $p = 0.0001$), and the corneal staining score was significantly reduced (−1.2 points; $p < 0.0001$) compared to baseline. These results are shown in greater detail in Table 2.

Table 2. Comparison of the tear breakup time (s), the Ocular Surface Disease Index (points), the Schirmer I test (mm), and corneal staining (points) from baseline to the last follow-up (FU: follow-up; MD: mean difference; SE: standard error; 95% CI: 95% confidence interval).

Endpoint	Baseline	Last FU	MD	SE	95% CI	T-Value	p
Tear breakup time	5.0 ± 3.3	6.1 ± 2.7	1.1	0.426	0.25 to 1.94	2.58	0.01
Ocular Surface Disease Index	32.9 ± 9.9	20.1 ± 6.5	−12.8	1.184	−15.13 to −10.46	−10.808	<0.0001
Schirmer I test	16.7 ± 4.3	18.5 ± 1.7	1.8	0.462	0.88 to 2.71	3.893	0.0001
Corneal Staining	2.3 ± 2.6	1.1 ± 0.9	−1.2	0.275	−1.74 to −0.65	−4.361	<0.0001

2.6. Honey-Related Treatment Strategies Compared to Other Treatments

No significant differences were found in terms of the tear breakup time ($p = 0.3$), the Ocular Surface Disease Index ($p = 0.4$), the Schirmer I test ($p = 0.3$), and corneal staining ($p = 0.3$) between the honey-related treatment and the control group (Figure 4).

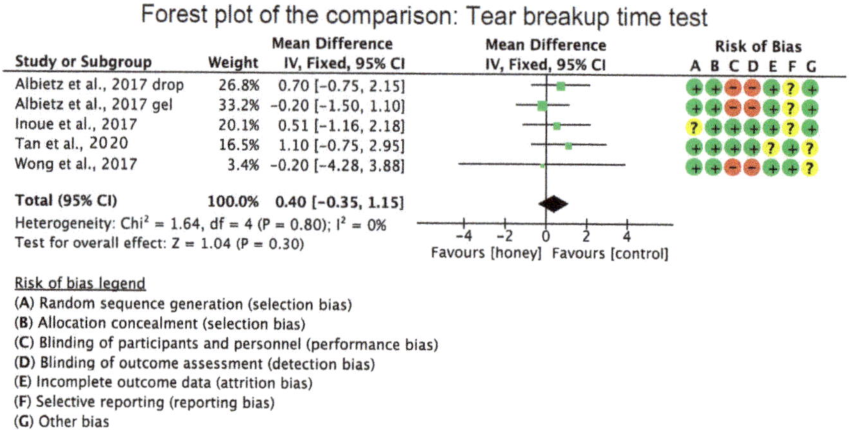

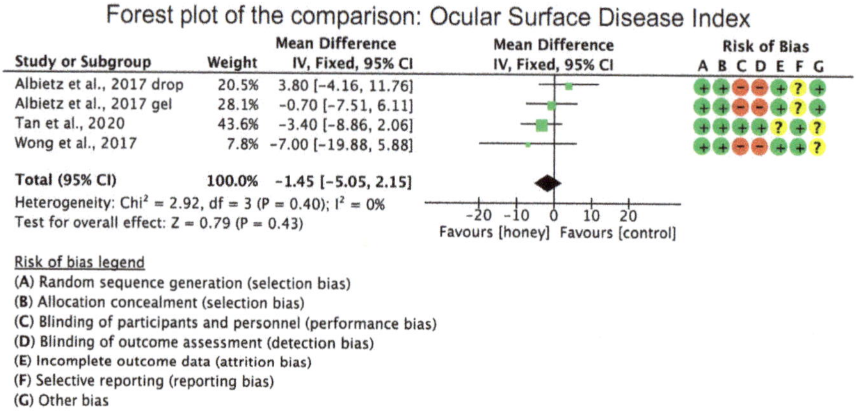

Figure 4. *Cont.*

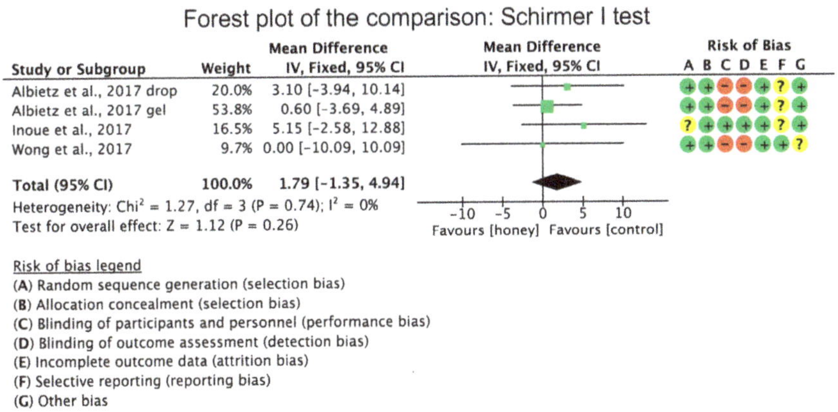

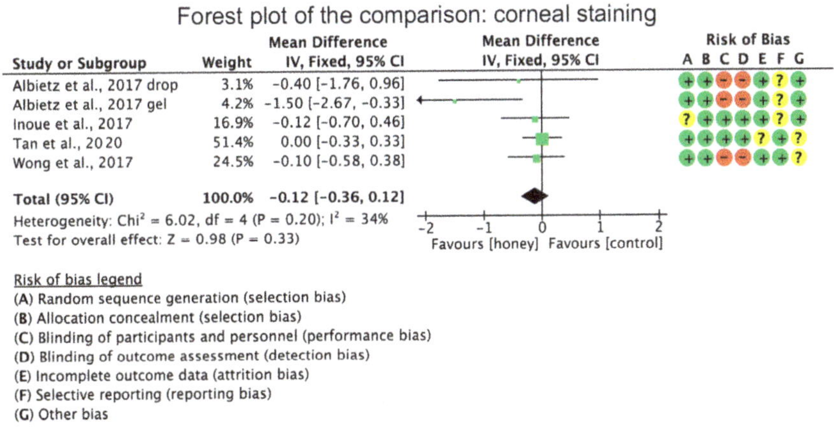

Figure 4. Results of the meta-analysis [27,29,36,38].

3. Discussion

According to the main findings of the present study, topical or systemic honey-related treatment strategies led to a significant increase in the tear breakup time and the Schirmer I test at the last follow-up compared to baseline in patients with DED. At the last follow-up, the Ocular Surface Disease Index score and corneal staining were significantly lower compared to the baseline in the honey-related treatment group. No differences in the tear breakup time, Schirmer I test, corneal staining, or Ocular Surface Disease Index scores between the honey-related treatment group and the control groups were identified. The proportion of females (53%) and age distribution in this study agree with previous publications [39,40].

Studies using both Manuka honey and Royal Jelly as a treatment in patients with DED were included in the present systematic review and meta-analysis. Manuka honey is a monofloral honey originating from the Manuka tree (*Leptospermum* sp.) [41]. Royal Jelly has been shown to have anti-bacterial, anti-inflammatory, and anti-fungal properties, and has been used to treat a variety of disorders in humans, including ocular diseases [42], as well as diabetes, or Alzheimer's disease [43]. Its exact mechanism of action is not completely understood. However, Royal Jelly has been reported to stimulate the mobilization of calcium ions via muscarinic signal transduction pathways in the lacrimal glands [21].

Recent studies showed that oxidative stress damages the ocular surface and plays an important role in DED [44]. Markers of oxidative stress, such as lipid peroxidase, myeloperoxidase, nitric oxide synthase, and reactive oxygen species were previously found in the tears, conjunctival cells, and conjunctival biopsies of patients suffering from DED [45]. Oxidative stress occurs when the balance between the level of reactive oxygen species and the level of protective enzymes is disrupted [46]. The ocular surface is constantly exposed to the burden of free radical stress caused by ultraviolet radiation and environmental pollution [8]. Honey has been demonstrated to show anti-oxidative properties as it causes free radicals to neutralize [22,47]. These anti-oxidant properties are mainly attributable to the flavonoids, carotenoids, and phenolic acids which are present in honey [48]. Flavonoids are a group of plant secondary metabolites which are known for their anti-oxidative, anti-inflammatory, anti-carcinogenic, and anti-mutagenic properties [49]. The phenolic acids contained in honey are capable of chelating ferrous ions and scavenging hydrogen peroxide [50]. Generally, anti-oxidants also have an anti-inflammatory effect given that oxygen free radicals are involved in several inflammatory conditions [51,52].

At the last follow-up, the tear breakup time was increased in the honey group compared to the control group. Recently, honey has been reported to promote the secretion of tears by the lacrimal gland [47]. A previous study demonstrated that orally supplied Royal Jelly promoted tear secretion in blink-suppressed dry eye animal models [47]. Furthermore, an increase in adenosine triphosphate (ATP) and mitochondrial function by modulation of the calcium signalling pathway has been demonstrated after oral administration of Royal Jelly, suggesting a restoration in the lacrimal production by the gland cells [47].

The efficacy of Manuka honey in reducing the bacterial colonization of the lid margin has been described in previous studies [36]. Moreover, a significant reduction in inflammatory markers after honey supplementation, such as matrix metallopeptidase 9, has been presumed [36]. DED from blepharitis is mainly attributed to bacterial side products rather than the bacteria themselves [53]. Thus, honey might reduce the susceptibility of DED patients to bacterial conjunctivitis and relieve the symptoms of DED by reducing the production of bacterial side products, e.g., bacterial lipases [54]. These bacterial lipases are believed to hydrolyse the lipids of the meibomian glands, thereby releasing free fatty acids which might destabilize the tear film and have toxic effects on the corneal epithelium [55]. Tear film hyperosmolarity has been shown to stimulate multiple inflammatory reactions on the ocular surface, which result in apoptotic cell death of conjunctival epithelium and goblet cells [28,56]. Decreasing goblet cell densities result in increased tear film evaporation, which is one important mechanism of DED [28,56]. However, the exact underlying mechanisms are still unclear.

Whereas no significant change in corneal staining was observed in the study by Tan et al. [38], Albietz and Schmid reported a significant reduction in interpalpebral corneal and conjunctival staining after Manuka honey [36]. These divergent results might be attributable to the different underlying grading scales: Tan et al. [38] graded the extent of staining for each quadrant using the Centre for Contact Lens Research Unit (CCLRU) grading scale [57] and averaged the results for the quadrants to obtain an overall score per eye [38], whereas Albietz et al. [36] used the Oxford Scheme [58] in their study [36]. Moreover, differences in baseline characteristics might explain the inhomogeneous results between the studies. In this regard, patients in the study by Albietz et al. [36] had a numerically higher Ocular Surface Disease Index score at baseline compared to patients in the study by Tan et al. [38] (38.2 vs. 33.7, respectively). Previously, honey has been demonstrated to stimulate angiogenesis, granulation, and epithelization [59]. In this context, it has been suggested that honey might stimulate cytokine production (e.g., tumour necrosis factor α or interleukin 6) from human monocytes [35]. However, the exact components of honey responsible for this effect and the precise mechanism of action are not yet fully understood [60]. Another suggestion on the efficacy of honey included the presence of microorganisms in honey, such as aerobic and anaerobic bacteria [61]. Hypothetically, the presence of microorganisms in honey explains its stimulation of immune cells [60,61].

However, recently, Tonks et al. identified a 5.8 kDA component of Manuka honey that is responsible for stimulating inflammatory responses including cytokine production in human monocytes via the Toll-like receptor 4 [60].

Some between-studies heterogeneities should be considered. Topical honey as a treatment for DED has been demonstrated to improve ocular comfort after 2 [27] to 13 weeks of follow-up [37]. Wong et al. investigated the effect of Manuka (*Leptospermum* sp.) honey eye drops in 24 patients with contact-lens-related DED [27]. They reported improvements in subjective symptomology as measured by the Ocular Surface Disease Index score in symptomatic patients. However, no improvements in objective signs, such as the Schirmer I test or tear breakup time, were demonstrated, which was attributed to the short follow-up period of 2 weeks by the authors [27]. Albietz et al. evaluated the efficacy of Manuka (*Leptospermum* sp.) combined with conventional therapy for DED, consisting of warm compresses, artificial tears, and lid massage, involving 114 patients. The authors reported significant improvement in corneal staining and meibum quality after therapy with Manuka. In addition, treatment with Manuka reduced the need for artificial tears [36]. Tan et al. [38] compared the efficacy of Manuka honey to artificial tears. The study included 46 patients with DED. After a follow-up of 4 weeks, patients treated with Manuka honey had significantly lower Ocular Surface Disease Index scores compared to the control group. Additionally, the authors reported a slight but not statistically significant increase in tear breakup time in the Manuka honey group at 4 weeks follow-up compared to baseline [38]. In a recent study by Craig et al. [37], the efficacy of an eye cream consisting of Manuka honey microemulsion on 53 patients with DED and blepharitis was evaluated [37]. After 3 months, topical Manuka honey resulted in significant improvements in subjective symptomology and tear breakup time [37]. Inoue et al. investigated the efficacy of Royal Jelly honey administration in 43 Japanese patients compared to a placebo for 8 weeks [29]. The authors found that the tear volume significantly increased following treatment with Royal Jelly honey. In patients with a baseline Schirmer I test value of $\leq$10 mm, a significant increase compared to baseline tear volume and also compared to the placebo group was witnessed [29]. No severe treatment-related adverse effects were reported in the included studies [27,36–38,62]. Minor adverse effects related to the topical honey eye drop or eye cream instillation included temporary stinging and discomfort in two of the included studies [36,37], while the other studies did not report any adverse events attributable to the topical honey treatment. To date, no further ongoing studies evaluating the efficacy of honey for DED are registered in the U.S. National Library of Medicine.

This study has several limitations. The limited study size was the most important limitation of the present study. Given the limited quantitative data available for inclusion, it was not possible to analyse different types of honey-related treatment strategies, such as Manuka honey or Royal Jelly, separately. Future comparative randomized controlled trials are warranted to investigate which type of honey might be most effective in patients with DED. The treatment protocols within the honey group were heterogeneous, including topical and oral honey administration and different honey types. Furthermore, different honey types which are derived from different plants might vary significantly in their composition and their anti-bacterial and anti-oxidant properties [63]. The control group was also heterogeneous: Conventional lubricant eye drops (Novartis International AG, Fort Worth, TX, USA) were used as a treatment in the control group by Wong et al. [27] and Tan et al. [38], and adjunctive conventional therapy including warm compresses, lid massage, and lubricants by Albietz et al. [36]. In the study by Inoue et al., patients in the control group received placebo tablets [29]. Craig et al. treated only one eye of their patients with Manuka honey microemulsion and left the second eye of their patients untreated as a control eye [37]. The heterogeneous length of the follow-up might also limit the reliability of our results. Different inclusion and exclusion criteria of the different studies were not accounted for. Future level I evidence studies should be undertaken to overcome current obstacles to clinical translation and study the role of topical honey treatment in DED more extensively. Moreover, future studies should focus on which cohort of DED patients can benefit from topical or systemic honey treatment compared to other treatment options for DED, such as artificial tears or anti-inflammatory agents.

4. Materials and Methods

4.1. Eligibility Criteria

All the clinical trials which investigated the efficacy of topical or oral application of honey-related treatment strategies for DED were accessed. According to the authors language capabilities, articles in English, German, Italian, French, and Spanish were eligible. According to the Oxford Centre of Evidence-Based Medicine [64], only level I evidence was considered. Reviews, opinions, letters, and editorials were not considered. Animals, in vitro, biomechanical, computational, and cadaveric studies were also not eligible. Only studies investigating patients affected by clinically manifest DED were eligible. Studies including patients with Sjögren's syndrome, graft vs. host disease, or Stevens–Johnson syndrome-related severe DED were not considered. Studies investigating the efficacy of honey-related treatment strategies in patients receiving punctal occlusion procedures were excluded. All types of honey-related treatment strategies as a treatment of DED were considered eligible. Studies combining honey-related treatment strategies with other treatments, except for conventional therapy including artificial tears, were excluded. Only studies which reported quantitative data under the endpoints of interest were eligible.

4.2. Search Strategy

This meta-analysis systematic review was conducted according to the Preferred Reporting Items for Systematic Reviews and Meta-Analyses: the 2020 PRISMA statement [65]. The PICO algorithm was preliminary established:

- P (Population): patients with DED;
- I (Intervention): Honey-related treatment strategies, including Manuka honey, Royal Jelly;
- C (Comparison): improvement at the last follow-up and compared with placebo or control group;
- O (Outcomes): Ocular Surface Disease Index; Tear breakup time test; Schirmer I test, corneal staining, adverse events.

In March 2023, the following databases were accessed: PubMed, Web of Science, Google Scholar, and Embase. No time constraints were used for the search. The following keywords were used in combination: dry eye disease, xerophthalmus, xeropthalmia, honey, Manuka honey, Royal Jelly, Leptospermum, Apis mellifera, management, therapy, Ocular Surface Disease Index; Tear breakup time test; Schirmer I test, corneal staining, aqueous-deficient dry eye disease, evaporative dry eye disease, lacrimal deficiency, lacrimal gland duct obstruction, drug-induced dry eye disease, vitamin A deficiency associated dry eye disease, contact lens wear associated dry eye disease, meibomian gland dysfunction.

4.3. Selection and Data Collection

Two authors (F.M. and J.P.) independently performed the database search. All the resulting titles were screened and, if suitable, the abstract of the articles was accessed. The full text of the abstracts which matched the topic of interest was accessed. A cross reference of the bibliography of the full-text articles was also screened for inclusion. Any disagreements were resolved by discussion, and a third author (N.M.) was involved in the final decision.

4.4. Data Items

Two authors (F.M. and J.P.) independently performed data extraction. The following data were extracted at baseline and at the last follow-up: Ocular Surface Disease Index [66], tear breakup time test [67], and Schirmer I test [68]. The primary outcome of interest was to investigate whether topical or oral honey-related treatment strategies improve the clinical outcome at the last follow-up compared to the baseline. The secondary outcome of interest was to compare honey-related therapy with placebo or artificial tears.

4.5. Study Risk of Bias Assessment

The between-studies risk of bias assessment was performed using the risk of bias tool of the Review Manager software (The Nordic Cochrane Collaboration, Copenhagen, Denmark). The following biases were evaluated by an independent author (J.P.): selection, performance, detection, attrition, reporting, and other sources of bias. The overall risk of publication bias was evaluated through the funnel plot. Asymmetry of the funnel plot is associated with a greater risk of publication bias.

4.6. Synthesis Methods

The statistical analysis was performed by the senior author (F.M.). To assess the improvement from the baseline to the last follow-up, the IBM SPSS software version 25 was used. Mean difference (MD), standard error (SE), T value and *t*-test were evaluated. For the comparisons, a meta-analysis was conducted using the Review Manager software (The Nordic Cochrane Collaboration, Copenhagen, Denmark) version 5.3. Data were analysed using the inverse variance and mean difference (MD) effect measure. The comparisons were performed with a fixed model effect as set-up. Heterogeneity was assessed through the Higgins-I^2 test. If the I^2 test was >50%, a random model effect was adopted. The confidence intervals (CI) were set at 95% in all analyses. Values of $p < 0.05$ were considered statistically significant. Forest plots were performed for each comparison.

5. Conclusions

According to the main findings of the present study, honey-related treatment strategies are an effective and feasible treatment option to improve symptoms and signs in patients with DED. Honey-related treatment strategies led to a significant increase in the tear breakup time and in the Schirmer I test and a significant reduction in the Ocular Surface Disease Index and corneal staining at the last follow-up. No significant differences were found in the tear breakup time, the Schirmer I test, corneal staining, or Ocular Surface Disease Index scores between the honey-related treatment and the control groups. No severe adverse effects were reported within the included studies. Future high-quality studies are needed to provide further evidence and to analyse the efficacy of different varieties of honey in the treatment of DED. Level I evidence studies are warranted to investigate the role of topical honey treatment in DED more extensively. In addition, future studies should determine which cohorts of DED patients could benefit from honey-related treatment options compared to other treatment options for DED, such as artificial tears or anti-inflammatory agents.

Author Contributions: Conceptualization, F.M. and J.P.; methodology, F.M. and N.M.; validation, M.F., P.W. and F.H.; formal analysis, F.M. and J.P.; writing—original draft preparation, J.P.; writing—review and editing, F.M., N.M. and P.W.; visualization, F.M.; supervision, F.M. and N.M. All authors have read and agreed to the published version of the manuscript.

Funding: This research received no external funding.

Institutional Review Board Statement: Not applicable.

Informed Consent Statement: Not applicable.

Data Availability Statement: Not applicable.

Conflicts of Interest: The authors declare no conflict of interest.

References

1. Craig, J.P.; Nelson, J.D.; Azar, D.T.; Belmonte, C.; Bron, A.J.; Chauhan, S.K.; de Paiva, C.S.; Gomes, J.A.P.; Hammitt, K.M.; Jones, L.; et al. TFOS DEWS II Report Executive Summary. *Ocul. Surf.* **2017**, *15*, 802–812. [CrossRef] [PubMed]
2. Craig, J.P.; Nichols, K.K.; Akpek, E.K.; Caffery, B.; Dua, H.S.; Joo, C.K.; Liu, Z.; Nelson, J.D.; Nichols, J.J.; Tsubota, K.; et al. TFOS DEWS II Definition and Classification Report. *Ocul. Surf.* **2017**, *15*, 276–283. [CrossRef] [PubMed]
3. Uchino, M.; Dogru, M.; Yagi, Y.; Goto, E.; Tomita, M.; Kon, T.; Saiki, M.; Matsumoto, Y.; Uchino, Y.; Yokoi, N.; et al. The features of dry eye disease in a Japanese elderly population. *Optom. Vis. Sci.* **2006**, *83*, 797–802. [CrossRef] [PubMed]
4. Nagino, K.; Sung, J.; Oyama, G.; Hayano, M.; Hattori, N.; Okumura, Y.; Fujio, K.; Akasaki, Y.; Huang, T.; Midorikawa-Inomata, A.; et al. Prevalence and characteristics of dry eye disease in Parkinson's disease: A systematic review and meta-analysis. *Sci. Rep.* **2022**, *12*, 18348. [CrossRef] [PubMed]
5. Hazra, D.; Yotsukura, E.; Torii, H.; Mori, K.; Maruyama, T.; Ogawa, M.; Hanyuda, A.; Tsubota, K.; Kurihara, T.; Negishi, K. Relation between dry eye and myopia based on tear film breakup time, higher order aberration, choroidal thickness, and axial length. *Sci. Rep.* **2022**, *12*, 10891. [CrossRef]
6. Javadi, M.A.; Feizi, S. Dry eye syndrome. *J. Ophthalmic Vis. Res.* **2011**, *6*, 192–198.
7. Alves, M.; Novaes, P.; Morraye, M.D.A.; Reinach, P.S.; Rocha, E.M. Is dry eye an environmental disease? *Arq. Bras. Oftalmol.* **2014**, *77*, 193–200. [CrossRef]
8. Seen, S.; Tong, L. Dry eye disease and oxidative stress. *Acta Ophthalmol.* **2018**, *96*, e412–e420. [CrossRef]
9. Bron, A.J.; de Paiva, C.S.; Chauhan, S.K.; Bonini, S.; Gabison, E.E.; Jain, S.; Knop, E.; Markoulli, M.; Ogawa, Y.; Perez, V.; et al. TFOS DEWS II pathophysiology report. *Ocul. Surf.* **2017**, *15*, 438–510. [CrossRef]
10. Martin, L.M.; Jeyabalan, N.; Tripathi, R.; Panigrahi, T.; Johnson, P.J.; Ghosh, A.; Mohan, R.R. Autophagy in corneal health and disease: A concise review. *Ocul. Surf.* **2019**, *17*, 186–197. [CrossRef]
11. Ohashi, Y.; Ishida, R.; Kojima, T.; Goto, E.; Matsumoto, Y.; Watanabe, K.; Ishida, N.; Nakata, K.; Takeuchi, T.; Tsubota, K. Abnormal protein profiles in tears with dry eye syndrome. *Am. J. Ophthalmol.* **2003**, *136*, 291–299. [CrossRef] [PubMed]
12. Downie, L.E.; Ng, S.M.; Lindsley, K.B.; Akpek, E.K. Omega-3 and omega-6 polyunsaturated fatty acids for dry eye disease. *Cochrane Database Syst. Rev.* **2019**, *12*, CD011016. [CrossRef] [PubMed]
13. Ervin, A.M.; Law, A.; Pucker, A.D. Punctal occlusion for dry eye syndrome: Summary of a Cochrane systematic review. *Br. J. Ophthalmol.* **2019**, *103*, 301–306. [CrossRef] [PubMed]
14. Zhou, X.Q.; Wei, R.L. Topical cyclosporine A in the treatment of dry eye: A systematic review and meta-analysis. *Cornea* **2014**, *33*, 760–767. [CrossRef]
15. Lee, H.K.; Ryu, I.H.; Seo, K.Y.; Hong, S.; Kim, H.C.; Kim, E.K. Topical 0.1% prednisolone lowers nerve growth factor expression in keratoconjunctivitis sicca patients. *Ophthalmology* **2006**, *113*, 198–205. [CrossRef]
16. Prinz, J.; Maffulli, N.; Fuest, M.; Walter, P.; Bell, A.; Migliorini, F. Efficacy of Topical Administration of Corticosteroids for the Management of Dry Eye Disease: Systematic Review and Meta-Analysis. *Life* **2022**, *12*, 1932. [CrossRef]
17. Lemp, M.A. Management of dry eye disease. *Am. J. Manag. Care* **2008**, *14*, S88–S101.
18. McGhee, C.N.; Dean, S.; Danesh-Meyer, H. Locally administered ocular corticosteroids: Benefits and risks. *Drug Saf.* **2002**, *25*, 33–55. [CrossRef]
19. Majtanova, N.; Cernak, M.; Majtan, J. Honey: A Natural Remedy for Eye Diseases. *Res. Complement. Med.* **2016**, *23*, 364–369. [CrossRef]
20. Carnahan, M.C.; Goldstein, D.A. Ocular complications of topical, peri-ocular, and systemic corticosteroids. *Curr. Opin. Ophthalmol.* **2000**, *11*, 478–483. [CrossRef]
21. Mittal, R.; Patel, S.; Galor, A. Alternative therapies for dry eye disease. *Curr. Opin. Ophthalmol.* **2021**, *32*, 348–361. [CrossRef] [PubMed]
22. Salehi, A.; Jabarzare, S.; Neurmohamadi, M.; Kheiri, S.; Rafieian-Kopaei, M. A double blind clinical trial on the efficacy of honey drop in vernal keratoconjunctivitis. *Evid. Based Complement. Altern. Med.* **2014**, *2014*, 287540. [CrossRef] [PubMed]
23. Bogdanov, S.; Jurendic, T.; Sieber, R.; Gallmann, P. Honey for nutrition and health: A review. *J. Am. Coll. Nutr.* **2008**, *27*, 677–689. [CrossRef] [PubMed]
24. Schneider, M.; Coyle, S.; Warnock, M.; Gow, I.; Fyfe, L. Anti-microbial activity and composition of manuka and portobello honey. *Phytother. Res.* **2013**, *27*, 1162–1168. [CrossRef]
25. da Silva, P.M.; Gauche, C.; Gonzaga, L.V.; Costa, A.C.; Fett, R. Honey: Chemical composition, stability and authenticity. *Food Chem.* **2016**, *196*, 309–323. [CrossRef] [PubMed]
26. Hills, S.P.; Mitchell, P.; Wells, C.; Russell, M. Honey Supplementation and Exercise: A Systematic Review. *Nutrients* **2019**, *11*, 1586. [CrossRef] [PubMed]
27. Wong, D.; Albietz, J.M.; Tran, H.; Du Toit, C.; Li, A.H.; Yun, T.; Han, J.; Schmid, K.L. Treatment of contact lens related dry eye with antibacterial honey. *Contact Lens Anterior Eye* **2017**, *40*, 389–393. [CrossRef]
28. Chong, K.K.; Lai, F.H.; Ho, M.; Luk, A.; Wong, B.W.; Young, A. Randomized trial on silicone intubation in endoscopic mechanical dacryocystorhinostomy (SEND) for primary nasolacrimal duct obstruction. *Ophthalmology* **2013**, *120*, 2139–2145. [CrossRef]
29. Inoue, S.; Kawashima, M.; Hisamura, R.; Imada, T.; Izuta, Y.; Nakamura, S.; Ito, M.; Tsubota, K. Clinical Evaluation of a Royal Jelly Supplementation for the Restoration of Dry Eye: A Prospective Randomized Double Blind Placebo Controlled Study and an Experimental Mouse Model. *PLoS ONE* **2017**, *12*, e0169069. [CrossRef]

30. Hermanns, R.; Mateescu, C.; Thrasyvoulou, A.; Tananaki, C.; Wagener, F.A.D.T.G.; Cremers, N.A.J. Defining the standards for medical grade honey. *J. Apic. Res.* **2020**, *59*, 125–135. [CrossRef]
31. Bashkaran, K.; Zunaina, E.; Bakiah, S.; Sulaiman, S.A.; Sirajudeen, K.; Naik, V. Anti-inflammatory and antioxidant effects of Tualang honey in alkali injury on the eyes of rabbits: Experimental animal study. *BMC Complement. Altern. Med.* **2011**, *11*, 90. [CrossRef] [PubMed]
32. Albietz, J.M.; Lenton, L.M. Standardised antibacterial Manuka honey in the management of persistent post-operative corneal oedema: A case series. *Clin. Exp. Optom.* **2015**, *98*, 464–472. [CrossRef] [PubMed]
33. Mansour, A.M.; Zein, W.; Haddad, R.; Khoury, J. Bullous keratopathy treated with honey. *Acta Ophthalmol. Scand.* **2004**, *82*, 312–313. [CrossRef] [PubMed]
34. Albietz, J.M.; Lenton, L.M. Late reactivation of herpes zoster keratitis results in band keratopathy. *Optom. Vis. Sci.* **2014**, *91*, e149–e155. [CrossRef]
35. Tonks, A.J.; Cooper, R.A.; Jones, K.P.; Blair, S.; Parton, J.; Tonks, A. Honey stimulates inflammatory cytokine production from monocytes. *Cytokine* **2003**, *21*, 242–247. [CrossRef]
36. Albietz, J.M.; Schmid, K.L. Randomised controlled trial of topical antibacterial Manuka (*Leptospermum species*) honey for evaporative dry eye due to meibomian gland dysfunction. *Clin. Exp. Optom.* **2017**, *100*, 603–615. [CrossRef]
37. Craig, J.P.; Cruzat, A.; Cheung, I.M.Y.; Watters, G.A.; Wang, M.T.M. Randomized masked trial of the clinical efficacy of MGO Manuka Honey microemulsion eye cream for the treatment of blepharitis. *Ocul. Surf.* **2020**, *18*, 170–177. [CrossRef]
38. Tan, J.; Jia, T.; Liao, R.; Stapleton, F. Effect of a formulated eye drop with Leptospermum spp honey on tear film properties. *Br. J. Ophthalmol.* **2020**, *104*, 1373–1377. [CrossRef]
39. Stapleton, F.; Alves, M.; Bunya, V.Y.; Jalbert, I.; Lekhanont, K.; Malet, F.; Na, K.S.; Schaumberg, D.; Uchino, M.; Vehof, J.; et al. TFOS DEWS II Epidemiology Report. *Ocul. Surf.* **2017**, *15*, 334–365. [CrossRef]
40. Betiku, A.O.; Oduyoye, O.O.; Jagun, O.O.; Olajide, O.S.; Adebusoye, S.O.; Aham-Onyebuchi, U.O. Prevalence and risk factors associated with dry eye disease among adults in a population-based setting in South-West Nigeria. *Niger. J. Clin. Pract.* **2022**, *25*, 354–360. [CrossRef]
41. Alvarez-Suarez, J.M.; Gasparrini, M.; Forbes-Hernández, T.Y.; Mazzoni, L.; Giampieri, F. The Composition and Biological Activity of Honey: A Focus on Manuka Honey. *Foods* **2014**, *3*, 420–432. [CrossRef] [PubMed]
42. Abd Rashid, N.; Mohammed, S.N.F.; Syed Abd Halim, S.A.; Ghafar, N.A.; Abdul Jalil, N.A. Therapeutic Potential of Honey and Propolis on Ocular Disease. *Pharmaceuticals* **2022**, *15*, 1419. [CrossRef] [PubMed]
43. Ahmad, S.; Campos, M.G.; Fratini, F.; Altaye, S.Z.; Li, J. New Insights into the Biological and Pharmaceutical Properties of Royal Jelly. *Int. J. Mol. Sci.* **2020**, *21*, 382. [CrossRef] [PubMed]
44. Uchino, Y.; Kawakita, T.; Miyazawa, M.; Ishii, T.; Onouchi, H.; Yasuda, K.; Ogawa, Y.; Shimmura, S.; Ishii, N.; Tsubota, K. Oxidative stress induced inflammation initiates functional decline of tear production. *PLoS ONE* **2012**, *7*, e45805. [CrossRef]
45. Navel, V.; Sapin, V.; Henrioux, F.; Blanchon, L.; Labbé, A.; Chiambaretta, F.; Baudouin, C.; Dutheil, F. Oxidative and antioxidative stress markers in dry eye disease: A systematic review and meta-analysis. *Acta Ophthalmol.* **2022**, *100*, 45–57. [CrossRef]
46. Dogru, M.; Kojima, T.; Simsek, C.; Tsubota, K. Potential Role of Oxidative Stress in Ocular Surface Inflammation and Dry Eye Disease. *Investig. Ophthalmol. Vis. Sci.* **2018**, *59*, DES163–DES168. [CrossRef]
47. Imada, T.; Nakamura, S.; Kitamura, N.; Shibuya, I.; Tsubota, K. Oral administration of royal jelly restores tear secretion capacity in rat blink-suppressed dry eye model by modulating lacrimal gland function. *PLoS ONE* **2014**, *9*, e106338. [CrossRef] [PubMed]
48. Ahmed, S.; Sulaiman, S.A.; Baig, A.A.; Ibrahim, M.; Liaqat, S.; Fatima, S.; Jabeen, S.; Shamim, N.; Othman, N.H. Honey as a Potential Natural Antioxidant Medicine: An Insight into Its Molecular Mechanisms of Action. *Oxid. Med. Cell. Longev.* **2018**, *2018*, 8367846. [CrossRef]
49. Panche, A.N.; Diwan, A.D.; Chandra, S.R. Flavonoids: An overview. *J. Nutr. Sci.* **2016**, *5*, e47. [CrossRef]
50. Cheng, N.; Wang, Y.; Cao, W. The Protective Effect of Whole Honey and Phenolic Extract on Oxidative DNA Damage in Mice Lymphocytes Using Comet Assay. *Plant. Foods Hum. Nutr.* **2017**, *72*, 388–395. [CrossRef]
51. Asgary, S.; Sahebkar, A.; Afshani, M.R.; Keshvari, M.; Haghjooyjavanmard, S.; Rafieian-Kopaei, M. Clinical evaluation of blood pressure lowering, endothelial function improving, hypolipidemic and anti-inflammatory effects of pomegranate juice in hypertensive subjects. *Phytother. Res.* **2014**, *28*, 193–199. [CrossRef] [PubMed]
52. Asgary, S.; Kelishadi, R.; Rafieian-Kopaei, M.; Najafi, S.; Najafi, M.; Sahebkar, A. Investigation of the lipid-modifying and antiinflammatory effects of *Cornus mas* L. supplementation on dyslipidemic children and adolescents. *Pediatr. Cardiol.* **2013**, *34*, 1729–1735. [CrossRef] [PubMed]
53. O'Brien, T.P. The role of bacteria in blepharitis. *Ocul. Surf.* **2009**, *7*, S21–S22. [CrossRef] [PubMed]
54. Albietz, J.M.; Lenton, L.M. Effect of antibacterial honey on the ocular flora in tear deficiency and meibomian gland disease. *Cornea* **2006**, *25*, 1012–1019. [CrossRef]
55. McCulley, J.P.; Dougherty, J.M. Bacterial aspects of chronic blepharitis. *Trans. Ophthalmol. Soc. U. K.* **1986**, *105 Pt 3*, 314–318. [PubMed]
56. Doughty, M.J. Contact lens wear and the goblet cells of the human conjunctiva-A review. *Contact Lens Anterior Eye* **2011**, *34*, 157–163. [CrossRef]
57. Terry, R.L.; Schnider, C.M.; Holden, B.A.; Cornish, R.; Grant, T.; Sweeney, D.; La Hood, D.; Back, A. CCLRU standards for success of daily and extended wear contact lenses. *Optom. Vis. Sci.* **1993**, *70*, 234–243. [CrossRef]

58. Bron, A.J.; Evans, V.E.; Smith, J.A. Grading of corneal and conjunctival staining in the context of other dry eye tests. *Cornea* **2003**, *22*, 640–650. [CrossRef]
59. Bergman, A.; Yanai, J.; Weiss, J.; Bell, D.; David, M.P. Acceleration of wound healing by topical application of honey. An animal model. *Am. J. Surg.* **1983**, *145*, 374–376. [CrossRef]
60. Tonks, A.J.; Dudley, E.; Porter, N.G.; Parton, J.; Brazier, J.; Smith, E.L.; Tonks, A. A 5.8-kDa component of manuka honey stimulates immune cells via TLR4. *J. Leukoc. Biol.* **2007**, *82*, 1147–1155. [CrossRef]
61. Snowdon, J.A.; Cliver, D.O. Microorganisms in honey. *Int. J. Food Microbiol.* **1996**, *31*, 1–26. [CrossRef] [PubMed]
62. Inoue, T.; Kawaji, T.; Inatani, M.; Kameda, T.; Yoshimura, N.; Tanihara, H. Simultaneous increases in multiple proinflammatory cytokines in the aqueous humor in pseudophakic glaucomatous eyes. *J. Cataract. Refract. Surg.* **2012**, *38*, 1389–1397. [CrossRef] [PubMed]
63. Irish, J.; Blair, S.; Carter, D.A. The antibacterial activity of honey derived from Australian flora. *PLoS ONE* **2011**, *6*, e18229. [CrossRef] [PubMed]
64. Howick, J.; Chalmers, I.; Glasziou, P.; Greenhalgh, T.; Heneghan, C.; Liberati, A.; Moschetti, I.; Phillips, B.; Thornton, H.; Goddard, O.; et al. The 2011 Oxford CEBM Levels of Evidence. *Oxf. Cent. Evid. Based Med.* **2011**, *1*, 1–3. Available online: https://www.cebm.net/index.aspx?o=5653 (accessed on 14 April 2023).
65. Page, M.J.; McKenzie, J.E.; Bossuyt, P.M.; Boutron, I.; Hoffmann, T.C.; Mulrow, C.D.; Shamseer, L.; Tetzlaff, J.M.; Akl, E.A.; Brennan, S.E.; et al. The PRISMA 2020 statement: An updated guideline for reporting systematic reviews. *BMJ* **2021**, *372*, n71. [CrossRef]
66. Walt, J.G.; Rowe, M.M.; Stern, K.L. Evaluating the functional impact of dry eye: The Ocular Surface Disease Index. *Drug Inf. J.* **1997**, *31*, b5.
67. Cho, P.; Leung, L.; Lam, A.; Choi, A. Tear break-up time: Clinical procedures and their effects. *Ophthalmic Physiol. Opt.* **1998**, *18*, 319–324. [CrossRef]
68. Cho, P.; Yap, M. Schirmer test. I. A review. *Optom. Vis. Sci.* **1993**, *70*, 152–156. [CrossRef]

pharmaceutics

Article

Rutin/Sulfobutylether-β-Cyclodextrin as a Promising Therapeutic Formulation for Ocular Infection

Federica De Gaetano [1], Martina Pastorello [1], Venerando Pistarà [2], Antonio Rescifina [2], Fatima Margani [3], Vincenzina Barbera [3], Cinzia Anna Ventura [1,*] and Andreana Marino [1,*]

1 Department of Chemical, Biological, Pharmaceutical and Environmental Sciences, University of Messina, Viale Ferdinando Stagno d'Alcontres 31, 98166 Messina, Italy; fedegaetano@unime.it (F.D.G.); martina.pastorello@studenti.unime.it (M.P.)
2 Department of Pharmaceutical and Health Sciences, University of Catania, Viale Andrea Doria 6, 95125 Catania, Italy; vpistara@unict.it (V.P.); arescifina@unict.it (A.R.)
3 Department of Chemistry, Materials and Chemical Engineering "G. Natta", Politecnico di Milano, Via Mancinelli 7, 20131 Milano, Italy; fatima.margani@polimi.it (F.M.); vincenzina.barbera@polimi.it (V.B.)
* Correspondence: caventura@unime.it (C.A.V.); anmarino@unime.it (A.M.)

Abstract: Ocular pathologies present significant challenges to achieving effective therapeutic results due to various anatomical and physiological barriers. Natural products such as flavonoids, alone or in association with allopathic drugs, present many therapeutic actions including anticancer, anti-inflammatory, and antibacterial action. However, their clinical employment is challenging for scientists due to their low water solubility. In this study, we designed a liquid formulation based on rutin/sulfobutylether-β-cyclodextrin (RTN/SBE-β-CD) inclusion complex for treating ocular infections. The correct stoichiometry and the accurate binding constant were determined by employing SupraFit software (2.5.120) in the UV-vis titration experiment. A deep physical–chemical characterization of the RTN/SBE-β-CD inclusion complex was also performed; it confirmed the predominant formation of a stable complex (K_c, 9660 M^{-1}) in a 1:1 molar ratio, with high water solubility that was 20 times (2.5 mg/mL) higher than the free molecule (0.125 mg/mL), permitting the dissolution of the solid complex within 30 min. NMR studies revealed the involvement of the bicyclic flavonoid moiety in the complexation, which was also confirmed by molecular modeling studies. In vitro, the antibacterial and antibiofilm activity of the formulation was assayed against *Staphylococcus aureus* and *Pseudomonas aeruginosa* strains. The results demonstrated a significant activity of the formulation than that of the free molecules.

Keywords: rutin; sulfobutylether-β-cyclodextrin; antibacterial activity; resistant strains; biofilm

Citation: De Gaetano, F.; Pastorello, M.; Pistarà, V.; Rescifina, A.; Margani, F.; Barbera, V.; Ventura, C.A.; Marino, A. Rutin/Sulfobutylether-β-Cyclodextrin as a Promising Therapeutic Formulation for Ocular Infection. *Pharmaceutics* **2024**, *16*, 233. https://doi.org/10.3390/pharmaceutics16020233

Academic Editor: Antonio María Rabasco Álvarez

Received: 11 January 2024
Revised: 26 January 2024
Accepted: 30 January 2024
Published: 5 February 2024

1. Introduction

Ocular infections are a worldwide health problem. If not treated properly, they can become worse, damaging the anatomic structure of the eye and leading to permanent vision loss or blindness [1].

Common ocular infections caused by microorganisms include conjunctivitis, keratitis, cellulitis, endophthalmitis, and dacryocystitis. Among these, keratitis is a devastating disease that is responsible for up to 2 million annual cases of blindness globally [2]. The main microorganisms causing ocular infections are bacteria [3]. Among these, *S. aureus* and *P. aeruginosa* are the most common pathogens [4]. *S. aureus* is a Gram-positive bacterium that is a leading cause of conjunctivitis, keratitis, and endophthalmitis [5]. This species is included in the ESKAPE group (*Enterococcus faecium*, *Staphylococcus aureus*, *Klebsiella pneumoniae*, *Acinetobacter baumannii*, *Pseudomonas aeruginosa*, and *Enterobacter* species). These bacteria are involved in infections and are categorized by multidrug resistance. Incidence of ocular infection caused by methicillin-resistant *S. aureus* (MRSA) has increased considerably over the last two decades [6] and this represents a significant global health concern mainly in hospital (HA-MRSA) and community settings (CA-MRSA) [5,6]. The Surveillance Network in the United States reported an increase in the percentage of MRSA among *S. aureus* ocular infections, from 29.5% in 2000 to 41.6% in 2005. In India, the incidence of MRSA increased from 9% in 2007 to 38% in 2017 [7]. Moreover, *S. aureus* can form biofilm which aggravates the problem of antimicrobial resistance. Biofilm is a structured consortium of bacteria embedded in a self-produced polymer matrix of polysaccharides, proteins, and DNA; it represents a physical barrier against drugs and host immune responses. *P. aeruginosa* is a Gram-negative bacterium included in the ESKAPE group, which is resistant to treatment with most antibiotics and causes vision-threatening ocular infections. Moreover, due to its predisposition to form biofilms, *P. aeruginosa* is the major cause of keratitis in contact-lens wearers [8]. In the United States, *P. aeruginosa* incidence may be as high as 70% for contact lens-associated keratitis. Treatment for several ocular surface diseases comprises eye drops containing antibiotics. However, this can stimulate changes in the healthy eye microbiota and contribute to increasing the resistance of pathogenic strains [9]. Currently, treatment for ocular surface infections involves the use of topical antibiotics such as fluoroquinolones, tetracycline, or chloramphenicol. Alternatively, fortified antibiotics (e.g., cefazolin with gentamicin or tobramycin) may be used in cases of severe infection [5,10,11].

As a response to rising antibiotic resistance, new therapeutic strategies are in development. Over the years, interest in plant extracts and their metabolites has risen within the scientific community [12,13]. Rutin (RTN) (Figure 1), which is a flavonoid isolated from plants or fruits, showed antibacterial activity against *S. aureus*, *A. baumannii*, and *P. aeruginosa* [14]. Some authors have suggested that RTN interferes with the membranes of *P. aeruginosa* and MRSA cells, causing the release of proteins and nucleic acids. Moreover, it has been demonstrated to decrease biofilm biomass of *P. aeruginosa* and MRSA catheter biofilms with a mechanism leading to the reduction of cell viability, exopolysaccharide, and extracellular DNA levels [15]. Furthermore, it has been demonstrated that RTN potentiates the antibacterial activity of different antibiotics against MRSA strains [4].

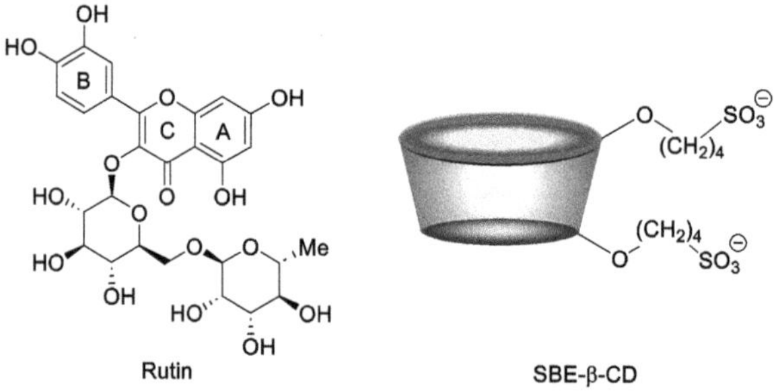

Figure 1. Molecular structure of RTN (**left**) and schematic structure of SBE-β-CD (**right**).

Despite these exciting attributes, unfavorable physical–chemical properties of RTN—particularly water solubility [16,17]—prevent its employment in therapy. It is highly insoluble in water and biological fluids in the doses in which it is to be administered, showing poor and erratic bioavailability [18]. Cyclodextrins (CDs) could be used to overcome this drawback. They are cyclic oligosaccharides that are able to complex apolar drugs and effectively improve their physicochemical properties, including water solubility [19–26] and biological effects [27–29].

A search of the literature shows that many studies have been performed concerning the preparation and physical–chemical characterization of the inclusion complexes between RTN and native or modified CDs [30,31]. In some cases, in vitro or in vivo biological activities were reported. For example, the complexation of RTN within native β-CD [32] and hydroxypropyl-β-CD (HP-β-CD) [33,34] improves its antioxidant and antimicrobial effects in vitro [34,35]. Furthermore, RTN/β-CD and RTN/dimethyl-β-CD showed improved antioxidant activity compared with free RTN in the DPPH free radical scavenging assay [36]. Recently, RTN/β-CD and RTN/HP-β-CD inclusion complexes have demonstrated good antiproliferative activity in different cultured cancer cells [37,38]. Oral administration of

RTN/HP-β-CD inclusion complex produced increased bioavailability of RTN from the gastrointestinal tracts of beagle dogs due to increased water solubility, faster dissolution rate, and gastrointestinal stability of the drug [39].

To the best of our knowledge, although substantial literature concerning the complexation of RTN with different modified CDs is available, very few papers describe the complexation of RTN with sulfobutyl-ether-β-CD (SBE-β-CD). Furthermore, none of these concern its antimicrobial and antibiofilm activity either in vitro or in vivo. Wu et al. [40] conducted a luminescence study to determine the association constant of RTN/SBE-β-CD inclusion complex and applied this technique to quantify RTN on urine samples. Gozcu et al. made a gel containing RTN/SBE-β-CD inclusion complex as a promising topical system [41], and Zhou et al. [42] reported a UV-vis spectroscopic characterization of the complex. However, neither were biological studies.

SBE-β-CD is an anionic modified CD (Figure 1) with higher water solubility and complexing ability than native β-CD or other modified β-CDs that are usually present in marketed pharmaceutical products. It shows high biocompatibility and non-toxicity, and is approved by the FDA for intramuscular (IM) and intravenous (IV) administration. Fifteen products are on the market today containing SBE-β-CD. This CD shows excellent complexing ability toward different drugs, significantly improving their solubility and dissolution rate and potentiating their biological effects [43]. The complexation of carbamazepine into SBE-β-CD enhances the antiepileptic activity in vivo compared with carbamazepine suspension, due to significant improvement of the drug solubility in gastric fluids, ameliorating absorption and oral bioavailability [44]. Curcumin/SBE-β-CD inclusion complex demonstrated superior antimicrobial activity against *Escherichia coli* and *Staphylococcus aureus* than free curcumin, showing good potential as a treatment option for urinary tract infections [45].

Based on these excellent properties, a more remarkable improvement of physical–chemical and biological properties of RTN could be expected using SBE-β-CD rather than other CDs. Thus, in this work, we developed a liquid formulation based on RTN/SBE-β-CD inclusion complex, which is able to improve the antibacterial and antibiofilm activity of RTN. The formulation is designed to be administered ophthalmically. The inclusion complex was prepared by freeze-drying and characterized by phase-solubility studies, UV-vis, and NMR spectroscopy. Thermogravimetric analysis and X-ray diffraction were performed on the inclusion complex in a solid state. Molecular modeling studies on the RTN/SBE-β-CD inclusion complex were conducted to evaluate the energetic and structural rationalization of the recognition process. Finally, the antibacterial properties of RTN/SBE-β-CD inclusion complex were assayed in comparison with those of free components, and complexed with SBE-β-CD by in vitro studies against *Staphylococcus aureus* and *Pseudomonas aeruginosa*.

2. Materials and Methods

2.1. Materials

Rutin (RTN, $C_{27}H_{30}O_{16}$, molecular weight, 610.5 g/mol) and levofloxacin hydrochloride (LVF, $C_{18}H_{20}FN_3O_4$, molecular weight (MW) 361.37 g/mol) were purchased from Sigma-Aldrich (St. Louis, MO, USA). Sulfobutyl-ether-β-cyclodextrin (SBE-β-CD, CAPTISOL®, average degree of substitution seven, average molecular weight, 2162 g/mol) was supplied by CyDex Pharmaceutical (Lenexa, KS, USA). Culture media were purchased from ThermoFisher (Oxoid, Milan, Italy). The other reagents were purchased from Sigma-Aldrich (Milan, Italy) unless otherwise specified in the text.

2.2. Preparation of RTN/SBE-β-CD Inclusion Complex and Physical Mixture

RTN/SBE-β-CD inclusion complex was prepared by lyophilization. Initially, 10 mg of RTN (1.64 M^{-3}) was weighed and solubilized in 2 mL of MeOH. Subsequently, 71 mg of SBE-β-CD (3.3 M^{-3}) was solubilized in 8 mL of H_2O and added to the methanol solution of RTN. The mixture was magnetically stirred at room temperature for 30 min. The obtained solution was freeze-dried for 72 h (VirtTis Benchtop K Instrument, SP Scientific, Gardiner, NY, USA).

RTN/SBE-β-CD physical mixture in a 1:2 molar ratio was obtained by carefully mixing an accurately weighed amount of drug and SBE-β-CD in a mortar, until the mixture was homogeneously colored.

2.3. UV-Vis Titration

Free RTN (0.09 mg, 0.03 M^{-3}) and increasing concentrations of SBE-β-CD (0.03, 0.09, 0.15, 0.3, 0.9, 1.5, 2.1, 3 × 10^{-3} M) were solubilized in a water/methanol mixture (80:20, *v*/*v*) and stirred in the dark at 500 rpm for 24 h, before the analysis. The solutions were analyzed by UV-vis spectroscopy in the spectral range 200–600 nm using a diode array spectrophotometer, StellarNet BLACK-Comet, Model C (Tampa, FL, USA).

2.4. Phase-Solubility Studies

Phase-solubility studies of the RTN/SBE-β-CD system were performed by the Higuchi and Connors method [46]. RTN was added to aqueous solutions containing increasing concentrations of SBE-β-CD (0–12 mM) at concentrations exceeding its intrinsic solubility. The obtained suspensions were left to stir in the dark in a thermostatic bath at 25.0 ± 0.5 °C (Telesystem 15.40, Thermo Scientific, Waltham, MA, USA). The bath was equipped with a temperature control unit (Telemodul 40C, Thermo Scientific, USA). After that, the suspensions were filtered through Sartorius Minisart-SRP 15-PTFE filters (0.22 µm, Bedford, MA, USA). The solutions were then diluted with methanol (all final solutions were water/methanol, 80/20, *v*/*v*) and analyzed spectrophotometrically to quantify RTN in solution. A calibration curve prepared in water/methanol solution (20/80, *v*/*v*) at a λmax of 256 nm, with concentrations ranging from 0.00090 to 0.036 mg/mL, was used and an R^2 value of 0.9953 was obtained.

The experiments were carried out in triplicate to obtain reliable results, and phase solubility diagrams were constructed. The concentration of SBE-β-CD is represented on the abscissas of these diagrams, while the concentration of RTN in solution is represented on the ordinates. Using the following Higuchi and Connors equation (Equation (1)) [46], the apparent 1:1 association constant (K_c) of the complex was calculated, where S_0 is the intrinsic water solubility of RTN:

$$K_c = \frac{\text{Slope}}{(1 - \text{Slope})S_0}, \tag{1}$$

2.5. Nuclear Magnetic Resonance Experiments

Samples containing equivalent concentrations (9 mM) of RTN, SBE-β-CD, and RTN/SBE-β-CD inclusion complex were added to a D_2O/CD_3OD (7/3, *v*/*v*) solution and transferred to 5 mm NMR tubes. A Varian Unity Inova 500 MHz (11.75 T) instrument was used for all spectra recorded at 300 K. The residual water peak (4.79 ppm) was used as the internal reference to avoid adding external ones that could interact with SBE-β-CD.

2.6. Molecular Modeling Studies

2.6.1. Structure Preparation

A 3D structure for the SBE-β-CD was not available, therefore, the structure was built according to our precedent study [47]. The 3D coordinates of the RTN molecule were downloaded from Pubchem (https://pubchem.ncbi.nlm.nih.gov/compound/Rutin, accessed on 10 January 2024).

2.6.2. Molecular Dynamics

The molecular dynamics (MD) simulation was made in explicit water using the YASARA Structure package (23.9.29) [48], according to previously reported procedures [49,50]. The RTN and SBE-β-CD force field parameters were generated using the GAFF2 [51] and AM1BCC [52] force fields as well as TIP3P for water. For Van der Waals forces (the default value used by AMBER), the cutoff was 10 Å [53], but no cutoff was used for electrostatic forces (the Particle Mesh Ewald method) [54]. Using procedures previously discussed in detail, the equations of movements were integrated with multiple time steps of 2.5 fs for bonded interactions and 5.0 fs for nonbonded interactions at a temperature of 298 K and a pressure of 1 atm (NPT ensemble) [55]. The finished system was around 30 × 36 × 32 Å3. To eliminate clashes, a brief MD simulation was performed solely on the solvent. Then, in order to remove conformational stress, the complete system was energy reduced using the steepest descent minimization. This was followed by a simulated annealing minimization until convergence (<0.01 kcal/mol Å). Ultimately, unrestricted MD simulations lasting 500 ns were run and the conformations of each system were recorded every 250 ps. The latest three ns averaged structures were taken into consideration for additional analysis after the solute RMSD as a function of simulation time was examined.

2.6.3. Binding Free Energy Calculation

The binding free energy was computed using the well-known and extensively applied molecular mechanics Poisson–Boltzmann surface area (MM/PBSA) approach [56] on the optimized MD structure acquired from the previous phase. YASARA adopted Nunthaboot's consolidated procedure for this process [57].

2.7. *Wide-Angle X-ray Diffraction (WAXD)*

WAXD patterns of RTN/SBE-β-CD inclusion complex were performed in comparison with free components and the physical mixture by using an automatic Bruker D8 Advance diffractometer (Bruker, Billerica, MA, USA), with nickel-filtered Cu–Kα radiation. The analyses were performed in reflection, in 4°–90° as the 2θ range, being 2θ the peak diffraction angle.

2.8. *Thermogravimetric Analysis (TGA)*

Thermal properties of the inclusion complex in comparison with the free components and RTN/SBE-β-CD physical mixture were investigated by using a Perkin Elmer STA 6000 instrument (PerkinElmer Inc., Waltham, MA, USA). All scans were performed under nitrogen. A weighed amount of each sample (5–10 mg) was heated from 30 °C to 300 °C at a heating rate of 10 °C min^{-1}, kept at 300 °C for 10 min, and then heated up to 550 °C at 20 °C min^{-1}. Samples were maintained at 550 °C for 15 min, then further heated up to 900 °C (heating rate of 10 °C/min) and kept at 900 °C for 3 min, then kept at 900 °C for 30 min under flowing air (60 mL/min).

2.9. *Fourier-Transform Infrared (FT-IR) Spectroscopy*

The FT-IR spectra of the inclusion complex, free components and the physical mixture were performed at 25 °C, with a wavenumber ranging from 4000 cm^{-1} to 400 cm^{-1}; this was done using a FT-IR Nicolet iS5 spectrometer (Nicolet Instrument Corporation, Madison, WI, USA).

2.10. *Scanning Electron Microscopy (SEM)*

The surface morphologies of free RTN, SBE-β-CD, the physical mixture, and their inclusion complex were investigated through scanning electron microscopy. SEM images were acquired using a Zeiss Evo 50 EP (Carl Zeiss SMT, Oberkochen, Germany) with an operating voltage of 15 kV. All samples were gold-coated using a sputtering system before imaging; a coating of roughly 10 nm was deposited.

2.11. *Determination of Water Solubility and Dissolution Profile of RTN/SBE-β-CD Inclusion Complex*

The solubility of RTN/SBE-β-CD inclusion complex was determined in the dark at 25.0 ± 0.5 °C. An excess of freeze-dried RTN/SBE-β-CD inclusion complex was dispersed into 10 mL of water. The suspension was kept under magnetic stirring for 24 h until the equilibrium was reached. At timed intervals a sample of suspension was collected, filtered and the RTN quantified by UV-vis spectroscopy (diode array spectrophotometer, StellarNet BLACK-Comet, Model C—Tampa, FL, USA).

Following the 44th United States Pharmacopoeia (USP), paddle method dissolution studies were conducted in the dark at 37.0 ± 0.5 °C, keeping the dissolution medium in a constant, smooth motion (100 rpm). Free RTN (150 mg) or a corresponding amount in the complex was suspended in 900 mL of water. At fixed times (15, 30, 45, 60, and 120 min), 1 mL aliquot was collected, filtered, and analyzed by UV-vis using a diode array spectrophotometer StellarNet BLACK-Comet, Model C (Tampa, FL, USA) to determine the concentration of RTN in the solution. The volume was kept constant by adding fresh preheated water, and the data were corrected according to the dilutions. Experiments were conducted in triplicate, and sink conditions were maintained for all the experiments.

2.12. *In Vitro Antibacterial and Antibiofilm Activity*

2.12.1. Strains

The following strains were used in this study: *Staphylococcus aureus* ATCC 6538, biofilm-producing reference strain [58], *S. aureus* ATCC 43300 (Methicillin resistant *S. aureus*-MRSA), *Pseudomonas aeruginosa* ATCC 9027, *P. aeruginosa* DSM 102273 (multidrug resistant). The strains were stored in the private collection of the Department of Chemical, Biological, Pharmaceutical and Environmental Sciences, University of Messina (Messina, Italy). They were stored at −70 °C in Microbanks™ (Pro-lab Diagnostics, Neston, UK).

2.12.2. Susceptibility Tests

The antibacterial activity of the RTN/SBE-β-CD inclusion complex was evaluated compared with free RTN and SBE-β-CD by determining the minimum inhibitory concentration (MIC) and the minimum bactericidal concentration (MBC) against the strains mentioned above. The MIC was assessed using the broth microdilution method, following the Clinical and Laboratory Standards Institute, with some modifications [59]. An overnight culture in Müeller–Hinton broth for each strain was adjusted to the required inoculum of 1×10^6 enumerate colony-forming units (CFU)/mL. Aliquots of 100 µL of each suspension were inoculated in a 96-well microtiter plate containing a serial 2-fold dilution of free RTN, free SBE-β-CD, RTN/SBE-β-CD inclusion complex or 100 µL medium (growth control). Negative controls (medium + samples) were included. Levofloxacin hydrochloride (LVF) was used as the positive drug control. The bacterial growth was indicated visually and by a developer of enzymatic activity (Triphenyl tetrazolium chloride 0.05%, TTC). This revealed bacterial growth, which showed as a purple color after 15 min heating at 37 °C. The maximum RTN concentration tested was 1250 µg/mL as soluble RTN/SBE-β-CD inclusion complex, 150 µg/mL for free RTN (maximum solubility) and 8875 µg/mL for free SBE-β-CD, corresponding to the amount present in the assayed inclusion complex. The MIC-values, representing the lowest concentration showing no visible bacterial growth, were obtained after 24 h of incubation at 37 ± 1 °C. The MBC was evaluated by pipetting 10 µL from each clear well onto Müeller–Hinton agar plates. After 24 h of incubation at 37 °C, MBC was read as the lowest concentration which resulted in killing 99.9% of the initial inoculum. All experiments were repeated in triplicate.

2.12.3. Effect on Biofilm Biomass and Viability

The antibiofilm effect was assessed, as described by Cramton et al. [60], with some modifications. Overnight cultures in Tryptic Soy Broth (TSB) with 1% glucose (TSBG) or without were diluted to standardize *S. aureus* or *P. aeruginosa* suspensions (1×10^6 CFU/mL), respectively. Aliquots of 100 µL were dispensed into each well of sterile flat-bottom 96-well polystyrene microtiter plates (Corning Inc., Corning, New York, NY, USA) in the presence of samples at sub-MIC concentrations (0.5 MIC) or 100 µL medium (positive control). Negative controls (medium + samples) were included. The microtiter plates were incubated for 24 h at 37 °C. The medium was then aspirated and the wells were rinsed twice with phosphate-buffered saline (PBS), and fixed by drying for 1 h. Once the wells were fully dry, 200 µL of 0.1% safranin was added for 5 min. The contents of the wells were then aspirated and, after rinsing with water, 200 µL of 30% acetic acid (*v*/*v*) was added to the wells for spectrophotometric analysis. The OD 492 nm value obtained for each strain without a sample was used as the control. The reduction percentage of biofilm biomass formation in the presence of different samples was calculated using the ratio between the values of OD 492 nm with and without samples, adopting the following formula:

$$[(\text{OD control} - \text{OD sample})/\text{OD control}) \times 100]$$

All experiments were repeated in triplicate. At the same time, the percentage of viable biomass was determined by the CFU counting method. Biofilm bacteria were scraped thoroughly from the wells with a pipet tip, with particular attention to the edges. The bacterial suspensions obtained were serially 10-fold diluted, plated on Tryptic Soy Agar plates, and grown for 24 h at 37 °C to enumerate CFU. Viability measures are derived from three separate experiments.

2.13. Statistical Analysis

Each measurement was repeated three times and the results were expressed as mean ± standard deviation (SD). Values were processed via one-way and two-way analysis of variance (ANOVA) followed by a Bonferroni post hoc test for multiple comparisons. A value of $p < 0.05$ was significant.

3. Results and Discussion

3.1. Studies of RTN/SBE-β-CD Characteristics

The interaction between SBE-β-CD and RTN has been extensively studied in solution and at solid state. RTN/SBE-β-CD inclusion complex was prepared by freeze-drying a hydroalcoholic solution containing RTN and SBE-β-CD in a 1:2 molar ratio. Twenty percent (*v*/*v*) of MeOH was added to allow complete solubilization of RTN, favoring the complexation. The excess of SBE-β-CD to 1:1 molar ratio was used to maintain the complex in solution.

3.1.1. UV-Vis Spectroscopy Studies

The host–guest interaction between RTN and SBE-β-CD was studied by UV-vis spectroscopy. In Figure 2, we showed the spectra of free RTN and in the presence of increasing concentrations of SBE-β-CD. RTN shows two very intense bands; the first at 256 nm (Band II) and the second at 351 nm (Band I) [32]. These are both attributed to the $\pi \rightarrow \pi^*$ transitions. Mabri et al. [61] attributed the band at 256 nm to the $\pi \rightarrow \pi^*$ electronic rearrangement of the phenyl group, and the band at 351 nm to the benzene ring of the pyrocatecholic moiety, which can be regarded as an acyl-disubstituted benzene chromophore. Increasing amounts of SBE-β-CD resulted in a significant variation of the UV-vis spectrum of RTN. Both absorption bands shifted progressively towards the blue (hypsochromic effect) and increased in intensity (Figure 2). The significant variation of the RTN spectrum observed in the presence of SBE-β-CD and the high value of the apparent association constant highlight variation of the local polarity of the RTN chromophores which pass from the hydrophilic environment into the apolar cavity of the macrocycle, with a corresponding perturbation of the electronic transition. Furthermore, we cannot exclude that complexation produces the breakdown of the intramolecular hydrogen bonds present in the RTN molecule between the C3-OH oxygen atom with the C4-OH proton of the A ring and between the C3-OH proton of the A ring with the rhamnosidic C2-OH oxygen atom [62], followed by an establishment of other hydrogen bonds between pyrocatecholic moiety of RTN and the sulfobutyl moiety of the CD.

The binding stoichiometries were analyzed by using SupraFit software (2.5.120) [63]. The results of the UV-vis titration were analyzed using a 1:1, 2:1/1:1, 1:1/1:2, and a 2:1/1:1/1:2 model as implemented in SupraFit. Each best-fit model was inspected using Monte Carlo simulation to identify the 1:1/1:2 (RTN/SBE-β-CD) as the best-fitted model with a $K_{1:1}$ of 32267 M^{-1} and a $K_{1:2}$ of 12 M^{-1} with an associated $DG_{binding}$ of −6.6 and −1.5 kcal/mol. Effectively, the almost exclusive complex in solution is the 1:1 one, whereas the 1:2 is present in a small amount at a high concentration of SBE-β-CD.

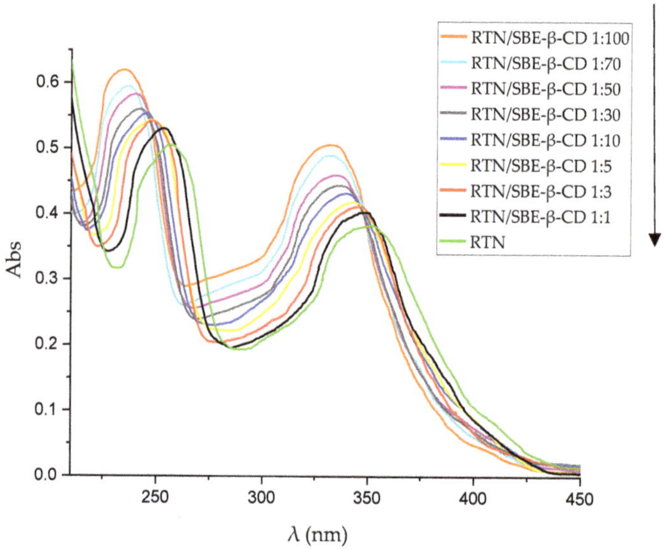

Figure 2. UV-vis spectra of free RTN and in the presence of an increasing amount of SBE-β-CD in water:MeOH 80:20 mixture (%, *v*/*v*). The experiments were carried out in triplicate.

3.1.2. Phase Solubility Studies

Figure 3 shows the phase solubility diagram obtained for RTN in the presence of increasing concentrations of SBE-β-CD. The graph obtained representing RTN concentration vs. SBE-β-CD concentration is of A_L type, showing that RTN/SBE-β-CD interaction leads to a soluble complex in the range of macrocycle concentrations considered. The slope of the graph is less than one, demonstrating the formation of a complex with 1:1 stoichiometry, and the association constant (K_c) determined following Higuchi and Connors was 9660 M^{-1}. This result is in line with UV-vis titration, which employs a more accurate method.

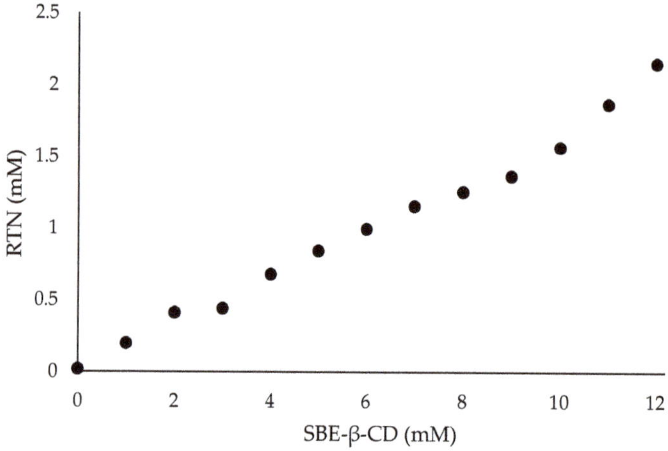

Figure 3. Phase solubility diagram of RTN/SBE-β-CD inclusion complex. The experiments were carried out in triplicate.

3.1.3. NMR Investigation

Nuclear magnetic resonance (NMR) is a fundamental spectroscopic technique to investigate the formation and geometry of inclusion complexes. The chemical and electronic environments of the protons are modified by the host–guest interactions; therefore, during the complexation, a chemically induced shift of the corresponding protons has been observed. Unfortunately, like most substituted CDs, SBE-β-CD is a statistical mixture of the different stereoisomers, with broad unresolved peaks; this makes it almost impossible to follow the chemical shifts of its protons, especially the H-3 and H-5 protons protruding into the CD cavity, even though these protons were identified through 2D COSY spectra [64]. All the RTN protons of the flavonoid moiety displayed chemical shifts between 6.30 and 7.67 ppm, which are free and more evident than the broad and unsolved peaks of SBE-β-CD proton (mainly at δ 3–4 ppm). Therefore, the RTN/SBE-β-CD inclusion complex formation was deduced from the chemical shift changes observed in ^{1}H NMR of the RTN aromatic protons previously measured in the free state. The enumeration of the RTN structure is shown in Figure 4, together with the stacked portions of the ^{1}H NMR spectra of RTN and RTN/SBE-β-CD inclusion complex. In Table 1, we reported the chemical shift of free and complexed RTN (RTN/SBE-β-CD 1:1 molar ratio).

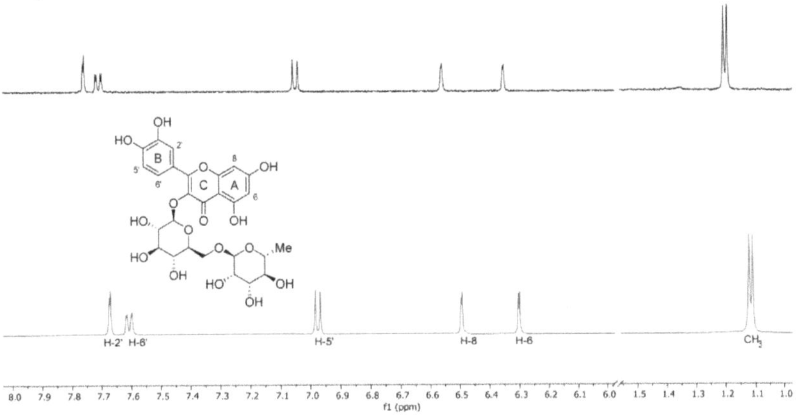

Figure 4. Stacked portions of the ^{1}H NMR spectra relative to the free RTN (blue line) and RTN/SBE-β-CD (black line) inclusion complex. Only those diagnostic signals relative to RTN are reported.

Table 1. ^{1}H NMR chemical shifts in δ and Δδ of RTN protons in the free state and RTN/SBE-β-CD 1:1 complex [9 mM in a 7:3 D_2O/MeOD solution]; for doublet or double-doublet, the reported δ refer to the centered signal.

Protons	RTN	RTN/SBE-β-CD	Δδ [a]
2′	7.67 (d)	7.76 (d)	0.09
5′	6.98 (d)	7.05 (d)	0.07
6′	7.61 (dd)	7.71 (dd)	0.10
6	6.30 (d)	6.35 (d)	0.05
8	6.49 (d)	6.56 (d)	1.07
CH_3	1.12 (d)	1.20 (d)	0.08

[a] $\Delta\delta = \delta_{complex} - \delta_{free}$.

The chemical shift changes of the RTN aromatic protons are diagnostics. The H-6 and H-8 protons of the RTN A ring resonate at 6.30 and 6.49 ppm, while H-2′, H-5′, and H-6′ B ring protons have chemical shifts at 7.67, 6.98, and 7.61 ppm, respectively. The inclusion of RTN in the SBE-β-CD hydrophobic cavity was confirmed by changes in the chemical shifts of the guest and host protons that were observed in the RTN/SBE-β-CD inclusion complex spectrum, in comparison with the chemical shift observed for the same protons in the free RTN.

In the RTN/SBE-β-CD spectrum of the complex (performed in a 7:3 D_2O/CD_3OD solution), significant changes were observed in the chemical shifts of H-8 RTN proton (Δδ 1.07) due to the proximity to the oxygen atom of the 1,4-glycosidic bonds between the seven glucopyranose units which constitute the SBE-β-CD molecule. Other interesting changes were observed for RTN protons H-6, H-2′, and H–5′ in the RTN/SBE-β-CD complex spectrum (Table 1). From these results, it can be assumed that the RTN benzopyranone skeleton was incorporated in the SBE-β-CD hydrophobic cavity (Figure 5).

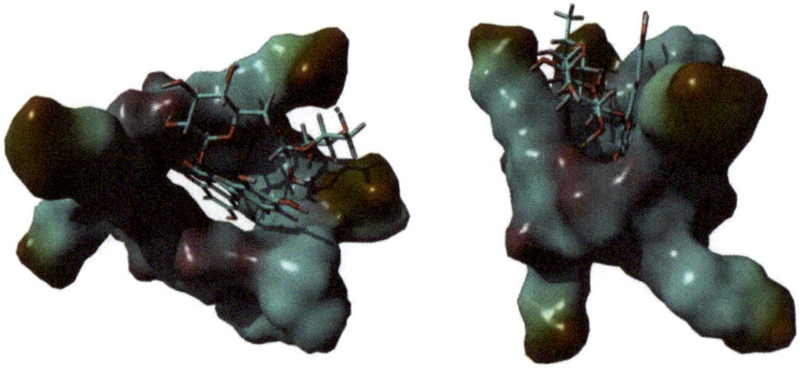

Figure 5. The 3D full minimized structure of RTN/SBE-β-CD inclusion complex. Top view (**left**) and side view (**right**). Hydrogen bonds were represented as a yellow dotted line.

The changes observed for H-2′, H-5′, and H–6′ protons of the RTN ring B indicate that this latter is probably in close contact with the sulfobutylether groups [19].

3.1.4. Molecular Modeling Studies

In order to investigate the RTN/SBE-β-CD host–guest interactions, we started the molecular modeling study docking the RTN into the SBE-β-CD hydrophobic cavity, as described in the Supplemenatary Materials (File S1). From the 10 most stable docked poses, the two that corresponded to the orientation of ring A or B within the hydrophobic cavity from the secondary edge were selected. These two complexes were subjected to a 500 ns molecular dynamics simulation. The analysis of the two simulations showed that after about 100 ns the molecule of RTN is stabilized into the SBE-β-CD cavity. Once inside the host molecule, the RTN establishes interactions that stabilize the complex and for the entire simulation time (500 ns) stays inside the CD, maintaining the same orientation. On all the trajectories of the MD simulation, we performed an MM/PBSA calculation to obtain the binding energy and, consequently, to select the most stable complex structures for both A and B ring orientations. Of these two optimized structures, ring A inside the RTN/SBE-β-CD hydrophobic cavity resulted in the most stability. This last structure, reported in Figure 5, is consistent with the complex geometry deduced by the NMR experiments. The A ring is fully inserted into the cavity and justifies the high shift registered for the H-8; even the C ring is partially inserted into the cavity, in line with the H2′ and H6′ shifts. Finally, the methyl group in one of the sugar rings is located between two of the seven sulfonic groups to deshield it; this also agrees with the magnitude of the low-field shift observed in NMR analysis. This structure is stabilized by two hydrogen bonds between two hydroxyl moieties of the sugar rings that interact with one of the alcoholic oxygens of the secondary rim and with one of the sulphonic oxygens, respectively.

3.1.5. WAXD, TGA, and FT-IR Analyses

The inclusion complex was characterized at solid state by X-ray diffractometry (WAXD), thermogravimetric analysis (TGA), and Fourier transform infrared spectroscopy (FT-IR).

WAXD patterns obtained for RTN/SBE-β-CD inclusion complex, free components, and RTN/SBE-β-CD physical mixture are shown in Figure 6. RTN shows an intense and sharp peak that evidences its crystalline nature. They were still present in the physical mixture but disappeared in the inclusion complex's spectrum. This latter showed a broad and diffuse signal without sharp crystalline peaks, indicating the amorphous nature of the complex due to the drug's inclusion within the SBE-β-CD cavity.

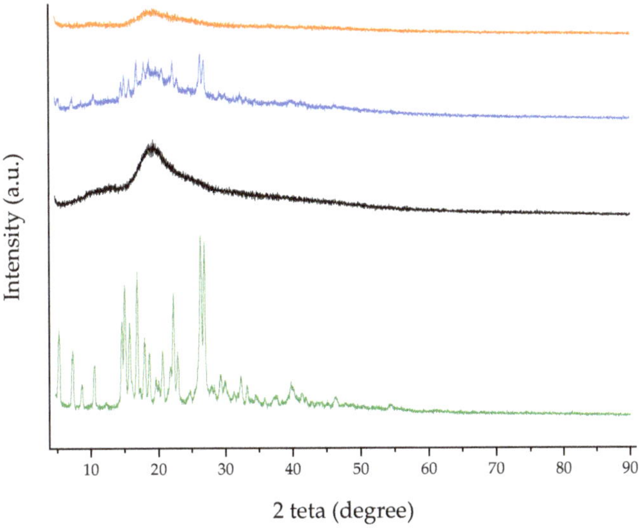

Figure 6. WAXD patterns of free RTN (green line), SBE-β-CD (black line), physical mixture (blue line), and inclusion complex (orange line).

The thermal properties of the RTN/SBE-β-CD inclusion complex, free RTN, SBE-β-CD, and the physical mixture were evaluated by TGA (Figure 7). For SBE-β-CD, the mass loss below 150 °C can be attributed to surface water evaporation associated with the macrocycle. For the RTN/SBE-β-CD inclusion complex, the mass loss in the 150–550 °C range may be related to internal water evaporation and SBE-β-CD or drug degradation. Furthermore, a slight modification of the degradation temperature of the macrocycle in the inclusion complex is highlighted, which would indeed suggest the formation of the inclusion complex in the solid phase. As can be seen, the thermal stability of RTN increases when complexed with SBE-β-CD.

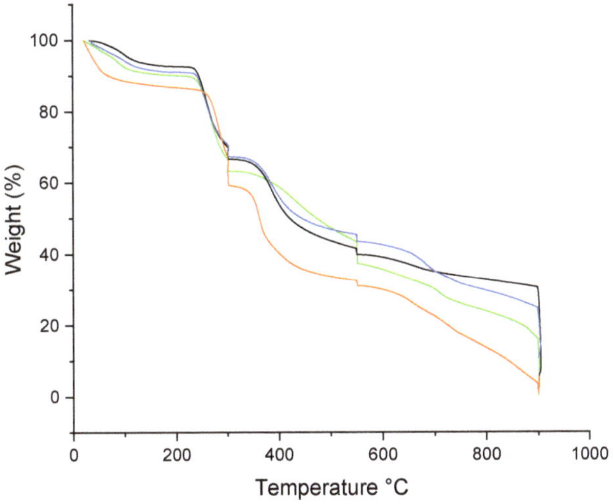

Figure 7. TGA curves of free RTN (green line), SBE-β-CD (black line), physical mixture (blue line), and inclusion complex (orange line).

Finally, FT-IR spectroscopy was used to verify the complexation. The variation of intensity, changes in wavenumbers, disappearance and/or magnification of the typical

FT-IR bands of the functional groups of the molecules suggest the formation of an inclusion complex [65]. The FT-IR spectra recorded at 25 °C of RTN/SBE-β-CD inclusion complex, free RTN and SBE-β-CD, and of the physical mixture are shown in Figure 8. The RTN spectrum is characterized by stretching vibrations of the hydroxyl groups, and intense bands are observable for the vibrations of the C=O, C=C, C-O, and C-O-C groups. Instead, the spectrum of SBE-β-CD has absorption bands for the hydroxyl groups, -CH and -CH_2, and for the C-O-C stretching vibration. In the inclusion complex, some IR drug bands are absent or reduced in intensity, suggesting that RTN is trapped in the macrocycle cavity.

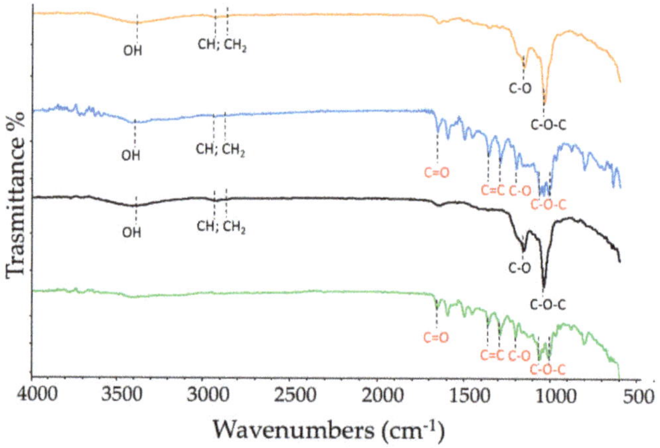

Figure 8. FT-IR spectra recorded at 25 °C of free RTN (green line), SBE-β-CD (black line) physical mixture (blue line), and inclusion complex (orange line). Characteristic peaks were labeled; the absorptions of RTN and SBE-β-CD functional groups are in red and black, respectively.

3.1.6. Scanning Electron Microscopy (SEM) Analysis

SEM is used in the solid-state characterization of the raw materials, and their corresponding physical mixtures and inclusion complexes [65]. This technique is inadequate to identify the formation mechanism of the complex, but it evidences morphological changes related to the interactions between the components [66]. The surface morphologies of free RTN, SBE-β-CD, the physical mixture, and the inclusion complex are shown in Figure 9a–d. Free RTN appeared with crystals of different sizes in rectangular blocks (Figure 9a), while the SBE-β-CD had an almost circular form with a perfectly smooth surface (Figure 9b). Both RTN and SBE-β-CD particles were still evident in the SEM image of the physical mixture. As shown in Figure 9c, the circular particles do not appear perfectly smooth, but a rough, irregular, and opaque surface characterizes this substrate. This different morphology suggests that the drug appears to adhere to the surface of SBE-β-CD in the physical mixture, slightly modifying its structure without interacting with it. On the other hand, the inclusion complex showed drastic changes in particle size and the shape of particles. The original morphology of the two pure compounds was lost, while a single solid structure is formed (Figure 9d). Thus, the very different shape and morphology can be considered as proof that a new structure was present.

3.2. Water Solubility and Dissolution Profile of RTN/SBE-β-CD Inclusion Complex

The inclusion of RTN into SBE-β-CD resulted in an approximately 20-fold increase in water solubility compared to the free drug (0.125 mg/mL in water) [48]. Due to the high solubility and complexing ability of the CD used in this study, the solubility increase of RTN is higher than that reported by other authors in the presence of different CDs [35,36]. Complete dissolution of the complex was observed in about 30 min, whereas only 10% of free RTN was dissolved in the same period of time and under the same conditions (Figure 10).

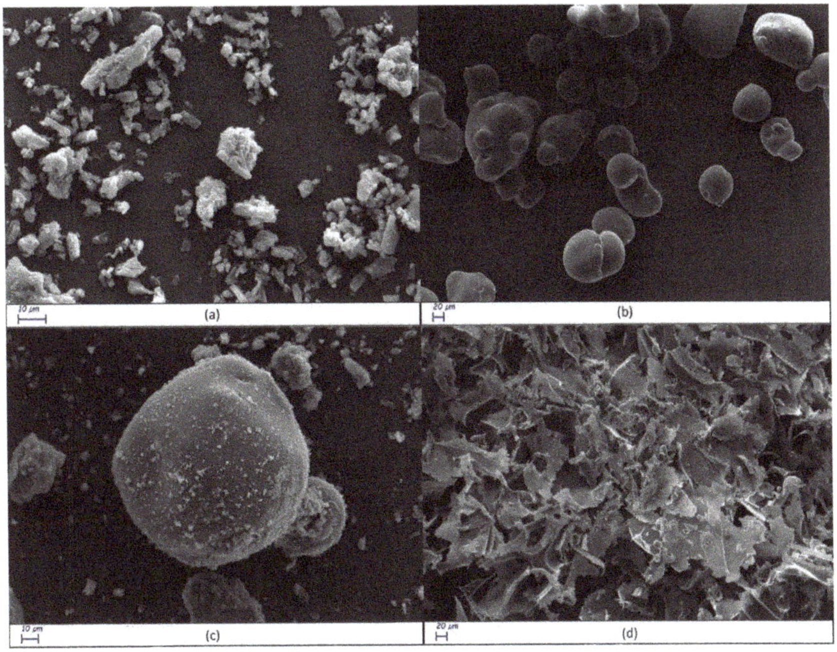

Figure 9. Scanning electron microscope (SEM) images of free RTN (**a**), SBE-β-CD (**b**), physical mixture (**c**), and inclusion complex (**d**) at different magnifications.

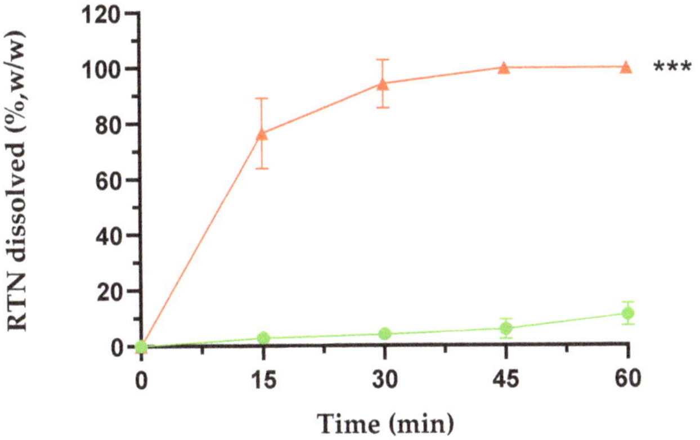

Figure 10. Dissolution profiles of free RTN (green line) and RTN/SBE-β-CD inclusion complex (orange line) in water at 25.0 ± 0.5 °C. All values of the inclusion complex are statistically significant compared to free RTN data (*** $p < 0.001$). The experiments were carried out in triplicate. The results are presented as the mean of three experiments ± standard deviation (SD). The error bar, if not shown, is inside the symbol.

3.3. *Antibacterial and Antibiofilm Activity*

3.3.1. Bacterial Susceptibility

The antibacterial activity of the RTN/SBE-β-CD inclusion complex compared to free RTN and SBE-β-CD was assayed against *S. aureus* and *P. aeruginosa*, including resistant strains. The activity of the samples was assayed by minimum inhibitory concentration (MIC) and minimum bactericidal concentration (MBC) methods. Due to its minimal solubility, free RTN was assayed at 150 μg/mL; higher concentrations rapidly precipitated in the culture medium. Several authors demonstrated the antibacterial activity of free RTN, although different MIC values were reported on the same strains [35,67]. Among the possible reasons, the different MIC values obtained may be due to solubility issues leading to poorly defined concentrations. When complexed with the macrocycle, RTN significantly increases its water solubility; thus, a higher concentration of complexed RTN (1250 μg/mL) can be assayed to the free drug. As reported in Table 2, free RTN showed bacteriostatic activity against *S. aureus* ATCC 6538 and *P. aeruginosa* ATCC 9027 with MIC values of 75 and 150 μg/mL, respectively. No activity was observed against resistant strains. As demonstrated by other authors, the RTN activity could be due to several mechanisms such as damage to the bacterial cell membrane [4] or inhibition of nucleic acid synthesis [68], efflux pumps [69], toxin formation and biofilm formation [70]. Free SBE-β-CD showed no activity against all the tested strains. Interesting results were obtained for the RTN/SBE-β-CD inclusion complex. The presence of macrocycle increased RTN effectiveness against all tested strains. Complexed RTN showed bactericidal activity against *S. aureus* ATCC 6538 and ATCC 43300 (MRSA) at a concentration of 4.88 μg/mL and against *P. aeruginosa* ATCC 9027 at 39.06 μg/mL. Furthermore, it showed bacteriostatic activity against *P. aeruginosa* DSM 102273 resistant strain with a MIC value of 1250 μg/mL. These results could depend not only on the increased solubility of RTN by the complexation, but also on the permeabilization of the bacterial wall produced by the macrocycle [28,71].

Table 2. Minimum inhibitory concentration (MIC) and minimum bactericidal concentration (MBC) of RTN/SBE-β-CD inclusion complex compared to free RTN.

Strains	Free RTN (μg/mL)	RTN/SBE-β-CD [a] (μg/mL)	LVF
S. aureus ATCC 6538			
MIC	75	1.22	0.5
MBC	150	4.88	1
S. aureus ATCC 43300			
MIC	—	1.22	0.008
MBC	—	4.88	0.031
P. aeruginosa ATCC 9027			
MIC	150	39.06	2
MBC	—	39.06	62.5
P. aeruginosa DSM 102273			
MIC	—	1250	125
MBC	—	—	500

[a] The concentration is referred to as the complexed RTN; —no activity. LVF (drug control).

3.3.2. Antibiofilm Effect

Biofilm is produced by microorganisms as an extracellular matrix and is composed of polysaccharides, secreted proteins, and extracellular DNA. It is considered an important virulence factor causing chronic infections [72]. *S. aureus* and *P. aeruginosa* are the most common bacterial pathogens associated with different types of eye surface infections including keratitis, dacryocystitis, blepharokeratoconjunctivitis, and conjunctivitis [11]. Chronic *S. aureus* and *P. aeruginosa* ocular infections associated with biofilms have become increasingly challenging to treat with current antimicrobials [11,73,74].

The activity of the RTN/SBE-β-CD inclusion complex compared to free RTN and SBE-β-CD against biofilm formation was measured by the crystal violet method and CFU assay. Free RTN and free SBE-β-CD showed no antibiofilm effect against all strains at 0.5 MIC concentration. The inclusion complex significantly decreased biofilm biomass production at 0.5 MIC against *S. aureus* ATCC 6538 (biofilm reduction 57%) and *S. aureus* MRSA (biofilm reduction 41%). The percentage of inhibition was found to be statistically significant compared with the negative control at $p < 0.05$ for *S. aureus* ATCC 6538 and at $p < 0.01$ for *S. aureus* MRSA (Figures 11a and 12a).

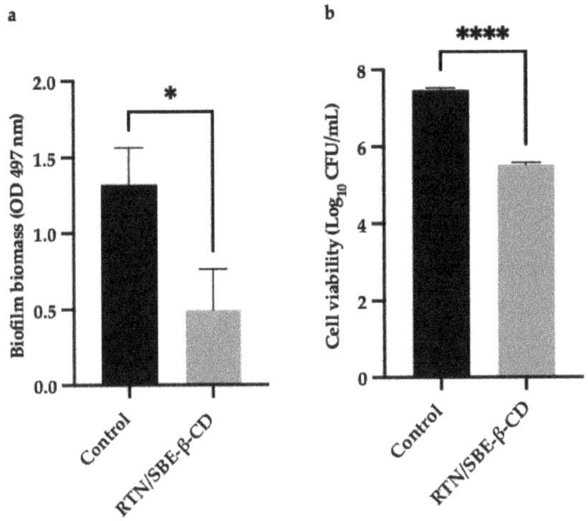

Figure 11. The results are expressed as mean ± SD. RTN/SBE-β-CD inclusion complex significantly reduced *S. aureus* ATCC 6538 biofilm formation at 0.5 MIC (0.61 μg/mL in RTN). (**a**) Biofilm biomass is expressed as crystal violet optical density (O.D. 497 nm) (* $p < 0.05$); (**b**) cell viability is expressed as Log_{10} CFU/mL (**** $p < 0.0001$).

Moreover, at 0.5 MIC the inclusion complex reduced the viability of *S. aureus* ATCC 6538 by 2 log_{10} units ($p < 0.0001$), and that of *S. aureus* MRSA by 3.6 log_{10} units ($p < 0.0001$) (Figures 11b and 12b).

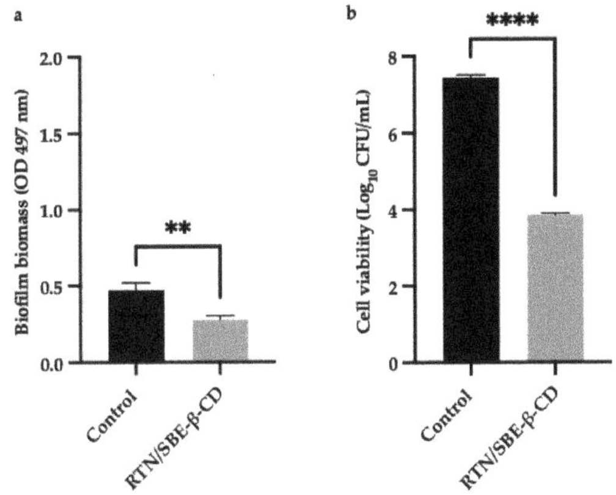

Figure 12. The results are expressed as mean ± SD. RTN/SBE-β-CD inclusion complex significantly reduced *S. aureus* ATCC 43300 (MRSA) biofilm formation at 0.5 MIC (0.61 μg/mL in RTN). (**a**) Biofilm biomass is expressed as crystal violet optical density (O.D. 497 nm) (** $p < 0.01$); (**b**) cell viability is expressed as Log_{10} CFU/mL (**** $p < 0.0001$).

However, RTN/SBE-β-CD inclusion complex showed no inhibitory effect on biofilm production against *P. aeruginosa* strains at 0.5 MIC, which is equivalent to 0.25 μg/mL and 62.5 μg/mL for *P. aeruginosa* ATCC 9027 and *P. aeruginosa* DSM 102273, respectively.

4. Conclusions

In this study, we demonstrated the ability of SBE-β-CD to complex the natural drug RTN to improve its water solubility and dissolution and potentiate its antibacterial effect. As in-solution and solid-state investigations demonstrated, a stable inclusion complex in a 1:1 molar ratio was formed. The complexation potentiates the antibacterial activity of RTN against Gram-positive and Gram-negative strains. Remarkably, the MIC and MBC of complexed RTN are, respectively, 60 times and 30 times higher than the free drug against *S. aureus* ATCC 6538. The complexed RTN shows similar high activity against *S. aureus* ATCC 43300 (MRSA), while free RTN shows no activity. The macrocycle increases the antibacterial activity of RTN, albeit less intense, towards the Gram-negative *P. aeruginosa* ATCC 9027. Furthermore, the inclusion complex has significant antibiofilm activity against *S. aureus* strains, reducing viability cells; while no antibiofilm activity was detected for free RTN.

Our results suggest that SBE-β-CD could be a suitable carrier for RTN, permitting the realization of liquid formulation for ophthalmic administration with antibacterial and antibiofilm properties, and representing a good starting point for our successive in vitro and in vivo investigations.

Supplementary Materials: The following supporting information can be downloaded at: https://www.mdpi.com/article/10.3390/pharmaceutics16020233/s1, File S1: Initial deployment of RTN for MD simulations and Free binding energy calculation.

Author Contributions: Conceptualization, A.M. and C.A.V.; methodology, A.M. and C.A.V.; software, A.R.; validation, A.R.; investigation, F.D.G., F.M., V.B., V.P., A.R. and M.P.; visualization, V.P. and A.R.; data curation, F.D.G., V.B., M.P., V.P. and A.R.; writing—original draft preparation, A.M., F.D.G., V.P. and A.R.; writing—review and editing, A.M., A.R., V.P. and C.A.V.; supervision, A.M. and C.A.V. All authors have read and agreed to the published version of the manuscript.

Funding: This research received no external funding.

Institutional Review Board Statement: Not applicable.

Informed Consent Statement: Not applicable.

Data Availability Statement: Data are contained within the article.

Conflicts of Interest: The authors declare no conflicts of interest.

References

1. Ayehubizu, Z.; Mulu, W.; Biadglegne, F. Common Bacterial Causes of External Ocular Infections, Associated Risk Factors and Antibiotic Resistance among Patients at Ophthalmology Unit of Felege Hiwot Referral Hospital, Northwest Ethiopia: A Cross-Sectional Study. *J. Ophthalmic Inflamm. Infect.* **2021**, *11*, 7. [CrossRef] [PubMed]
2. Ting, D.S.J.; Ho, C.S.; Deshmukh, R.; Said, D.G.; Dua, H.S. Infectious Keratitis: An Update on Epidemiology, Causative Microorganisms, Risk Factors, and Antimicrobial Resistance. *Eye* **2021**, *35*, 1084–1101. [CrossRef] [PubMed]
3. Petrillo, F.; Pignataro, D.; Di Lella, F.M.; Reibaldi, M.; Fallico, M.; Castellino, N.; Parisi, G.; Trotta, M.C.; D'Amico, M.; Santella, B.; et al. Antimicrobial Susceptibility Patterns and Resistance Trends of *Staphylococcus aureus* and Coagulase-Negative Staphylococci Strains Isolated from Ocular Infections. *Antibiotics* **2021**, *10*, 527. [CrossRef] [PubMed]
4. Amin, M.U.; Khurram, M.; Khattak, B.; Khan, J. Antibiotic Additive and Synergistic Action of Rutin, Morin and Quercetin against Methicillin Resistant *Staphylococcus aureus*. *BMC Complement. Altern. Med.* **2015**, *15*, 59. [CrossRef] [PubMed]
5. Afzal, M.; Vijay, A.K.; Stapleton, F.; Willcox, M.D.P. Susceptibility of Ocular *Staphylococcus aureus* to Antibiotics and Multipurpose Disinfecting Solutions. *Antibiotics* **2021**, *10*, 1203. [CrossRef] [PubMed]
6. Bispo, P.J.M.; Ung, L.; Chodosh, J.; Gilmore, M.S. Hospital-Associated Multidrug-Resistant MRSA Lineages Are Trophic to the Ocular Surface and Cause Severe Microbial Keratitis. *Front. Public Health* **2020**, *8*, 204. [CrossRef]
7. Nithya, V.; Rathinam, S.; Siva Ganesa Karthikeyan, R.; Lalitha, P. A Ten Year Study of Prevalence, Antimicrobial Susceptibility Pattern, and Genotypic Characterization of Methicillin Resistant *Staphylococcus aureus* Causing Ocular Infections in a Tertiary Eye Care Hospital in South India. *Infect. Genet. Evol.* **2019**, *69*, 203–210. [CrossRef]
8. Elhardt, C.; Wolf, A.; Wertheimer, C.M. Successful Treatment of Multidrug-Resistant *Pseudomonas aeruginosa* Keratitis with Meropenem Eye Drops—A Case Report. *J. Ophthalmic Inflamm. Infect.* **2023**, *13*, 40. [CrossRef]
9. McGhee, C.N.J.; Dean, S.; Danesh-Meyer, H. Locally Administered Ocular Corticosteroids: Benefits and Risks. *Drug Saf.* **2002**, *25*, 33–55. [CrossRef]
10. Kowalski, R.P.; Nayyar, S.V.; Romanowski, E.G.; Jhanji, V. Anti-Infective Treatment and Resistance Is Rarely Problematic with Eye Infections. *Antibiotics* **2022**, *11*, 204. [CrossRef]
11. Shah, S.; Wozniak, R.A.F. *Staphylococcus aureus* and *Pseudomonas aeruginosa* Infectious Keratitis: Key Bacterial Mechanisms That Mediate Pathogenesis and Emerging Therapeutics. *Front. Cell. Infect. Microbiol.* **2023**, *13*, 1250257. [CrossRef] [PubMed]
12. Bonincontro, G.; Scuderi, S.A.; Marino, A.; Simonetti, G. Synergistic Effect of Plant Compounds in Combination with Conventional Antimicrobials against Biofilm of *Staphylococcus aureus*, *Pseudomonas aeruginosa*, and *Candida* spp. *Pharmaceuticals* **2023**, *16*, 1531. [CrossRef] [PubMed]

13. Di Marzio, L.; Ventura, C.A.; Cosco, D.; Paolino, D.; Di Stefano, A.; Stancanelli, R.; Tommasini, S.; Cannavà, C.; Celia, C.; Fresta, M. Nanotherapeutics for Anti-Inflammatory Delivery. *J. Drug Deliv. Sci. Technol.* **2016**, *32*, 174–191. [CrossRef]
14. Memar, M.Y.; Yekani, M.; Sharifi, S.; Dizaj, S.M. Antibacterial and Biofilm Inhibitory Effects of Rutin Nanocrystals. *Biointerface Res. Appl. Chem.* **2022**, *13*, 132. [CrossRef]
15. Ivanov, M.; Novović, K.; Malešević, M.; Dinić, M.; Stojković, D.; Jovčić, B.; Soković, M. Polyphenols as Inhibitors of Antibiotic Resistant Bacteria-Mechanisms Underlying Rutin Interference with Bacterial Virulence. *Pharmaceuticals* **2022**, *15*, 385. [CrossRef] [PubMed]
16. Pedriali, C.A.; Fernandes, A.U.; Bernusso, L.D.C.; Polakiewicz, B. The Synthesis of a Water-Soluble Derivative of Rutin as an Antiradical Agent. *Quím. Nova* **2008**, *31*, 2147–2151. [CrossRef]
17. Khalifa, T.I.; Muhtadi, F.J.; Hassan, M.M.A. Rutin. In *Analytical Profiles of Drug Substances*; Florey, K., Ed.; Academic Press: Cambridge, MA, USA, 1983; Volume 12, pp. 623–681.
18. Gullón, B.; Lú-Chau, T.A.; Moreira, M.T.; Lema, J.M.; Eibes, G. Rutin: A Review on Extraction, Identification and Purification Methods, Biological Activities and Approaches to Enhance Its Bioavailability. *Trends Food Sci. Technol.* **2017**, *67*, 220–235. [CrossRef]
19. De Gaetano, F.; Margani, F.; Barbera, V.; D'Angelo, V.; Germanò, M.P.; Pistarà, V.; Ventura, C.A. Characterization and In Vivo Antiangiogenic Activity Evaluation of Morin-Based Cyclodextrin Inclusion Complexes. *Pharmaceutics* **2023**, *15*, 2209. [CrossRef]
20. De Gaetano, F.; Cristiano, M.C.; Paolino, D.; Celesti, C.; Iannazzo, D.; Pistarà, V.; Iraci, N.; Ventura, C.A. Bicalutamide Anticancer Activity Enhancement by Formulation of Soluble Inclusion Complexes with Cyclodextrins. *Biomolecules* **2022**, *12*, 1716. [CrossRef]
21. De Gaetano, F.; Scala, A.; Celesti, C.; Lambertsen Larsen, K.; Genovese, F.; Bongiorno, C.; Leggio, L.; Iraci, N.; Iraci, N.; Mazzaglia, A.; et al. Amphiphilic Cyclodextrin Nanoparticles as Delivery System for Idebenone: A Preformulation Study. *Molecules* **2023**, *28*, 3023. [CrossRef]
22. Musumeci, T.; Bonaccorso, A.; De Gaetano, F.; Larsen, K.L.; Pignatello, R.; Mazzaglia, A.; Puglisi, G.; Ventura, C.A. A Physico-Chemical Study on Amphiphilic Cyclodextrin/Liposomes Nanoassemblies with Drug Carrier Potential. *J. Liposome Res.* **2020**, *30*, 407–416. [CrossRef]
23. Gao, S.; Zong, L.; Zhang, Y.; Zhang, Y.; Guo, X.; Guo, G.; Zhao, L.; Ye, F.; Fu, Y. Antifungal Pentachloronitrobenzene/Hydroxypropyl-Beta-Cyclodextrin Inclusion Complex Nanofibers by Electrospun with No Polymer: Fabrication and Characterization. *J. Clean. Prod.* **2023**, *413*, 137499. [CrossRef]
24. Zhang, Y.; Li, F.; Guo, G.; Xiu, Y.; Yan, H.; Zhao, L.; Gao, S.; Ye, F.; Fu, Y. Preparation and Characterization of Betulin/Methyl-Beta-Cyclodextrin Inclusion Complex Electrospun Nanofiber: Improving the Properties of Betulin. *Ind. Crops Prod.* **2024**, *209*, 117974. [CrossRef]
25. Wang, Z.; Zou, W.; Liu, L.; Wang, M.; Li, F.; Shen, W. Characterization and Bacteriostatic Effects of β-Cyclodextrin/Quercetin Inclusion Compound Nanofilms Prepared by Electrospinning. *Food Chem.* **2021**, *338*, 127980. [CrossRef]
26. Paladini, G.; Caridi, F.; Crupi, V.; De Gaetano, F.; Majolino, D.; Tommasini, S.; Ventura, C.A.; Venuti, V.; Stancanelli, R. Temperature-Dependent Dynamical Evolution in Coum/SBE-β-CD Inclusion Complexes Revealed by Two-Dimensional FTIR Correlation Spectroscopy (2D-COS). *Molecules* **2021**, *26*, 3749. [CrossRef]
27. Matencio, A.; Hoti, G.; Monfared, Y.; Rezayat, A.; Pedrazzo, A.; Caldera, F.; Trotta, F. Cyclodextrin Monomers and Polymers for Drug Activity Enhancement. *Polymers* **2021**, *13*, 1684. [CrossRef]
28. Saha, P.; Rafe, M.R. Cyclodextrin: A Prospective Nanocarrier for the Delivery of Antibacterial Agents against Bacteria That Are Resistant to Antibiotics. *Heliyon* **2023**, *9*, e19287. [CrossRef]
29. Zhang, G.; Yuan, C.; Sun, Y. Effect of Selective Encapsulation of Hydroxypropyl-β-Cyclodextrin on Components and Antibacterial Properties of Star Anise Essential Oil. *Molecules* **2018**, *23*, 1126. [CrossRef]
30. Haiyun, D.; Jianbin, C.; Guomei, Z.; Shaomin, S.; Jinhao, P. Preparation and Spectral Investigation on Inclusion Complex of β-Cyclodextrin with Rutin. *Spectrochim. Acta Part. A Mol. Biomol. Spectrosc.* **2003**, *59*, 3421–3429. [CrossRef]
31. Chang, C.; Song, M.; Ma, M.; Song, J.; Cao, F.; Qin, Q. Preparation, Characterization and Molecular Dynamics Simulation of Rutin–Cyclodextrin Inclusion Complexes. *Molecules* **2023**, *28*, 955. [CrossRef]
32. Calabrò, M.L.; Tommasini, S.; Donato, P.; Stancanelli, R.; Raneri, D.; Catania, S.; Costa, C.; Villari, V.; Ficarra, P.; Ficarra, R. The Rutin/β-Cyclodextrin Interactions in Fully Aqueous Solution: Spectroscopic Studies and Biological Assays. *J. Pharm. Biomed. Anal.* **2005**, *36*, 1019–1027. [CrossRef]
33. Nguyen, T.A.; Liu, B.; Zhao, J.; Thomas, D.S.; Hook, J.M. An Investigation into the Supramolecular Structure, Solubility, Stability and Antioxidant Activity of Rutin/Cyclodextrin Inclusion Complex. *Food Chem.* **2013**, *136*, 186–192. [CrossRef]
34. Naeem, A.; Yu, C.; Zang, Z.; Zhu, W.; Deng, X.; Guan, Y. Synthesis and Evaluation of Rutin–Hydroxypropyl β-Cyclodextrin Inclusion Complexes Embedded in Xanthan Gum-Based (HPMC-g-AMPS) Hydrogels for Oral Controlled Drug Delivery. *Antioxidants* **2023**, *12*, 552. [CrossRef]
35. Paczkowska, M.; Mizera, M.; Piotrowska, H.; Szymanowska-Powałowska, D.; Lewandowska, K.; Goscianska, J.; Pietrzak, R.; Bednarski, W.; Majka, Z.; Cielecka-Piontek, J. Complex of Rutin with β-Cyclodextrin as Potential Delivery System. *PLoS ONE* **2015**, *10*, e0120858. [CrossRef]
36. Liu, J.; Zhang, S.; Zhao, X.; Lu, Y.; Song, M.; Wu, S. Molecular Simulation and Experimental Study on the Inclusion of Rutin with β-Cyclodextrin and Its Derivative. *J. Mol. Struct.* **2022**, *1254*, 132359. [CrossRef]

37. Araruna, M.K.; Brito, S.A.; Morais-Braga, M.F.; Santos, K.K.; Souza, T.M.; Leite, T.R.; Costa, J.G.; Coutinho, H.D. Coutinho Evaluation of Antibiotic & Antibiotic Modifying Activity of Pilocarpine & Rutin. *Indian J. Med. Res.* **2012**, *135*, 252–254.
38. Corina, D.; Florina, B.; Iulia, P.; Cristina, D.; Rita, A.; Alexandra, P.; Virgil, P.; Hancianu, M.; Daliana, M.; Codruta, S. Rutin and Its Cyclodextrin Inclusion Complexes: Physico-Chemical Evaluation and in Vitro Activity on B164A5 Murine Melanoma Cell Line. *Curr. Pharm. Biotechnol.* **2018**, *18*, 1067–1077. [CrossRef]
39. Miyake, K.; Arima, H.; Hirayama, F.; Yamamoto, M.; Horikawa, T.; Sumiyoshi, H.; Noda, S.; Uekama, K. Improvement of Solubility and Oral Bioavailability of Rutin by Complexation with 2-Hydroxypropyl-Beta-Cyclodextrin. *Pharm. Dev. Technol.* **2000**, *5*, 399–407. [CrossRef]
40. Wu, M.; Song, Z.; Zhang, J. A Luminescence Study of the Interaction of Sulfobutylether-β-Cyclodextrin with Rutin. *Drug Metab. Lett.* **2011**, *5*, 259–266. [CrossRef]
41. GÖZCÜ, S.; POLAT, K.H. Thermosensitive In Situ Gelling System for Dermal Drug Delivery of Rutin. *Turk. J. Pharm. Sci.* **2023**, *20*, 78–83. [CrossRef]
42. Zhou, C.J.; Li, L.F.; Liu, Y.; Wen, S.P.; Guo, Y.E.; Niu, X.G. Study on the Inclusion Complex of Rutin/Sulfobutylether-β-Cyclodextrin. *Adv. Mater. Res.* **2012**, *455–456*, 1177–1181. [CrossRef]
43. Das, O.; Ghate, V.M.; Lewis, S.A. Utility of Sulfobutyl Ether Beta-Cyclodextrin Inclusion Complexes in Drug Delivery: A Review. *Indian J. Pharm. Sci.* **2019**, *81*, 589–600. [CrossRef]
44. Jain, A.S.; Date, A.A.; Pissurlenkar, R.R.S.; Coutinho, E.C.; Nagarsenker, M.S. Sulfobutyl Ether7 β-Cyclodextrin (SBE7 β-CD) Carbamazepine Complex: Preparation, Characterization, Molecular Modeling, and Evaluation of In Vivo Anti-Epileptic Activity. *AAPS PharmSciTech* **2011**, *12*, 1163–1175. [CrossRef]
45. Sravani, A.B.; Shenoy, K.M.; Chandrika, B.; Kumar, B.H.; Kini, S.G.; Pai, K.S.R.; Lewis, S.A. Curcumin-Sulfobutyl-Ether Beta Cyclodextrin Inclusion Complex: Preparation, Spectral Characterization, Molecular Modeling, and Antimicrobial Activity. *J. Biomol. Struct. Dyn.* **2023**, 1–16. [CrossRef]
46. Higuchi, T.; Connors, K.A. Phase Solubility Techniques. *Adv. Anal. Chem. Instrum.* **1965**, *4*, 117–212. Available online: https://www.scirp.org/reference/ReferencesPapers?ReferenceID=170636 (accessed on 3 May 2023).
47. Rescifina, A.; Surdo, E.; Cardile, V.; Avola, R.; Eleonora Graziano, A.C.; Stancanelli, R.; Tommasini, S.; Pistarà, V.; Ventura, C.A. Gemcitabine Anticancer Activity Enhancement by Water Soluble Celecoxib/Sulfobutyl Ether-β-Cyclodextrin Inclusion Complex. *Carbohydr. Polym.* **2019**, *206*, 792–800. [CrossRef]
48. Krieger, E.; Vriend, G. YASARA View—Molecular Graphics for All Devices—From Smartphones to Workstations. *Bioinformatics* **2014**, *30*, 2981–2982. [CrossRef]
49. Gentile, D.; Floresta, G.; Patamia, V.; Chiaramonte, R.; Mauro, G.L.; Rescifina, A.; Vecchio, M. An Integrated Pharmacophore/Docking/3D-QSAR Approach to Screening a Large Library of Products in Search of Future Botulinum Neurotoxin A Inhibitors. *Int. J. Mol. Sci.* **2020**, *21*, 9470. [CrossRef]
50. Floresta, G.; Patamia, V.; Gentile, D.; Molteni, F.; Santamato, A.; Rescifina, A.; Vecchio, M. Repurposing of FDA-Approved Drugs for Treating Iatrogenic Botulism: A Paired 3D-QSAR/Docking Approach†. *ChemMedChem* **2020**, *15*, 256–262. [CrossRef]
51. Wang, J.; Wolf, R.M.; Caldwell, J.W.; Kollman, P.A.; Case, D.A. Development and Testing of a General Amber Force Field. *J. Comput. Chem.* **2004**, *25*, 1157–1174. [CrossRef]
52. Jakalian, A.; Jack, D.B.; Bayly, C.I. Fast, Efficient Generation of High-Quality Atomic Charges. AM1-BCC Model: II. Parameterization and Validation. *J. Comput. Chem.* **2002**, *23*, 1623–1641. [CrossRef]
53. Hornak, V.; Abel, R.; Okur, A.; Strockbine, B.; Roitberg, A.; Simmerling, C. Comparison of Multiple Amber Force Fields and Development of Improved Protein Backbone Parameters. *Proteins* **2006**, *65*, 712–725. [CrossRef]
54. Essmann, U.; Perera, L.; Berkowitz, M.L.; Darden, T.; Lee, H.; Pedersen, L.G. A Smooth Particle Mesh Ewald Method. *J. Chem. Phys.* **1995**, *103*, 8577–8593. [CrossRef]
55. Krieger, E.; Vriend, G. New Ways to Boost Molecular Dynamics Simulations. *J. Comput. Chem.* **2015**, *36*, 996–1007. [CrossRef]
56. Genheden, S.; Ryde, U. The MM/PBSA and MM/GBSA Methods to Estimate Ligand-Binding Affinities. *Expert. Opin. Drug Discov.* **2015**, *10*, 449–461. [CrossRef]
57. Wongpituk, P.; Nutho, B.; Panman, W.; Kungwan, N.; Wolschann, P.; Rungrotmongkol, T.; Nunthaboot, N. Structural Dynamics and Binding Free Energy of Neral-Cyclodextrins Inclusion Complexes: Molecular Dynamics Simulation. *Mol. Simul.* **2017**, *43*, 1356–1363. [CrossRef]
58. Azzam, A.; Shawky, R.M.; El-Mahdy, T.S. Sub-Inhibitory Concentrations of Ceftriaxone Induce Morphological Alterations and PIA-Independent Biofilm Formation in *Staphylococcus aureus*. *Braz. J. Microbiol.* **2023**. [CrossRef]
59. Weinstein, M.P.; Patel, J.B. *Methods for Dilution Antimicrobial Susceptibility Tests for Bacteria That Grow Aerobically: M07-A11*, 11th ed.; Clinical and Laboratory Standards Institute: Wayne, PA, USA, 2018; ISBN 978-1-56238-836-2.
60. Cramton, S.E.; Gerke, C.; Schnell, N.F.; Nichols, W.W.; Götz, F. The Intercellular Adhesion (Ica) Locus Is Present in *Staphylococcus aureus* and Is Required for Biofilm Formation. *Infect. Immun.* **1999**, *67*, 5427–5433. [CrossRef]
61. Mabry, T.; Markham, K.R.; Thomas, M.B. *The Systematic Identification of Flavonoids*; Springer Science & Business Media: Berlin/Heidelberg, Germany, 2012; ISBN 978-3-642-88458-0.
62. Payán-Gómez, S.A.; Flores-Holguín, N.; Pérez-Hernández, A.; Piñón-Miramontes, M.; Glossman-Mitnik, D. Computational Molecular Characterization of the Flavonoid Rutin. *Chem. Cent. J.* **2010**, *4*, 12. [CrossRef]

63. Hübler, C. SupraFit—An Open Source Qt Based Fitting Application to Determine Stability Constants from Titration Experiments. *Chem.–Methods* **2022**, *2*, e202200006. [CrossRef]
64. De Gaetano, F.; Marino, A.; Marchetta, A.; Bongiorno, C.; Zagami, R.; Cristiano, M.C.; Paolino, D.; Pistarà, V.; Ventura, C.A. Development of Chitosan/Cyclodextrin Nanospheres for Levofloxacin Ocular Delivery. *Pharmaceutics* **2021**, *13*, 1293. [CrossRef]
65. Mura, P. Analytical Techniques for Characterization of Cyclodextrin Complexes in the Solid State: A Review. *J. Pharm. Biomed. Anal.* **2015**, *113*, 226–238. [CrossRef]
66. Kringel, D.H.; Antunes, M.D.; Klein, B.; Crizel, R.L.; Wagner, R.; de Oliveira, R.P.; Dias, A.R.G.; Zavareze, E.D.R. Production, Characterization, and Stability of Orange or Eucalyptus Essential Oil/β-Cyclodextrin Inclusion Complex. *J. Food Sci.* **2017**, *82*, 2598–2605. [CrossRef]
67. Miklasińska-Majdanik, M.; Kępa, M.; Wąsik, T.J.; Zapletal-Pudełko, K.; Klim, M.; Wojtyczka, R.D. The Direction of the Antibacterial Effect of Rutin Hydrate and Amikacin. *Antibiotics* **2023**, *12*, 1469. [CrossRef]
68. Bernard, F.X.; Sablé, S.; Cameron, B.; Provost, J.; Desnottes, J.F.; Crouzet, J.; Blanche, F. Glycosylated Flavones as Selective Inhibitors of Topoisomerase IV. *Antimicrob. Agents Chemother.* **1997**, *41*, 992–998. [CrossRef]
69. Jhanji, R.; Bhati, V.; Singh, A.; Kumar, A. Phytomolecules against Bacterial Biofilm and Efflux Pump: An in Silico and in Vitro Study. *J. Biomol. Struct. Dyn.* **2020**, *38*, 5500–5512. [CrossRef]
70. Wang, Z.; Ding, Z.; Li, Z.; Ding, Y.; Jiang, F.; Liu, J. Antioxidant and Antibacterial Study of 10 Flavonoids Revealed Rutin as a Potential Antibiofilm Agent in *Klebsiella pneumoniae* Strains Isolated from Hospitalized Patients. *Microb. Pathog.* **2021**, *159*, 105121. [CrossRef]
71. Wong, C.E.; Dolzhenko, A.V.; Lee, S.M.; Young, D.J. Cyclodextrins: A Weapon in the Fight Against Antimicrobial Resistance. *J. Mol. Eng. Mater.* **2017**, *05*, 1740006. [CrossRef]
72. Diriba, K.; Kassa, T.; Alemu, Y.; Bekele, S. In Vitro Biofilm Formation and Antibiotic Susceptibility Patterns of Bacteria from Suspected External Eye Infected Patients Attending Ophthalmology Clinic, Southwest Ethiopia. *Int. J. Microbiol.* **2020**, *2020*, 8472395. [CrossRef]
73. Verderosa, A.D.; Totsika, M.; Fairfull-Smith, K.E. Bacterial Biofilm Eradication Agents: A Current Review. *Front. Chem.* **2019**, *7*, 824. [CrossRef]
74. Vazquez, N.M.; Mariani, F.; Torres, P.S.; Moreno, S.; Galván, E.M. Cell Death and Biomass Reduction in Biofilms of Multidrug Resistant Extended Spectrum β-Lactamase-Producing Uropathogenic *Escherichia coli* Isolates by 1,8-Cineole. *PLoS ONE* **2020**, *15*, e0241978. [CrossRef] [PubMed]

pharmaceutics

MDPI

Article

Formulating Resveratrol and Melatonin Self-Nanoemulsifying Drug Delivery Systems (SNEDDS) for Ocular Administration Using Design of Experiments

Elide Zingale [1,2], Angela Bonaccorso [1,2], Agata Grazia D'Amico [3], Rosamaria Lombardo [1], Velia D'Agata [4], Jarkko Rautio [5] and Rosario Pignatello [1,2,*]

1 Laboratory of Drug Delivery Technology, Department of Drug and Health Sciences, University of Catania, Viale A. Doria 6, 95125 Catania, Italy; elide.zingale@phd.unict.it (E.Z.); angela.bonaccorso@unict.it (A.B.); rosamaria-lombardo@libero.it (R.L.)
2 NANOMED—Research Centre for Nanomedicine and Pharmaceutical Nanotechnology, Department of Drug and Health Sciences, University of Catania, 95125 Catania, Italy
3 Department of Drug and Health Sciences, Section of Systems Biology, University of Catania, Viale A. Doria 6, 95125 Catania, Italy; agata.damico@unict.it
4 Department of Biomedical and Biotechnological Sciences, Section of Anatomy, Histology and Movement Sciences, University of Catania, 95100 Catania, Italy; vdagata@unict.it
5 School of Pharmacy, University of Eastern Finland, Yliopistonranta 1C, 70210 Kuopio, Finland; jarkko.rautio@uef.fi
* Correspondence: rosario.pignatello@unict.it

Abstract: Recent studies have demonstrated that Sirtuin-1 (SIRT-1)-activating molecules exert a protective role in degenerative ocular diseases. However, these molecules hardly reach the back of the eye due to poor solubility in aqueous environments and low bioavailability after topical application on the eye's surface. Such hindrances, combined with stability issues, call for the need for innovative delivery strategies. Within this context, the development of self-nanoemulsifying drug delivery systems (SNEDDS) for SIRT-1 delivery can represent a promising approach. The aim of the work was to design and optimize SNEDDS for the ocular delivery of two natural SIRT-1 agonists, resveratrol (RSV) and melatonin (MEL), with potential implications for treating diabetic retinopathy. Pre-formulation studies were performed by a Design of Experiment (DoE) approach to construct the ternary phase diagram. The optimization phase was carried out using Response Surface Methodology (RSM). Four types of SNEDDS consisting of different surfactants (Tween® 80, Tween® 20, Solutol® HS15, and Cremophor® EL) were optimized to achieve the best physico-chemical parameters for ocular application. Stability tests indicated that SNEDDS produced with Tween® 80 was the formulation that best preserved the stability of molecules, and so it was, therefore, selected for further technological studies. The optimized formulation was prepared with Capryol® PGMC, Tween® 80, and Transcutol® P and loaded with RSV or MEL. The SNEDDS were evaluated for other parameters, such as the mean size (found to be <50 nm), size homogeneity (PDI < 0.2), emulsion time (around 40 s), transparency, drug content (>90%), mucoadhesion strength, in vitro drug release, pH and osmolarity, stability to dilution, and cloud point. Finally, an in vitro evaluation was performed on a rabbit corneal epithelial cell line (SIRC) to assess their cytocompatibility. The overall results suggest that SNEDDS can be used as promising nanocarriers for the ocular drug delivery of RSV and MEL.

Keywords: SNEDDS; ocular delivery; SIRT-1; stability; experimental design; surfactants; oils

Citation: Zingale, E.; Bonaccorso, A.; D'Amico, A.G.; Lombardo, R.; D'Agata, V.; Rautio, J.; Pignatello, R. Formulating Resveratrol and Melatonin Self-Nanoemulsifying Drug Delivery Systems (SNEDDS) for Ocular Administration Using Design of Experiments. *Pharmaceutics* **2024**, *16*, 125. https://doi.org/10.3390/pharmaceutics16010125

Academic Editor: Francisco Javier Otero-Espinar

Received: 29 November 2023
Revised: 12 January 2024
Accepted: 16 January 2024
Published: 18 January 2024

1. Introduction

Many degenerative ocular diseases such as cataracts, macular degeneration, diabetic retinopathy (DR), glaucoma, and optic neuritis are associated with a downregulation of Sirtuin-1 (SIRT-1) [1–6]. Looking specifically at posterior eye diseases, the role of SIRT-1 in DR has been extensively studied, but the complex molecular interactions are not fully understood. However, in recent years, numerous studies have demonstrated a strong link between SIRT-1 expression and the development of DR. In advanced pathological conditions, hyperglycemia lowers intracellular NAD+ levels and reduces SIRT-1 expression. SIRT-1 is a histone deacetylase protein involved in numerous pathways related to inflammation and oxidative stress. An over-repression of SIRT-1 can suppress inflammation in various tissues, whereas its deletion causes an increase in inflammation locally. By acting on the mediators of inflammation, e.g., through the suppression of NF-kB, SIRT-1 can modulate and reduce the inflammatory response [2]. Indeed, it becomes a therapeutic target for oxidative stress-associated diseases that have been extensively studied. Among them, DR, age-related macular degeneration (AMD), and glaucoma are the most studied conditions in relation to the downregulation of this enzyme.

Some natural compounds have been shown to be potent activators of SIRT-1, inducing beneficial effects that demonstrate SIRT-1 as a potential target against the inflammation process [7]. For instance, resveratrol (RVS) is able to activate SIRT-1 allosterically; however, its clinical utility is compromised by poor water solubility, instability, and scarce bioavailability [8,9]. RSV protects the ocular tissues from degeneration, including the retinal tissue, by promoting the SIRT-1 pathway [10,11]. Melatonin (MEL) is another excellent regulator of SIRT-1 as its administration induces an upregulation of the enzyme levels. Its role as a modulator of SIRT-1 has been observed in tissues in the testes, ovaries, heart, and nervous system [12–15].

MEL activity on SIRT-1 has also been linked to protection at an ocular level. MEL supplementation demonstrated a protective effect on the retina in an elderly diabetic rat model. The protective effect of MEL supplementation occurs by increasing both retinal antioxidant activity and retinal SIRT-1 gene expression [16]. Most treatments for ocular disorders involve the oral administration of MEL. Its low bioavailability, however, distresses its therapeutic efficacy. Only a low amount of the administered drug reaches the target sites; thus, larger doses and repeated administrations are required.

In this context, discussing nanotechnological systems to improve the efficacy of these two molecules, as well as other natural SIRT-1 agonists, appears to be an innovative approach. Among the latest generation of colloidal carriers, in situ nanoemulsifying systems (SNEDDS) seem to be highly promising but still insufficiently studied. No studies in the literature concern the development of SNEDDS for delivering SIRT-1 agonists into the eye. SNEDDS can be considered an "advanced" formulation compared to micro- and nanoemulsions since they are emulsified directly in situ, avoiding drug loss during storage [17]. SNEDDS are very simple formulations consisting of three components in an anhydrous mixture: oil, surfactant, and co-surfactant (or co-solvent). When considering ocular delivery, with the known technological constraints outlined by pharmacopeias, the choice of the starting materials and the construction of a ternary plot are crucial factors for obtaining formulations appropriate for an industrial scale-up [18,19]. The present work is based on the optimization of a SNEDDS platform for the topical ophthalmic delivery of RSV and MEL. To the best of our knowledge, there is no study published on MEL-loaded SNEDDS (MEL-SNEDDS) and only a few publications about RSV-loaded SNEDDS (RSV-SNEDDS), but none of them are related to the ocular field; therefore, this work can be considered a novelty in the area of nanotechnological application to therapy.

RSV- and MEL-SNEDDS were optimized using a Quality-by-Design (QbD) approach, first for the identification of the nanoemulsion zone and then for the optimization of the final formulation. Four different formulations were studied based on the type of surfactant: Tween® 80, Tween® 20, Cremophor® EL, and Solutol® HS15, respectively. Once the blank systems in terms of physico-chemical properties were optimized, they were loaded with RSV and MEL, respectively, resulting in RSV-SNEDDS and MEL-SNEDDS. The stability of the formulations allowed the identification of the optimal system, which was determined to be the one produced using Tween® 80. This formulation was subsequently selected for further characterization. The systems were always prepared by reconstituting the anhydrous pre-concentrated SNEDDS (pre-SNEDDS) mixtures with simulated tear fluid

(STF, pH 7.4) to mimic the conditions post-ocular instillation. A small dilution volume, a suitable temperature, and gentle agitation were chosen to produce the nanoemulsions, which were then fully characterized from a technological point of view, focusing on the requirements for ophthalmic topical formulations. Finally, cytotoxicity on rabbit corneal cells (SIRC) was assessed following a Short-Time Exposure Test (STE) protocol.

2. Materials and Methods

2.1. Materials

Mygliol® 812 from IOI Oleo GmbH (Witten, Germany), isopropylmyristate (IPM) from A.C.E.F (Fiorenzuola d'Arda, Italy), Tegin® O (glyceryl oleate), Capryol® PGMC (Propylene glycol mono and dicaprylate NF), and Capryol® 90 (propylene glycol monocaprylate NF) donated by Gattefossé SAS (Saint-Priest, France), castor oil from Sigma (Schnelldorf, Germany) were initially tested to assess the solubility of the model drugs in different oily vehicles. For the preparation of the SNEDDS, the following surfactants were used: Tween® 80 (polysorbate 80), Tween® 20 (polysorbate 20), and Cremophor® EL (castor oil polyoxyethylene ether) were purchased from Merck (Darmstadt, Germany); Solutol® HS15 (Kolliphor® HS15, polyethylene glycol (15)-hydroxystearate) was gifted by BASF (Ludwigshafen am Rhein, Germany). Transcutol®, (2-(2-ethoxyethoxy)ethanol) gifted by Gattefossé SAS (Saint-Priest, France) was used as the co-surfactant. MEL (purity ≥98% by HPLC) was purchased from Merck (Darmstadt, Germany); RSV [trans-3,4′,5-Trihydroxystilbene; hydroalcoholic extract from Polygonum cuspidatum, Siebold et Zucc., roots; purity 99.0% by HPLC] was produced by Giellepi SpA (Seregno, Italy) and kindly gifted by Labomar SpA (Istrana, Italy). Supplementary Table S1 resumes the physico-chemical properties of the two drugs.

2.2. Solubility in Different Oil

Solubility studies were performed by UV spectroscopy (UH5300 UV–visible spectrophotometer, Hitachi, Chiyoda, Japan) to evaluate the solubility of RSV and MEL in different oils (see Section 2.1). An excess amount of RSV was added to 1 mL of each oil and mixed for 24 h at room temperature (r.t.). Samples were then centrifuged at 25 °C for 1 h at 10,000 rpm. The supernatant was separated, and RSV was quantified after appropriate dilutions with methanol, using a standard calibration curve at λ = 306 nm, which was linear in the concentration range 1.527–20.36 µg/mL (R^2 = 0.9992). The same procedure was adopted for MEL, which was quantified in the samples against a standard calibration curve at λ = 224 nm, which was linear in the range of concentrations 12.844–0.803 µg/mL (R^2 = 0.9985).

2.3. Development of SNEDDSs Employing the QbD Approach

2.3.1. Ternary Phase Construction: Choice of Oil

A prototype panel of 14 formulations of blank SNEDDS was prepared by mixing oil, surfactant, and co-surfactant for each 8 tested mixtures: Capryol 90/Tween 80/Transcutol P, Capryol PGMC/Tween 80/Transcutol P, Capryol 90/Tween 20/Transcutol P, Capryol PGMC/Tween 20/Transcutol P, Capryol 90/Cremophor EL/Transcutol P, Capryol PGMC/Cremophor EL/Transcutol P, Capryol 90/Solutol HS15/Transcutol P, and Capryol PGMC/Solutol HS15/Transcutol P. The weight ratio of each component varied from 10% to 80%. All mixtures (in a total amount of 1 g) were prepared by stirring until the three phases were completely homogeneous. The prepared pre-SNEDDS was mixed in a 1:10 volume ratio with freshly prepared simulated tear fluid (STF, composed of 0.68 g NaCl, 0.22 g $NaHCO_3$, 0.008 g $CaCl_2 \cdot 2H_2O$, 0.14 g KCl, and distilled deionized water to 100 mL) and the ternary phase diagram was obtained by measuring the % transmittance of the obtained mixture using a UV–Visible Spectrometer at 650 nm, using distilled water as the reference. Ternary phase diagrams were drawn using the Design of Experiment (DoE) software (Design Expert® 13.0, Stat-Ease Inc., Minneapolis, MN, USA). Simplex Lattice Design was used to perform this analysis, in which the emulsions obtained were classified as SNEDDS according to a clear and transparent nanoemulsion formation. The variables and responses of the design are described in Table 1.

Table 1. Variables of Simplex Lattice Design for pseudo-ternary phase diagram.

Component	Units	Type	Minimum	Maximum
A (oil)	% (*w/w*)	Mixture	10	80
B (surfactant)	% (*w/w*)	Mixture	10	80
C (co-surfactant)	% (*w/w*)	Mixture	10	80
Constraints			Total (A + B + C) = 100	
Transmittance	T%	Response		

2.3.2. Construction of the Design Space

Once the oil had been chosen and the emulsion zone was understood through the construction of ternary graphs, the formulation was optimized by assembling an experimental design using I-Optimal design (Design Expert® 13.0, Stat-Ease Inc., Minneapolis, MN, USA). The numerical variables entered were oil concentration (% *w/w*) (X_1), surfactant concentration (% *w/w*) (X_2), and co-surfactant concentration (% *w/w*) (X_3). For each one, a minimum and a maximum level were chosen, as reported in Table 2. The effect of the surfactant type (Tween® 80, Tween® 20, Cremophor® EL, and Solutol® HS15) as categorical variable (X_4) was also investigated on globule size (nm) (Y_1), time of emulsification (s) (Y_2), and % transmittance (Y_3) after reconstitution of SNEDDS with STF (in 1:10 volume ratio). The type of oil and co-surfactant were constant for all the experiments. A constraint was added to the design, i.e., the sum of the terms should be equal to 100. Table 2 summarizes the factor and their levels and the responses used to build the experimental domain.

Table 2. Variables of the Design Space.

Factors	Name	Units	Type	Levels	
				Low	High
X_1	Oil concn.	% (*w/w*)	Numeric	10	30
X_2	Surfactant concn.	% (*w/w*)	Numeric	10	70
X_3	Co-surfactant concn.	% (*w/w*)	Numeric	10	70
X_4	Surfactant type		Categoric		Tween® 80 Tween® 20 Cremophor® EL Solutol® HS15
Constraints: $X_1 + X_2 + X_3 = 100$					
Y_1	Size	nm			
Y_2	Time of emulsification	s			
Y_3	Transmittance	%			

2.3.3. Characterization of SNEDDS (Particle Size, Time of Emulsification and % Transmittance)

The preconcentrate formulation was diluted with STF (pH 7.4) at a 1:10 volume ratio under soft stirring at 30 rpm and at 35 °C to resemble the corneal surface conditions and eyelid blinking. The formed nanoemulsion was checked for mean particle size (Z-ave), time of emulsification, and % transmittance as responses of the DoE. Further characterization parameters are reported below.

Z-Ave was measured by Photon correlation spectroscopy (PCS, Zetasizer Nano S90; Malvern Instruments, Malvern, UK) at a 90° angle of detection, at 25 °C with a 4 mW He-Ne laser operating at 633 nm. All measurements were performed in triplicate, and the results were expressed as mean ± standard deviation (SD).

Time of self-emulsification was monitored by adding SNEDDDS to STF until the formation of a clear, transparent, blueish-tinted nanoemulsion was visually appreciable. The time for transparent blueish tint appearance was registered with a chronometer and noted.

The formed nanoemulsions were also checked for % transmittance to determine the optical clarity using a–Visible Spectrometer set at 650 nm, using distilled water as the reference. Each measurement was made in triplicate.

2.3.4. Optimization of SNEDDS

SNEDDS optimization was performed using the "desirability tool" provided by the Design-Expert® 13.0 software(Stat-Ease Inc., Minneapolis, MN, USA). The desirability parameter was considered for three responses included in the experimental design: Z-Ave, time of emulsification, and % transmittance. The desirability values ranged from 0 (undesirable) to 1 (desirable). The levels of all independent variables were then automatically combined to identify the conditions within the experimental optimal domain. Four blank formulations were optimized for each surfactant (A = Tween® 80; B = Tween® 20; C = Cremophor® EL; D = Solutol® HS15).

2.4. Preparation of RSV-SNEDDS and MEL-SNEDDS

RSV-SNEDDS (AR, BR, CR, DR, where A, B, C, D indicate the different surfactants and R indicates the addition of RSV) were prepared by mixing the oil (Capryol® PGMC), respective surfactant (A = Tween® 80; B = Tween® 20; C = Cremophor® EL, and D = Solutol® HS15), and cosurfactant (Transcutol® P) at predetermined amounts, defined by optimization, until reaching a transparent and homogeneous solution. An appropriate amount of RSV (2 mg/g) was then added, and the blend was mixed at room temperature using a magnetic stirrer until complete dissolution of RSV. The prepared formulations were stored for further studies out of the light. The same procedure was used to prepare MEL-SNEDDS in order to achieve four different formulations (AM, BM, CM, DM) with 2 mg/g of MEL in the mixtures.

2.5. Characterization of Optimized SNEDDS

SNEDDS were reconstituted with a ten-fold volume of STF under faint stirring (about 30 rpm) prior to characterization to simulate the blinking phenomenon and mimic their behavior in the ocular environment after administration. The Z-ave, polydispersity index (PDI), and zeta potential (ZP) values of SNEDDS after reconstitution were measured by PCS analysis, as previously described (Section 2.3.3). Analogously, the time of self-emulsification and optical clarity (% transmittance) were measured as described for the non-optimized systems (Section 2.3.3).

2.6. Stability Evaluation

Stability studies were performed following the ICH Q1A (R2) guidelines (Stability testing of new drug substances and products) [20]. All samples (SNEDDS, RSV-SNEDDS, and MEL-SNEDDS) were evaluated after storage at different conditions (4 °C, 25 ± 2 °C/60 ± 5% R.H, and 40 ± 2 °C/75% ± 5% R.H.) in a climate chamber (Blinder GmbH, Tuttlingen, Germany). Z-ave, PDI, and ZP were measured every month and up to 3 months, as previously described.

2.7. Stability in Ocular Environment

To evaluate the stability of SNEDDS in the ocular environment, the pre-SNEDDS were diluted in a ratio of 1 to 10 with STF and placed in a climatic chamber at 37 °C. At time intervals (5, 10, 15, 20, 30, 60, 120, and 180 min), they were analyzed for size, PDI, and % transmittance.

2.8. pH, Osmolarity, and Viscosity Determination

The pH of SNEDDS formulations was measured at 25 °C by a Mettler Toledo pH-meter (Columbus, OH, USA). The instrument was calibrated using standard Mettler Toledo buffer solutions (pH 4.01 ± 0.02; 7.00 ± 0.02, and 10.00 ± 0.02; slope 99.8%). Each measurement was performed in triplicate. The osmolality (mOsm/Kg) of the samples was determined using a cryoscopic osmometer (Osmomat, mod. 030-D, Gonotec, Berlin, Germany). Deionized water (consistent with the 0 mOsmol point) and a 300 mOsmol/L calibration standard (consistent with the 300 mOsmol point) were used for a 2-point calibration. Each sample was analyzed in triplicate.

Dynamic viscosity of SNEDDS preconcentrates was obtained by rheological measurements with a rheometer (Haake Mars, ThermoFisher Scientific, Darmstadt, Germany). A C35/1° Ti-plate measuring system was used. The measurement parameters were as follows: shear stress 1–50 Pa, frequency 1 Hz, temperature 25 ± 0.5 °C.

2.9. FT-IR Analysis

FT-IR spectrophotometer (Perkin-Elmer Spectrum RX I, Waltham, MA, USA) was employed for the measurement of pure materials (Capryol® PGMC, Transcutol® P, Tween® 80, RSV, and MEL), blank SNEDDS, RSV-SNEDDS, and MEL-SNEDDS. The tool was equipped with an attenuated total reflectance (ATR) accessory, a diamond window, and zinc selenide crystal (diamond/ZnSe). For each sample, 64 scans were collected at room temperature over the 4000–600 cm^{-1} range at a resolution of 4 cm^{-1}. Any background absorption was subtracted before each analysis.

2.10. Mucoadhesion Study

The mucoadhesion study was performed with the formulation produced with Tween® 80 (A). Pre-SNEDDS were reconstituted with STF (1:10 by volume), and the formed nanoemulsion was incubated with porcine mucin (0.1%, *w/v*) dispersion (1:1, *v/v*) in STF at 37 °C. Mean globule size, % transmittance, and ZP were measured after 0, 30 min, 1, 2, and 24 h of incubation.

2.11. Drug Entrapment Efficiency (EE%)

RSV-SNEDDS and MEL-SNEDDS (1 mL) with a concentration of each drug of 2 mg/g were centrifuged for 30 min at r.t and at 10,000 rpm. The supernatant was suitably diluted with methanol and analyzed by UV spectrophotometry. The drugs were quantified at a wavelength of 306 nm for RSV and 224 nm for MEL. EE% was calculated as follows for each sample:

$$EE\% = (\text{total } \mu g \text{ drug} - \mu g \text{ of drug in the supernatant})/(\text{total } \mu g \text{ drug}) \times 100$$

2.12. Cloud Point Measurements

The cloud point typically refers to the temperature at which a mixture of surfactants undergoes a phase transition, leading to the formation of a cloudy or turbid appearance due to the separation of the emulsion components. This corresponds to the breaking of the emulsion, and it is visually noticeable because the nanoemulsion becomes turbid. The analysis was carried out as follows: different dilutions of SNEDDS/STF were prepared (1:10, 1:50, 1:100, 1:200, 1:300, *v/v*). Each formulation was then placed in a thermostat bath, and the temperature gradually raised. When the formulation became turbid, the temperature was recorded, and the sample was subjected to turbidimetric UV analysis at

650 nm to confirm the change in appearance [21]. The breaking of the nanoemulsion was corroborated by the measurement of Z-ave and PDI changes.

2.13. High-Performance Liquid Chromatography (HPLC) Method for the Quantification of MEL

HPLC analysis was performed using an Agilent 1100 binary pump (Agilent Technologies Inc., Wilmington, DE, USA), a 1100 micro vacuum degasser, a HP 1050 Autosampler, and a HP 1050 variable wavelength detector (operated at 235 nm). The chromatographic separation was achieved on a Supelco Supelcosil™ LC-SI analytical column (4.6 mm × 250 mm, 5 µm) (Supelco Inc., Bellefonte, PA, USA) by an isocratic elution of a formic acid 0.1% (*v/v*) solution in Milli-Q® water and a formic acid methanol solution (0.1%, *v/v*) (40:60, *v/v*). Effluent was monitored at a wavelength of 278.4 nm, with a flow rate of 1 mL/min; the injection volume was 5 µL, retention time of MEL was 3.5 min. The column was maintained at 45.0 ± 0.2 °C throughout the whole analysis.

The standard calibration curves were prepared at different dilutions of MEL in Milli-Q® water/methanol (1:1, *v/v*). The linear regression coefficient determined in the range 0.5–200 µg/mL was 0.9999.

2.14. High-Performance Liquid Chromatography (HPLC) Method for the Quantification of RSV

HPLC analysis was performed using an Agilent 1100 binary pump (Agilent Technologies Inc., Wilmington, DE, USA), a 1100 micro vacuum degasser, a HP 1050 Autosampler, and a HP 1050 variable wavelength detector (operated at 235 nm). The chromatographic separations were achieved on a ZORBAX® Eclipse XDB-C18 (2.1 mm × 100 mm, 1.8 µm) (Agilent, USA) by using isocratic elution of Milli-Q® water and acetonitrile (75:25, *v/v*). Effluent was monitored at a wavelength of 310 nm, with a flow rate of 0.3 mL/min; the injection volume was 5 µL; retention time of RSV was 5.2 min. The column was maintained at 45 °C throughout the analysis.

RSV standard calibration curves were prepared in Milli-Q® water/EtOH (20% *v/v*) with a linear regression coefficient determined in the range 0.1–100 µg/mL was 0.9989. All procedures were carried out to protect the sample from light.

2.15. In Vitro Release Test

The in vitro release profile of MEL-SNEDDS and RSV-SNEDDS in STF, pH 7.4, was performed through a dialysis bag method. One milliliter samples were transferred into a dialysis tube (Spectrum™ Spectra/Por™ membranes, MWCO 3.5 kDa; Fisher Scientific Italia, Segrate, Milan, Italy). The bag was incubated in 4 mL of medium and maintained under magnetic stirring at 37 °C for up to 8 h. At predetermined time points, 2 mL of the release solution was withdrawn and replaced with the same volume of fresh medium. The taken specimens were immediately put into liquid nitrogen and freeze-dried (BuchiLyovaporTM L-200 Freeze Dryer, Fisher Scientific Italia, Segrate, Milan, Italy) for 24 h at 0.1 mbar.

In order to extract MEL, each dried sample was dissolved in 0.5 mL of Milli-Q® water/methanol (1:1, *v/v*) by vortexing for 5 min. The sample was then centrifuged at 10,000× *g* at 4 °C for 30 min to remove the lipid matrix residue, and the supernatant was collected and injected into the HPLC to measure the MEL content. The experiment and HPLC analyses were performed in duplicate. The concentration of MEL was quantified as reported in Section 2.11.

To extract RSV, each dried sample was dissolved in 0.3 mL of Milli-Q® water/ethanol (1:5, *v/v*) by vortexing for 5 min. The sample was then centrifuged at 10,000× *g* at 4 °C for 30 min to remove the SNEDDS matrix residue, and the supernatant was collected and injected into the HPLC to measure the RSV content. The whole procedure was carried out, protecting the sample from light. The experiments and the HPLC analyses were performed in duplicate. The concentration of RSV was quantified as reported in Section 2.12.

The in vitro release data of SNEDDS were analyzed according to various kinetic models:

Zero-order model: $R = Kot$

First-order model: $R = 1 - e - kt$

Higuchi model: R = KH t1/2
Hixson–Crowell model: Wo1/3 − Wt1/3 = KHCt
Korsmeyer–Peppas model: R = kKP tn

The amount of the MEL and RSV released at time t; ko, k, kH, KHC, and kKp (k are the rate constants for the different above models) was expressed by R. Wo is the initial amount of MEL/RSV, and Wt is the amount of drug at time t; n is the release exponent in the Korsmeyer–Peppas model [22]. The model with the highest correlation coefficient (R2) was selected to describe the mechanism of MEL and RSV release. Calculations were made on the linear part of the release curves (from 0.5 h forward).

2.16. Cell Cultures and Viability Assay (MTT)

The test was performed following the short-time exposure test (STE) [23,24]. The Statens Serum Institut Rabbit Cornea (SIRC) epithelial cells (ATCC CCL-60) were grown in specific medium, Eagle's Minimum Essential Medium (ATCC 30-2003TM), complemented with 10% fetal bovine serum (FBS) and 1% penicillin–streptomycin (P/S) and maintained at 37 °C and 5% CO_2, as previously described [25]. Fresh medium was replaced every day, and when the confluence was reached, the cells were seeded into 96-well plates at a density of 1×10^4 cells/well in 100 µL of medium for 24 h. Subsequently, the cells were treated with different concentrations of SNEDDS, RSV-SNEDDS and MEL-SNEDDS in a medium supplemented with 1% FBS for 5 min. Then, the viability assay was performed by adding 100 µL of 3-[4,5-dimethylthiazol-2-yl]-2,5-diphenyltetrazolium bromide (MTT) (ACROS Organics, Antwerp, Belgium) solution for 3 h at 37 °C and 5% CO_2, as previously described [26]. At the end of incubation, the supernatant was removed and replaced with 100 µL of DMSO in order to dissolve the formazan salts produced by mitochondria. The amount of formazan formed by the cleavage of the yellow tetrazolium salt MTT, proportional to the number of viable cells, was measured by using a microplate reader (Biotek Synergy-HT, Winooski, VT, USA) at 550–600 nm. Six replicate wells were used for each group, and at least three separate experiments were performed.

2.17. Statistical Analysis

Characterization data are representative of three separate experiments, and statistical analysis was carried out by two-way ANOVA followed by Dunnett's test. For the mucoadhesion study, statistical analysis was performed by Graphpad Prism 9.5.0 (GraphPad Software, Inc., San Diego, CA, USA) through two-way ANOVA and Šídák's multiple comparisons tests. For the MTT assay, results are representative of at least three independent experiments, and values are expressed as a percentage of control (** $p < 0.01$ or *** $p < 0.001$ vs. STF, as determined by one-way ANOVA followed by Tukey–Kramer post hoc test).

3. Results and Discussion

3.1. Solubility of Drugs in Various Oils

The solubility of RSV and MEL was determined to evaluate which oil better solubilized the active compounds. The set of tested oils was selected based on those most commonly used in the literature for the preparation of SNEDDS (Figure 1). Among the six assayed oils, Capryol® PGMC showed the highest solubility (9.92 ± 1.30 mg/mL for RSV and 23.18 ± 0.88 mg/mL for MEL). Capryol® PGMS was followed by Capryol® 90 with the capacity to solubilize 4.47 ± 1.07 mg/mL of RSV and 15.86 ± 1.70 of MEL. The choice of the oily vehicle is a crucial step; indeed, the formulation must consist of components that solubilize the drug and form a monophasic mixture when shaken together. Furthermore, Capryol® 90 and, even more, PGMC possess the ability to spontaneously form clear emulsions when mixed with surfactants with high HLB, such as polysorbates (Tween®). Both have been extensively investigated for the development of nanoemulsion and SNEDDS, as well as microemulsions and SMEDDS [27–30]. The emulsion formed must be clear and limpid and must not allow the drug to precipitate [31]. Therefore, the choice of the oil in which the drug is most soluble is highly relevant. These two oils were chosen to continue the study with the search for the emulsion zone using the ternary graph.

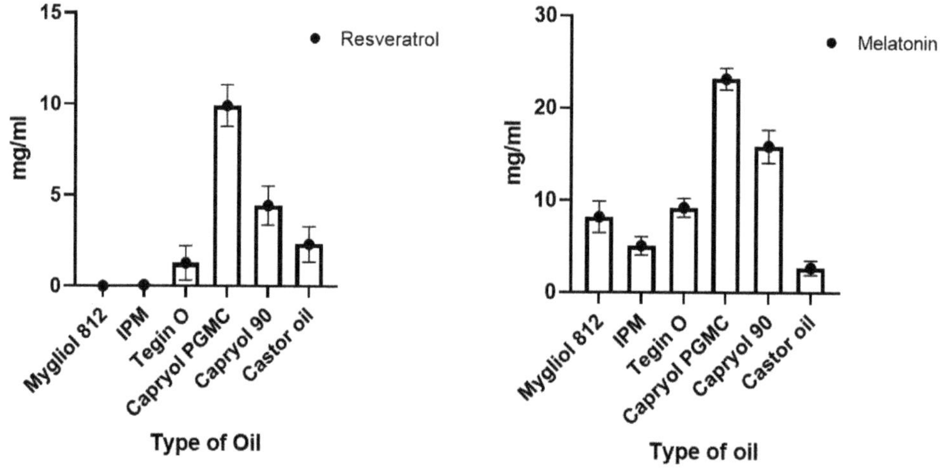

Figure 1. Solubility of RSV and MEL in different oils.

3.2. Ternary Plot Diagram Construction

The ratio between the phases varied in each experiment, keeping the sum of the three phases constant at 1 g in the final SNEDDS. The % transmittance was evaluated in a range from 0.1 to 100% for the various emulsions produced. The blue zone indicated an emulsion with a high % transmittance, followed by the green, orange, and finally red zones, which indicated increasingly lower transmittances down to 0.1 (red zone). Obtaining a transmittance close to 100% suggested a globule size below 100 nm. As Figure 2 shows, Capryol® PGMC allowed to produce emulsions with a high degree of transmittance. When comparing the graphs, it is possible to see a higher concentration of blue areas in the graphs produced with Capryol® PGMC. Both are propylene glycol mono- and diesters of caprylic acid (C8) but with different fractions of monoesters [32]. This slightly different composition, combined with a different behavior with the various surfactants, gave rise to differences in terms of spontaneous nanoemulsification in favor of Capryol® PGMC. It had already demonstrated its superiority over Capryol® 90 in terms of self-nanoemulsification efficiency in many mixtures with different surfactants [33].

3.3. Construction of the Experimental Design

The blank SNEDDS were first optimized with the experimental design. Forty-two runs were formulated to obtain all possible combinations with the four surfactants. For the construction of the experimental design, the following numerical variables were chosen: oil concentration (% *w/w*), surfactant concentration (% *w/w*), and co-surfactant concentration (% *w/w*). This is a crucial pre-formulation point. Choosing in which ratios the three phases should co-exist allows the final goal to be achieved: a homogenous formulation that emulsifies in a short time without giving the presence of drug precipitate. Finally, the type of surfactant was chosen as the categorical variable. Four surfactants with a common characteristic, i.e., hydrophilicity (HLB > 12), were tested, and they were included in the design as they favor the occurrence of O/A emulsions. Tween® 80 (HLB = 15), Tween® 20 (HLB = 16.7), Cremophor®-EL (HLB = 13), and Solutol® HS15 (HLB = 15) are non-ionic surfactants, and they are considered less toxic and more cytocompatible than ionic surfactants [34]. They also had a very good ability to emulsify Capryol® PGMC. In fact, the possibility of quick emulsification in contact with small volumes of an aqueous fluid, such as in the ocular surface, is possible using a surfactant with a high HLB. The choice of testing four surfactants was linked to the consideration that the emulsification ability of each surfactant is typically influenced not only by the HLB and structure but also by their physical behavior once mixed with the other two components [35].

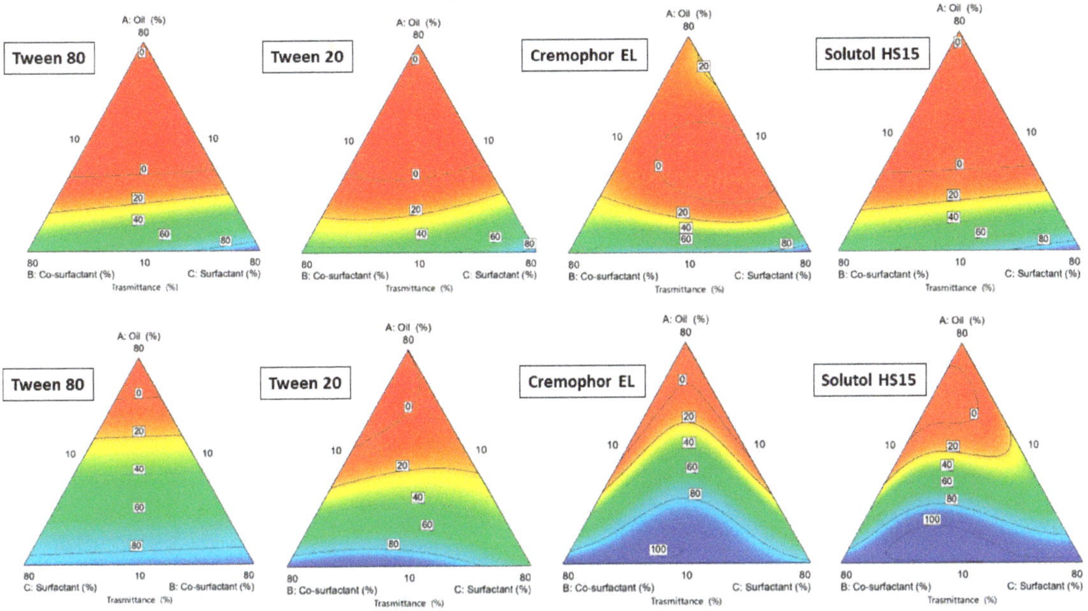

Figure 2. Ternary plot diagrams obtained by the mixtures of Transcutol® P, different surfactants and Capryol® 90 (upper row) and Capryol® PGMC (bottom row).

3.3.1. Effect of Independent Variables on Globule Size

DoE involves creating a structured plan for understanding the relationship between the independent variables (factors) and dependent variables (responses) in a system. Once all the experiments suggested by the software are completed, it provides polynomial equations, one for each response, to determine the influence of each factor in the response and the interaction between factors and responses. The equation below represents the influence of each factor on the size of SNEDDS (1). This was obtained once all the formulations of SNEDDS were prepared and analyzed for particle size. The obtained globule size for all experiments was in the range 13.29 ± 0.135–455.1 ± 15.36 nm.

$$\text{Size } (Y_1) = 152.98044384037 + 111.97043203167\, X_1 + 84.068897927114\, X_3 - 5.413763606443\, X4\,[1] + 21.113050603648\, X4\,[2] - 48.03416483216\, X1{\times}4\,[1] + 8.8903231966525\, X1X4\,[2] + 45.844330806972\, X12 \quad (1)$$

The ANOVA analysis of the full regression models showed that only some factors were statistically significant; thus, statistically non-significant terms were removed except for terms needed for hierarchy in the reduced regression model. The quality of the fit of the experimental data using the reduced quadratic models was assessed based on several statistical criteria. Taking into account the R^2 parameter, the quadratic model was considered the most significant since Adjusted R^2, given by the software, was close to Predicted R^2. Moreover, the generated model F-value of 9.77 implies the model is significant. The term B, which refers to co-surfactant concentration, was excluded by the model because it had no significant influence on globule size. When both oil and surfactant concentrations were increased, globule size decreased due to the oil's dominant influence over the surfactant. Indeed, oil concentration appeared to be the factor most influential on the mean size response, with an estimated coefficient equal to +111.97. A positive coefficient revealed a direct relationship between the variable and the response. As shown by the response surface graphs, an increase in oil concentration produced larger particles (Figure 3). Smaller particle sizes were observed when using Tween® 80, as represented in response surface graphs (Figure 3). Tween 80® allows for better stabilization of nanoemulsions, forming a protective layer around the micelles and preventing their aggregation. It also has a controlling role in the whole emulsification process, reducing the surface energy and leading to the inhibition of crystal growth during the entire process [36]. The square bracket in polynomial Equation (1) indicates an optional third parameter associated with the level of that factor implied in the polynomial regression. For example, the influence associated with the type of surfactant depends mainly on the first level with Tween® 80 and on the second level and thus on Tween® 20 (a result that perfectly corroborates the response surface plots below).

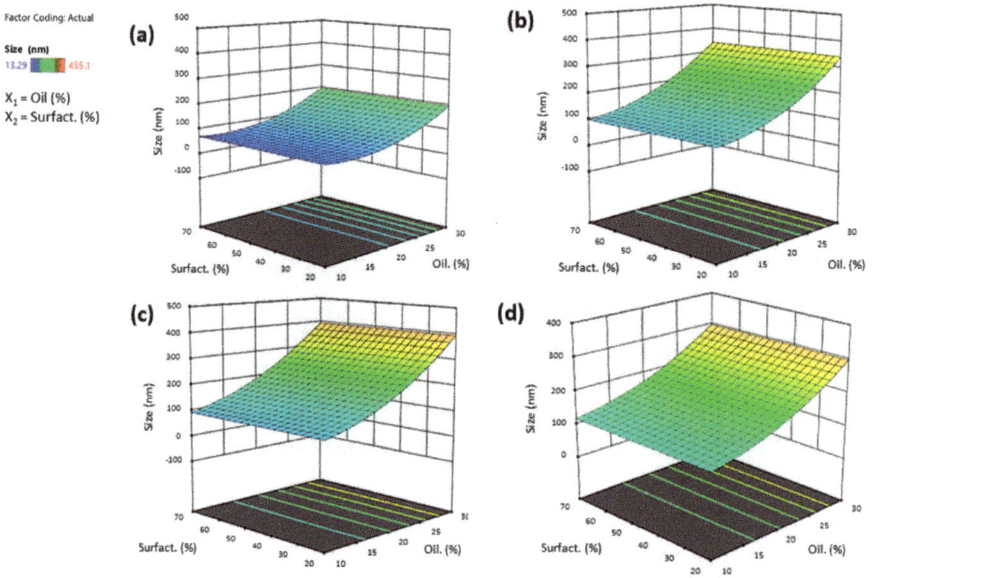

Figure 3. Three-dimensional surface of the effect of independent variables (surfactant vs. oil concentration) on the globule size of SNEDDS after reconstitution with STF (1:10 by volume) using Tween® 80 (**a**), Tween® 20 (**b**), Cremophor® EL (**c**), or Solutol® HS15 (**d**).

3.3.2. Effect of Independent Variables on Time of Emulsification

Once the values are inserted in the software, it generates a polynomial Equation (2) that relates the influence of each factor with the time of emulsification derived from all SNEDDS prepared. The obtained time of emulsification for all experiments was in the range of 31 ± 1.2–134 ± 5.50 s. As demonstrated in the polynomial equation, the surfactant concentration and the interaction between surfactant type and its concentration were identified as the most influential factors regarding the time of emulsification response.

$$\text{Time of emulsification} = 75.162927762315 + 0.12557087841826\,X_1 + 23.558956914706\,X_2 + 12.877171801241\,X4\,[1] + 5.5936332662947\,X4\,[2] + 0.43202022289143\,X1X4\,[1] + -8.844328114505\,X1X4\,[2] + 20.231882039157\,X2X4\,[1] + 13.526675893769\,X2X4\,[2] \quad (2)$$

As suggested by the software, the reduced 2FI model was considered significant since Adjusted R^2 was close to Predicted R^2. The generated F-value of 9.30 for this model implies the model is significant. Some factors were deleted by the model since they were considered not significant. One of them was the co-surfactant concentration, whose influence was considered not significant in changing the time of emulsification parameter.

Factors X_2 had a positive influence on this response (+25.66). An increasing amount of surfactant increased the emulsion time. The right surfactant concentration allows accessibility to the oil/water interface, reducing interfacial tension and thus the possibility of obtaining an emulsion in a short time. But when the surfactant is excessive, the formulation becomes viscous, and the moment fluid comes into contact with the SNEDDS, the emulsion time of the latter increases. It is worth noting from the graphs that the interaction between surfactant type and oil is important (Figure 4). In the case of both Tween® 20 and 80, the emulsion time increased with increasing surfactant concentration, without any influence from the oil concentration. In the case of Cremophor® and Solutol® HS 15, instead, the increase in oil concentration must also be taken into account: the emulsion time increased when the surfactant amount decreased, and the oil concentration increased at the same time. The formation of a mixture that was more viscous (such as with Tween® 80 and Tween® 20) could slow down the movement of the liquid between the phases and result in the formation of droplets for a longer time. Higher viscosities tend to slow down the emulsification rate, as reported by Nasr et al. [37].

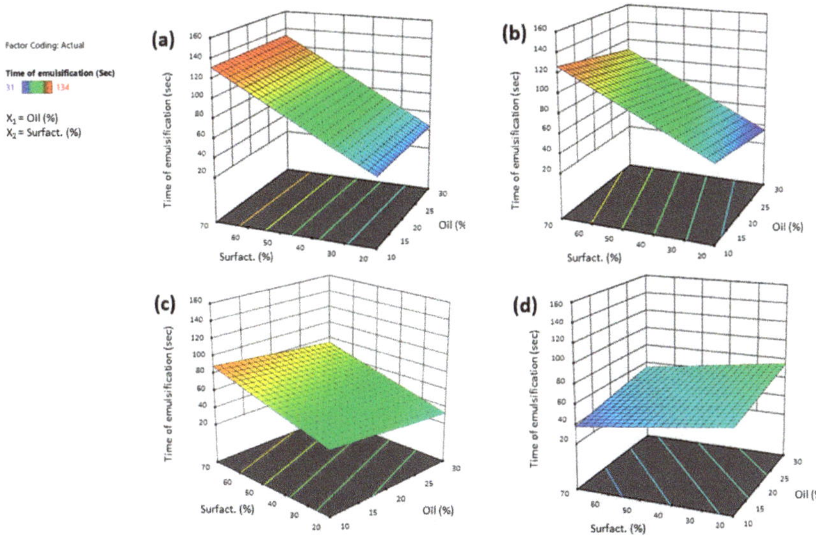

Figure 4. Three-dimensional surface of the effect of independent variables (surfactant vs. oil concentration) on the time of emulsification of SNEDDS after reconstitution with STF (1:10 by volume) using Tween® 80 (**a**), Tween® 20 (**b**), Cremophor® EL (**c**), or Solutol® HS15 (**d**).

3.3.3. Effect of Independent Variables on Transmittance%

The obtained % transmittance for all experiments was in the range 0.1–100 ± 0.10%. Just as in the case of size, for transmittance, the most influential factor was the amount of oil. Transmittance and particle size are closely linked: a high optical clarity (90–100%) stands for globules with a size smaller than 50 nm. In contrast, a low transmittance indicates that the emulsion formed is not clear and will certainly contain particles of the order of more than 100 nm.

As for other responses, the equation below (3) represents the quantitative effect of the process variables (oil, surfactant, and co-surfactant) and their interaction on the % transmittance. In this case, all the factors investigated exerted a significant influence on the response. The linear model (F-value of 20.94) was considered significant, with Adjusted R2 being close to Predicted R2 and, as the equation below shows, the most influential factor was oil concentration.

$$\text{Transmittance} = 38.873268681425 - 36.562914111227\,X_1 + 11.233423582655\,X_2 - 26.931299436827\,X_3 + 26.002042325709\,X4\,[1] - 12.538357360177\,X4\,[2] \quad (3)$$

Given the negative estimated coefficient (−36.56) of X_1, the relationship between % transmittance and oil was indirect: higher oil concentrations produced milky nanoemulsions with low transmittance (~0.1%), which, in turn, was synonymous with the presence of larger globules (Figure 5). The coefficient of the co-surfactant was also negative, meaning that with increasing concentrations of the co-surfactant, the transmittance value decreased. Formulations with a high percentage of Transcutol® P gave emulsions with a milky appearance, with transmittance values less than 30%. This could be attributed to the low HLB of Transcutol® P, around 4–5, that allowed rapid emulsification in combination with Tween® 80 but produced milky emulsions. Indeed, Transcutol® P is sometimes used as an oil phase for the development of SNEDDS; and, as discussed above, an increase in the oil phase generated a higher transmittance.

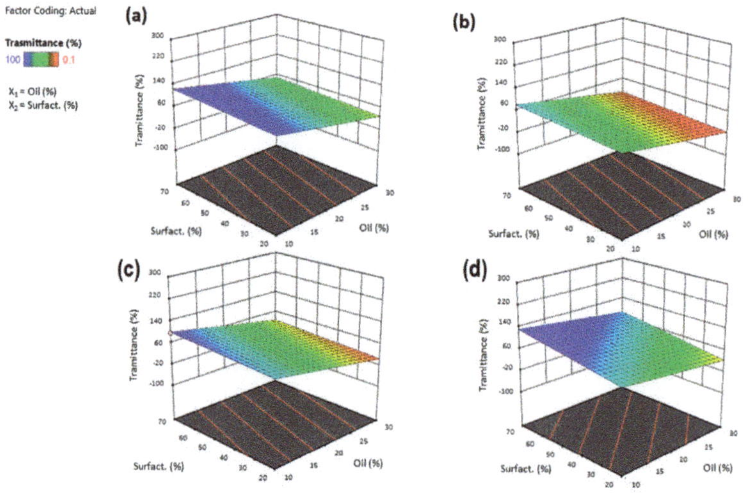

Figure 5. Three-dimensional surface of the effect of independent variables (surfactant vs. oil concentration) on the % transmittance of SNEDDS after reconstitution with STF (1:10 by volume) using Tween® 80 (**a**), Tween® 20 (**b**), Cremophor® EL (**c**), or Solutol® HS15 (**d**).

3.4. Optimization Phase

For the optimization of SNEDDS, different criteria were set to suit the ocular administration by topical instillation. Therefore, it was decided to (i) minimize the oil concentration, as it affected both size and transmittance; (ii) increase the surfactant concentration, as this choice produced smaller sizes; (iii) minimize the concentration of co-surfactant, given its influence on % transmittance and clarity of the nanoemulsions.

The surfactant type remained in the range to have more options to optimize the formulations: a small size was preferable, as it would improve the diffusion towards the deeper structures of the eye globe.

Preferably, a time of less than 20 s would be perfect since SNEDDS, once applied on the ocular surface, must emulsify with the tear fluid very quickly. A long time would not allow the SNEDDS to emulsify before being drained away. Finally, high transmittance was important since this would prevent blurred vision when the formulation was instilled. The selected optimization criteria are shown in Table 3.

Table 3. Optimization criteria for SNEDDS production.

Factors and Responses		Goal	Lower Limit	Upper Limit
X_1	Oil concn. % (*w/w*)	Minimize	10	30
X_2	Surfactant concn. % (*w/w*)	Maximize	20	70
X_3	Co-surfactant concn. % (*w/w*)	Minimize	20	70
X_4	Type of surfactant	In range	Tween® 80, Tween® 20, Cremophor® EL, Solutol® HS15	
Y_1	Mean particle size (nm)	Close to 20 nm	13.29	455.1
Y_2	Time of emulsification (s)	Minimize	31	134
Y_3	% Transmittance	Maximize	0.1	100

Once the optimization criteria were chosen, the software generated a set of optimized formulations, which were sorted according to desirability values. Desirability gives an idea of how well the predicted formulation fits with the chosen parameters. It ranges from a value of 0 to 1. Four formulations with the highest desirability were selected, one for each surfactant, in order to assess the stability of the active ingredients in each of them (Table 4).

Table 4. Optimized formulation according to the desirability parameter.

Sample	Type of Oil	Oil Concn. %	Surfactant Concn. %	Co-Surfactant Concn. %	Desirability
A	Tween® 80	15.041	55.181	28.211	0.886
B	Tween® 20	15.456	52.471	30.133	0.723
C	Cremophor® EL	14.351	58.025	23.358	0.761
D	Solutol® HS15	14.351	58.025	23.358	0.868

The produced four formulations were characterized in terms of size, emulsification time, and % transmittance (Table 5). After calculating the % error between the predicted response and that obtained experimentally, an error of less than 10% was registered for all responses. The chosen model could thus be considered highly predictive for the formulation of SNEDDS [38].

Table 5. Experimental values of size, % transmittance, and time of emulsification for optimized SNEDDS.

Sample	Size (nm) ± SD	% Transmittance	Time of Emulsification (s)
A	13.26 ± 0.07	100	12.04
B	127.29 ± 1.12	88	12.18
C	11.29 ± 0.11	100	17.85
D	18.82 ± 0.41	100	15.76

3.5. Characterization of SNEDDS, RSV-SNEDDS, and MEL-SNEDDS

MEL and RSV were loaded into the SNEDDS in order to achieve a therapeutic concentration of drugs after reconstitution. Literature data indicate that MEL at 10^{-4} μM attenuates oxidative stress and inflammation of Müller cells via activating the SIRT-1 pathway [39,40]. RSV at 100 μM increases SIRT-1 overexpression in retinal pigment epithelium [41,42].

Technological and physico-chemical parameters remained unchanged when the formulations were loaded with drugs with respect to the blank systems (Figure 6). Furthermore, no precipitate was observed after the formation of the extemporaneous nanoemulsion. The resultant small droplet size would provide a large interfacial surface area for drug release and absorption. The results obtained in terms of size seemed optimal. The passage from the corneal surface to the vitreous humor is allowed for molecules smaller than 500 nm since the mesh size of the bovine vitreous has been estimated at ~550 nm. However, to allow diffusion without minimal steric hindrance and to obtain formulations that do not cause irritation or blurred vision upon administration, a size less than 200 nm is preferable [43]. Furthermore, the slightly negative charge of the SNEDDS obtained and their small size, especially in the case of systems A, C, and D, allowed them to move toward the retina. Studies demonstrated that small-sized (≈50 nm) PEG-coated anionic liposomes showed the most extensive cellular distribution and localization in the retina [44]. All the produced SNEDDS had a very small size, slightly higher in the case of SNEDDS formed with Tween® 20. A PDI of less than 0.3 always indicated a good homogeneity of the formulation. The slightly negative ZP was attributable to the materials used; however, none of the SNEDDS displayed a net charge and were very close to neutral.

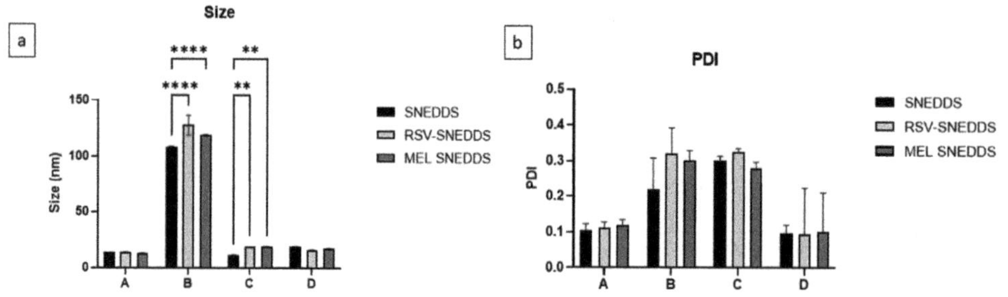

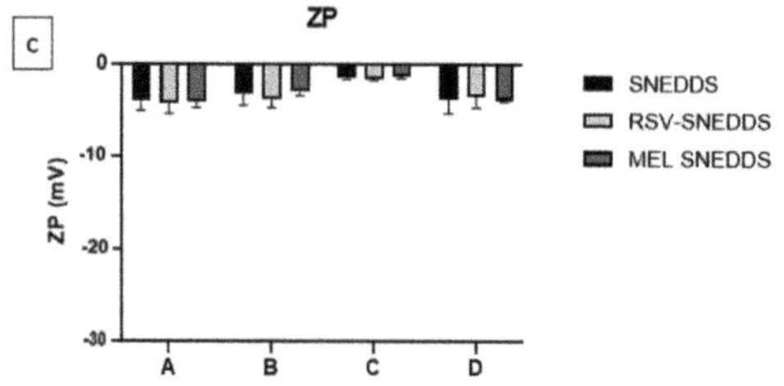

d

Samples		Entrapment efficiency (%)
A	AM	100
	AR	100
B	BM	100
	BR	98
C	CM	100
	CR	100
D	DM	98
	DR	98

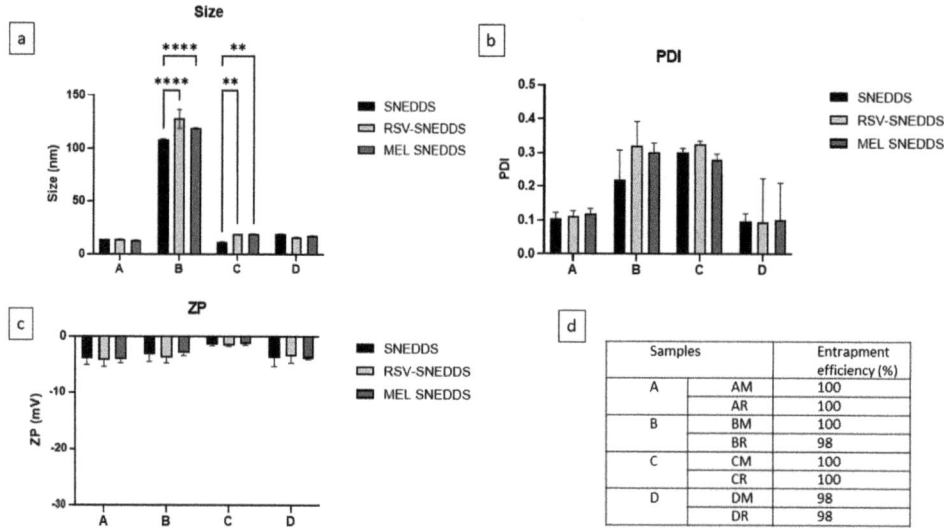

Figure 6. Characterization of SNEDDS in terms of (**a**) size, (**b**) PDI and (**c**) ZP before and after loading with RSV and MEL; (**d**) Entrapment efficiency (EE%) of drug-loaded samples A, B, C, and D. ** $p < 0.01$, **** $p < 0.0001$.

The entrapment efficiency of SNEDDS loaded with RSV (AR, BR, CR, DR) or MEL (AM, BM, CM, DM) was high for all samples. No precipitate was observed after dilution with STF as proof that all the active ingredient was encapsulated and retained in the lipid mixtures. The pH and osmolarity values were assessed upon dilution with STF; the small dilution gave an idea of the actual SNEDDS values. All SNEDDS showed pH values between 6.9 and 7.5 and osmolarity in the range of 0.281 to 0.320 Osm/kg after reconstitution with STF (1:10 by volume). These values could be considered optimal for an ophthalmic liquid formulation that should be non-irritating once applied [45]. Higher or lower values of osmolarity could cause irritation and extensive lachrymation, provoking a rapid wash-out of the solution and consequently a poor drug local bioavailability [46].

The values of viscosity obtained for formulations A, AR, and AM were in the range of 15–58 mPa as a function of time. A viscosity value up to 50 mPa-s is generally considered tolerated for an ocular formulation. Thus, the tested SNEDDS appears to be suitable for ocular administration in terms of viscosity without presumption of impairment of normal visual function.

3.6. Stability in Simulated Ocular Environment

Characterization of SNEDDS in the potential ocular environment can be useful for evaluating their potential behavior in vitro and in vivo. The temperature, the pH, and the ions present in the tear fluid could influence the interaction of the systems with the cellular compartment [47]. Therefore, the colloidal stability of the SNEDDS placed in contact with a potential ocular environment (STF, 37 °C in a climatic chamber) was evaluated for a maximum time of 180 min. At specific various time intervals, they were analyzed in terms of Z-ave, PDI, and % transmittance. Significant changes would indicate an instability of the systems. Figure 7 highlighted high stability for all formulations except for C and B. At 37 °C, the latter formulation exhibited an increase in size and % transmittance over time, turning milky already after 5–10 min. The increase in size observed in both formulations may be attributed to an aggregation phenomenon, suggesting minimal stability within three hours. Formulations A and D exhibit considerable stability throughout the analysis period. The absence of particle aggregation is crucial as this phenomenon could potentially induce irritative effects, leading to rapid drainage of the systems before interacting with the ocular surface, thereby compromising the effectiveness of the system.

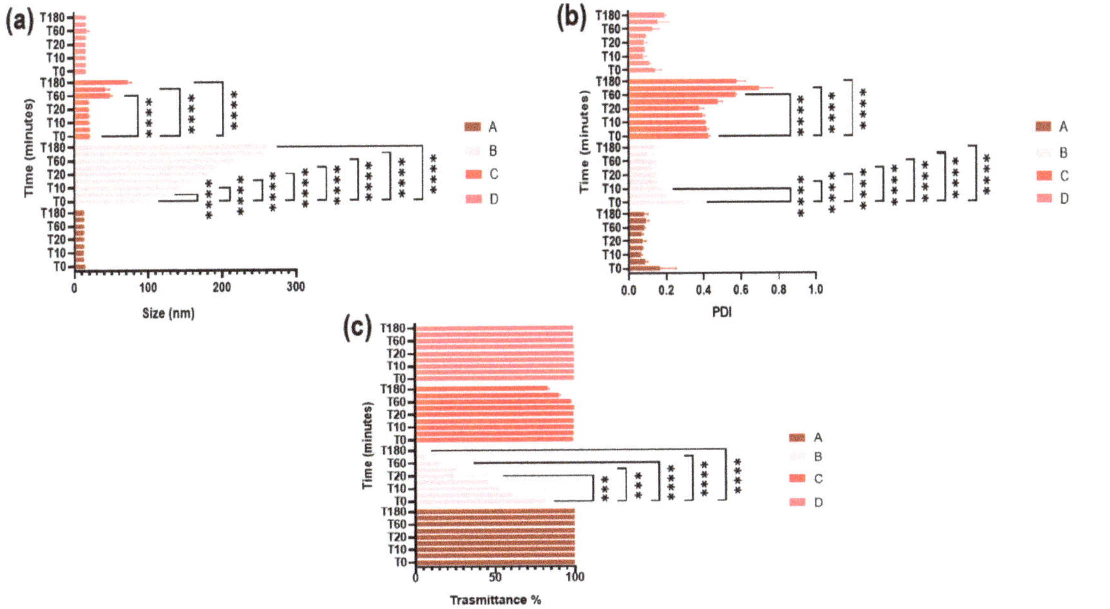

Figure 7. Stability in ocular environment of formulations A, B, C and D in terms of (**a**) size, (**b**) PDI and (**c**) % transmittance (*** $p < 0.001$ or **** $p < 0.0001$ vs. T0, as determined by two-way ANOVA followed by Dunnett's multiple comparisons test).

3.7. SNEDDS Stability Evaluation

The stability study of the SNEDDS was carried out according to the ICH guidelines for the stability testing of new drug substances and products [20] under different storage conditions. Like all new drug products, nanomedicines should demonstrate constancy of physico-chemical and microbiological parameters under suitable thermal and humidity storage conditions and durations prior to their registration [48]. When nanomedicines do not contain or are not decorated with biotechnological molecules but incorporate only a drug and/or an imaging agent, as in the present work, stability testing can follow the indications of the ICH guidelines Q1A (R2) and Q1C (in the case of new dosage forms of already registered products) [48].

Drug-loaded SNEDDS were, therefore, placed at three different temperatures: 4 °C, 25 °C (at 60% R.H.), and 40 °C (at 75% R.H.). SNEDDS loaded with MEL showed no sign of visual instability; RSV-SNEDDS instead showed a strong degradation of RSV already after one week at 25 °C, but especially at 40 °C, as suggested by the development of a yellow color in the vials (Figure 8b). The instability could be definitely associated with the encapsulated RSV since, as Figure 8a shows, the corresponding blank SNEDDS did not show the same alterations until 3 months of storage.

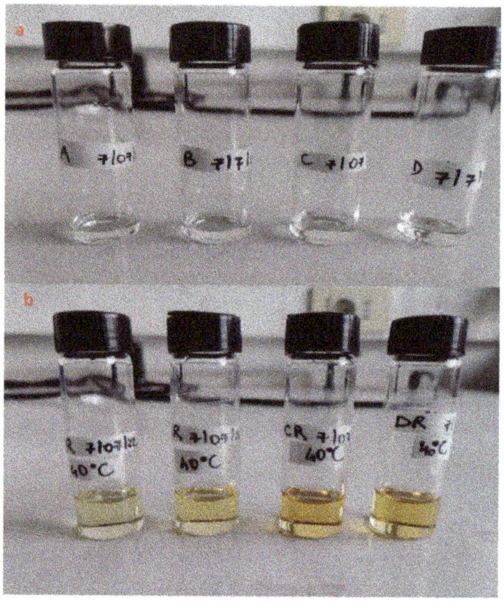

Figure 8. (**a**) Blank SNEDDS after 6 months after storage at 40 °C and (**b**) RSV-SNEDDS after one week of storage at the same temperature.

Blank SNEDDS can be defined as stable systems since formulations that do not show significant changes at 40 °C for at least 6 months (accelerated stability conditions) can be defined as stable for a hypothetical time frame of at least one year [20]. Literature studies confirm the stability of RSV at temperatures between 4 °C and −20 °C and also confirm the high possibility of degradation at temperatures above 25 °C [49,50]. High temperature favored oxidation, epimerization, hydrolysis, and/or polymerization of stilbenes [51]. The increase in temperature induces a change in the appearance of the formulation with a typical color change that is evident as the temperature rises (40 °C > 25 °C). Indeed, oxidation of RSV at high temperatures produces a change in the molecule that leads to a light yellow to dark yellow color. This degradation was also influenced by the materials used, as shown in Figure 8b [52]. The color change produced during storage at high temperatures is due to the degradation of RSV. The degradation of RSV produces aromatic degradation under products that absorb at wavelengths above 300 nm that can be monitored with UV-visible and are potentially responsible for the color change in the formulation. This is a phenomenon that is much more noticeable when exposing the RSV to light but is still visible when the RSV is exposed to high temperatures [53,54]. To reduce RSV alteration, the formulations were supplemented with an antioxidant agent, namely vitamin E TPGS or ascorbic acid, and their stability was monitored at 25 and 40 °C. As shown in Figure 9, the use of antioxidants increased the shelf life of the RSV-SNEDDS during a 3-month period.

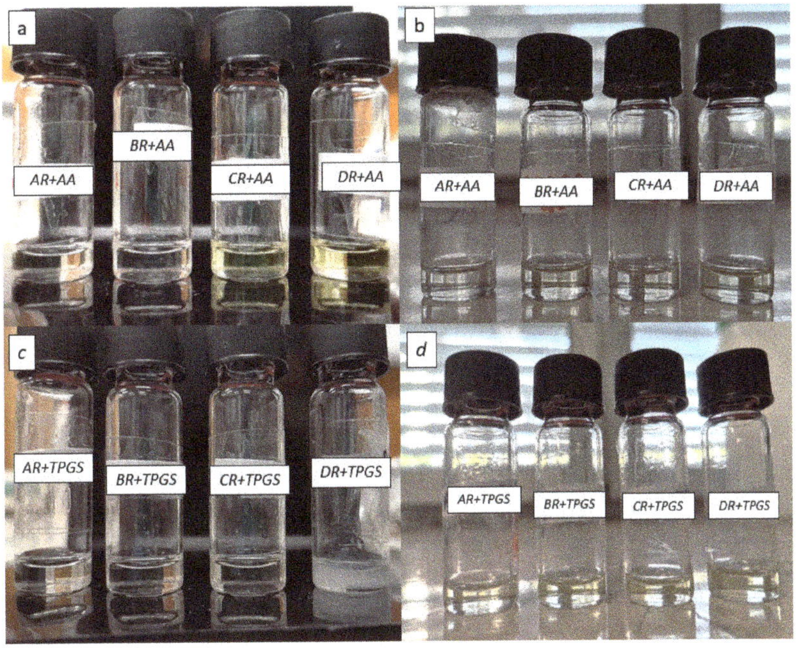

Figure 9. RSV-SNEDDS after 3 months of storage (**a**) with ascorbic acid at 25 °C and (**b**) at 40 °C, or (**c**) with TPGS at 25 °C and (**d**) at 40 °C.

As revealed by Figure 9, formulation A was much more physically stable with the addition of both antioxidants under the conditions tested. Tween® 80, as a surfactant combined with an antioxidant compound, was able to prevent the degradation of RSV, as also reported by Das et al. [52]. Therefore, this formulation was chosen for the subsequent studies. In addition, stability studies showed that formulations C and D underwent gelation at the temperature of 4 °C, with increased size and PDI. Formulation B, despite being moderately stable, is the formulation that gives the largest size with increasing transmittance over time. Its instability is not suitable for ocular administration. The unloaded formulation A was subjected to stability studies under the same storage conditions. As shown in Figure 10, it was stable for up to 3 months, showing no signs of destabilization in terms of size, PDI, and ZP. The unchanging parameters for a long period highlight the high robustness of formulation A, even under accelerated conditions. The AR formulation (RSV-loaded A formulation) supplemented with an antioxidant was evaluated in terms of size, ZP, PDI, and % transmittance (cf. Table inside Figure 10), giving excellent preservation results to corroborate the visual results presented above (Figure 9). MEL-SNEDDS gave the same results also for formulations B, C, and D. Formulation A, loaded with MEL (AM), was the most stable for up to 3 months at 4 °C without antioxidant addition and at 25 and 40 °C with the addition of a small percentage (0.015% *w/w*) of TPGS or ascorbic acid. It did not show significant destabilization phenomena or signs of MEL precipitation. The size, PDI, and ZP remained unchanged for the whole tested period.

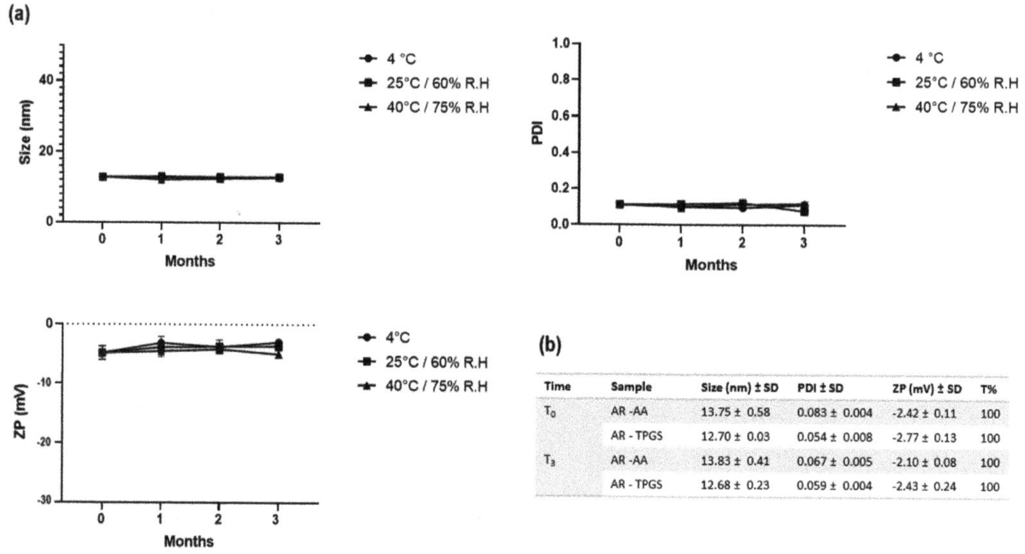

Time	Sample	Size (nm) ± SD	PDI ± SD	ZP (mV) ± SD	T%
T_0	AR -AA	13.75 ± 0.58	0.083 ± 0.004	-2.42 ± 0.11	100
	AR - TPGS	12.70 ± 0.03	0.054 ± 0.008	-2.77 ± 0.13	100
T_3	AR -AA	13.83 ± 0.41	0.067 ± 0.005	-2.10 ± 0.08	100
	AR - TPGS	12.68 ± 0.23	0.059 ± 0.004	-2.43 ± 0.24	100

Figure 10. (**a**) Stability of SNEDDS at different storage conditions in terms of size, PDI and ZP. (**b**) Stability after 3 months of AR added with TPGS or ascorbic acid (AA) at concentration of 0.015% *w/w*.

Measurement of Cloud Point

The cloud point represents the temperature at which an emulsion becomes cloudy and breaks down. It is important to assess whether a nanoemulsion maintains its physical stability at the body site of administration. For ocular application, the emulsion must remain stable and not break down at 35 °C, the temperature of the ocular surface. At temperatures above the cloud point, an irreversible phase separation occurs due to dehydration of the formulation. This can inhibit the efficiency of the system, induce expulsion of the drug from the formed micelles, with its precipitation, and thus affect the drug absorption and efficacy overall.

Table 6 shows that the emulsion formed after reconstitution of SNEDDS A with different ratios of STF had a cloud point above 40 °C at all the dilutions tested. This was corroborated by the size and PDI value, measured just after the dilution and gathered in the same table. The results demonstrated excellent temperature stability up to 47 °C in the case of a small dilution, as might occur on the ocular surface, and even greater stability at higher dilutions, which might be important for other routes of administration.

Table 6. Temperature, size and PDI of different dilutions of SNEDDS/STF subjected to cloud point measurement.

Ratio SNEDDS/STF	Temperature (°C)	Size (nm) ± SD	PDI
1:10	47.2	210 ± 17.5	0.263 ± 0.090
1:50	60.5	201.1 ± 11.73	0.311 ± 0.049
1:100	70.0	120.1 ± 5.208	0.289 ± 0.024
1:200	79.9	443.8 ± 286	0.575 ± 0.601
1:300	82.2	1228.6 ± 16.09	0.561 ± 0.105

3.8. FT-IR Spectroscopy

To study any possible interaction between the drugs and components of the samples, FT-IR spectroscopic analysis was applied to the neat ingredients and to blank formulation A and formulation A loaded with RSV or MEL (AR and AM, respectively) (Figures 11 and 12).

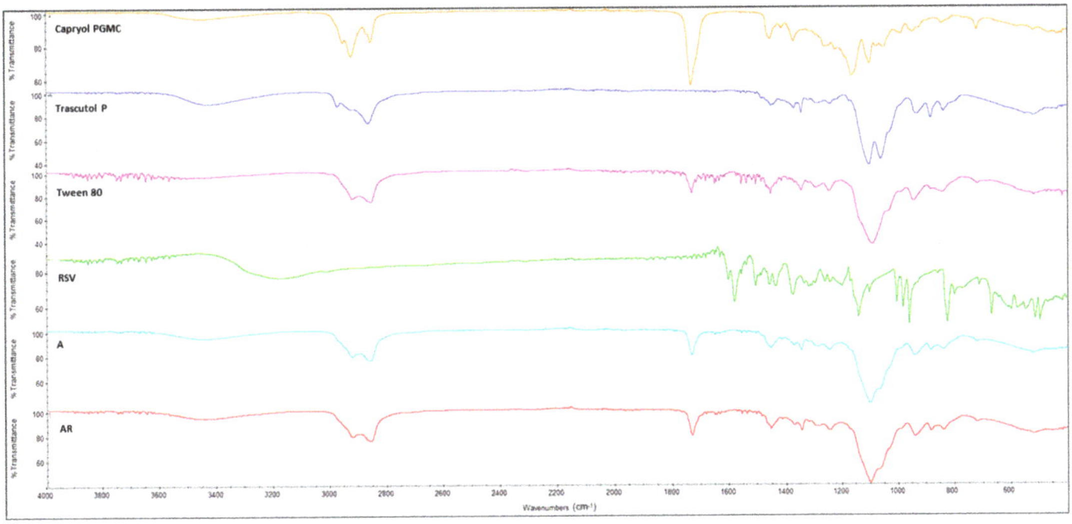

Figure 11. FTIR spectra of pure SNEDDS components and blank (A) and RSV-loaded (AR) nanocarriers.

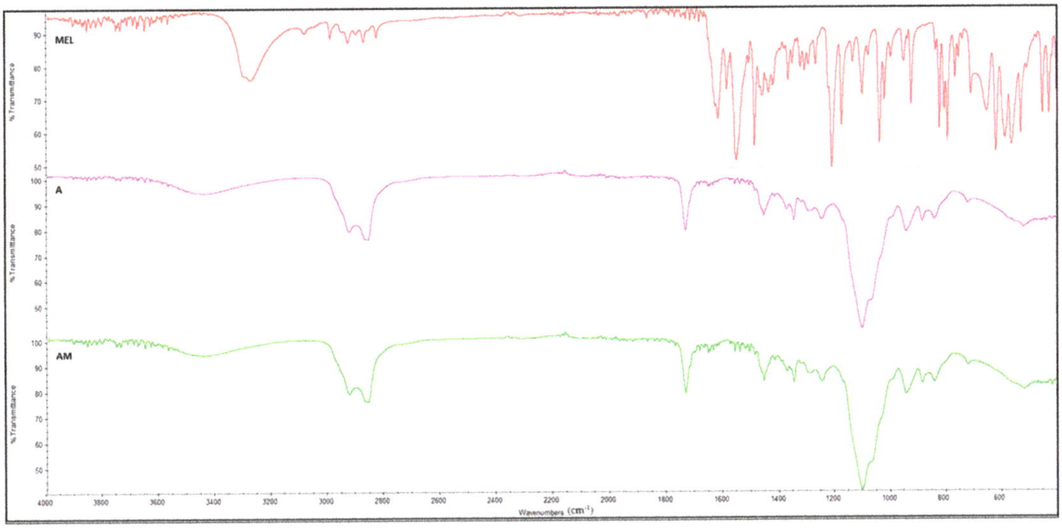

Figure 12. FTIR Spectra for MEL, blank SNEDDS (A) and MEL-loaded SNEDDS (AM).

Figure 11 delineates the primary peaks of the used materials. They exhibit compatibility with each other, as evidenced by formulation A wherein the characteristic peaks of Capryol® PGMC at 3447 cm^{-1} (O-H) and 1735 cm^{-1} (C=O) are distinctly visible, along with the aliphatic C-H carbon peaks between 2995–2856 cm^{-1}, specific of Transcutol® P and Tween® 80. Moreover, the latter surfactant displayed a peak at approximately 1700 cm^{-1} (HOH bending) and another at 1096 cm^{-1} (C-O), both of which reappeared in the spectrum of formulation A. Despite slight shifts with minor significance, all components maintain their intrinsic characteristics within the blank formulation. The RSV-SNEDDS specimen exhibits a spectrum that was superimposable with the one of blank SNEDDS, encompassing all previously observed peaks. However, distinct RSV peaks, such as the one at 3177.63 cm^{-1} (corresponding to OH functional groups) and the peak around 1580 cm^{-1}, are absent in the loaded formulation. This outcome, combined with the resemblance to the blank SNEDDS spectrum, suggests the effective encapsulation of RSV within the formulation [55]. Moreover, the absence of characteristic RSV peaks in the spectrum of AR formulation implies that the drug was situated inside the emulsion micelles rather than on their surface.

The NH stretching peak belonging to MEL at 3273.55 cm^{-1} was not observed in the spectrum of formulation AM (Figure 12), which completely overlaps with the unloaded formulation A. The peaks observed corresponded to those derived from the raw materials Capryol® PGMC, Transcutol® P, and Tween® 80, already shown in Figure 11, also indicating, in this case, the complete entrapment of MEL within the micelles of the AM emulsion [56].

3.9. Mucoadhesion Study

To assess the mucoadhesive properties of SNEDDS, the interaction with mucin was evaluated over a period of 3 h by measuring the absorbance of SNEDDS/mucin mixtures at 650 nm and any change in size and ZP values.

As Figure 13 shows, there was a slight but significant interaction with mucin. Actually, the components of SNEDDS were not mucoadhesive materials and did not possess a net charge that could interact electrostatically with the negative charges of the protein. An increase in size and absorbance was apparent already after 15 min of contact with mucin and was maintained for the next 3 h. Mucin was absorbed into the lipid micelles, which led to the registered increase in size and, in turn, in turbidity. The increase in particle size was not followed by significant aggregation phenomena since PDI values remained ≤0.4. The turbidity measurement was found to be significant at all time points. However, the formulation maintained its transparency, as absorbance values were found to be ≤0.2, which is suited for ocular administration [57].

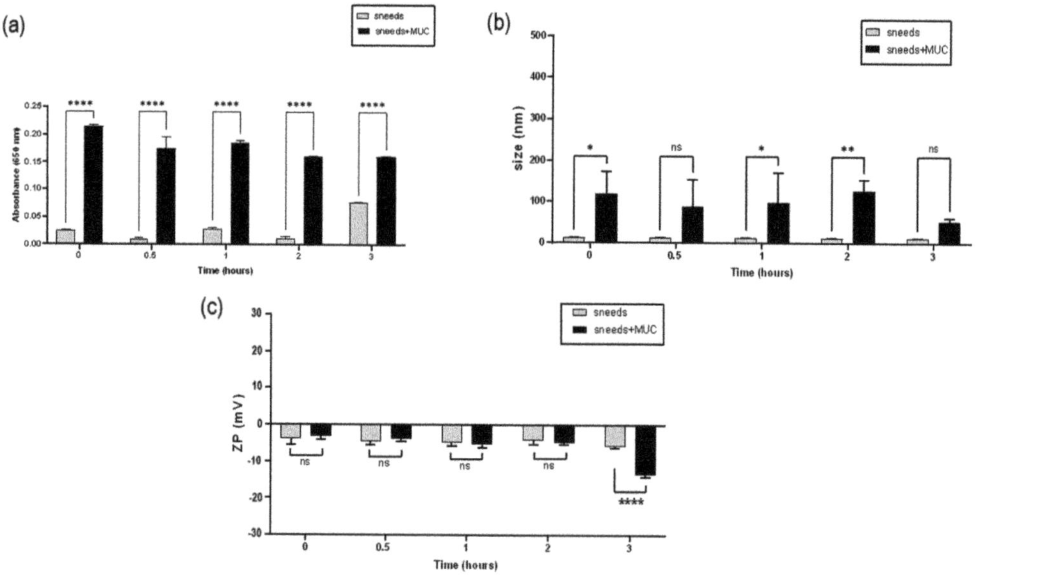

Figure 13. (**a**) Absorbance, (**b**) mean size and (**c**) ZP values of formulation A before (SNEDDS) and after different times of incubation with mucin dispersion in STF at 37 °C (SNEDDS+MUC). * $p < 0.05$, ** $p < 0.01$, **** $p < 0.0001$, ns = not significant.

A stronger interaction could be proven by a change in the ZP value of the colloidal system once in contact with mucin [58]. In this case, it was evident that the interaction was not very strong and occurred noticeably after 3 h of contact. The use of ingredients with mucoadhesive potential or lipid materials with a positive charge could reinforce the interaction with mucin [59,60]. Mucoadhesive properties could improve the residence time of a formulation on the corneal surface. This is important since SNEDDS form very small globules, in the order of about 50 nm, after their dilution with the tear fluid. Such small particles can easily be carried away by the tear flow. By improving the interaction between the formulation and the mucin present on the ocular surface, the residence time can be ameliorated.

3.10. In Vitro Release in Simulated Ocular Environment

The cumulative release rate was calculated according to the released RSV and MEL compared to the total initial drug amounts. It is not simply to evaluate the effective release from a SNEDDS formulation. When SNEDDS comes in contact with the tear fluid, different entities are formed, including the free molecular state of the drug, the drug inside the nanoemulsion droplets, and the drug in the micellar solution [61]. In this case, both drugs seemed to have a good encapsulation within the systems, as suggested by the low release up to 6 h (Figure 14).

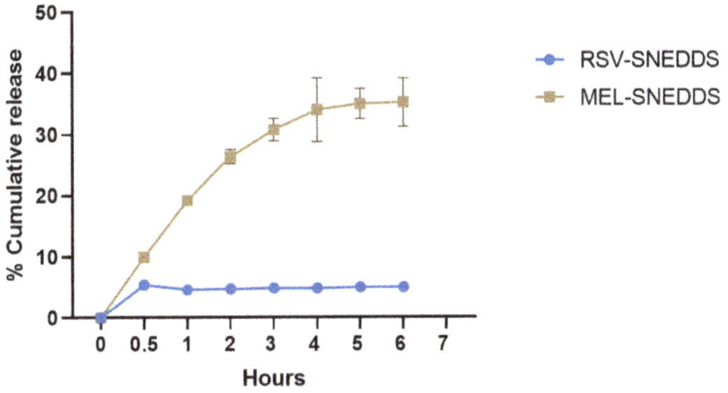

Figure 14. Cumulative release of RSV and MEL from AR and AM, respectively, in simulated ocular environment.

The release test was performed in STF at 35 °C, monitoring the drug release for 6 h. As can be observed, the very lipophilic RSV was retained by the lipid matrix and was released to a maximum of 5% in a constant manner. The outer medium also probably became saturated, giving a very low-release profile. Many studies prefer to use a medium added with a surfactant, e.g., Tween® 80 at 2.5%, to raise the release up to 100% [62].

MEL followed a different pattern, its amphiphilic nature allowing a faster release over time, with a peak at 4 h with 35% of the released drug. The low and constant release of these drugs by SNEDDS formulations could be useful for a prolonged release.

The release rate constant was estimated from the slope of the different curves, and regression values (R^2) were obtained. Table 7 shows that the in vitro MEL release from SNEDDS was best described by both the Higuchi equation ($R^2 = 0.8685$) and the Korsmeyer–Peppas equation ($R^2 = 0.8863$). The former equation indicates that the drug release occurred via diffusion through the dispersed globules in a constant and controlled manner [63]. The second equation showed a diffusional release exponent parameter, indicated with n, which was 0.414. This suggests a quasi-Fickian diffusion profile (when $n < 0.45$) of MEL release [64]. Regarding the in vitro RSV release, this was best described by Korsmeyer–Peppas equation ($R^2 = 0.9736$) with $n = 0.084$, indicating again a quasi-Fickian diffusion profile [64].

Table 7. Regression coefficient values (R^2) for different release kinetic models obtained from the in vitro release profiles of loaded SNEDDS in STF. The calculations were made on the linear part of the release curves (from 0.5 h forward).

Sample	Zero Order	First Order	Higuchi	Hixson–Crowell	Korsmeyer–Peppas
MEL	0.7465	0.6142	0.8685	0.7692	0.8863
RSV	0.0116	0.0072	0.0456	0.0117	0.9736

3.11. Short Time Exposure Test (STE)

The STE test was used to assess the cytotoxicity of the formulated systems. This test, described by Takahashi et al., can be applied when formulations to be tested contain large percentages of surfactant(s). The test was performed on cells of the corneal epithelium, such as SIRCs, for a time of 5 min [23,24]. The evaluation of cytotoxicity was carried out by means of an MTT test. First, an analysis was made on the blank formulation (A) at different dilutions (Figure 15a). The dilution of 1:100 was thus chosen for further studies.

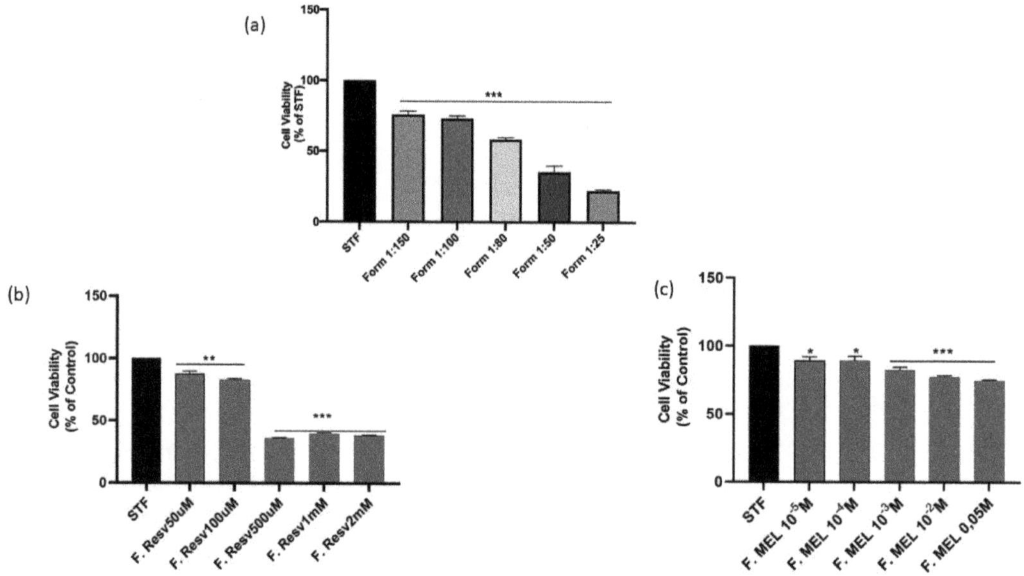

Figure 15. Effect of (**a**) blank formulation treatment on SIRC cell viability; (**b**) Cell viability of SIRC cultured in STF, representing the control group, or treated with different concentrations of AR (50 μM, 100 μM, 500 μM, 1 mM or 2 mM) for 5 min, or (**c**) with different concentrations of AM (10^{-5} M, 10^{-4} M, 10^{-3} M, 10^{-2} M, 0.05 M). * $p < 0.05$, ** $p < 0.01$, *** $p < 0.001$.

As Figure 15 shows, the concentrations tested on a 1:100 SNEDDS/STF dilution were 5 for the formulation with RSV (AR) and 5 for the formulation with MEL (AM). The choice of concentrations ranged from a minimum of the therapeutic drug concentration up to a maximum of 100 times the therapeutic drug concentration. RSV at concentrations of 50 μM and 100 μM was protective in retinal cells exposed to hypertension-derived damage through the regulation of a SIRT-1-related pathway [41]. MEL at a concentration of 10^{-4} M inhibited the activation of Müller cells (support for the retinal pigment epithelium) and the production of pro-inflammatory cytokines in a model of diabetic retinopathy through the upregulation of a SIRT-1 pathway [39,40]. It is well known that less than 5% of the dose reaches the back of the eye, so a concentrated formulation is preferable for better efficacy. All AM concentrations were compatible and non-toxic to SIRCs under the used test conditions. AR was cytotoxic at the highest concentrations, from 500 μM upwards [65,66].

4. Conclusions

The aim of this study was to design systems, using a statistical approach, with technological properties and characteristics suitable for topical ocular administration. The rationale of the study was to design SNEDDS for the delivery of SIRT-1 agonists in ocular degenerative diseases characterized by a downregulation of the enzyme. RSV and MEL were chosen as model drugs, both being well known for their effect in regulating the SIRT-1 pathway in inflammatory states of ocular tissues, in particular of the retina.

Four formulations with four different surfactants (Tween® 80, Tween® 20, Cremophor® EL, and Solutol® HS15) were optimized and characterized in terms of mean size, PDI, ZP, pH, osmolarity, emulsion time, and transmittance (clearness). All these parameters were found to be compatible with a possible ocular administration. The SNEDDS formulations were loaded with RSV and MEL, giving excellent encapsulation results.

The formulation consisting of Capryol® PGMC, Transcutol® P, and Tween® 80 was chosen for its higher physical stability for the subsequent studies. A slight mucoadhesive capacity was found after incubation with mucin in a simulated ocular environment. The formulations of RSV-SNEDDS and MEL-SNEDDS proved to be cytocompatible with cells of the corneal epithelium.

The results of this work demonstrate that the use of a DoE approach can enable the optimization of formulations suitable for ocular administration that must encapsulate highly lipophilic drugs, increasing their apparent solubility in water. Further, in vivo studies are ongoing to evaluate the mechanism of diffusion of drugs towards the posterior eye segment and the pharmacological activity of the loaded nanocarriers.

Supplementary Materials: The following supporting information can be downloaded at https://www.mdpi.com/article/10.3390/pharmaceutics16010125/s1, Supplementary Table S1. Physicochemical properties of melatonin and resveratrol.

Author Contributions: Conceptualization, E.Z. and R.P.; methodology, E.Z., A.B. and A.G.D.; software, A.B.; validation, E.Z., J.R. and R.P.; formal analysis, E.Z., V.D. and A.B.; investigation, E.Z., R.L. and A.G.D.; resources, R.P.; data curation, E.Z.; writing—original draft preparation, E.Z.; writing—review and editing, R.P., A.B., R.L., J.R. and V.D.; supervision, R.P. All authors have read and agreed to the published version of the manuscript.

Funding: This research received no external funding.

Institutional Review Board Statement: Not applicable.

Informed Consent Statement: Not applicable.

Data Availability Statement: Data are contained within the article and supplementary materials.

Acknowledgments: E. Z. was partially supported by the PhD course in Neurosciences at the University of Catania.

Conflicts of Interest: The authors declare no conflicts of interest.

References

1. Zhou, M.; Luo, J.; Zhang, H. Role of Sirtuin 1 in the Pathogenesis of Ocular Disease (Review). *Int. J. Mol. Med.* **2018**, *42*, 13–20. [CrossRef] [PubMed]
2. Wu, Q.-J.; Zhang, T.-N.; Chen, H.-H.; Yu, X.-F.; Lv, J.-L.; Liu, Y.-Y.; Liu, Y.-S.; Zheng, G.; Zhao, J.-Q.; Wei, Y.-F.; et al. The Sirtuin Family in Health and Disease. *Signal Transduct. Target. Ther.* **2022**, *7*, 402. [CrossRef] [PubMed]
3. Yao, Q.; Zhou, Y.; Yang, Y.; Cai, L.; Xu, L.; Han, X.; Guo, Y.; Li, P.A. Activation of Sirtuin1 by Lyceum Barbarum Polysaccharides in Protection against Diabetic Cataract. *J. Ethnopharmacol.* **2020**, *261*, 113165. [CrossRef] [PubMed]
4. Golestaneh, N.; Chu, Y.; Cheng, S.K.; Cao, H.; Poliakov, E.; Berinstein, D.M. Repressed SIRT1/PGC-1α Pathway and Mitochondrial Disintegration in iPSC-Derived RPE Disease Model of Age-Related Macular Degeneration. *J. Transl. Med.* **2016**, *14*, 344. [CrossRef]
5. Yaman, D.; Takmaz, T.; Yüksel, N.; Dinçer, S.A.; Şahin, F.İ. Evaluation of Silent Information Regulator T (SIRT) 1 and Forkhead Box O (FOXO) Transcription Factor 1 and 3a Genes in Glaucoma. *Mol. Biol. Rep.* **2020**, *47*, 9337–9344. [CrossRef]
6. Mimura, T.; Kaji, Y.; Noma, H.; Funatsu, H.; Okamoto, S. The Role of SIRT1 in Ocular Aging. *Exp. Eye Res.* **2013**, *116*, 17–26. [CrossRef]

7. DiNicolantonio, J.J.; McCarty, M.F.; O'Keefe, J.H. Nutraceutical Activation of Sirt1: A Review. *Open Heart* **2022**, *9*, e002171. [CrossRef] [PubMed]
8. Pop, R.; Daescu, A.; Rugina, D.; Pintea, A. Resveratrol: Its Path from Isolation to Therapeutic Action in Eye Diseases. *Antioxidants* **2022**, *11*, 2447. [CrossRef]
9. Huang, Y.; Lu, J.; Zhan, L.; Wang, M.; Shi, R.; Yuan, X.; Gao, X.; Liu, X.; Zang, J.; Liu, W.; et al. Resveratrol-Induced Sirt1 Phosphorylation by LKB1 Mediates Mitochondrial Metabolism. *J. Biol. Chem.* **2021**, *297*, 100929. [CrossRef]
10. Wu, Y.; Pang, Y.; Wei, W.; Shao, A.; Deng, C.; Li, X.; Chang, H.; Hu, P.; Liu, X.; Zhang, X. Resveratrol Protects Retinal Ganglion Cell Axons through Regulation of the SIRT1-JNK Pathway. *Exp. Eye Res.* **2020**, *200*, 108249. [CrossRef]
11. Zhang, H.; He, S.; Spee, C.; Ishikawa, K.; Hinton, D.R. SIRT1 Mediated Inhibition of VEGF/VEGFR2 Signaling by Resveratrol and Its Relevance to Choroidal Neovascularization. *Cytokine* **2015**, *76*, 549–552. [CrossRef] [PubMed]
12. Kumar, J.; Haldar, C.; Verma, R. Melatonin Ameliorates LPS-Induced Testicular Nitro-Oxidative Stress (iNOS/TNFα) and Inflammation (NF-kB/COX-2) via Modulation of SIRT-1. *Reprod. Sci.* **2021**, *28*, 3417–3430. [CrossRef]
13. Pal, S.; Haldar, C.; Verma, R. Melatonin Attenuates LPS-Induced Ovarian Toxicity via Modulation of SIRT-1, PI3K/pAkt, pErk1/2 and NFκB/COX-2 Expressions. *Toxicol. Appl. Pharmacol.* **2022**, *451*, 116173. [CrossRef] [PubMed]
14. Savran, M.; Asci, H.; Ozmen, O.; Erzurumlu, Y.; Savas, H.; Sonmez, Y.; Sahin, Y. Melatonin Protects the Heart and Endothelium against High Fructose Corn Syrup Consumption–Induced Cardiovascular Toxicity via SIRT-1 Signaling. *Hum. Exp. Toxicol.* **2019**, *38*, 1212–1223. [CrossRef] [PubMed]
15. Carloni, S.; Albertini, M.C.; Galluzzi, L.; Buonocore, G.; Proietti, F.; Balduini, W. Melatonin Reduces Endoplasmic Reticulum Stress and Preserves Sirtuin 1 Expression in Neuronal Cells of Newborn Rats after Hypoxia–Ischemia. *J. Pineal Res.* **2014**, *57*, 192–199. [CrossRef]
16. Atacak, A.; Baltaci, S.B.; Akgun-Unal, N.; Mogulkoc, R.; Baltaci, A.K. Melatonin Protects Retinal Tissue Damage in Streptozotocin-Induced Aged Rats. *Arch. Gerontol. Geriatr.* **2023**, *112*, 105035. [CrossRef]
17. Rehman, F.U.; Shah, K.U.; Shah, S.U.; Khan, I.U.; Khan, G.M.; Khan, A. From Nanoemulsions to Self-Nanoemulsions, with Recent Advances in Self-Nanoemulsifying Drug Delivery Systems (SNEDDS). *Expert. Opin. Drug Deliv.* **2017**, *14*, 1325–1340. [CrossRef]
18. Rasoanirina, B.N.V.; Lassoued, M.A.; Miladi, K.; Razafindrakoto, Z.; Chaâbane-Banaoues, R.; Ramanitrahasimbola, D.; Cornet, M.; Sfar, S. Self-Nanoemulsifying Drug Delivery System to Improve Transcorneal Permeability of Voriconazole: In-Vivo Studies. *J. Pharm. Pharmacol.* **2020**, *72*, 889–896. [CrossRef]
19. Singh, G. Resveratrol: Nanocarrier-based delivery systems to enhance its therapeutic potential. *Nanomedicine* **2020**, *15*, 28. [CrossRef]
20. ICH Q1A (R2) Guideline: 'Stability Testing of New Drug Substances and Products'. Available online: https://ich.org/page/quality-guidelines (accessed on 31 December 2023).
21. Singh, G.; Pai, R.S. *Trans*-Resveratrol Self-Nano-Emulsifying Drug Delivery System (SNEDDS) with Enhanced Bioavailability Potential: Optimization, Pharmacokinetics and in Situ Single Pass Intestinal Perfusion (SPIP) Studies. *Drug Deliv.* **2015**, *22*, 522–530. [CrossRef]
22. Lombardo, R.; Ruponen, M.; Rautio, J.; Ghelardini, C.; Di Cesare Mannelli, L.; Calosi, L.; Bani, D.; Lampinen, R.; Kanninen, K.M.; Koivisto, A.M.; et al. Development of Lyophilised Eudragit® Retard Nanoparticles for the Sustained Release of Clozapine via Intranasal Administration. *Pharmaceutics* **2023**, *15*, 1554. [CrossRef]
23. Takahashi, Y.; Koike, M.; Honda, H.; Ito, Y.; Sakaguchi, H.; Suzuki, H.; Nishiyama, N. Development of the Short Time Exposure (STE) Test: An in Vitro Eye Irritation Test Using SIRC Cells. *Toxicol. Vitr.* **2008**, *22*, 760–770. [CrossRef]
24. Takahashi, Y.; Hayashi, K.; Abo, T.; Koike, M.; Sakaguchi, H.; Nishiyama, N. The Short Time Exposure (STE) Test for Predicting Eye Irritation Potential: Intra-Laboratory Reproducibility and Correspondence to Globally Harmonized System (GHS) and EU Eye Irritation Classification for 109 Chemicals. *Toxicol. Vitr.* **2011**, *25*, 1425–1434. [CrossRef]
25. Maugeri, G.; D'Amico, A.G.; Giunta, S.; Giallongo, C.; Tibullo, D.; Bucolo, C.; Saccone, S.; Federico, C.; Scollo, D.; Longo, A.; et al. Activity-Dependent Neuroprotective Protein (ADNP)-Derived Peptide (NAP) Counteracts UV-B Radiation-Induced ROS Formation in Corneal Epithelium. *Antioxidants* **2022**, *11*, 128. [CrossRef] [PubMed]
26. Fallica, A.N.; Sorrenti, V.; D'Amico, A.G.; Salerno, L.; Romeo, G.; Intagliata, S.; Consoli, V.; Floresta, G.; Rescifina, A.; D'Agata, V.; et al. Discovery of Novel Acetamide-Based Heme Oxygenase-1 Inhibitors with Potent In Vitro Antiproliferative Activity. *J. Med. Chem.* **2021**, *64*, 13373–13393. [CrossRef] [PubMed]
27. Borhade, V.; Pathak, S.; Sharma, S.; Patravale, V. Clotrimazole Nanoemulsion for Malaria Chemotherapy. Part I: Preformulation Studies, Formulation Design and Physicochemical Evaluation. *Int. J. Pharm.* **2012**, *431*, 138–148. [CrossRef] [PubMed]
28. Lee, J.-H.; Lee, G.-W. Formulation Approaches for Improving the Dissolution Behavior and Bioavailability of Tolvaptan Using SMEDDS. *Pharmaceutics* **2022**, *14*, 415. [CrossRef]
29. Seo, Y.G.; Kim, D.W.; Yousaf, A.M.; Park, J.H.; Chang, P.-S.; Baek, H.H.; Lim, S.-J.; Kim, J.O.; Yong, C.S.; Choi, H.-G. Solid Self-Nanoemulsifying Drug Delivery System (SNEDDS) for Enhanced Oral Bioavailability of Poorly Water-Soluble Tacrolimus: Physicochemical Characterisation and Pharmacokinetics. *J. Microencapsul.* **2015**, *32*, 503–510. [CrossRef]
30. Ahmed, B.; Rizwanullah, M.; Mir, S.R.; Akhtar, M.S.; Amin, S. Development of Cannabidiol Nanoemulsion for Direct Nose to Brain Delivery: Statistical Optimization, in Vitro and in Vivo Evaluation. *Biomed. Mater.* **2022**, *17*, 065009. [CrossRef]

31. Buya, A.B.; Terrasi, R.; Mbinze, J.K.; Muccioli, G.G.; Beloqui, A.; Memvanga, P.B.; Préat, V. Quality-by-Design-Based Development of a Voxelotor Self-Nanoemulsifying Drug-Delivery System with Improved Biopharmaceutical Attributes. *Pharmaceutics* **2021**, *13*, 1388. [CrossRef]
32. Silva, A.E.; Barratt, G.; Chéron, M.; Egito, E.S.T. Development of Oil-in-Water Microemulsions for the Oral Delivery of Amphotericin B. *Int. J. Pharm.* **2013**, *454*, 641–648. [CrossRef]
33. Shakeel, F.; Haq, N.; Alanazi, F.K.; Alsarra, I.A. Impact of Various Nonionic Surfactants on Self-Nanoemulsification Efficiency of Two Grades of Capryol (Capryol-90 and Capryol-PGMC). *J. Mol. Liq.* **2013**, *182*, 57–63. [CrossRef]
34. Leonardi, A.; Bucolo, C.; Romano, G.L.; Platania, C.B.M.; Drago, F.; Puglisi, G.; Pignatello, R. Influence of Different Surfactants on the Technological Properties and in Vivo Ocular Tolerability of Lipid Nanoparticles. *Int. J. Pharm.* **2014**, *470*, 133–140. [CrossRef]
35. Buya, A.B.; Ucakar, B.; Beloqui, A.; Memvanga, P.B.; Préat, V. Design and Evaluation of Self-Nanoemulsifying Drug Delivery Systems (SNEDDSs) for Senicapoc. *Int. J. Pharm.* **2020**, *580*, 119180. [CrossRef] [PubMed]
36. Sukmawati, A.; Utami, W.; Yuliani, R.; Da'i, M.; Nafarin, A. Effect of Tween 80 on Nanoparticle Preparation of Modified Chitosan for Targeted Delivery of Combination Doxorubicin and Curcumin Analogue. *IOP Conf. Ser. Mater. Sci. Eng.* **2018**, *311*, 012024. [CrossRef]
37. Nasr, A.; Gardouh, A.; Ghonaim, H.; Abdelghany, E.; Ghorab, M. Effect of oils, surfactants and cosurfactants on phase behavior and physicochemical properties of self-nanoemulsifying drug delivery system (SNEDDS) for irbesartan and olmesartan. *Int. J. Appl. Pharm.* **2016**, *8*, 13–24.
38. Bonaccorso, A.; Carbone, C.; Tomasello, B.; Italiani, P.; Musumeci, T.; Puglisi, G.; Pignatello, R. Optimization of Dextran Sulfate/Poly-l-Lysine Based Nanogels Polyelectrolyte Complex for Intranasal Ovalbumin Delivery. *J. Drug Deliv. Sci. Technol.* **2021**, *65*, 102678. [CrossRef]
39. Tu, Y.; Zhu, M.; Wang, Z.; Wang, K.; Chen, L.; Liu, W.; Shi, Q.; Zhao, Q.; Sun, Y.; Wang, X.; et al. Melatonin Inhibits Müller Cell Activation and Pro-inflammatory Cytokine Production via Upregulating the MEG3/miR-204/Sirt1 Axis in Experimental Diabetic Retinopathy. *J. Cell Physiol.* **2020**, *235*, 8724–8735. [CrossRef] [PubMed]
40. Tu, Y.; Song, E.; Wang, Z.; Ji, N.; Zhu, L.; Wang, K.; Sun, H.; Zhang, Y.; Zhu, Q.; Liu, X.; et al. Melatonin Attenuates Oxidative Stress and Inflammation of Müller Cells in Diabetic Retinopathy via Activating the Sirt1 Pathway. *Biomed. Pharmacother.* **2021**, *137*, 111274. [CrossRef]
41. Ishikawa, K.; He, S.; Terasaki, H.; Nazari, H.; Zhang, H.; Spee, C.; Kannan, R.; Hinton, D.R. Resveratrol Inhibits Epithelial-Mesenchymal Transition of Retinal Pigment Epithelium and Development of Proliferative Vitreoretinopathy. *Sci. Rep.* **2015**, *5*, 16386. [CrossRef]
42. Cao, K.; Ishida, T.; Fang, Y.; Shinohara, K.; Li, X.; Nagaoka, N.; Ohno-Matsui, K.; Yoshida, T. Protection of the Retinal Ganglion Cells: Intravitreal Injection of Resveratrol in Mouse Model of Ocular Hypertension. *Invest. Ophthalmol. Vis. Sci.* **2020**, *61*, 13. [CrossRef]
43. Käsdorf, B.T.; Arends, F.; Lieleg, O. Diffusion Regulation in the Vitreous Humor. *Biophys. J.* **2015**, *109*, 2171–2181. [CrossRef]
44. Tavakoli, S.; Peynshaert, K.; Lajunen, T.; Devoldere, J.; Del Amo, E.M.; Ruponen, M.; De Smedt, S.C.; Remaut, K.; Urtti, A. Ocular Barriers to Retinal Delivery of Intravitreal Liposomes: Impact of Vitreoretinal Interface. *J. Control Release* **2020**, *328*, 952–961. [CrossRef] [PubMed]
45. Hanieh, P.N.; Bonaccorso, A.; Zingale, E.; Cimarelli, S.; Souto, E.B.; Rinaldi, F.; Marianecci, C.; Pignatello, R.; Carafa, M. Almond Oil O/W Nanoemulsions: Potential Application for Ocular Delivery. *J. Drug Deliv. Sci. Technol.* **2022**, *72*, 103424. [CrossRef]
46. Zhang, R.; Yang, J.; Luo, Q.; Shi, J.; Xu, H.; Zhang, J. Preparation and in Vitro and in Vivo Evaluation of an Isoliquiritigenin-Loaded Ophthalmic Nanoemulsion for the Treatment of Corneal Neovascularization. *Drug Deliv.* **2022**, *29*, 2217–2233. [CrossRef] [PubMed]
47. Bonaccorso, A.; Gigliobianco, M.R.; Lombardo, R.; Pellitteri, R.; Di Martino, P.; Mancuso, A.; Musumeci, T. Nanonized Carbamazepine for Nose-to-Brain Delivery: Pharmaceutical Formulation Development. *Pharm. Dev. Technol.* **2023**, *28*, 248–263. [CrossRef]
48. Muthu, M.S.; Feng, S.-S. Pharmaceutical stability aspects of nanomedicines. *Nanomedicine* **2009**, *4*, 857–860. [CrossRef] [PubMed]
49. Zupančič, Š.; Lavrič, Z.; Kristl, J. Stability and Solubility of Trans-Resveratrol Are Strongly Influenced by pH and Temperature. *Eur. J. Pharm. Biopharm.* **2015**, *93*, 196–204. [CrossRef]
50. Sessa, M.; Tsao, R.; Liu, R.; Ferrari, G.; Donsì, F. Evaluation of the Stability and Antioxidant Activity of Nanoencapsulated Resveratrol during in Vitro Digestion. *J. Agric. Food Chem.* **2011**, *59*, 12352–12360. [CrossRef]
51. Ferreyra, S.; Bottini, R.; Fontana, A. Temperature and Light Conditions Affect Stability of Phenolic Compounds of Stored Grape Cane Extracts. *Food Chem.* **2023**, *405*, 134718. [CrossRef] [PubMed]
52. Das, S.; Lee, S.H.; Chow, P.S.; Macbeath, C. Microemulsion Composed of Combination of Skin Beneficial Oils as Vehicle: Development of Resveratrol-Loaded Microemulsion Based Formulations for Skin Care Applications. *Colloids Surf. B Biointerfaces* **2020**, *194*, 111161. [CrossRef]
53. Agustin-Salazar, S.; Gamez-Meza, N.; Medina-Juàrez, L.À.; Soto-Valdez, H.; Cerruti, P. From Nutraceutics to Materials: Effect of Resveratrol on the Stability of Polylactide. *ACS Sustain. Chem. Eng.* **2014**, *2*, 1534–1542. [CrossRef]
54. Bancuta, O.R.; Chilian, A.; Bancuta, I.; Setnescu, R.; Setnescu, T.; Ion, R.M. Thermal Characterization of Resveratrol. *Rev. Chim.* **2018**, *69*, 1346–1351. [CrossRef]

55. Lin, Y.C.; Hu, S.C.S.; Huang, P.H.; Lin, T.C.; Yen, F.L. Electrospun resveratrol-loaded polyvinylpyrrolidone/cyclodextrin nanofibers and their biomedical applications. *Pharmaceutics* **2020**, *12*, 552. [CrossRef] [PubMed]
56. Topal, B.; Altındal, D.Ç.; Gümüşderelioğlu, M. Melatonin/HPβCD complex: Microwave synthesis, integration with chitosan scaffolds and inhibitory effects on MG-63CELLS. *Int. J. Pharm.* **2015**, *496*, 801–811. [CrossRef] [PubMed]
57. Akhtar, M.S.; Mandal, S.K.; Malik, A.; Choudhary, A.; Agarwal, S.; Sarkar, S.; Dey, S. Nano micelle: Novel Approach for Targeted Ocular Drug Delivery System. *Egypt. J. Chem.* **2022**, *65*, 337–355. [CrossRef]
58. Corsaro, R.; Lombardo, R.; Ghelardini, C.; Di Cesare Mannelli, L.; Bani, D.; Bonaccorso, A.; Pignatello, R. Development of Eudragit® Nanoparticles for Intranasal Drug Delivery: Preliminary Technological and Toxicological Evaluation. *Appl. Sci.* **2022**, *12*, 2373. [CrossRef]
59. Bonaccorso, A.; Pepe, V.; Zappulla, C.; Cimino, C.; Pricoco, A.; Puglisi, G.; Giuliano, F.; Pignatello, R.; Carbone, C. Sorafenib Repurposing for Ophthalmic Delivery by Lipid Nanoparticles: A Preliminary Study. *Pharmaceutics* **2021**, *13*, 1956. [CrossRef]
60. Cimino, C.; Leotta, C.G.; Marrazzo, A.; Musumeci, T.; Pitari, G.M.; Pignatello, R.; Bonaccorso, A.; Amata, E.; Barbaraci, C.; Carbone, C. Nanostructured Lipid Carrier for the Ophthalmic Delivery of Haloperidol Metabolite II Valproate Ester (±)-MRJF22: A Potential Strategy in the Treatment of Uveal Melanoma. *J. Drug Deliv. Sci. Technol.* **2023**, *87*, 104811. [CrossRef]
61. Vikash, B.; Shashi; Pandey, N.K.; Kumar, B.; Wadhwa, S.; Goutam, U.; Alam, A.; Al-Otaibi, F.; Chaubey, P.; Mustafa, G.; et al. Formulation and Evaluation of Ocular Self-Nanoemulsifying Drug Delivery System of Brimonidine Tartrate. *J. Drug Deliv. Sci. Technol.* **2023**, *81*, 104226. [CrossRef]
62. Gu, H.; Chen, P.; Liu, X.; Lian, Y.; Xi, J.; Li, J.; Song, J.; Li, X. Trimethylated Chitosan-Coated Flexible Liposomes with Resveratrol for Topical Drug Delivery to Reduce Blue-Light-Induced Retinal Damage. *Int. J. Biol. Macromol.* **2023**, *252*, 126480. [CrossRef]
63. Paul, D.R. Elaborations on the Higuchi Model for Drug Delivery. *Int. J. Pharm.* **2011**, *418*, 13–17. [CrossRef] [PubMed]
64. Ekenna, I.C.; Abali, S.O. Comparison of the Use of Kinetic Model Plots and DD Solver Software to Evaluate the Drug Release from Griseofulvin Tablets. *J. Drug Deliv. Ther.* **2022**, *12*, 5–13. [CrossRef]
65. Rüweler, M.; Gülden, M.; Maser, E.; Murias, M.; Seibert, H. Cytotoxic, Cytoprotective and Antioxidant Activities of Resveratrol and Analogues in C6 Astroglioma Cells in Vitro. *Chem. Biol. Interact.* **2009**, *182*, 128–135. [CrossRef]
66. Soo, E.; Thakur, S.; Qu, Z.; Jambhrunkar, S.; Parekh, H.S.; Popat, A. Enhancing Delivery and Cytotoxicity of Resveratrol through a Dual Nanoencapsulation Approach. *J. Colloid. Interface Sci.* **2016**, *462*, 368–374. [CrossRef]

pharmaceutics

Article

Fabrication and Characterization of an Enzyme-Triggered, Therapeutic-Releasing Hydrogel Bandage Contact Lens Material

Susmita Bose [1], Chau-Minh Phan [1,2,*], Muhammad Rizwan [3], John Waylon Tse [3], Evelyn Yim [3] and Lyndon Jones [1,2]

1 Centre for Ocular Research & Education (CORE), School of Optometry and Vision Science, University of Waterloo, 200 University Avenue West, Waterloo, ON N2L 3G1, Canada; s3bose@uwaterloo.ca (S.B.); lyndon.jones@uwaterloo.ca (L.J.)
2 Centre for Eye and Vision Research (CEVR), 17W Hong Kong Science Park, Hong Kong, China
3 Chemical Engineering, University of Waterloo, 200 University Avenue West, Waterloo, ON N2L 3G1, Canada; muh.rizwan@utoronto.ca (M.R.); tse.jwt@gmail.com (J.W.T.); eyim@uwaterloo.ca (E.Y.)
* Correspondence: c2phan@uwaterloo.ca; Tel.: +1-519-8884567 (ext. 36547)

Abstract: Purpose: The purpose of this study was to develop an enzyme-triggered, therapeutic-releasing bandage contact lens material using a unique gelatin methacrylate formulation (GelMA+). Methods: Two GelMA+ formulations, 20% *w/v*, and 30% *w/v* concentrations, were prepared through UV polymerization. The physical properties of the material, including porosity, tensile strain, and swelling ratio, were characterized. The enzymatic degradation of the material was assessed in the presence of matrix metalloproteinase-9 (MMP-9) at concentrations ranging from 0 to 300 μg/mL. Cell viability, cell growth, and cytotoxicity on the GelMA+ gels were evaluated using the AlamarBlue™ assay and the LIVE/DEAD™ Viability/Cytotoxicity kit staining with immortalized human corneal epithelial cells over 5 days. For drug release analysis, the 30% *w/v* gels were loaded with 3 μg of bovine lactoferrin (BLF) as a model drug, and its release was examined over 5 days under various MMP-9 concentrations. Results: The 30% *w/v* GelMA+ demonstrated higher crosslinking density, increased tensile strength, smaller pore size, and lower swelling ratio ($p < 0.05$). In contrast, the 20% *w/v* GelMA+ degraded at a significantly faster rate ($p < 0.001$), reaching almost complete degradation within 48 h in the presence of 300 μg/mL of MMP-9. No signs of cytotoxic effects were observed in the live/dead staining assay for either concentration after 5 days. However, the 30% *w/v* GelMA+ exhibited significantly higher cell viability ($p < 0.05$). The 30% *w/v* GelMA+ demonstrated sustained release of the BLF over 5 days. The release rate of BLF increased significantly with higher concentrations of MMP-9 ($p < 0.001$), corresponding to the degradation rate of the gels. Discussion: The release of BLF from GelMA+ gels was driven by a combination of diffusion and degradation of the material by MMP-9 enzymes. This work demonstrated that a GelMA+-based material that releases a therapeutic agent can be triggered by enzymes found in the tear fluid.

Keywords: bandage contact lens; corneal wounding; gelatin methacrylate; GelMA+; MMP-9

Citation: Bose, S.; Phan, C.-M.; Rizwan, M.; Tse, J.W.; Yim, E.; Jones, L. Fabrication and Characterization of an Enzyme-Triggered, Therapeutic-Releasing Hydrogel Bandage Contact Lens Material. *Pharmaceutics* **2024**, *16*, 26. https://doi.org/10.3390/pharmaceutics16010026

Academic Editors: Rosario Pignatello, Hugo Almeida, Debora Santonocito and Carmelo Puglia

Received: 5 December 2023
Revised: 19 December 2023
Accepted: 21 December 2023
Published: 24 December 2023

1. Introduction

Corneal injury and subsequent damage to the corneal epithelium can lead to corneal scarring, vision loss, and potentially blindness. An estimated 1.5 to 2.0 million cases of monocular blindness are caused by ocular trauma and corneal ulceration annually [1]. Historically, the standard treatment for a corneal abrasion is the insertion of a lubricant onto the ocular surface, followed by patching the eye to prevent blinking, permitting the epithelium to heal under the patch. However, the use of an eye patch leads to frustration for the patient due to the loss of binocular vision. Furthermore, if the eye patch is not worn appropriately, then it can lead to delays in epithelial recovery, and it is also cumbersome for clinicians to assess the wound healing progress as this requires the removal of the patch [2,3]. Since the advent of more oxygen-transmissible silicone hydrogel materials in the late 1990's, the standard of care for managing a corneal abrasion has switched to the use of bandage contact lenses (BCLs), in which a soft lens is typically worn for 7–10 days without removal [4–7].

The use of BCLs overcomes the aforementioned problems by allowing the patient to retain binocular vision while undergoing treatment, and clinicians can easily track the wound healing progression without having to remove the lens, as they can view the eye through the transparent lens material [2,3,8–10]. Unfortunately, current BCLs alone do not outperform ocular lubricants in terms of efficacy or speed of recovery, as they lack the ocular surface factors or therapeutics that are essential to aid ocular surface repair. Therefore, it would be beneficial if BCLs could also deliver topical therapeutic agents concurrently to the surface of the eye while in situ [11]. A soft BCL consists of hydrophilic polymers that can absorb large volumes of fluid [12,13]. As a result, these materials can also absorb and release soluble compounds, such as drugs, from their gel matrix [14]. However, previous studies have shown that commercial contact lens materials are unable to maintain sustained drug release, and the vast majority of adsorbed drugs are released within the first few hours of exposure to the eye, thus not providing a desirable release profile [15–19]. Modifications to current materials are needed to improve the release kinetics of currently available BCLs.

Among the various types of hydrogels available, gelatin is one of the most common polymers used in biomedical applications [20]. It is an amphoteric protein [20,21]. derived from the hydrolysis of collagen [22], a naturally occurring polymer in the human cornea [23]. It is a water-soluble, non-cytotoxic polymer with low immunogenicity, and is biodegradable and highly biocompatible [24–26]. Additionally, it contains many bioactive sequences, such as arginine-glycine-aspartic acid, which can facilitate cell attachment and adhesion [20,27,28], making it an ideal material for developing devices used in corneal wound healing [27]. Not surprisingly, gelatin-based hydrogels have been widely used in drug delivery and tissue engineering applications [29–31]. However, unmodified gelatin is relatively weak mechanically, making it a poor material for use as a BCL. These mechanical disadvantages of gelatin-based hydrogels can be overcome by chemical modifications or by integrating them with other monomers or polymers [20,32,33]. Gelatin methacrylate (GelMA), a derivative of porcine-derived gelatin, is produced by substituting the free amine groups of gelatin with methacrylate anhydride [20]. This polymer can be photo-crosslinked with a photoinitiator to produce a stronger permanent gel on exposure to ultraviolet (UV) radiation [20].

A previous publication showed that GelMA can be converted to GelMA+ by forming a gel at 4 °C before the UV crosslinking step [34]. The resulting gel has eight times higher mechanical strength than that of conventional GelMA [34]. The gelation step leads to the construction of triple helix and physical networks, which enhances the crosslinking density and produces a more homogenous microstructure [34].

An important feature of GelMA and its derivatives is the presence of matrix metalloproteinase-sensitive sites, which allows the gel to be biodegraded by matrix metalloproteinase (MMP) enzymes [35–37]. Several in vitro studies have shown that GelMA can be degraded in the presence of MMPs [36,37]. Of note with respect to the use of GelMA in the ocular environment is that elevated levels of MMP enzymes are observed following a corneal wound, in particular MMP-2 (72 kDa type IV collagenase) and MMP-9 (92 kDa type IV collagenase) [38–41]. Therefore, it would be possible to use GelMA as a primary polymer in an enzyme-triggered drug delivery system in which the release trigger is exposure to an MMP enzyme. The GelMA can be used to entrap drugs, drug nanoparticles, or therapeutics, which are then released when the gel is degraded by the MMPs present at the wound site. This study aimed to evaluate the release of a wound-healing therapeutic, bovine lactoferrin (BLF), from GelMA+ materials in the presence of MMP-9.

2. Materials and Methods

2.1. Materials

Gelatin Type A, BLF (80 kDa), methacrylic anhydride, and Irgacure 2959 were obtained from Sigma–Aldrich (St. Louis, MO, USA). MMP-9 was obtained from Gibco Thermo Fisher Scientific (Grand Island, NY, USA). The BLF ELISA kit was obtained from Bethyl Laboratories Inc. (Montgomery, TX, USA). The Spectrum™ Spectra/Por™ 4 RC Dialysis Membrane Tubing 12,000 to 14,000 Dalton MWCO was purchased from Fisher Scientific (Carlsbad, CA, USA). The EpiGRO™ Human Ocular Epithelia Complete Media kit was obtained from Millipore Sigma (Burlington, MA, USA). The LIVE/DEAD™ Viability/Cytotoxicity Kit for mammalian cells and the AlamarBlue™ Cell Viability Reagent were purchased from Invitrogen™ by Thermo Fisher Scientific (Eugene, OR, USA).

2.2. Gelatin Methacrylate Synthesis

The method for the synthesis of GelMA+ has been previously described [34]. In brief, 5 g of gelatin (type A) was dissolved in 50 mL of phosphate-buffered saline 1× (PBS) (10% *w*/*v*) with continuous magnetic stirring at 50–60 °C until the gelatin dissolved. 10 mL of methacrylic anhydride (20% *v*/*v*) was then added dropwise at 50–60 °C with continuous magnetic stirring and the reaction continued for 1 h. The resulting mixture was diluted with PBS and dialyzed in deionized (DI) water for 5 days at 40 °C using 12–14 kDa cut-off dialysis membrane tubes. The GelMA solution was then frozen at −80 °C and lyophilized.

2.3. Preparation of GelMA+ Hydrogels and BLF-Loaded GelMA+ Hydrogels

Lyophilized GelMA was mixed in a 1× PBS solution containing the photo-initiator 0.5% *w*/*v* Irgacure 2959 to obtain mixtures with 20% and 30% *w*/*v* of GelMA. The mixture was incubated at 60 °C for 48 h and centrifuged for 10 min at 5000 rpm. The mixtures were further incubated for 30 min at 60 °C before being carefully pipetted into an acrylic mould to create circular disks (thickness~0.65 mm, diameter~6 mm). The samples were then incubated at 4 °C for 1 h, before being exposed to UV radiation (360–420 nm) at an intensity of 32 mW/cm^2 and polymerized in a Dymax ultraviolet curing chamber (Torrington, CT, USA) for 5 min to create GelMA+ gels. For the BLF-loaded GelMA+ hydrogels, 60 µL of 50 µg/mL of BLF was added to the mixture after the 48 h incubation period at 60 °C, then centrifuged for 10 min at 5000 rpm. Afterwards, the same procedure for the preparation of the GelMA+ hydrogel was followed (see Figure 1).

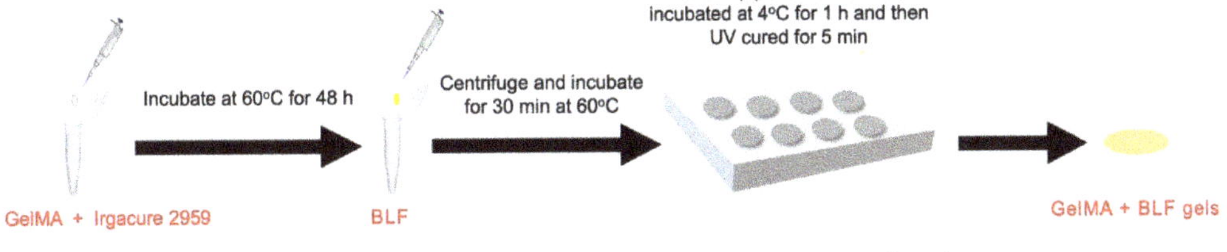

Figure 1. Preparation schematic for BLF-loaded GelMa+ hydrogels.

2.4. Physical Characterization

2.4.1. Scanning Electron Microscopy

The pore size and surface morphology of the various gels were observed using an environmental scanning electron microscope (ESEM-FEI QUANTA™ 250) manufactured by Field Electron and Ion Company (Hillsboro, OR, USA). The gels were kept in 1× PBS at room temperature (22–24 °C) to ensure complete swelling and to enable a clear picture of the morphology of the GelMA+ gels. The samples were observed under an accelerating voltage of 20 kV, in a low vacuum mode with a chamber pressure of 0.8 mbar. The electron beam energy was 20 keV. The sample surface was imaged with two detectors simultaneously: a large field detector to detect secondary electrons, which is more morphology sensitive, and a backscattering electron detector to detect backscattered electrons, which is more concentration sensitive.

2.4.2. Enzymatic Degradation of the GelMA+ Hydrogels

The degradation of the 20% w/v and 30% w/v GelMA+ hydrogels was studied in the presence of varying concentrations of MMP-9. The MMP-9 concentrations were 0, 10, 50, 100, 300 (µg/mL). The circular disk-shaped GelMA+ samples were weighed to determine their initial weight (W_0) and then placed in 2 mL of varying MMP-9 concentration solutions in a 24-well plate at 37 °C. The GelMA+ gels were then reweighed at predetermined time intervals (0 h, 4 h, 8 h, 12 h, 24 h, 48 h, 96 h, 144 h) to determine weight changes over time (W_t). Before weighing, the gels were gently blotted using lens paper to remove any excess moisture. The MMP-9 solutions were replaced every day to maintain enzymatic activity. The percentage degradation was calculated using Equation (1).

$$\text{Percent Degradation} = \frac{W_0 - W_t}{W_0} \times 100\% \qquad (1)$$

2.4.3. Swelling Percentage and Water Content of the GelMA+ Hydrogels

To determine their swelling properties, the GelMA+ samples were incubated in 2 mL of PBS at 37 °C for 24 h. After 24 h, the samples were blotted dry using lens paper and weighed (W_s). The same samples were then freeze-dried and weighed (W_d). The percent swelling was calculated using Equation (2). The water content of the gels was measured similarly. Water content was calculated using Equation (3).

$$\text{Percent Swelling} = \frac{W_s - W_d}{W_d} \times 100\% \qquad (2)$$

$$\text{Water Content} = \frac{W_s - W_d}{W_s} \times 100\% \qquad (3)$$

2.4.4. Mechanical Properties of the GelMA+ Hydrogels

The stiffness of the GelMA+ hydrogels was assessed using a Mandel–Shimadzu (AGS-X) tensile testing unit (Shimadzu Corp., Kyoto, Japan) at room temperature (22 °C to 24 °C). The GelMA+ samples were moulded in a rectangular shape of 7 cm by 1 cm by 0.7 cm (length × width × thickness) and then soaked in PBS for 24 h at room temperature. The samples were clamped with two steel clamps 5 mm apart, with Kim wipe tissues used to hold the edges of the gels to prevent the gels from breaking at the edge of the clamp and to prevent slippage. The rectangular-shaped gels were stretched at a rate of 1 mm/min to the breaking point with a load of 500 N. Young's modulus was calculated from the slope of the linear region of the stress-strain curve.

2.4.5. Optical Transmittance of the GelMA+ Hydrogels

The optical transmittance of gels with and without BLF was measured via a UV spectrophotometer (Biotek Citation 5; Winooski, VT, USA). The gels were placed in PBS in a 48-well plate and the measurements were performed through a wavelength range of 450–700 nm.

2.4.6. In Vitro Release of Bovine Lactoferrin (BLF)

The in vitro release of BLF from 30% w/v GelMA+ gels was undertaken in the presence of varying concentrations of MMP-9 (0; 100; 300 µg/mL) at 37 °C. The samples were washed in 2 mL of PBS for 1 h to remove any loosely bound BLF. At t = 0, 1, 12, 24, 48, 72, 96, and 120 h, the samples were analyzed using the BLF ELISA kit. In brief, 100 µL of the test sample and the standard were added to the 96-well ELISA plate. HRP (streptavidin-conjugated horseradish peroxidase) and TMB (3,3′,5,5′-tetramethylbenzidine) reagents from the kit were added to each well to produce a colorimetric reaction. The change in yellow colour, proportional to the lactoferrin present in the sample, was measured at 450 nm absorbance using a UV spectrophotometer (BioTek Cytation 5; Winooski, VT, USA).

2.5. Biological Characterizations

2.5.1. Cell Culture

The human papilloma virus (HPV) immortalized human corneal epithelial (HCEC) cell line was obtained as frozen from the Centre for Ocular Research & Education (CORE), School of Optometry and Vision Science at the University of Waterloo. The cells were cultured in tissue culture treated Corning® cell culture flasks (Millipore Sigma, MA, USA) with a canted neck plug seal cap and a surface area of 25 cm^2. The nutrient media consisted of EpiGRO™ Human Ocular Epithelia Complete Media along with supplements of L-Glutamine, Epifactor O, Epifactor P, Epinephrine, rh Insulin, Apo transferrin, and Hydrocortisone hemisuccinate (Millipore Sigma, MA, USA). The cells were seeded at a ratio of 1:2 and grown in an incubator at 37 °C and 5% carbon dioxide.

2.5.2. Cell Culture in the Presence of GelMA+ Hydrogels

Once the HCEC cells reached 90% confluency, they were seeded on 48-well VWR Tissue Culture (VWR International, Radnor, PA, USA) treated plates at a cell density of 5×10^4 cells/cm^2. The cells were grown in the nutrient media, as described above. Freshly prepared and sterile (UV sterilized) GelMA+ hydrogels of both the 20% *w/v* and 30% *w/v* formulations were placed carefully onto the cells in each well and incubated at 37 °C and 5% carbon dioxide. The disc-shaped gels were washed with sterile PBS for 4 min inside the cell culture hood prior to exposure to the cells. The gels were washed four times in 5 mL of fresh sterile PBS for 1 min each time to ensure that any unreacted photo crosslinker was removed. On the 5th day, the cell growth on the hydrogels was evaluated.

2.5.3. Cell Mortality Assay

The AlamarBlue™ cell viability assay (Thermo Fischer Scientific, Eugene, OR, USA) was conducted after 1, 5, and 7 days of incubation of the GelMA+ hydrogels with the immortalized HCEC cells. Freshly prepared and sterile (UV sterilized) GelMA+ hydrogels of both the 20% *w/v* and 30% *w/v* formulations were placed carefully onto the cells in each well and incubated at 37 °C and 5% carbon dioxide. The disc-shaped gels were washed with sterile PBS for 4 min inside the cell culture hood prior to exposure to the cells. The gels were washed four times in 5 mL of fresh sterile PBS for 1 min each time to remove any unreacted photocrosslinker. At each time point, the cell culture media was removed and then 0.5 mL of 10% *v/v* of the AlamarBlue™ cell viability reagent prepared with serum-free DMEM/F12 media was added to each well. The resulting solution was then incubated at 37 °C and 5% carbon dioxide for 4 h. 100 µL of the solution from each well was transferred to a new 96-well plate. The fluorescence was measured (excitation 540 nm, emission 590 nm) using the BioTek Citation 5 (BioTek, Winooski, VT, USA).

2.5.4. Live/Dead Assay

The cells were cultured and incubated in the presence of the GelMA+ hydrogels as previously described for 5 days. The media was changed on alternate days. Freshly prepared and UV-sterilized GelMA+ hydrogels were placed carefully onto the cells in each well and incubated at 37 °C and 5% carbon dioxide. Before placement onto the cells, the disc-shaped gels were washed to remove any unreacted photocrosslinker as described. The LIVE/DEAD™ Viability/Cytotoxicity kit (Thermo Fischer Scientific, Eugene, OR, USA) was used to stain the cells and the procedure was performed as described by the manufacturer. 20 µL of 2 mM of EthD-1 was added to 10 mL of sterile PBS, resulting in a 4 µM EthD-1 solution. 5 µL of 4 mM calcein AM stock solution to the 10 mL EthD1 solution. The solution was vortexed to ensure thorough mixing. The growth media was withdrawn from the wells of the 48-well plate containing the cells and the resulting approximately 2 µM Calcein AM and 4 µM EthD-1 solution was then added directly to cells containing the GelMA+ gels. The cells were incubated with dye at room temperature (22–24 °C) for 20–30 min. Images were obtained with Citation 5 (BioTek, Winooski, VT, USA) via fluorescence microscopy on the 5th day.

2.5.5. Statistical Analysis

Statistical analysis and graphs were plotted using GraphPad Prism 6 software (GraphPad, La Jolla, CA, USA). An analysis of variance (ANOVA) and a post-hoc Tukey's test were performed when necessary to determine the statistical significance between different conditions. A p-value of <0.05 was considered significant.

3. Results

3.1. Physical Characterization

3.1.1. Scanning Electron Microscopy Images

Figure 2 demonstrates the surface morphology and pore size of the GelMA+ hydrogels at concentrations of 20% *w/v* and 30% *w/v* via SEM. The images provide a visual representation of the internal porous structure of both GelMA+ formulations. In Figure 2A, the morphology of the pre-polymerized GelMA exhibits a highly porous surface, with estimated pore sizes ranging from 150 μm to 300 μm. Figure 2B,C exhibit the internal porous structures of the 20% and 30% *w/v* GelMA+ hydrogels, respectively. The surface of the 20% *w/v* GelMA+ exhibits a porous texture, characterized by pore sizes ranging from 30 μm to 90 μm. In contrast, the 30% *w/v* GelMA+ surface is more compact, with pore sizes measuring between 0.078 μm and 0.8 μm.

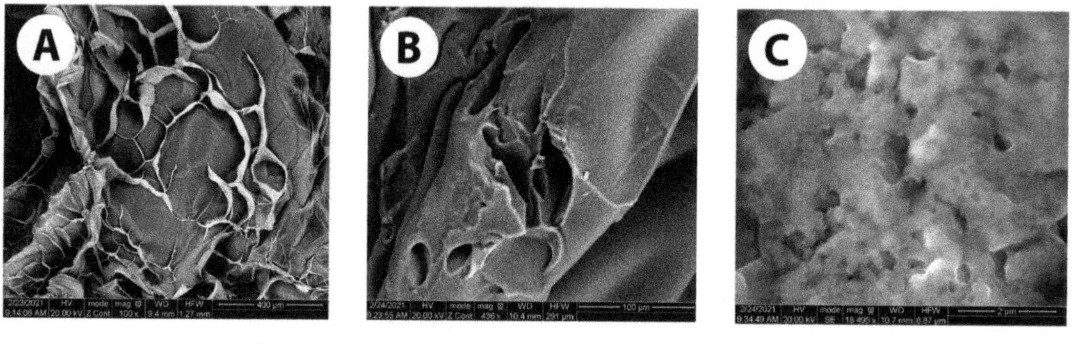

Figure 2. SEM images of (**A**) pre-polymerised GelMA (**B**) 20% *w/v* GelMA+ hydrogel and (**C**) 30% *w/v* GelMA+ hydrogel.

3.1.2. Enzymatic Degradation of GelMA+ Hydrogel

Figure 3 shows the degradation of the GelMA hydrogels in MMP-9 over 144 h (6 days). Figure 3A,B shows the degradation profile of GelMA+ in the presence of different MMP-9 concentration solutions. For both formulations of GelMA+ gels, the degradation rate increased with increasing concentrations of MMP-9 ($p < 0.0001$). The 20% *w/v* GelMA+ gels degraded faster than the 30% *w/v* GelMA+ gels ($p < 0.001$). On the second day (48 h), the circular-shaped 20% *w/v* GelMA+ gels completely degraded in the presence of 300 μg/mL of MMP-9 without any gel remnants. In contrast, the 30% *w/v* GelMA+ gels took almost 144 h to degrade approximately 95% of their original weight, leaving behind only a thin piece of the original gel.

3.1.3. Swelling Profile and Water Content of GelMA+ Hydrogel

Table 1 shows the swelling ratio and the water content of 20% *w/v* and 30% *w/v* GelMA+ hydrogels ($n = 4$). Both formulations of GelMA+ substantially were swelled over 24 h in the presence of PBS to ensure that an equilibrium was achieved. After 24 h, it was observed that the 20% *w/v* GelMA+ gels swelled more ($p < 0.05$) than the 30% *w/v* GelMA+.

The water content of 20% *w*/*v* GelMA+ gels was significantly higher as compared to 30% *w*/*v* GelMA+ gels ($p < 0.05$).

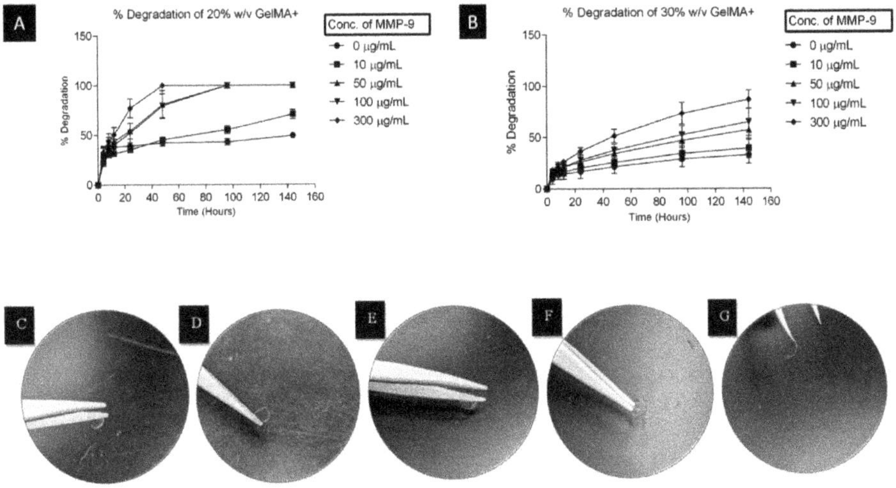

Figure 3. Degradation profile of (**A**) 20% *w*/*v* GelMA+ hydrogel in varying MMP-9 concentrations, (**B**) 30% *w*/*v* GelMA+ hydrogel in varying MMP-9 concentrations, (**C**) the shape of 20% *w*/*v* GelMA+ hydrogel in PBS after 48 h, (**D**) the shape of 20% *w*/*v* GelMA+ hydrogel in 100 µg/mL of MMP-9 after 48 h, (**E**) the shape of 30% *w*/*v* GelMA+ hydrogel in PBS after 144 h, (**F**) the shape of 30% *w*/*v* GelMA+ hydrogel in 100 µg/mL of MMP-9 after 144 h, (**G**) the shape of 30% *w*/*v* GelMA+ hydrogel in 300 µg/mL of MMP-9 after 144 h. The degradation was conducted at 37 °C.

Table 1. Percent swelling, water content, tensile strain, and Young's modulus of both GelMA+ formulations.

Formulation	20% GelMA+	30% GelMA+
% Swelling	303.69 ± 6.95	234.68 ± 8.98
Water content (%)	74.85 ± 0.67	70.85 ± 1.81
Tensile strain (kPa)	133.06 ± 8.98	181.85 ± 25.25
Young modulus (MPa)	2.04 ± 0.16	2.80 ± 0.74

3.1.4. Tensile Test

Table 1 shows the influence of the increasing GelMA+ concentration on the tensile strain and Young's Modulus ($n = 3$). The higher GelMA+ concentration increased the tensile strain values ($p < 0.05$). The 20% *w*/*v* GelMA+ gels were softer with a Young's modulus value of 2.04 MPa. The 30% *w*/*v* GelMA+ gels were stiffer with Young's modulus value of 2.80 MPa with reduced elongation at breakpoints.

3.1.5. Optical Transmittance

The optical clarity ($n = 5$) of both the blank 20% *w*/*v* GelMA+ and 30% *w*/*v* GelMA+ gels and BLF-loaded GelMA+ gels (Figure 4) were measured between 450–700 nm using the Citation 5UV spectrophotometer. The transmittances of the 30% *w*/*v* GelMA+ decreased significantly ($p < 0.0001$) as opposed to 20% *w*/*v* GelMA+. The blank 20% *w*/*v* GelMA+ gels exhibited approximately 90% transmittance at 450 nm. At 630 nm, the transmittance of 20% *w*/*v* GelMA+ was 95.59 ± 1.80%. At 450 nm, the blank 30% *w*/*v* GelMA+ gels exhibited 86.07 ± 3.88% transmittance, and at 630 nm, the transmittance was 92.69 ± 2.96%. The 20% *w*/*v* GelMA+ gels loaded with BLF exhibited 83.61 ± 3.47% transmittance at 450 nm. At 630 nm, the transmittance of the same gel was 90.82 ± 3.06%. At 450 nm, the

BLF-loaded 30% w/v GelMA+ gels exhibited 78.15 ± 2.64% transmittance, and at 630 nm, the transmittance was 89.49 ± 1.29%.

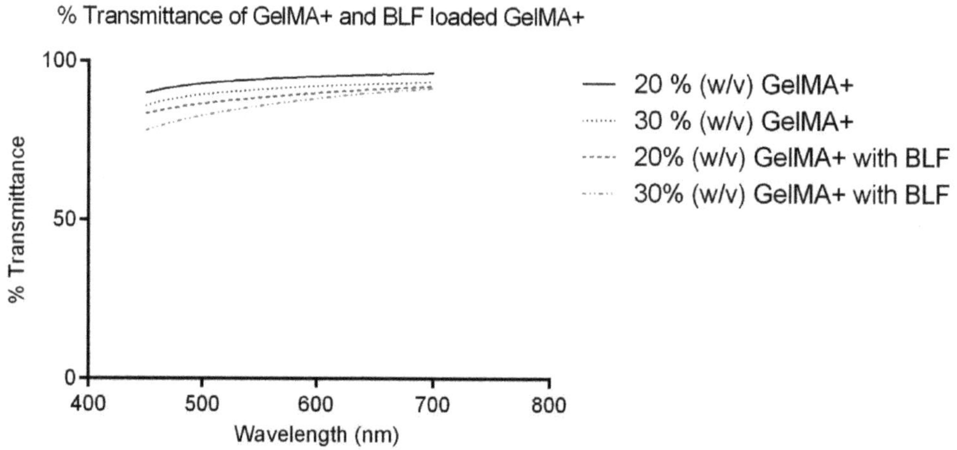

Figure 4. Optical transmittance of GelMA+ gels and BLF-loaded GelMA+ gels measured at a wavelength range of 450 nm to 700 nm.

3.1.6. In Vitro Release of Bovine Lactoferrin

The cumulative percent in vitro release kinetics of the BLF ($n = 4$) is shown in Figure 5. The release of BLF from the 30% w/v GelMA+ hydrogel matrix significantly increased with increasing concentration of MMP-9 ($p < 0.0001$). The amount of BLF released increased over time for all MMP-9 concentrations ($p < 0.0001$). Due to the initial washing of the gels for an hour, there was no burst release observed. The results show that the release of BLF from the gels was primarily driven by the enzyme present in the solution.

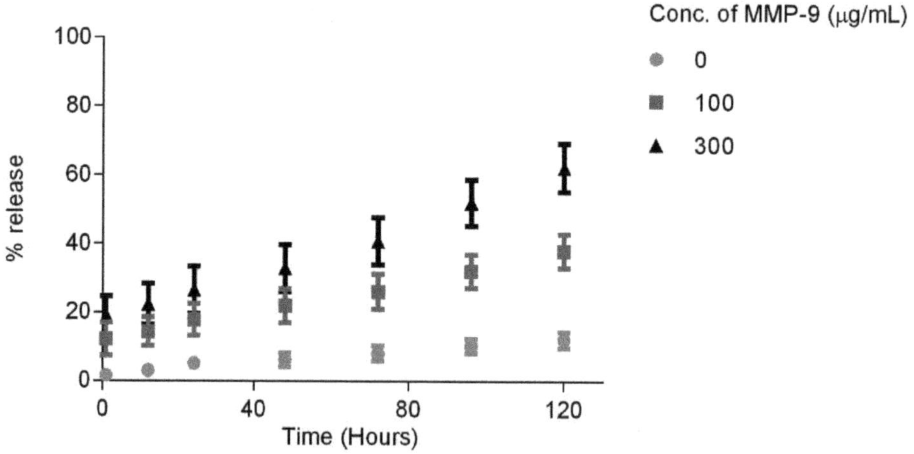

Figure 5. In vitro release of Bovine Lactoferrin from 30% w/v GelMA+ in the presence of varying MMP-9 concentrations at 37 °C.

3.2. Biological Characterization

3.2.1. Cell Growth on GelMA+ Gels

Figure 6 the growth and attachment of the immortalized HCEC cells in the presence of both the formulations of GelMA+ gels ($n = 4$). With 30% w/v GelMA+ gels, a greater amount of cell growth and attachment was observed as compared to 20% w/v GelMA+.

The images were observed phase-contrast microscopy with a 20× objective. The images were captured on the 5th day using Zeiss AxioVision Software (White Plains, NY, USA).

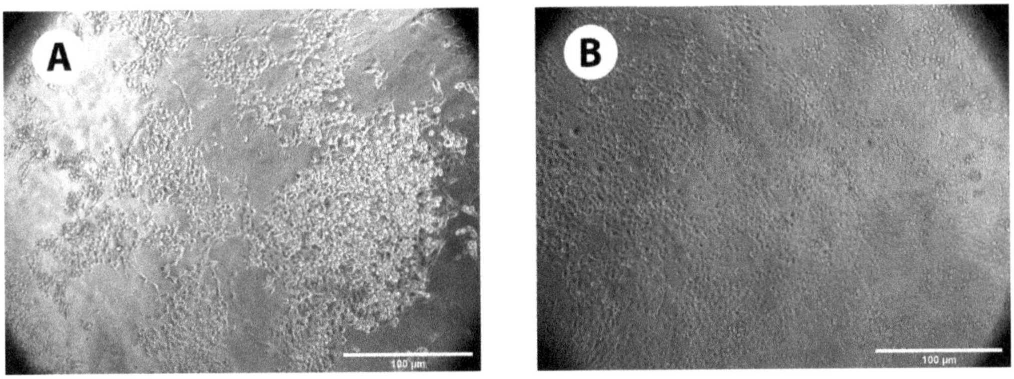

Figure 6. (**A**) Growth of immortalized HCEC cells on 20% w/v GelMA+ gels, (**B**) Growth of immortalized HCEC cells on 30% w/v GelMA+ gels. On the 5th day, the cell growth on the respective hydrogels was observed.

3.2.2. Cell Mortality Assay

Figure 7 shows the percentage of cells viable on the GelMA+ hydrogels (n = 4) on the 1, 5, and 7 days of incubation as measured by the AlamarBlue^{TM} assay. The cell viability was compared to the control, where the cells were grown in the absence of the GelMA+ gels, only in the presence of EpiGrow media. On the 7th day, 20% w/v GelMA+ hydrogel showed 80% cell viability, whereas the 30% w/v GelMA+ showed almost 95% cell viability.

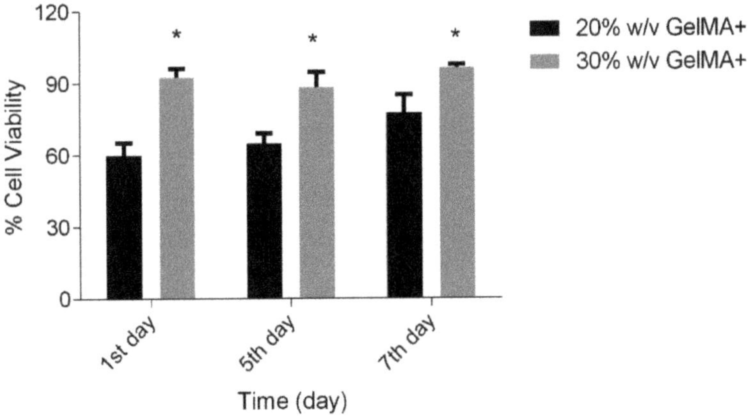

Figure 7. Percentage of HCEC cell viability in the presence of 20% w/v and 30% w/v GelMA+ respectively in comparison to control. * $p < 0.05$.

3.2.3. Live/Dead Assay

Figure 8A–C show the live and dead cell distribution after 5 days in the culture media control (no GelMA+), cells incubated with 20% w/v GelMA+ and cells incubated with 30% w/v GelMA+ (n = 4). The experiments were repeated on different days. Cells that were stained green (Calcein-AM) were live cells whereas the cells that were stained red (EthD-1) were dead cells. For both the formulations of GelMA+, a large number of cells remained alive with no signs of cytotoxicity (as evident from the green colour of Calcein-AM) when compared to the control after 5 days.

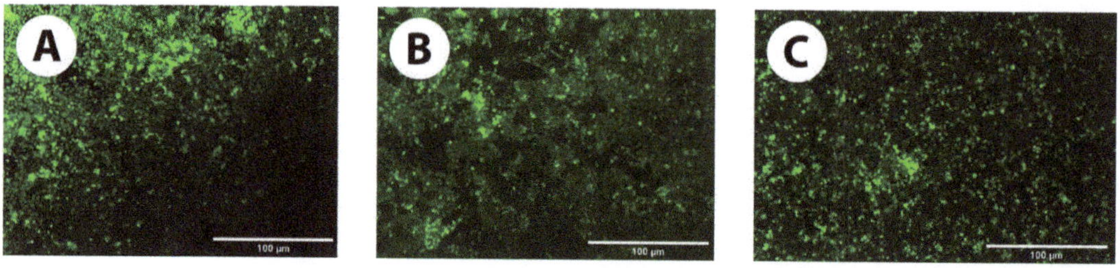

Figure 8. Live/Dead HCEC cells distribution on (**A**) Control (No GelMA+), (**B**) 20% *w/v* GelMA+, (**C**) 30% *w/v* GelMA+. The green-coloured (calcein AM) dots denote the presence of live cells and the red-coloured dots (EthD-1) denote the presence of dead cells. These images were captured after 5 days of incubation of the HCECs on the respective GelMA+. The images show the higher number of live cells in the presence of GelMA+ which is comparable to the control.

4. Discussion

GelMA hydrogels have been previously used in various biomedical devices [42–45], but the material lacks the mechanical strength required for high wear-tear applications, such as for use on the eye [34]. In a previous study, the modification of a conventional GelMA hydrogel using a sequential hybrid crosslinking process was described, involving both physical and chemical crosslinking, to improve the mechanical properties of the resulting material [34]. The new material, GelMA+, demonstrated an 8-fold increase in mechanical strength as compared to GelMA. The extra incubation period leads to improved triple helix and physical network formation leading to enhanced crosslinking. The resulting GelMA+ material has significantly improved mechanical strength and exhibits slower biodegradation kinetics (both in vitro and in vivo) than GelMA [34].

The physical characterization (porosity, tensile modulus, and water swelling) and biological parameters (cell viability and spreading) of GelMA hydrogels are important to determine the suitability of these hydrogel polymers for different biomedical applications. The SEM images (Figure 2) showed the porous nature of the GelMA+ hydrogel. The porosity of the hydrogel affects both the drug uptake and release [46,47]. Previous studies on GelMA have shown the porous nature of the hydrogel, with pore sizes ranging from 50 μm to 77 μm [48,49]. The pore size of the fully crosslinked GelMA+ was considerably less compared to the pre-polymerized GelMA. The pore size of pre-polymerized GelMA was around 150 μm to 300 μm, whereas the pore size for 20% and 30% *w/v* GelMA+ were around 30–90 μm and 0.078–0.8 μm respectively. With an increase in the concentration of the polymer, there was an increase in the crosslink density, which was also observed in previous studies [50,51]. The increase in cross-linking density concurrently leads to a decrease in the pore size.

Both the formulations showed a considerably high tensile strength. The 30% *w/v* GelMA+ was stiffer, with a tensile strain of 181.85 $\pm$ 25.25 kPa, as compared to the 20% *w/v* GelMA which had a tensile strain of 133.06 $\pm$ 8.98 kPa (see Table 1). The higher modulus can be attributed to an increase in crosslink density, which limits the material's ability to deform. These high tensile values are important to maintain the original shape and physical dimensions of any contact lens or ocular drug-delivering insert made for exposure to the ocular surface, which would be exposed to blinking [52]. The 30% *w/v* GelMA+ was stiffer, with a Young's modulus of 2.8 MPa, as compared to the 20% *w/v* GelMA, which had a tensile modulus of 2.0 MPa (Table 1). This shows that the mechanical property of the GelMA+ hydrogel could be effectively regulated by increasing the GelMA+ concentration. To prepare GelMA+ gels with tensile moduli values of commercial soft contact lens materials, which are typically around 0.3 to 0.6 MPa [53], further tuning of the GelMA+ material is needed.

Hydrogels consist of hydrophilic polymeric networks capable of imbibing large amounts of water [54,55]. A previous study demonstrated that hydrogels with smaller pore sizes have lower swelling ratios [56]. As expected (Table 1), the 20% *w/v* GelMA+, with its lower cross-link density and larger pore sizes, swelled more than the 30% *w/v* GelMA+. Crosslink density also affected the rate of degradation of the GelMA+ gels. In this study, the degradation was also shown to be dependent on the presence of collagenase enzymes such as MMPs, with increasing amounts of MMP-9 concentration increasing the degradation rate (Figure 3). The 20% *w/v* GelMA+ was completely degraded in the 300 μg/mL MMP-9 in 2 days, without any remnant of the original polymer. However, the 30% *w/v* GelMA+ took almost 6 days to degrade to 95% of the original polymer in the same MMP-9 concentration. The results suggest that increasing the GelMA+ cross-link density can be used to extend the degradation time for the GelMA+ hydrogels by MMP enzymes. Figure 3C–G shows the shape of the gels during the stages of degradation. In Figure 3B,D, it was observed that the edges of the circular gels remained after degradation. This can be attributed to the shape of the mould in which the gels were formed, which is thicker on the edges than the centre. Based on this study, the 30% *w/v* GelMA+ would be an ideal candidate for encapsulation of drugs and therapeutics.

The transmittance of contact lenses should be above 90% for optical clarity [57]. It is evident from Figure 4 that the transmittance of both blank GelMA+ formulations is above 90% in the visible light range. However, the 30% *w/v* GelMA+ gels exhibited lower ($p < 0.0001$) transmittance compared to 20% *w/v* GelMA+. This is likely due to the higher concentration of polymer in the 30% *w/v* GelMA+ [58]. With BLF-loaded GelMA+ gels, the transmittance values were lower than the blank gels (Figure 4) owing to the presence of BLF molecules in the GelMA+ matrix. Commercial soft contact lenses have a central thickness ranging from 0.06 mm to 0.24 mm [59]. The GelMA+ gels in this study have a thickness of around 0.65 mm. The transmittance value of both the blank and BLF-loaded GelMA+ formulations would increase if the gels were made thinner [60].

Several papers have shown that GelMA is a favourable biopolymer for cell growth [49,61–64] and hence proliferation and cytotoxicity tests were conducted to evaluate the biocompatibility of GelMA+. Figure 6A,B indicated that the HCEC thrived and proliferated in the presence of GelMA+, with greater cell growth on the 30% *w/v* GelMA+ hydrogel compared to 20% *w/v* GelMA+. It was hypothesized that at higher GelMA+ concentrations, there are more cell-attachment sites (Arg-Gly-Asp (RGD)). The greater spreading of GelMA+ may also be associated with the material's increased stiffness, which is required as an adequate surface/matrix for HCEC growth [65]. In line with the Alamar Blue data observed in the cell growth on GelMA+ gels (Figure 7), more cells were viable in the presence of 30% *w/v* GelMA+ gels ($p < 0.0001$). indicating that the cells preferred the presence of GelMA+. The Live/Dead cell assay (Figure 8A–C) indicated that neither formulation was cytotoxic to the HCEC cells. A large number of cells were viable for a period of 5 days with very few dead cells, as indicated by the red dots (EthD-1) in the live/dead cell assay images. For both formulations of GelMA+, a considerably large number of cells remained alive with almost no signs of cytotoxicity. Overall, these results indicated that the immortalized HCEC could proliferate over 5 days on all GelMA+ hydrogels, with greater attachment and proliferation on 30% *w/v* GelMA+.

Based on the porosity of the GelMA+ gels, a high molecular weight compound would be an ideal candidate for entrapment and release from the gel when degraded by collagenase enzymes. It was hypothesized that smaller molecules could simply diffuse from the gels at a faster rate than the rate of degradation. For this study, BLF was used as a model therapeutic for wound healing, which has a molecular weight of around 80 kDA [66]. Lactoferrin, an iron-binding monomeric glycoprotein [67], is produced by the epithelial cells of different mammalian organs and found in several secretions, including milk, saliva, tears [68], digestive secretions, nasal secretions, colostrum, and vaginal fluids, with colostrum and milk producing the highest amount of lactoferrin. It can be obtained from several mammalian species [69–71]. BLF has been reported to promote wound healing [66,72–74] and has shown promising results in the closure of alkali-wounded corneal epithelial cells [66,72]. It has been shown that the C-lobe of BLF is primarily responsible for the healing of wounded corneal epithelial cells [75].

MMPs play an important role in wound healing and inflammation [76]. These enzymes are responsible for the cleaving and remodelling of epithelial basement components and tight junction proteins [77,78]. MMPs are proteolytic enzymes that are produced where ocular surfaces are stressed [79,80]. The presence of pro MMP-9 in the tears of healthy patients was found at around 20.32 ± 5.21 ng/mL. However, patients suffering from conjunctivochalasis had MMP-9 concentrations around 223.4 ± 74.53 ng/mL [81]. In another study, active MMP-9 among healthy patients was reported at 8.39 ± 4.70 ng/mL, while patients suffering from severe dysfunctional tear syndrome showed a very high MMP-9 activity of 381.24 ± 142.83 ng/mL [82]. The presence of MMP-9 on the ocular surface can be utilized to enhance the release of active therapeutic agents from GelMA+ materials, and subsequently aid in corneal wound healing. Here, as a proof of concept, a higher level of enzymatic concentration than that typically found on the ocular surface was chosen to trigger the release of BLF from 30% *w*/*v* GelMA+ gels to demonstrate the correlation between the enzymatic concentration and the release of the therapeutic agent. However, more work will be needed to design materials that exhibit the same degradation kinetics at physiological concentrations of MMP9s.

As the 30% *w*/*v* GelMA+ was found to be a favourable candidate for the wound healing material, it was chosen as the hydrogel polymer to study the triggered release of BLF dispersed in its matrix over a period 5 days in the presence of varying MMP-9 concentrations. The GelMA+ was able to release BLF over the specified study period in an increasing manner (Figure 5). The release kinetics of BLF from the gels did not show a burst release within the first hour, which is normally observed in drug release studies from hydrogels [15,18,19,83]. It was hypothesized that the initial wash step for an hour removed most of the loosely bound BLF on the surface or sub-surface of the gels, which was around 14% of the total therapeutic concentration, which could have contributed to a burst release. In the absence of MMP-9, only 12.06 ± 3.41% of the total BLF was released after 120 h, which was due to passive diffusion. The overall results showed that the release of the BLF is dependent on both diffusion and enzyme concentration but with a higher impact from the latter. Thus, it is possible to control the release of the drug therapeutic from the GelMA+ by adjusting the polymer and enzyme concentration. Depending on the enzymes available at the wounded site, the GelMA+ gels can be formulated similarly so that they degrade completely in situ, releasing the therapeutic or drug to assist in wound healing.

One advantage of an enzyme-degradable biomaterial is that it does need to be removed while it degrades in situ. It can be used for sustained and controlled drug delivery to deliver drugs to the site of action in the body [84,85]. As observed from the BLF release profile, the release of the therapeutic agent is directly proportional to the presence of MMP-9. This implies that the drug release will respond to the wound's severity. Large wounds will have higher MMP levels [86,87] and this in turn will degrade the GelMA+ faster, leading to a higher release of the therapeutic agents. The main disadvantage of a GelMA+ bandage contact lens is that it would cause vision problems as it degrades. One alternative is to incorporate this material as a contact lens skirt or ring implant or formulate the material as an ocular insert that is inserted under the lower lid, where slow degradation would not impact vision but would release the therapeutic of interest.

5. Conclusions

This study investigated the use of GelMA+ gels at different concentrations (20% and 30% *w*/*v*) as potential materials for therapeutic bandage contact lenses or ocular inserts to treat recurrent corneal erosion or other ocular surface injuries. GelMA+ gels demonstrated degradation in the presence of MMP-9, an enzyme upregulated during corneal wounds. The release of BLF from the GelMA+ gel was facilitated by MMP-9. These findings suggest that GelMA+ gels hold promise as a biomaterial to promote corneal wound healing. Further research can explore ways to optimize the gel properties for faster degradation at lower, physiologically relevant MMP-9 concentrations.

Author Contributions: Conceptualization, S.B., C.-M.P., M.R., J.W.T., E.Y. and L.J.; Methodology, S.B., C.-M.P., E.Y. and L.J.; Validation, S.B. and C.-M.P.; Formal analysis, S.B.; Investigation, S.B.; Resources, E.Y. and L.J.; Writing—original draft, S.B. and C.-M.P.; Writing—review and editing, S.B., C.-M.P., M.R., E.Y. and L.J.; Supervision, C.-M.P. and L.J.; Funding acquisition, L.J. All authors have read and agreed to the published version of the manuscript.

Funding: This project was supported and funded by the Ontario Research Fund and the InnoHK initiative and the Hong Kong Special Administrative Region Government.

Institutional Review Board Statement: Not applicable.

Informed Consent Statement: Not applicable.

Data Availability Statement: The data can be shared up on request.

Conflicts of Interest: Over the past 3 years, CORE has received research support or lectureship honoraria from the following companies: Alcon, Azura Ophthalmics, Bausch Health, CooperVision, Essilor, Hoya, i-Med Pharma, J&J Vision, Menicon, Novartis, Ophtecs, Oté Pharma, Santen, SightGlass, SightSage, Topcon, and Visioneering. Lyndon Jones is also a consultant and/or serves on an advisory board for Alcon, CooperVision, J&J Vision, Novartis, and Ophtecs.

References

1. Whitcher, J.P.; Srinivasan, M.; Upadhyay, M.P. Corneal Blindness: A Global Perspective. *Bull. World Health Organ.* **2001**, *79*, 214–221. [PubMed]
2. Ross, M.; Deschenes, J. Practice Patterns in the Interdisciplinary Management of Corneal Abrasions. *Can. J. Ophthalmol.* **2017**, *52*, 548–551. [CrossRef] [PubMed]
3. Schrader, S.; Wedel, T.; Moll, R.; Geerling, G. Combination of Serum Eye Drops with Hydrogel Bandage Contact Lenses in the Treatment of Persistent Epithelial Defects. *Graefe Arch. Clin. Exp. Ophthalmol.* **2006**, *244*, 1345–1349. [CrossRef] [PubMed]
4. Arora, R.; Jain, S.; Monga, S.; Narayanan, R.; Raina, U.K.; Mehta, D.K. Efficacy of Continuous Wear Purevision Contact Lenses for Therapeutic Use. *Contact Lens Anterior Eye* **2004**, *27*, 39–43. [CrossRef] [PubMed]
5. Blackmore, S.J. The Use of Contact Lenses in the Treatment of Persistent Epithelial Defects. *Contact Lens Anterior Eye* **2010**, *33*, 239–244. [CrossRef] [PubMed]
6. Sun, Y.-C.; Inamoto, Y.; Wang, R.-K.; Lee, S.-J.; Hung, K.-F.; Shen, T.-T. The Disposable Bandage Soft Contact Lenses Therapy and Anterior Segment Optical Coherence Tomography for Management of Ocular Graft-Versus-Host Disease. *BMC Ophthalmol.* **2021**, *21*, 271. [CrossRef]
7. Mangan, M.S.; Tekcan, H.; Yurttaser Ocak, S. Efficacy of Bandage Contact Lenses Versus Eye Patching in Early Postoperative Period of Müller's Muscle-Conjunctival Resection. *Ophthalmic Res.* **2021**, *64*, 139–144. [CrossRef]
8. Busin, M.; Spitznas, M. Sustained Gentamicin Release by Presoaked Medicated Bandage Contact Lenses. *Ophthalmology* **1988**, *95*, 796–798. [CrossRef]
9. Donnenfeld, E.D.; Selkin, B.A.; Perry, H.D.; Moadel, K.; Selkin, G.T.; Cohen, A.J.; Sperber, L.T. Controlled Evaluation of a Bandage Contact Lens and a Topical Nonsteroidal Anti-Inflammatory Drug in Treating Traumatic Corneal Abrasions. *Ophthalmology* **1995**, *102*, 979–984. [CrossRef]
10. Kanpolat, A.; Ucakhan, O.O. Therapeutic Use of Focus Night & Day Contact Lenses. *Cornea* **2003**, *22*, 726–734.
11. Ahad, M.A.; Anandan, M.; Tah, V.; Dhingra, S.; Leyland, M. Randomized Controlled Study of Ocular Lubrication Versus Bandage Contact Lens in the Primary Treatment of Recurrent Corneal Erosion Syndrome. *Cornea* **2013**, *32*, 1311–1314. [CrossRef] [PubMed]
12. Ahmadi, F.; Oveisi, Z.; Samani, S.M.; Amoozgar, Z. Chitosan Based Hydrogels: Characteristics and Pharmaceutical Applications. *Res. Pharm. Sci.* **2015**, *10*, 1–16. [PubMed]
13. Kashyap, N.; Kumar, N.; Kumar, M.N. Hydrogels for Pharmaceutical and Biomedical Applications. *Crit. Rev. Ther. Drug Carr. Syst.* **2005**, *22*, 107–149. [CrossRef] [PubMed]
14. Hoare, T.R.; Kohane, D.S. Hydrogels in Drug Delivery: Progress and Challenges. *Polymer* **2008**, *49*, 1993–2007. [CrossRef]
15. Bajgrowicz, M.; Phan, C.M.; Subbaraman, L.N.; Jones, L. Release of Ciprofloxacin and Moxifloxacin from Daily Disposable Contact Lenses from an in Vitro Eye Model. *Investig. Ophthalmol. Vis. Sci.* **2015**, *56*, 2234–2242. [CrossRef]
16. Hui, A.; Bajgrowicz-Cieslak, M.; Phan, C.M.; Jones, L. In Vitro Release of Two Anti-Muscarinic Drugs from Soft Contact Lenses. *Clin. Ophthalmol.* **2017**, *11*, 1657–1665. [CrossRef]
17. Maulvi, F.A.; Soni, T.G.; Shah, D.O. A Review on Therapeutic Contact Lenses for Ocular Drug Delivery. *Drug Deliv.* **2016**, *23*, 3017–3026. [CrossRef]
18. Phan, C.M.; Subbaraman, L.; Liu, S.; Gu, F.; Jones, L. In Vitro Uptake and Release of Natamycin Dex-B-Pla Nanoparticles from Model Contact Lens Materials. *J. Biomater. Sci. Polym. Ed.* **2014**, *25*, 18–31. [CrossRef]

19. Phan, C.M.; Subbaraman, L.N.; Jones, L. In Vitro Uptake and Release of Natamycin from Conventional and Silicone Hydrogel Contact Lens Materials. *Eye Contact Lens* **2013**, *39*, 162–168. [CrossRef]
20. Yue, K.; Trujillo-de Santiago, G.; Alvarez, M.M.; Tamayol, A.; Annabi, N.; Khademhosseini, A. Synthesis, Properties, and Biomedical Applications of Gelatin Methacryloyl (Gelma) Hydrogels. *Biomaterials* **2015**, *73*, 254–271. [CrossRef]
21. Koshy, S.T.; Desai, R.M.; Joly, P.; Li, J.; Bagrodia, R.K.; Lewin, S.A.; Joshi, N.S.; Mooney, D.J. Click-Crosslinked Injectable Gelatin Hydrogels. *Adv. Healthc. Mater.* **2016**, *5*, 541–547. [CrossRef] [PubMed]
22. Ward, A.J.; Courts, A. *The Science and Technology of Gelatin*; Academic Press: Cambridge, MA, USA, 1977.
23. Zimmermann, D.R.; Trüeb, B.; Winterhalter, K.H.; Witmer, R.; Fischer, R.W. Type Vi Collagen is a Major Component of the Human Cornea. *FEBS Lett.* **1986**, *197*, 55–58. [CrossRef] [PubMed]
24. Barbetta, A.; Dentini, M.; Zannoni, E.M.; De Stefano, M.E. Tailoring the Porosity and Morphology of Gelatin-Methacrylate Polyhipe Scaffolds for Tissue Engineering Applications. *Langmuir* **2005**, *21*, 12333–12341. [CrossRef] [PubMed]
25. Chen, Y.C.; Lin, R.Z.; Qi, H.; Yang, Y.; Bae, H.; Melero-Martin, J.M.; Khademhosseini, A. Functional Human Vascular Network Generated in Photocrosslinkable Gelatin Methacrylate Hydrogels. *Adv. Funct. Mater.* **2012**, *22*, 2027–2039. [CrossRef] [PubMed]
26. Singh, D.; Tripathi, A.; Nayak, V.; Kumar, A. Proliferation of Chondrocytes on a 3-D Modelled Macroporous Poly(Hydroxyethyl Methacrylate)-Gelatin Cryogel. *J. Biomater. Sci. Polym. Ed.* **2011**, *22*, 1733–1751. [CrossRef] [PubMed]
27. Gómez-Guillén, M.C.; Turnay, J.; Fernández-Dıaz, M.; Ulmo, N.; Lizarbe, M.A.; Montero, P. Structural and Physical Properties of Gelatin Extracted from Different Marine Species: A Comparative Study. *Food Hydrocoll.* **2002**, *16*, 25–34. [CrossRef]
28. Nichol, J.W.; Koshy, S.T.; Bae, H.; Hwang, C.M.; Yamanlar, S.; Khademhosseini, A. Cell-Laden Microengineered Gelatin Methacrylate Hydrogels. *Biomaterials* **2010**, *31*, 5536–5544. [CrossRef]
29. Gnavi, S.; di Blasio, L.; Tonda-Turo, C.; Mancardi, A.; Primo, L.; Ciardelli, G.; Gambarotta, G.; Geuna, S.; Perroteau, I. Gelatin-Based Hydrogel for Vascular Endothelial Growth Factor Release in Peripheral Nerve Tissue Engineering. *J. Tissue Eng. Regen. Med.* **2017**, *11*, 459–470. [CrossRef]
30. Sharifi, S.; Islam, M.M.; Sharifi, H.; Islam, R.; Koza, D.; Reyes-Ortega, F.; Alba-Molina, D.; Nilsson, P.H.; Dohlman, C.H.; Mollnes, T.E.; et al. Tuning Gelatin-Based Hydrogel Towards Bioadhesive Ocular Tissue Engineering Applications. *Bioact. Mater.* **2021**, *6*, 3947–3961. [CrossRef]
31. Tronci, G.; Neffe, A.T.; Pierce, B.F.; Lendlein, A. An Entropy–Elastic Gelatin-Based Hydrogel System. *J. Mater. Chem.* **2010**, *20*, 8875–8884. [CrossRef]
32. Maitra, J.; Shukla, V.K. Cross-Linking in Hydrogels—A Review. *Am. J. Polym. Sci.* **2014**, *4*, 25–31.
33. Jia, X.; Kiick, K.L. Hybrid Multicomponent Hydrogels for Tissue Engineering. *Macromol. Biosci.* **2009**, *9*, 140–156. [CrossRef] [PubMed]
34. Rizwan, M.; Peh, G.S.; Ang, H.-P.; Lwin, N.C.; Adnan, K.; Mehta, J.S.; Tan, W.S.; Yim, E.K. Sequentially-Crosslinked Bioactive Hydrogels as Nano-Patterned Substrates with Customizable Stiffness and Degradation for Corneal Tissue Engineering Applications. *Biomaterials* **2017**, *120*, 139–154. [CrossRef] [PubMed]
35. Van den Steen, P.E.; Dubois, B.; Nelissen, I.; Rudd, P.M.; Dwek, R.A.; Opdenakker, G. Biochemistry and Molecular Biology of Gelatinase B or Matrix Metalloproteinase-9 (Mmp-9). *Crit. Rev. Biochem. Mol. Biol.* **2002**, *37*, 375–536. [CrossRef]
36. Xu, F.; Inci, F.; Mullick, O.; Gurkan, U.A.; Sung, Y.; Kavaz, D.; Li, B.; Denkbas, E.B.; Demirci, U. Release of Magnetic Nanoparticles from Cell-Encapsulating Biodegradable Nanobiomaterials. *ACS Nano* **2012**, *6*, 6640–6649. [CrossRef]
37. Xiao, W.; He, J.; Nichol, J.W.; Wang, L.; Hutson, C.B.; Wang, B.; Du, Y.; Fan, H.; Khademhosseini, A. Synthesis and Characterization of Photocrosslinkable Gelatin and Silk Fibroin Interpenetrating Polymer Network Hydrogels. *Acta Biomater.* **2011**, *7*, 2384–2393. [CrossRef]
38. Sivak, J.M.; Fini, M.E. Mmps in the Eye: Emerging Roles for Matrix Metalloproteinases in Ocular Physiology. *Prog. Retin. Eye Res.* **2002**, *21*, 1–14. [CrossRef]
39. Matsubara, M.; Girard, M.T.; Kublin, C.L.; Cintron, C.; Fini, M.E. Differential Roles for Two Gelatinolytic Enzymes of the Matrix Metalloproteinase Family in the Remodelling Cornea. *Dev. Biol.* **1991**, *147*, 425–439. [CrossRef]
40. Mulholland, B.; Tuft, S.J.; Khaw, P.T. Matrix Metalloproteinase Distribution During Early Corneal Wound Healing. *Eye* **2005**, *19*, 584–588. [CrossRef]
41. Fini, M.E.; Girard, M.T.; Matsubara, M. Collagenolytic/Gelatinolytic Enzymes in Corneal Wound Healing. *Acta Ophthalmol.* **1992**, *70* (Suppl. 1985), 26–33. [CrossRef]
42. Derakhshanfar, S.; Mbeleck, R.; Xu, K.; Zhang, X.; Zhong, W.; Xing, M. 3d Bioprinting for Biomedical Devices and Tissue Engineering: A Review of Recent Trends and Advances. *Bioact. Mater.* **2018**, *3*, 144–156. [CrossRef] [PubMed]
43. Kim, S.-Y.; Choi, A.-J.; Park, J.-E.; Jang, Y.-S.; Lee, M.-H. Antibacterial Activity and Biocompatibility with the Concentration of Ginger Fraction in Biodegradable Gelatin Methacryloyl (Gelma) Hydrogel Coating for Medical Implants. *Polymers* **2022**, *14*, 5317. [CrossRef] [PubMed]
44. Feng, M.; Hu, S.; Qin, W.; Tang, Y.; Guo, R.; Han, L. Bioprinting of a Blue Light-Cross-Linked Biodegradable Hydrogel Encapsulating Amniotic Mesenchymal Stem Cells for Intrauterine Adhesion Prevention. *ACS Omega* **2021**, *6*, 23067–23075. [CrossRef] [PubMed]
45. Wang, J.-H.; Tsai, C.-W.; Tsai, N.-Y.; Chiang, C.-Y.; Lin, R.-S.; Pereira, R.-F.; Li, Y.-C.-E. An Injectable, Dual Crosslinkable Hybrid Pectin Methacrylate (Pecma)/Gelatin Methacryloyl (Gelma) Hydrogel for Skin Hemostasis Applications. *Int. J. Biol. Macromol.* **2021**, *185*, 441–450. [CrossRef] [PubMed]

46. Ukmar, T.; Maver, U.; Planinsek, O.; Kaučič, V.; Gaberšček, M.; Godec, A. Understanding Controlled Drug Release from Mesoporous Silicates: Theory and Experiment. *J. Control. Release* **2011**, *155*, 409–417. [CrossRef]
47. Siboro, S.A.; Anugrah, D.S.; Ramesh, K.; Park, S.H.; Kim, H.R.; Lim, K.T. Tunable Porosity of Covalently Crosslinked Alginate-Based Hydrogels and Its Significance in Drug Release Behavior. *Carbohydr. Polym.* **2021**, *260*, 117779. [CrossRef]
48. Noshadi, I.; Hong, S.; Sullivan, K.E.; Sani, E.S.; Portillo-Lara, R.; Tamayol, A.; Shin, S.R.; Gao, A.E.; Stoppel, W.L.; Black, L.D., III; et al. In Vitro and in Vivo Analysis of Visible Light Crosslinkable Gelatin Methacryloyl (Gelma) Hydrogels. *Biomater. Sci.* **2017**, *5*, 2093–2105. [CrossRef]
49. ur Rehman, S.R.; Augustine, R.; Zahid, A.A.; Ahmed, R.; Tariq, M.; Hasan, A. Reduced Graphene Oxide Incorporated Gelma Hydrogel Promotes Angiogenesis for Wound Healing Applications. *Int. J. Nanomed.* **2019**, *14*, 9603. [CrossRef]
50. Yang, J.; Wang, F.; Tan, T. Controlling Degradation and Physical Properties of Chemical Sand Fixing Agent-Poly (Aspartic Acid) by Crosslinking Density and Composites. *J. Appl. Polym. Sci.* **2009**, *111*, 1557–1563. [CrossRef]
51. Peng, Z.; Chen, F. Hydroxyethyl Cellulose-Based Hydrogels with Various Pore Sizes Prepared by Freeze-Drying. *J. Macromol. Sci. Part B Phys.* **2010**, *50*, 340–349. [CrossRef]
52. Tranoudis, I.; Efron, N. Tensile Properties of Soft Contact Lens Materials. *Contact Lens Anterior Eye* **2004**, *27*, 177–191. [CrossRef] [PubMed]
53. Bhamra, T.S.; Tighe, B.J. Mechanical Properties of Contact Lenses: The Contribution of Measurement Techniques and Clinical Feedback to 50 Years of Materials Development. *Contact Lens Anterior Eye* **2017**, *40*, 70–81. [CrossRef] [PubMed]
54. Peppas, N.A.; Hoffman, A.S. Hydrogels. In *Biomaterials Science*; Wagner, W.R., Sakiyama-Elbert, S.E., Zhang, G., Yaszemski, M.J., Eds.; Academic Press: Cambridge, MA, USA, 2020; pp. 153–166.
55. Wang, Y.; Nian, G.; Kim, J.; Suo, Z. Polyacrylamide Hydrogels. Vi. Synthesis-Property Relation. *J. Mech. Phys. Solids* **2023**, *170*, 105099. [CrossRef]
56. Yacob, N.; Hashim, K. Morphological Effect on Swelling Behaviour of Hydrogel. *AIP Conf. Proc.* **2014**, *1584*, 153–159.
57. Wang, Z.; Li, X.; Zhang, X.; Sheng, R.; Lin, Q.; Song, W.; Hao, L. Novel Contact Lenses Embedded with Drug-Loaded Zwitterionic Nanogels for Extended Ophthalmic Drug Delivery. *Nanomaterials* **2021**, *11*, 2328. [CrossRef] [PubMed]
58. Gupta, S.; Goswami, S.; Sinha, A. A Combined Effect of Freeze--Thaw Cycles and Polymer Concentration on the Structure and Mechanical Properties of Transparent Pva Gels. *Biomed. Mater.* **2012**, *7*, 015006. [CrossRef] [PubMed]
59. Lira, M.; Pereira, C.; Real Oliveira, M.E.; Castanheira, E.M. Importance of Contact Lens Power and Thickness in Oxygen Transmissibility. *Contact Lens Anterior Eye* **2015**, *38*, 120–126. [CrossRef]
60. Kapfelsberger, A.; Eckstein, J.; von Ahrentschildt, A.; Bischoff, J.; Marx, S.; Sickenberger, W. Ultraviolet and Visible Transmittance of Soft Contact Lenses with and without Ultraviolet Blockers. *Optom. Vis. Sci.* **2021**, *98*, 1270–1278. [CrossRef]
61. Wang, H.; Zhou, L.; Liao, J.; Tan, Y.; Ouyang, K.; Ning, C.; Ni, G.; Tan, G. Cell-Laden Photocrosslinked Gelma-Dexma Copolymer Hydrogels with Tunable Mechanical Properties for Tissue Engineering. *J. Mater. Sci. Mater. Med.* **2014**, *25*, 2173–2183. [CrossRef]
62. Augustine, R.; Hasan, A.; Dalvi, Y.B.; Rehman, S.R.U.; Varghese, R.; Unni, R.N.; Yalcin, H.C.; Alfkey, R.; Thomas, S.; Al Moustafa, A.E. Growth Factor Loaded In Situ Photocrosslinkable Poly(3-Hydroxybutyrate-Co-3-Hydroxyvalerate)/Gelatin Methacryloyl Hybrid Patch for Diabetic Wound Healing. *Mater. Sci. Eng. C-Mater. Biol. Appl.* **2021**, *118*, 111519. [CrossRef]
63. Fathi, A.; Lee, S.; Breen, A.; Shirazi, A.N.; Valtchev, P.; Dehghani, F. Enhancing the Mechanical Properties and Physical Stability of Biomimetic Polymer Hydrogels for Micro-Patterning and Tissue Engineering Applications. *Eur. Polym. J.* **2014**, *59*, 161–170. [CrossRef]
64. Liu, B.; Wang, Y.; Miao, Y.; Zhang, X.; Fan, Z.; Singh, G.; Zhang, X.; Xu, K.; Li, B.; Hu, Z.; et al. Hydrogen Bonds Autonomously Powered Gelatin Methacrylate Hydrogels with Super-Elasticity, Self-Heal and Underwater Self-Adhesion for Sutureless Skin and Stomach Surgery and E-Skin. *Biomaterials* **2018**, *171*, 83–96. [CrossRef] [PubMed]
65. Sun, Y.; Deng, R.; Ren, X.; Zhang, K.; Li, J. 2d Gelatin Methacrylate Hydrogels with Tunable Stiffness for Investigating Cell Behaviors. *ACS Appl. Bio Mater.* **2018**, *2*, 570–576. [CrossRef] [PubMed]
66. Pattamatta, U.; Willcox, M.; Stapleton, F.; Cole, N.; Garrett, Q. Bovine Lactoferrin Stimulates Human Corneal Epithelial Alkali Wound Healing in Vitro. *Investig. Ophthalmol. Vis. Sci.* **2009**, *50*, 1636–1643. [CrossRef] [PubMed]
67. Groves, M.L. The Isolation of a Red Protein from Milk2. *J. Am. Chem. Soc.* **1960**, *82*, 3345–3350. [CrossRef]
68. Flanagan, J.L.; Willcox, M.D. Role of Lactoferrin in the Tear Film. *Biochimie* **2009**, *91*, 35–43. [CrossRef] [PubMed]
69. Gruden, S.; Poklar Ulrih, N. Diverse Mechanisms of Antimicrobial Activities of Lactoferrins, Lactoferricins, and Other Lactoferrin-Derived Peptides. *Int. J. Mol. Sci.* **2021**, *22*, 11264. [CrossRef]
70. Masson, P.L.; Heremans, J.F. Lactoferrin in Milk from Different Species. *Comp. Biochem. Physiol. Part B* **1971**, *39*, 119–129. [CrossRef]
71. Masson, P.; Heremans, J.; Dive, C. An Iron-Binding Protein Common to Many External Secretions. *Clin. Chim. Acta* **1966**, *14*, 735–739. [CrossRef]
72. Tang, L.; Wu, J.J.; Ma, Q.; Cui, T.; Andreopoulos, F.M.; Gil, J.; Valdes, J.; Davis, S.C.; Li, J. Human Lactoferrin Stimulates Skin Keratinocyte Function and Wound Re-Epithelialization. *Br. J. Dermatol.* **2010**, *163*, 38–47. [CrossRef]
73. Engelmayer, J.; Blezinger, P.; Varadhachary, A. Talactoferrin Stimulates Wound Healing with Modulation of Inflammation. *J. Surg. Res.* **2008**, *149*, 278–286. [CrossRef] [PubMed]

74. Mouritzen, M.V.; Petkovic, M.; Qvist, K.; Poulsen, S.S.; Alarico, S.; Leal, E.C.; Dalgaard, L.T.; Empadinhas, N.; Carvalho, E.; Jenssen, H. Improved Diabetic Wound Healing by Lfcinb Is Associated with Relevant Changes in the Skin Immune Response and Microbiota. *Mol. Ther. Methods Clin. Dev.* **2021**, *20*, 726–739. [CrossRef] [PubMed]
75. Ashby, B.; Garrett, Q.; Willcox, M. Bovine Lactoferrin Structures Promoting Corneal Epithelial Wound Healing in Vitro. *Investig. Ophthalmol. Vis. Sci.* **2011**, *52*, 2719–2726. [CrossRef] [PubMed]
76. Li, D.Q.; Pflugfelder, S.C. Matrix Metalloproteinases in Corneal Inflammation. *Ocul. Surf.* **2005**, *3*, S198–S202. [CrossRef] [PubMed]
77. Behzadian, M.A.; Wang, X.L.; Windsor, L.J.; Ghaly, N.; Caldwell, R.B. Tgf-Beta Increases Retinal Endothelial Cell Permeability by Increasing Mmp-9: Possible Role of Glial Cells in Endothelial Barrier Function. *Investig. Ophthalmol. Vis. Sci.* **2001**, *42*, 853–859.
78. Sternlicht, M.D.; Werb, Z. How Matrix Metalloproteinases Regulate Cell Behavior. *Annu. Rev. Cell Dev. Biol.* **2001**, *17*, 463–516. [CrossRef] [PubMed]
79. Pflugfelder, S.C. Antiinflammatory Therapy for Dry Eye. *Am. J. Ophthalmol.* **2004**, *137*, 337–342. [CrossRef]
80. Afonso, A.A.; Sobrin, L.; Monroy, D.C.; Selzer, M.; Lokeshwar, B.; Pflugfelder, S.C. Tear Fluid Gelatinase B Activity Correlates with Il-1alpha Concentration and Fluorescein Clearance in Ocular Rosacea. *Investig. Ophthalmol. Vis. Sci.* **1999**, *40*, 2506–2512.
81. Acera, A.; Vecino, E.; Duran, J.A. Tear Mmp-9 Levels as a Marker of Ocular Surface Inflammation in Conjunctivochalasis. *Investig. Ophthalmol. Vis. Sci.* **2013**, *54*, 8285–8291. [CrossRef]
82. Chotikavanich, S.; de Paiva, C.S.; Chen, J.J.; Bian, F.; Farley, W.J.; Pflugfelder, S.C. Production and Activity of Matrix Metalloproteinase-9 on the Ocular Surface Increase in Dysfunctional Tear Syndrome. *Investig. Ophthalmol. Vis. Sci.* **2009**, *50*, 3203–3209. [CrossRef]
83. Tse, J. Gelatin Methacrylate as a Controlled Release Vehicle for Treatment of Recurrent Corneal Erosion. Master's Thesis, University of Waterloo, Waterloo, ON, Canada, 2018.
84. Langer, R. Drug Delivery. Drugs on Target. *Science* **2001**, *293*, 58–59. [CrossRef] [PubMed]
85. Ulijn, R.V. Enzyme-Responsive Materials: A New Class of Smart Biomaterials. *J. Mater. Chem.* **2006**, *16*, 2217–2225. [CrossRef]
86. Da Silva, A.A.; Leal-Junior, E.C.; Alves, A.C.; Rambo, C.S.; Dos Santos, S.A.; Vieira, R.P.; De Carvalho, P.D. Wound-Healing Effects of Low-Level Laser Therapy in Diabetic Rats Involve the Modulation of Mmp-2 and Mmp-9 and the Redistribution of Collagen Types I and Iii. *J. Cosmet. Laser Ther.* **2013**, *15*, 210–216. [CrossRef] [PubMed]
87. Eichler, W.; Bechtel, J.M.; Schumacher, J.; Wermelt, J.A.; Klotz, K.F.; Bartels, C. A Rise of Mmp-2 and Mmp-9 in Bronchoalveolar Lavage Fluid Is Associated with Acute Lung Injury after Cardiopulmonary Bypass in a Swine Model. *Perfusion* **2003**, *18*, 107–113. [CrossRef]

pharmaceutics

Article

Celecoxib/Cyclodextrin Eye Drop Microsuspensions: Evaluation of In Vitro Cytotoxicity and Anti-VEGF Efficacy for Retinal Diseases

Phatsawee Jansook [1,2,*], Hay Man Saung Hnin Soe [1], Rathapon Asasutjarit [3], Theingi Tun [1], Hay Marn Hnin [1], Phyo Darli Maw [1], Tanapong Watchararot [1] and Thorsteinn Loftsson [4]

1 Faculty of Pharmaceutical Sciences, Chulalongkorn University, Bangkok 10330, Thailand; haymansaunghninsoe@gmail.com (H.M.S.H.S.); theingitun.tgt1793@gmail.com (T.T.); haymarn793@gmail.com (H.M.H.); phyodarlimaw1994@gmail.com (P.D.M.); tanapongbiggie@hotmail.com (T.W.)
2 Cyclodextrin Application and Nanotechnology-Based Delivery Systems Research Unit, Chulalongkorn University, Bangkok 10330, Thailand
3 Thammasat University Research Unit in Drug, Health Product Development and Application (DHP-DA), Department of Pharmaceutical Sciences, Faculty of Pharmacy, Thammasat University, Pathum Thani 12120, Thailand; rathapon@tu.ac.th
4 Faculty of Pharmaceutical Sciences, University of Iceland, Hofsvallagata 53, IS-107 Reykjavik, Iceland; thorstlo@hi.is
* Correspondence: phatsawee.j@chula.ac.th; Tel.: +66-2-218-8273

Abstract: Celecoxib (CCB), a cyclooxygenase-2 inhibitor, is capable of reducing oxidative stress and vascular endothelial growth factor (VEGF) expression in retinal cells and has been shown to be effective in the treatment of diabetic retinopathy and age-related macular degeneration. However, the ocular bioavailability of CCB is hampered due to its very low aqueous solubility. In a previous study, we developed 0.5% (*w*/*v*) aqueous CCB eye drop microsuspensions (MS) containing randomly methylated β-cyclodextrin (RMβCD) or γ-cyclodextrin (γCD) and hyaluronic acid (HA) as ternary CCB/CD/HA nanoaggregates. Both formulations exhibited good physicochemical properties. Therefore, we further investigated their cytotoxicity and efficacy in a human retina cell line in this study. At a CCB concentration of 1000 μg/mL, both CCB/RMβCD and CCB/γCD eye drop MS showed low hemolysis activity (11.1 ± 0.3% or 4.9 ± 0.2%, respectively). They revealed no signs of causing irritation and were nontoxic to retinal pigment epithelial cells. Moreover, the CCB eye drop MS exhibited significant anti-VEGF activity by reducing VEGF mRNA and protein levels compared to CCB suspended in phosphate buffer saline. The ex vivo transscleral diffusion demonstrated that a high quantity of CCB (112.47 ± 37.27 μg/mL) from CCB/γCD eye drop MS was deposited in the porcine sclera. Our new findings suggest that CCB/CD eye drop MS could be safely delivered to the ocular tissues and demonstrate promising eye drop formulations for retinal disease treatment.

Keywords: cyclodextrin; celecoxib; eye drop; microsuspensions; cytotoxicity; anti-VEGF

Citation: Jansook, P.; Soe, H.M.S.H.; Asasutjarit, R.; Tun, T.; Hnin, H.M.; Maw, P.D.; Watchararot, T.; Loftsson, T. Celecoxib/Cyclodextrin Eye Drop Microsuspensions: Evaluation of In Vitro Cytotoxicity and Anti-VEGF Efficacy for Retinal Diseases. *Pharmaceutics* **2023**, *15*, 2689. https://doi.org/10.3390/pharmaceutics15122689

Academic Editors: Ruggero Bettini, Monica M. Jablonski, Rosario Pignatello, Hugo Almeida, Debora Santonocito and Carmelo Puglia

Received: 12 October 2023
Revised: 14 November 2023
Accepted: 26 November 2023
Published: 28 November 2023

1. Introduction

Age-related macular degeneration (AMD) and diabetic retinopathy (DR) are emerging as global health issues that are leading causes of irreversible blindness and visual impairment [1,2]. The prevalence of both conditions is expected to rise over time and approximately 288 million people will be affected with AMD by 2040 and 191 million people with DR by 2030 [2,3]. Indeed, vascular endothelial growth factor (VEGF) is a common factor involved in the pathophysiology of both DR and AMD [4]. Excessive VEGF expression in the retina causes vascular leakage and choroidal neovascularization, which mean the formation of new, abnormal blood vessels in the choroid and subretinal region [5,6], ultimately causing a breakdown of the blood–ocular barrier and allowing the influx of fluids and macromolecules from the blood into the retina, resulting in central vision impairment [7]. Laser photocoagulation and vitrectomy have been the gold standard therapy for decades. Additionally, the systematic use of anti-inflammatory, antiangiogenesis, and antihypertensive agents, antioxidants, and hypoglycemic agents has been reported as beneficial in managing AMD and DR [8–10]. In recent years, researchers have increasingly focused on strategies targeting VEGF [11].

Celecoxib (CCB), a selective cyclooxygenase-2 inhibitor, has shown anti-inflammatory, anti-VEGF, and antiproliferative effects on the retina cells [4]. CCB reduces VEGF secretion from retinal pigment epithelium (RPE) and exhibits antiproliferative effects on RPE and the choroid endothelium. These unique properties make CCB a potential drug candidate for the treatment of AMD and DR [4]. Recently, oral administration of CCB has been proven to reduce vascular leakage and retinal VEGF mRNA expression in diabetic rat models. However, achieving therapeutic levels in the eyes requires a very high oral dose (50 mg/kg twice daily), leading to systemic side effects and toxicity [12]. Although invasive intravitreal injections can provide effective drug levels in the targeted retina, this approach is often complicated by endophthalmitis and retinal detachment, particularly after multiple injections [13]. Likewise, intraocular and periocular injections also carry a high risk of tissue damage and ocular infections [14].

To address these challenges, in a previous study, we developed noninvasive eye drop microsuspensions (MS) containing CCB and cyclodextrin (CD) [15]. Our findings revealed that randomly methylated β-cyclodextrin (RMβCD) or γ-cyclodextrin (γCD) had a strong complex forming affinity to CCB, and the addition of a biocompatible polymer enhanced CD solubilization through ternary complex formation [15]. The developed aqueous 0.5% (*w*/*v*) CCB eye drop MS, containing RMβCD or γCD and hyaluronic acid (HA), exhibited favorable physicochemical properties, including pH, osmolality, and viscosity, along with good mucoadhesion. Moreover, they exhibited a high permeation flux across various tested membranes [16]. In the present study, we conducted further investigations into the safety of our developed CCB/CD eye drop MS using in vitro hemolysis, the hen's egg test-chorioallantoic membrane, cell viability, and short-time exposure tests. Additionally, the anti-VEGF effects (both protein and mRNA levels) in human retinal cell line were assessed using a western blot assay and a real-time polymerase chain reaction assay to evaluate the efficacy of the drug. Finally, we investigated the ex vivo transscleral diffusion of CCB/CD eye drop MS through porcine sclera.

2. Materials and Methods

2.1. Materials

Celecoxib (CCB) was kindly donated by Unison Laboratories Co., Ltd., (Bangkok, Thailand). Randomly methylated β-cyclodextrin (RMβCD) with molar substitution of 1.8 (MW 1312 Da) was purchased from Wacker Chemie (Munich, Germany) and γ-cyclodextrin (γCD) was kindly gifted by Ashland (Wilmington, DE, USA). Hyaluronic acid (HA), MW 1–1.4 MDa was from Soliance (Pomacle, France); ethylenediaminetetraacetic acid disodium salt dihydrate (EDTA) and sodium chloride (NaCl) were from Ajax Finechem Pty Ltd. (Taren Point, Australia); and benzalkonium chloride (BAC) was from Sigma–Aldrich (St. Louis, MO, USA). All other chemicals used were of analytical reagent grade purity. Milli-Q (Millipore, Billerica, MA, USA) water was used for the preparation of all solutions. The Statens Seruminstitut Rabbit Cornea (SIRC) and human retinal pigment epithelial (ARPE-19) cell lines were purchased from American Type Culture Collection (ATCC) (Manassas, VA, USA). All reagents used in cell culture were purchased from Invitrogen (Thermo Fisher Scientific, Waltham, MA, USA).

2.2. Preparation and Characterizations of CCB Eye Drop Microsuspensions (MS)

Previously, preparation of the CCB/RMβCD MS and CCB/γCD MS eye drops and their characterization has been described [16]. A 0.5% (*w*/*v*) solution of CCB was suspended in an aqueous CD solution (7.5% *w*/*v* RMβCD or 10% *w*/*v* γCD). Then, 0.1% (*w*/*v*) EDTA and

0.02% (*w*/*v*) BAC were added to the suspension. A mixer mill (RETSCH® MM400, Haan, Germany) with 2 mm zirconium beads was used to reduce the size of the aqueous CCB eye drop suspensions and the process was performed at 25 Hz for 30 min. Subsequently, 0.5% (*w*/*v*) HA was added and mixed until it was completely dissolved. The pH of the resulting CCB eye drop MS was adjusted to 7.4 with sodium hydroxide (NaOH) and tonicity was adjusted with NaCl. The suspension was further sonicated in an ultrasonic bath (GT Sonic, China) at 70 °C for 1 h, and finally, water for injection was added to obtain the desired volume. CCB ophthalmic MS containing RMβCD or γCD were designated as CCB/RMβCD MS and CCB/γCD MS, respectively. These CCB eye drop MS contain micro- and nanoparticles of free CCB, solid CCB/CD complexes, and dissolved CCB/CD nanoaggregates. The particle size of CCB/RMβCD MS and CCB/γCD MS is less than 8 μm, which has been previously reported as acceptable and nonirritating to the eye [16].

The appearance of CCB eye drop MS was visually inspected, and the pH value was measured using a pH meter (METTLER TOLEDO™, SevenCompact S220-Basic, GmbH, Giessen, Germany) at room temperature. The osmolality was measured in an osmometer (OSMOMAT 3000 basic, Genotec GmbH, Berlin, Germany) using the freezing point depression principle at room temperature. A viscometer (Sine-wave Vibro SV-10, A&D Company, Tokyo, Japan) was used to determine the viscosity of each formulation. The surface tension of the formulation was measured by using a dynamic contact angle meter and tensiometer (DCAT 21, Dataphysics instrument GmbH, Filderstadt, Germany) via a Wilhelmy plate. The re-dispersion time, i.e., the time required to obtain a uniform suspension, was determined after the vial was placed in an upright position and motionless for 5 days. A mechanical shaker (Stuart Scientific, Nottingham, UK) was used to roll the container in a horizontal position at 75 rpm and time for the achievement of the homogenously suspended formulation was recorded. Total CCB content and dissolved content were analyzed using reversed-phase high-performance liquid chromatography (HPLC), as detailed in our previous report [16]. Each measurement was conducted in triplicate, and the results are expressed as the mean values ± standard deviation (SD).

2.3. Hemolysis Activity

Sheep blood was supplied by the Faculty of Veterinary Science, Chulalongkorn University. Initially, the blood sample was centrifuged at 4000 rpm for 20 min. The supernatant and the buffy coat were discarded via pipetting. The erythrocytes (RBCs) were washed three times with phosphate buffer saline (PBS, pH 7.4) and then resuspended. It was noted that the hematocrit value of RBCs in PBS was 40%. After appropriate dilution, RBCs were counted using a hemocytometer (Boeco, Hamburg, Germany). Following this, CCB eye drop MS was added to the suspended RBCs and diluted with PBS to achieve a final CCB concentration range of 25–1000 μg/mL. The samples were agitated in a shaking incubator at 37 °C and 100 rpm for 30 min and then transferred in an ice bath to stop hemolysis. Finally, the samples were centrifuged at 3000 rpm for 5 min, and the supernatant was analyzed for free hemoglobin concentration at 576 nm using a UV–VIS spectrophotometer (Model UV-1601, Shimadzu, Tokyo, Japan) [17]. The percentage of hemolyzed RBC (% hemolysis) was determined using the following equation.

$$\%\ \text{Hemolysis} = \frac{(\text{Abs} - \text{Abs}_0)}{(\text{Abs}_{100} - \text{Abs}_0)} \times 100 \quad (1)$$

where Abs, Abs_0, and Abs_{100} were the absorbances for the sample, control with PBS, and control with distilled water, respectively.

2.4. Irritation Study by Hen's Egg Test-Chorioallantoic Membrane (HET-CAM)

The cytocompatibility of CCB/RMβCD MS and CCB/γCD MS were determined using the HET-CAM assay [18]. Firstly, fertile broiler chicken eggs were hatched at 38.0 ± 0.5 °C with a relative humidity of 58.0 ± 2.0% for 9 days in an automatic rotation incubator. The rotation of the incubator was stopped on day 8 to position the air sac in the wider part of the egg for an additional day. On day 9, the outer eggshell was carefully removed, and then 300 µL of CCB eye drop MS was directly applied onto the chorioallantoic membrane. The irritation potential was observed at fixed time intervals of 0.5, 2, and 5 min. In this study, 0.1% (*w*/*v*) NaOH solution served as a positive control (C+), and 0.9% (*w*/*v*) NaCl solution served as a negative control (C−). The irritation scores (IS) ranging from 0 to 21, were recorded according to Luepke (1985) [19], and irritation was classified as follows: (I) hemorrhage (vessels bleeding), (II) vascular lysis (disintegration of blood vessel) and (III) coagulation (intra- and/or extravascular denaturation of protein). The experiment was performed in triplicate.

2.5. *In Vitro Cytotoxicity Study*

2.5.1. Short-Time Exposure (STE)

SIRC cells were used for performing the STE test to determine the cytotoxic effect of chemicals on corneal epithelium damage and eye irritation potential [20]. Briefly, SIRC cells (ATCC, Manassas, VA, USA) were grown in a complete medium and incubated at 37 °C in a 5% carbon dioxide (CO_2) humidified air incubator. The complete medium used in this study consisted of Eagle's Minimum Essential Medium (EMEM; ATCC, Manassas, VA, USA), 10% fetal bovine serum (FBS), and 1% penicillin/streptomycin solution. The cells were seeded in 96-well plates at a density of 1×10^5 cells/well/100 µL and allowed to grow at 37 °C for 24 h. Subsequently, the cells were treated with 200 µL of formulations, i.e., CCB/RMβCD MS and CCB/γCD MS and their respective blanks, at concentrations of 5% and 0.05% in normal saline. The blanks of each formulation consist of excipients, except for the CCB, and follow the procedure of preparation as described in Section 2.2. Blanks of CCB/RMβCD MS and CCB/γCD MS were designated as blank RMβCD MS and blank γCD MS, respectively. The coefficient of variation (%CV) of SIRC cells was evaluated after a 5 min exposure, and ocular irritation was graded using scores of 1, 2, and 3 to indicate minimal, moderate, and severe conditions, respectively. Then, the total eye irritation score was calculated by summing the scores obtained from both 5% and 0.05% of each test [20].

2.5.2. Cell Viability (CV) Test

The methyl thiazolyl-diphenyl-tetrazolium bromide (MTT) assay was employed to further investigate in vitro cytotoxicity [21,22] and to provide information for determining drug efficacy. CCB/RMβCD MS, CCB/γCD MS, and their respective blanks were tested to determine the toxicity in the ARPE-19 cell line (ATCC, Manassas, VA, USA). ARPE-19 cells express angiogenic factor, i.e., VEGF in retinal diseases [23]. In brief, the cells were grown in Dulbecco's modified Eagle's medium F12 (DMEM/F12; ATCC, Manassas, VA, USA), supplemented with 10% FBS and 1% penicillin/streptomycin solution, and maintained at 37 °C in a 5% CO_2 humidified air incubator. Cells were seeded in 96-well plates at a density of 1×10^4 cells/well/100 µL. Next, cells were treated by adding 100 µL of the test sample at concentrations ranging from 12.5 to 500 µg/mL to each well. After 24 h of incubation, cells were rinsed twice with PBS (pH 7.4). Subsequently, MTT solution in PBS (pH 7.4) was added to each well and incubated for 4 h. Formazan crystals were dissolved in isopropanol (100 µL/well) with 0.04 M HCl. The optical density (OD) in each well was measured at 570 nm using Fluostar Omega microplate reader (BMG Labtech, Ortenberg, Germany). The %CV was then computed according to Equation (2). A test sample was considered lethal to the cells when the %CV was less than 70%.

$$\mathrm{CV}\ (\%) = \frac{\mathrm{OD_{sample}}}{\mathrm{OD_{control}}} \times 100 \quad (2)$$

where OD_{sample} means the OD of media in each well that contains the cells treated with the drug sample, and MTT solution, and $OD_{control}$ means the OD media without drug samples.

2.6. Anti-VEGF Activity

2.6.1. Hypoxia Exposure

Cobalt chloride ($CoCl_2$) was employed to simulate a hypoxic state by inducing the activity of hypoxia-inducible factor 1-alpha (HIF-1α), leading to the release of VEGF-A in retinal epithelial cells [24]. Our preliminary data demonstrated that a concentration of 100 μM $CoCl_2$ was not toxic to ARPE-19 cells. Prior to $CoCl_2$ exposure, the cells were cultured to establish a confluent monolayer in a complete medium. Subsequently, the culture medium was replaced with fresh medium containing 100 μM $CoCl_2$. After a 24 h induction period, the medium containing $CoCl_2$ was removed, and the cells were further incubated with samples (i.e., CCB in PBS, CCB/RMβCD MS, CCB/γCD MS, and their respective blanks). The well without treatment was replaced by the medium and designated as a negative control.

2.6.2. Western Blot

A western blot assay was carried out to assess the anti-VEGF activity at the protein level [25]. After 24 h treatment with samples, ARPE-19 cells were washed with PBS and lysed. The protein was extracted by adding radioimmunoprecipitation assay buffer (10×, cat no. 9806S; Cell Signaling Technology, Danvers, MA, USA), supplemented with a protease inhibitor cocktail (100×, cat. no. 5871; Cell Signaling Technology, Danvers, MA, USA). The lysed cells were then centrifuged at 4 °C, 12,000 rpm for 5 min, and the supernatant was collected. The protein concentration was determined using a microplate reader (Fluostar Omega, BMG Labtech, Ortenberg, Germany). A standard amount of protein was mixed with loading dye (cat. no. R1151; Thermo Scientific™, Waltham, MA, USA) and heated for 5 min at 95 °C. This mixture was subjected to sodium dodecyl sulfate polyacrylamide gel electrophoresis and then transferred to a nitrocellulose membrane (Bio-Rad Laboratories, Benicia, CA, USA). After blocking with 5% skimmed milk for 1 h, the membrane was incubated with a primary antibody, VEGF-A (1:1000; cat. no. ab67214615; Abcam, Cambridge, UK), overnight at 4 °C, followed by incubation with the secondary antibody, i.e., horseradish peroxidase-conjugated goat anti-rabbit IgG antibody (1:3000; cat. no. ab6721; Abcam, Cambridge, UK) for 1 h at room temperature. Protein bands were visualized after extensive washing with enhanced chemiluminescence substrate (cat. no. ab65623; Abcam, Cambridge, UK) using the ChemiDoc Imaging System (ChemiDoc™, Bio-Rad Laboratories Inc., Benicia, CA, USA). To verify the equal loading of the proteins, membranes were stripped, reblocked, and reprobed to detect beta-actin (β-actin; 1:1000; cat. no. ab6721; Abcam, Cambridge, UK). The quantification of bands on membrane was carried out using densitometry analysis through ImageJ software version 1.54 (National Institute of Health, http://rsb.info.nih.gov/ij/ [accessed on 15 January 2023]). The integrated optical density (IOD) of each band was calculated and normalized by β-actin as described [26]. All experiments were conducted in triplicate.

2.6.3. Real-Time Polymerase Chain Reaction (RT-PCR)

The suppression of VEGF-A levels in mRNA was determined by RT-PCR. After 24 h treatment of samples, ARPE-19 cells were washed with PBS. Then, total RNA extraction was performed utilizing the AURUM total RNA Mini Kit with DNase digestion (Bio-Rad, Laboratories Inc., Benicia, CA, USA), following the recommended procedure provided by the manufacturer. First-strand cDNA was generated from 1 μg of total RNA using the iScript cDNA Synthesis Kit (Bio-Rad, Laboratories Inc., Benicia, CA, USA). Quantitative real-time PCR (qPCR) was conducted using SYBR Green on the iQ5 Multicolor Real-time PCR Detection System (Bio-Rad, Laboratories Inc., Benicia, CA, USA). The VEGF primer (PrimePCR™ SYBR® Green Assay: VEGF-A, Human, Bio-Rad, Laboratories Inc., Benicia, CA, USA) was used as the target gene, while a mixture of forward primer 18sRNA-5584 (GTAACCCGTTGAACCCCATT) and reverse primer 18sRNA-5734 (CCATCCAATCGGTAGTAGCG) was used for reference genes. The final reaction mixture consisted of 1 μL of each primer, 0.5 μL of cDNA, and 5 μL of iTaq Universal SYBR Green Supermix (Bio-Rad, Laboratories Inc., Benicia, CA, USA), with the remaining mixture volume adjusted to 10 μL using RNase-free water. All reactions were conducted in triplicate. RT-PCR was carried out in a thermal cycler (CFX96™ Real-Time System, Bio-Rad, Laboratories Inc., Benicia, CA, USA) with an initial 3 min hot start denaturation step at 95 °C, followed by 40 cycles at 95 °C for 2 s and at 60 °C for 20 s. Throughout the reaction, fluorescence, and consequently the quantity of PCR products, were continuously monitored via CFX Maestro™ software version 2.3 (Bio-Rad, Laboratories Inc., Benicia, CA, USA). The samples were compared using the relative cycle threshold (Ct) method. After normalization, the levels of increase or decrease were determined with respect to controls, using the formula $2^{-\Delta\Delta Ct}$, where ΔCt is (gene of interest Ct) − (reference gene Ct), and ΔΔ Ct is (ΔCt experimental) − (ΔCt control) [26,27].

2.7. Ex Vivo Porcine Transscleral Permeation of CCB

The ex vivo ocular permeation study was conducted using vertical Franz diffusion cells (NK laboratory, Bangkok, Thailand) across the porcine sclera. The receptor phase consisted of 2.0% (*w*/*v*) γCD in PBS (pH 7.4). γCD was added to the receptor phase to maintain a sink condition. A volume of 1.5 mL of CCB/γCD MS was placed in the donor compartment, and the system was maintained at 35 ± 0.5 °C with continuous agitation at 750 rpm throughout the test. CCB in PBS suspension served as a reference formulation. At specific time points, i.e., 1, 2, and 4 h, the sclera was removed and washed three times with ultrapure water and PBS. The amount of CCB retained in each sclera was extracted by cutting them into small pieces and sonicating them in methanol for 30 min. Subsequently, the concentration of CCB was analyzed using the validated HPLC method described in our previous report [16].

2.8. Statistical Analysis

All quantitative data were presented as mean ± standard deviation (SD). The statistical analysis was conducted using SPSS version 16.0 software. Initially, the normality of the data distribution was assessed using the Shapiro–Wilk test. The results indicated a normal distribution of the data, justifying the use of a one-way ANOVA for the analysis. Subsequently, we performed a one-way ANOVA followed by Tukey's post-hoc test. Statistical significance was set at a *p*-value of 0.05.

3. Results and Discussion

3.1. Physicochemical Characteristics of CCB Eye Drop MS

Table 1 displays the physicochemical characteristics of CCB eye drop MS. These CCB eye drop MS exhibited milky white suspensions. The pH values for both CCB eye drop formulations were determined to be 7.40 after adjustment with sodium hydroxide, which is well tolerated by the eye [28]. The tonicity of the formulations was adjusted by NaCl to be isotonic (260–330 mOsm/kg). The viscosities of these CCB ophthalmic preparations are close to the upper limit of the optimal range, which falls between 15 and 25 cps [29]. This maximum viscosity is able to enhance drug contact time with the ocular surface and keeps the particles well suspended. The surface tension of CCB/RMβCD MS fell within the normal physiological range of lacrimal fluid's surface tension (40–46 mN/m) [30], whereas CCB/γCD MS exhibited slightly higher surface tension than the physiological range. Surface tension exceeding the physiological range is associated with dry eyes and can lead to tear film instability [31]. Both of the developed CCB eye drop MS were easily redispersed, ensuring the uniform dispersion of solid drug particles in the aqueous vehicle.

It is worth noting that the fraction of CCB dissolved in the aqueous CCB eye drop MS containing RMβCD was significantly higher compared to that containing γCD (approximately 32 times higher). On the other hand, in the formulation containing RMβCD 49% of the drug was in the solid fraction (free CCB and solid CCB/CD complex), whereas this figure was 98% in the formulation containing γCD. All of these physicochemical parameters aligned with previous studies and met the acceptance criteria.

Table 1. Physicochemical parameters of CCB eye drop MS.

Parameters	CCB/RMβCD MS	CCB/γCD MS
Appearance	Milky white suspension	Milky white suspension
pH	7.40 ± 0.06	7.39 ± 0.02
Osmolality (mOsmol/kg)	299.67 ± 2.08	301.00 ± 2.00
Viscosity (cPs) [a]	22.76 ± 1.53	27.53 ± 1.72
Surface tension (mN/m) [a]	45.32 ± 0.15	48.35 ± 2.07
Redispersion time (s)	28.00 ± 2.65	20.67 ± 1.15
Total drug content (%)	102.51 ± 0.07	96.34 ± 0.78
Dissolved CCB content (%)	51.44 ± 4.11	1.61 ± 0.12

[a] determined at 25 °C.

3.2. *In Vitro Hemolytic Activity*

The % hemolysis of CCB/RMβCD and CCB/γCD MS is depicted in Figure 1 and can be regarded in a dose-dependent manner. A higher % hemolysis was observed in CCB/RMβCD eye drop MS compared to that in CCB/γCD eye drop MS. It was observed that the hemolysis of CCB/RMβCD MS (11.1 ± 0.3%) was two times higher than that of CCB/γCD MS (4.9 ± 0.2%) at a CCB concentration of 1000 μg/mL. At this CCB concentration, RMβCD was used at a concentration of 1.5% (*w*/*v*), while γCD was used at a concentration of 2% (*w*/*v*).

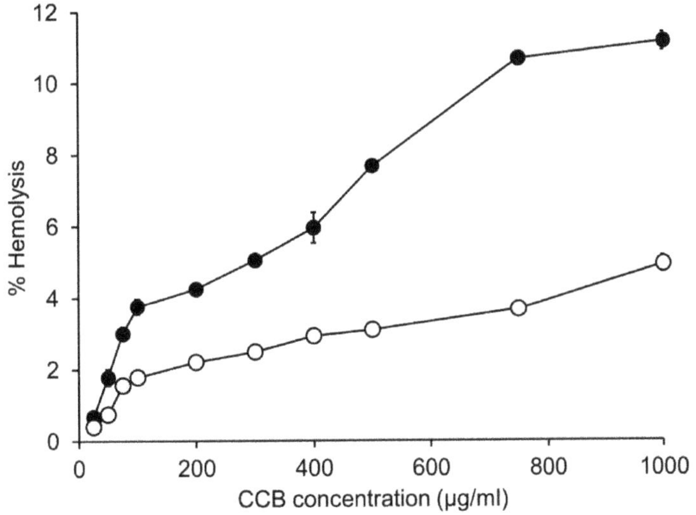

Figure 1. In vitro hemolytic study of sheep red blood cells at the various concentrations of CCB in eye drop MS: CCB/RMβCD MS (•), CCB/γCD MS (○). Data are presented as mean ± S.D., *n* = 3. Note that the error bars are smaller than the symbols' sizes.

Based on previous investigations of in vitro permeation of CCB in eye drop MS through semipermeable and scleral membranes, the permeation flux of CCB from CCB/RMβCD eye drop MS was 29 and 50 times higher than from CCB/γCD eye drop MS, respectively. This difference was attributed to the higher dissolved fraction of CCB in CCB/RMβCD MS, which contributed to drug release regulation and a greater likelihood of binding with the RBC membrane, resulting in increased toxicity. In fact, RMβCD is a lipophilic CD and has a strong affinity to cholesterol. Therefore, it has the ability to extract cholesterol from blood cell membranes, leading to hemolysis even at low concentrations [32].

3.3. Hen's Egg Test-Chorioallantoic Membrane (HET-CAM)

The HET-CAM test is an alternative test to the Draize test, which is used to evaluate the potential eye irritancy of ocular formulations [33]. The IS values of the CCB/CD eye drop MS were evaluated and compared with those of the positive and negative controls. This HET-CAM experiment can be considered valid because the positive control exhibited an IS value of 17.0 ± 0.0 (Figure 2b), indicating severe irritation, while the negative control showed an IS of 0, demonstrating no irritation (Figure 2a). Applying CCB/RMβCD MS and CCB/γCD MS did not produce any visible signs of irritation or vascular damage, indicating that the developed CCB eye drop MS were safe for ocular drug delivery (Figure 2c,d). Therefore, both CCB eye drop MS were considered suitable for further in vitro cytotoxicity assays.

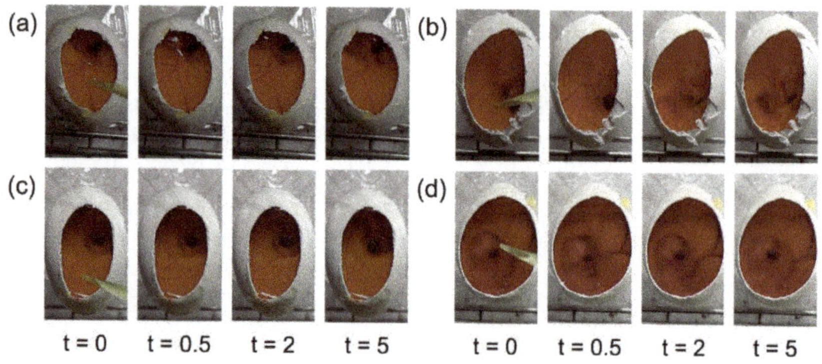

Figure 2. Photographs of HET-CAM at 0, 0.5, 2 and 5 min postinstillation at room temperature: (**a**) 0.9% NaCl (negative control); (**b**) 0.1 M NaOH (positive control); (**c**) CCB/RMβCD MS; and (**d**) CCB/γCD MS.

3.4. Short-Time Exposure (STE) Test

The STE test was conducted to assess the cytotoxicity of CCB eye drop MS and to provide eye irritation information similar to that provided by the Draize test conducted on rabbits [19]. Table 2 displays the %CV of SIRC cells after 5 min exposure to 5% and 0.05% CCB eye drop MS, and the scores represent the degree of eye discomfort. The overall score for ocular irritation potential associated with CCB eye drop MS was found to be 1. This indicates that treatment with both CCB eye drop MS and their respective blanks resulted in % CV exceeding 80%. Based on these results, both CCB/CD eye drop MS were classified as mild irritants and considered suitable for ocular drug delivery.

Table 2. Scores obtained from the STE test of CCB eye drop MS (mean ± S.D., n = 4).

Concentrations of Test Samples	Test Samples	%CV of SIRC Cells	Criteria for Scoring	Obtained Scores
(I) 5%	Blank RMβCD MS	92.95 ± 1.70		0
	Blank γCD MS	94.51 ± 2.76	If CV > 70%: scored = 0	0
	CCB/RMβCD MS	77.96 ± 4.57	If CV ≤ 70%: scored = 1	0
	CCB/γCD MS	84.88 ± 3.15		0
(II) 0.05%	Blank RMβCD MS	99.30 ± 1.29		1
	Blank γCD MS	99.68 ± 1.00	If CV > 70%: scored = 1	1
	CCB/RMβCD MS	89.74 ± 2.21	If CV ≤ 70%: scored = 2	1
	CCB/γCD MS	91.22 ± 1.41		1
Total score (I and II)				
Blank RMβCD MS				1
Blank γCD MS				1
CCB/RMβCD MS				1
CCB/γCD MS				1

3.5. Cell Viability (CV) Test

The in vitro cytotoxicity of CCB/RMβCD MS and CCB/γCD MS on the ARPE-19 cells was further determined using the MTT assay, which was considered cytotoxic when % CV was less than 70% [34,35]. Both CCB/CD eye drop MS and their respective blanks were incubated with ARPE-19 cells at concentrations ranging from 12.5 to 500 μg/mL for 24 h. In all cases, CCB eye drop MS exhibited slightly higher cytotoxicity than their respective blanks. Additionally, the CCB/γCD MS showed lower toxicity compared to CCB/RMβCD MS. CCB/RMβCD MS showed a cytotoxic effect to ARPE-19 cells, with % CV falling below 70% at a CCB concentration of 250 μg/mL, whereas CCB/γCD MS exhibited toxicity only at a CCB concentration of 500 μg/mL (two-fold concentration) (Figure 3). On the other hand, according to the CD concentrations in both drug-free and CCB/CD MS conditions, RMβCD at the concentration of 0.375% (*w*/*v*) and γCD at the concentration of 1% (*w*/*v*) were toxic to ARPE-19 cells. It was confirmed that the lipophilic nature of RMβCD can interact with the cell membrane and induce cell death, consistent with the in vitro hemolysis assay results. From these resulting data, CCB eye drop MS at 100 μg/mL was selected as a safe concentration for further drug efficacy studies.

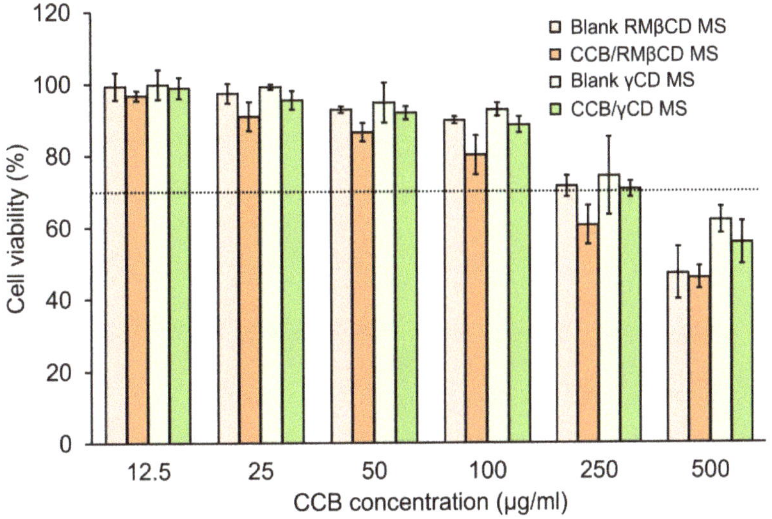

Figure 3. Viability of ARPE-19 cells after 24 h incubation with CCB/RMβCD MS, CCB/γCD MS and their respective blanks. Data are presented as mean ± S.D., *n* = 3.

3.6. Western Blotting Assay and Real-Time Polymerase Chain Reaction (RT-PCR)

The ARPE-19 cells were subjected to hypoxia with $CoCl_2$ for 24 h and then incubated with CCB/CD eye drop MS, their respective blanks, or CCB in PBS. The protein levels and VEGF-A mRNA were examined in the cells using western blot and RT-PCR assays. Pierce et al. (1995) [36] demonstrated that VEGF-A mRNA levels, followed by VEGF protein, increase in a mouse model with relative retinal hypoxia. In Figure 4A, the variation in β-actin band intensity is likely due to the membrane stripping process, which was carried out after VEGF protein detection and subsequent re-probing of the membrane for β-actin, potentially resulting in some protein loss and variable band intensities. However, each sample contained an equal total protein content (100 μg/well) loaded into the wells before running gel electrophoresis, and the quantitative protein expression calculations were determined based on relative protein intensities normalized to the control. In Figure 4B, we found that CCB suspended in PBS had a slight effect on VEGF-A levels, possibly due to the low aqueous solubility of CCB. Surprisingly, drug-free CD-based MS exhibited a lowering effect on VEGF-A protein levels after treatment. In these drug-free CD-based

MS, the concentration of γCD was 0.2% (*w*/*v*), while RMβCD was present at 0.15% (*w*/*v*). Therefore, we speculate that the excipients in eye drop formulations partially suppress hypoxia-induced VEGF expression in ARPE-19 cells. There is a report demonstrating that the injection of sodium hyaluronate inhibited the expression of vascular endothelial growth factor receptor-2 (VEGFR-2), but it did not have any impact on reducing the expression of VEGF mRNA in cartilage [37]. Additionally, the incorporation of CCB in these CD-based eye drop formulations significantly suppressed VEGF-A expression ($p < 0.05$). Sun et al. (2017) [38] investigated the signaling mechanism involved in regulating the hypoxia-induced expression of HIF-1α and VEGF through the PI3K/AKT pathway in RPE cells and found that CCB treatment suppressed the activation of this pathway and diminished the protein levels of HIF-1α and VEGF.

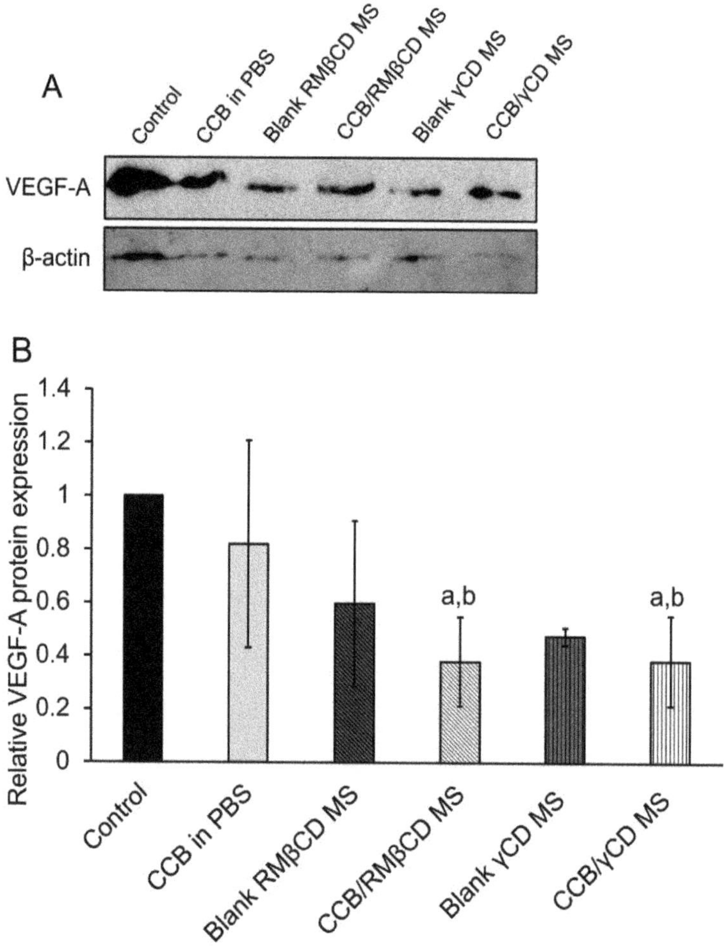

Figure 4. Western blot analysis of VEGF-A protein levels (**A**). β-actin was used as a loading control. Densitometry analysis of VEGF-A protein levels at 100 μg/mL CCB (**B**). Data are presented as mean ± S.D., $n = 3$. [a]: $p < 0.05$ compared with the values of hypoxic control group and [b]: $p < 0.05$ compared with the values of CCB in PBS group.

The VEGF-A mRNA levels after treatment with CCB eye drop MS were observed by RT-PCR. In comparison to CCB suspended in PBS, significant suppression of VEGF-A mRNA levels in both CCB/CD eye drop MS ($p < 0.05$, Figure 5) was observed. This reduction can be attributed to the high CCB loading and the CCB/CD nanoaggregates, which provide better intracellular uptake than free CCB in PBS. There was an insignificant difference in anti-VEGF efficacy between these two CCB/CD eye drop MS ($p > 0.05$). Therefore, CCB/CD eye drop MS has the potential to deliver CCB to the retina for AMD and DR treatment. Based on the results of the cytotoxicity studies, CCB/γCD MS exhibited less hemolytic activity and lower cytotoxicity to the ARPE-19 cells compared with CCB/RMβCD MS, and thus, it was selected for further investigation.

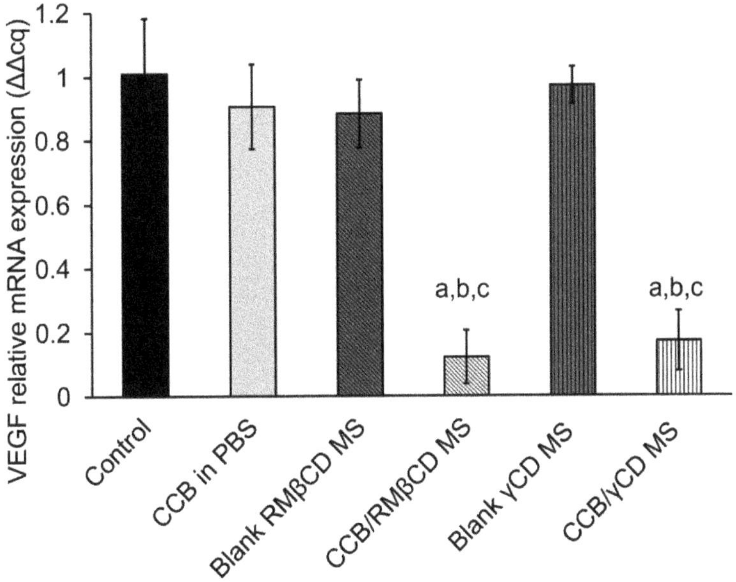

Figure 5. Expression of VEGF-A mRNA in hypoxic ARPE-19 cells. VEGF mRNA levels were determined by RT-PCR at 100 μg/mL CCB. Data are presented as mean ± SD, $n = 3$. ^{a}: $p < 0.05$ compared with the values of hypoxic control group, ^{b}: $p < 0.05$ compared with the values of CCB in PBS group, and ^{c}: $p < 0.05$ compared with their respective blank MS group.

3.7. Ex Vivo Transscleral Diffusion Studies

Figure 6 displays the results of ex vivo transscleral diffusion of CCB (CCB in PBS or CCB/γCD MS) through the porcine sclera. After 1 h, the amount of CCB diffused from CCB/γCD MS into sclera tissue was found to be 11.31 ± 4.11 μg/mL, while in the case of CCB in PBS, it was undetected. The diffusion of CCB was observed to increase over time in the cases of both CCB/γCD MS and CCB in PBS. After 4 h, CCB/γCD MS showed a significantly higher amount of CCB retained in sclera tissue (112.47 ± 37.27 μg/mL) compared to CCB in PBS (1.51 ± 0.29 μg/mL) ($p < 0.05$). This improvement (approximately 74 times higher than CCB in PBS) might be attributed to (1) increasing the aqueous solubility of CCB through the CCB/γCD inclusion complex; (2) the addition of HA, a mucoadhesive polymer, which adheres to the sclera membrane surface and provides sustained CCB release; and (3) increasing the contact area through the formation of nano and small microparticles (i.e., increasing the surface area via particle size reduction), resulting in an increased quantity of CCB deposited in the deeper scleral tissues.

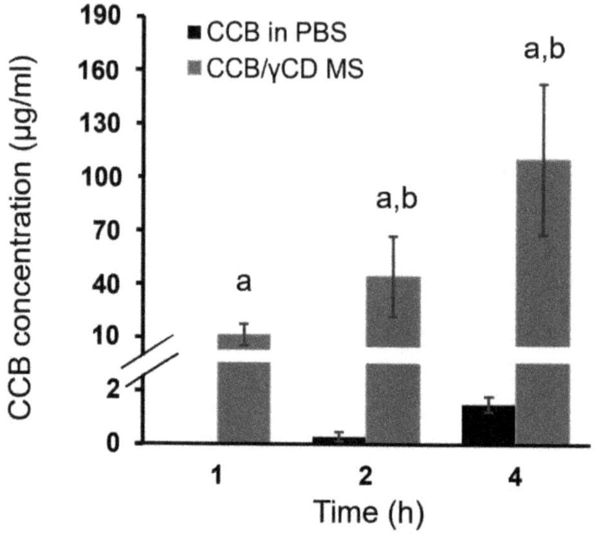

Figure 6. Ex vivo transscleral diffusion of CCB suspended in PBS and CCB from CCB/γCD MS through the porcine sclera. Data are presented as mean ± SD, n = 3–4; [a]: $p < 0.05$ compared with the values of CCB in PBS, and [b]: $p < 0.05$ compared with the values in different time intervals.

4. Conclusions

This study confirmed that our developed CCB/CD eye drop MS can be reproducible for manufacturing with reliable physicochemical characteristics. Both CCB/RMβCD MS and CCB/γCD MS are well tolerated by the eyes, with low hemolytic activity, cytocompatibility with corneal and retinal cell lines, and no signs of irritation. Due to the favorable toxicological profiles of γCD, CCB in γCD-based MS exhibited lower toxicity than the eye drops containing RMβCD. Regarding our CD-based technology, the diffusion of CCB into scleral tissue was successfully achieved. Our CCB/CD eye drop MS demonstrates that CCB has anti-VEGF efficacy, effectively reducing VEGF protein and mRNA levels in hypoxic RPE cells. Based on these findings, it is reasonable to propose that our developed eye drop MS containing ternary CCB/CD/HA complexes has promising properties for the potential treatment of AMD and DR, and this warrants further investigation through in vivo studies.

Author Contributions: Conceptualization, P.J.; investigation, H.M.S.H.S., R.A., T.T., T.W., P.D.M. and H.M.H.; resources, T.W., P.J. and R.A.; writing—original draft preparation, H.M.S.H.S., H.M.H., T.T. and P.J.; writing—review and editing, P.J., R.A. and T.L.; supervision, T.L. All authors have read and agreed to the published version of the manuscript.

Funding: This research was funded by the Thailand Science Research and Innovation Fund Chulalongkorn University; the Asahi Glass Foundation (Grant number RES_67_000_3300_000); the Thammasat University Research Unit in Drug, Health Product Development and Application (DHP-DA) (Project ID. 6305001); the Second Century Fund (C2F) of Chulalongkorn University; and the Office of Academic Affairs, Chulalongkorn University.

Institutional Review Board Statement: Not applicable.

Informed Consent Statement: Not applicable.

Data Availability Statement: Data are contained within the article.

Conflicts of Interest: The authors declare no conflict of interest.

References

1. Colijn, J.M.; Buitendijk, G.H.S.; Prokofyeva, E.; Alves, D.; Cachulo, M.L.; Khawaja, A.P.; Cougnard-Gregoire, A.; Merle, B.M.J.; Korb, C.; Erke, M.G.; et al. Prevalence of age-related macular degeneration in europe: The past and the future. *Ophthalmology* **2017**, *124*, 1753–1763. [CrossRef] [PubMed]
2. Zheng, Y.; He, M.; Congdon, N. The worldwide epidemic of diabetic retinopathy. *Indian J. Ophthalmol.* **2012**, *60*, 428. [PubMed]
3. Wong, W.L.; Su, X.; Li, X.; Cheung, C.M.G.; Klein, R.; Cheng, C.-Y.; Wong, T.Y. Global prevalence of age-related macular degeneration and disease burden projection for 2020 and 2040: A systematic review and meta-analysis. *Lancet Glob. Health* **2014**, *2*, e106–e116. [CrossRef] [PubMed]
4. Amrite, A.; Pugazhenthi, V.; Cheruvu, N.; Kompella, U. Delivery of celecoxib for treating diseases of the eye: Influence of pigment and diabetes. *Expert Opin. Drug Deliv.* **2010**, *7*, 631–645. [CrossRef] [PubMed]
5. Kliffen, M.; Sharma, H.S.; Mooy, C.M.; Kerkvliet, S.; de Jong, P.T. Increased expression of angiogenic growth factors in age-related maculopathy. *Br. J. Ophthalmol.* **1997**, *81*, 154–162. [CrossRef]
6. Adamis, A.P.; Miller, J.W.; Bernal, M.-T.; D'Amico, D.J.; Folkman, J.; Yeo, T.-K.; Yeo, K.-T. Increased vascular endothelial growth factor levels in the vitreous of eyes with proliferative diabetic retinopathy. *Am. J. Ophthalmol.* **1994**, *118*, 445–450. [CrossRef]
7. Freund, K.B.; Yannuzzi, L.A.; Sorenson, J.A. Age-related macular degeneration and choroidal neovascularization. *Am. J. Ophthalmol.* **1993**, *115*, 786–791. [CrossRef]
8. Ciulla, T.A.; Amador, A.G.; Zinman, B. Diabetic retinopathy and diabetic macular edema: Pathophysiology, screening, and novel therapies. *Diabetes Care* **2003**, *26*, 2653–2664. [CrossRef]
9. Hughes, P.M.; Olejnik, O.; Chang-Lin, J.-E.; Wilson, C.G. Topical and systemic drug delivery to the posterior segments. *Adv. Drug Deliv. Rev.* **2005**, *57*, 2010–2032. [CrossRef]
10. Lu, L.; Jiang, Y.; Jaganathan, R.; Hao, Y. Current advances in pharmacotherapy and technology for diabetic retinopathy: A systematic review. *J. Ophthalmol.* **2018**, *2018*, 1694187.
11. Rusciano, D.; Bagnoli, P. Pharmacotherapy and nutritional supplements for neovascular eye diseases. *Medicina* **2023**, *59*, 1334. [CrossRef] [PubMed]
12. Ayalasomayajula, S.P.; Kompella, U.B. Celecoxib, a selective cyclooxygenase-2 inhibitor, inhibits retinal vascular endothelial growth factor expression and vascular leakage in a streptozotocin-induced diabetic rat model. *Eur. J. Pharmacol.* **2003**, *458*, 283–289. [CrossRef] [PubMed]
13. Raghava, S.; Hammond, M.; Kompella, U.B. Periocular routes for retinal drug delivery. *Expert Opin. Drug Deliv.* **2004**, *1*, 99–114. [CrossRef] [PubMed]
14. Lee, S.-B.; Geroski, D.H.; Prausnitz, M.R.; Edelhauser, H.F. Drug delivery through the sclera: Effects of thickness, hydration, and sustained release systems. *Exp. Eye Res.* **2004**, *78*, 599–607. [CrossRef] [PubMed]
15. Jansook, P.; Kulsirachote, P.; Loftsson, T. Cyclodextrin solubilization of celecoxib: Solid and solution state characterization. *J. Incl. Phenom. Macrocycl. Chem.* **2018**, *90*, 75–88. [CrossRef]
16. Jansook, P.; Kulsirachote, P.; Asasutjarit, R.; Loftsson, T. Development of celecoxib eye drop solution and microsuspension: A comparative investigation of binary and ternary cyclodextrin complexes. *Carbohydr. Polym.* **2019**, *225*, 115209. [CrossRef] [PubMed]
17. Jansook, P.; Maw, P.D.; Soe, H.M.S.H.; Chuangchunsong, R.; Saiborisuth, K.; Payonitikarn, N.; Autthateinchai, R.; Pruksakorn, P. Development of amphotericin B nanosuspensions for fungal keratitis therapy: Effect of self-assembled γ-cyclodextrin. *J. Pharm. Investig.* **2020**, *50*, 513–525. [CrossRef]
18. Interagency Coordinating Committee on the Validation of Alternative Methods (ICCVAM). *ICCVAM-Recommended Test Method Protocol: Hen's Egg Test—Chorioallantoic Membrane (HET-CAM) Test Method*; Tech. Rep. 10-7553; NIH Publication: Research Triangle Park, NC, USA, 2010.
19. Luepke, N. Hen's egg chorioallantoic membrane test for irritation potential. *Food Chem. Toxicol.* **1985**, *23*, 287–291. [CrossRef]
20. Takahashi, Y.; Koike, M.; Honda, H.; Ito, Y.; Sakaguchi, H.; Suzuki, H.; Nishiyama, N. Development of the short time exposure (STE) test: An in vitro eye irritation test using SIRC cells. *Toxicol. In Vitro* **2008**, *22*, 760–770. [CrossRef]
21. Manconi, M.; Manca, M.L.; Valenti, D.; Escribano, E.; Hillaireau, H.; Fadda, A.M.; Fattal, E. Chitosan and hyaluronan coated liposomes for pulmonary administration of curcumin. *Int. J. Pharm.* **2017**, *525*, 203–210. [CrossRef]
22. Asasutjarit, R.; Managit, C.; Phanaksri, T.; Treesuppharat, W.; Fuongfuchat, A. Formulation development and in vitro evaluation of transferrin-conjugated liposomes as a carrier of ganciclovir targeting the retina. *Int. J. Pharm.* **2020**, *577*, 119084. [CrossRef] [PubMed]
23. Ford, K.M.; Saint-Geniez, M.; Walshe, T.; Zahr, A.; D'Amore, P.A. Expression and role of VEGF in the adult retinal pigment epithelium. *Investig. Ophthalmol. Vis. Sci.* **2011**, *52*, 9478–9487. [CrossRef] [PubMed]
24. Cervellati, F.; Cervellati, C.; Romani, A.; Cremonini, E.; Sticozzi, C.; Belmonte, G.; Pessina, F.; Valacchi, G. Hypoxia induces cell damage via oxidative stress in retinal epithelial cells. *Free Radic. Res.* **2014**, *48*, 303–312. [CrossRef] [PubMed]
25. Puddu, A.; Sanguineti, R.; Traverso, C.E.; Viviani, G.L.; Nicolò, M. Response to anti-VEGF-A treatment of retinal pigment epithelial cells in vitro. *Eur. J. Ophthalmol.* **2016**, *26*, 425–430. [CrossRef] [PubMed]
26. Soe, H.M.S.H.; Maw, P.D.; Asasutjarit, R.; Loftsson, T.; Jansook, P. Tacrolimus/hydroxypropyl-β-cyclodextrin-loaded nanoemulsions stabilized by Zein-Soluplus® nanoparticles for retinal diseases. *J. Drug Deliv. Sci. Technol.* **2023**, *88*, 104936. [CrossRef]
27. Yuan, J.S.; Reed, A.; Chen, F.; Stewart, C.N. Statistical analysis of real-time PCR data. *BMC Bioinform.* **2006**, *7*, 85. [CrossRef]

28. Kramer, I.; Haber, M.; Duis, A. Requirements concerning antiseptics for periorbital, orbital and intraorbital application: Formulation requirements for the ophthalmic use of antiseptics. In *Antiseptic Prophylaxis and Therapy in Ocular Infections*; Kramer, A., Behrens-Baumann, W., Eds.; Karger Publishers Inc.: Basel, Switzerland, 2002; pp. 85–116.
29. Aldrich, D.S.; Bach, C.M.; Brown, W.; Chambers, W.; Fleitman, J.; Hunt, D.; Marques, M.R.C.; Mille, Y.; Mitra, A.K.; Platzer, S.M.; et al. Ophthalmic Preparations. 2003. Available online: http://www.triphasepharmasolutions.com/Resources/USP%2520Ophthalmic%2520Preparations.pdf (accessed on 18 January 2023).
30. Nagyová, B.; Tiffany, J.M. Components responsible for the surface tension of human tears. *Curr. Eye Res.* **1999**, *19*, 4–11. [CrossRef]
31. Hotujac Grgurević, M.; Juretić, M.; Hafner, A.; Lovrić, J.; Pepić, I. Tear fluid-eye drops compatibility assessment using surface tension. *Drug Dev. Ind. Pharm.* **2017**, *43*, 275–282. [CrossRef]
32. Szejtli, J. Past, present and futute of cyclodextrin research. *Pure Appl. Chem.* **2004**, *76*, 1825–1845. [CrossRef]
33. McKenzie, B.; Kay, G.; Matthews, K.H.; Knott, R.M.; Cairns, D. The hen's egg chorioallantoic membrane (HET-CAM) test to predict the ophthalmic irritation potential of a cysteamine-containing gel: Quantification using Photoshop® and ImageJ. *Int. J. Pharm.* **2015**, *490*, 1–8. [CrossRef]
34. Romagna, G.; Allifranchini, E.; Bocchietto, E.; Todeschi, S.; Esposito, M.; Farsalinos, K.E. Cytotoxicity evaluation of electronic cigarette vapor extract on cultured mammalian fibroblasts (ClearStream-LIFE): Comparison with tobacco cigarette smoke extract. *Inhal. Toxicol.* **2013**, *25*, 354–361. [CrossRef] [PubMed]
35. Yun, J.-W.; Hailian, Q.; Na, Y.; Kang, B.-C.; Yoon, J.-H.; Cho, E.-Y.; Lee, M.; Kim, D.-E.; Bae, S.; Seok, S.H.; et al. Exploration and comparison of in vitro eye irritation tests with the ISO standard in vivo rabbit test for the evaluation of the ocular irritancy of contact lenses. *Toxicol. In Vitro* **2016**, *37*, 79–87. [CrossRef] [PubMed]
36. Pierce, E.A.; Avery, R.L.; Foley, E.D.; Aiello, L.P.; Smith, L.E. Vascular endothelial growth factor/vascular permeability factor expression in a mouse model of retinal neovascularization. *Proc. Natl. Acad. Sci. USA* **1995**, *92*, 905–909. [CrossRef] [PubMed]
37. Ilochonwu, B.C.; Urtti, A.; Hennink, W.E.; Vermonden, T. Intravitreal hydrogels for sustained release of therapeutic proteins. *J. Control. Release* **2020**, *326*, 419–441. [CrossRef]
38. Sun, Y.-Z.; Cai, N.; Liu, N.-N. Celecoxib Down-Regulates the hypoxia-induced expression of HIF-1α and VEGF through the PI3K/AKT pathway in retinal pigment epithelial cells. *Cell. Physiol. Biochem.* **2017**, *44*, 1640–1650. [CrossRef]

pharmaceutics

MDPI

Article

A Rapid Screening Platform for Simultaneous Evaluation of Biodegradation and Therapeutic Release of an Ocular Hydrogel

Brandon Ho [1,2], Chau-Minh Phan [1,2,*], Piyush Garg [1], Parvin Shokrollahi [1] and Lyndon Jones [1,2]

1 Centre for Ocular Research & Education (CORE), School of Optometry & Vision Science, University of Waterloo, 200 University Avenue West, Waterloo, ON N2L 3G1, Canada; brandon.ho@uwaterloo.ca (B.H.); piyush.garg@uwaterloo.ca (P.G.); p.shokrollahi@uwaterloo.ca (P.S.); lyndon.jones@uwaterloo.ca (L.J.)
2 Centre for Eye and Vision Research (CEVR), 17W Hong Kong Science Park, Hong Kong
* Correspondence: c2phan@uwaterloo.ca

Abstract: This study attempts to address the challenge of accurately measuring the degradation of biodegradable hydrogels, which are frequently employed in drug delivery for controlled and sustained release. The traditional method utilizes a mass-loss approach, which is cumbersome and time consuming. The aim of this study was to develop an innovative screening platform using a millifluidic device coupled with automated image analysis to measure the degradation of Gelatin methacrylate (GelMA) and the subsequent release of an entrapped wetting agent, polyvinyl alcohol (PVA). Gel samples were placed within circular wells on a custom millifluidic chip and stained with a red dye for enhanced visualization. A camera module captured time-lapse images of the gels throughout their degradation. An image-analysis algorithm was used to translate the image data into degradation rates. Simultaneously, the eluate from the chip was collected to quantify the amount of GelMA degraded and PVA released at various time points. The visual method was validated by comparing it with the mass-loss approach ($R = 0.91$), as well as the amount of GelMA eluted ($R = 0.97$). The degradation of the GelMA gels was also facilitated with matrix metalloproteinases 9. Notably, as the gels degraded, there was an increase in the amount of PVA released. Overall, these results support the use of the screening platform to assess hydrogel degradation and the subsequent release of entrapped therapeutic compounds.

Keywords: millifluidics; image analysis; biodegradation; hydrogels; ocular drug delivery

Citation: Ho, B.; Phan, C.-M.; Garg, P.; Shokrollahi, P.; Jones, L. A Rapid Screening Platform for Simultaneous Evaluation of Biodegradation and Therapeutic Release of an Ocular Hydrogel. *Pharmaceutics* **2023**, *15*, 2625. https://doi.org/10.3390/pharmaceutics15112625

Academic Editors: Rosario Pignatello, Hugo Almeida, Carmelo Puglia and Debora Santonocito

Received: 31 October 2023
Revised: 10 November 2023
Accepted: 13 November 2023
Published: 15 November 2023

1. Introduction

Despite advancements in ocular drug delivery, the eye's complex physiological barriers continue to pose challenges for sustained and controlled drug release. Drugs and therapeutics administered topically have very low bioavailability due to tear-fluid turnover, nonspecific absorption and blinking [1–3]. As a result, novel therapeutic approaches for topical applications such as nanoparticles, liposomes, gels and novel hydrogels are being developed. These technologies aim to increase the drug retention time, overcome ocular barriers and improve bioavailability [4–8].

Among the novel drug-delivery methods are biodegradable hydrogels, which are designed to release entrapped drugs or therapeutics as the gel degrades in situ. Studies have demonstrated that drugs released from degradable materials can be controlled and sustained over several days [9–12]. In comparison to other drug-delivery approaches, the release of therapeutics from degradable materials, assuming that the therapeutic is entrapped, largely depends on the degradation rate rather than just passive diffusion [9]. Consequently, it is possible to achieve drug-release kinetics by using biodegradable hydrogels that approach the ideal zero-order release [11,12].

The primary challenge in developing biodegradable hydrogels for drug delivery lies in accurately measuring their degradation over time, while also simultaneously being able to evaluate the drug-release kinetics. Standard approaches to assess the biodegradation of hydrogels are either by volume or mass loss, the latter of which is more common [13–15]. When assessing mass loss, researchers measure the weight of the dried gel at a specified time point [14,15]. This procedure is exceptionally cumbersome and time consuming because a dried gel from one time point cannot be reused for subsequent measurements. Moreover, the generated dataset would contain significant variability because the same gels cannot be assessed repeatedly over time. Furthermore, the mass-loss method of measuring degradation would not allow researchers to simultaneously monitor drug release.

To properly evaluate the biodegradation of an ocular device or its drug-release kinetics, it is essential to also simulate key factors of the ocular environment, such as the ocular temperature, tear flow and low tear volume. However, most drug-release kinetics for ocular drug delivery are typically performed in a static vial at room temperature [16,17]. This setup may not simulate the eye's dynamic biological conditions, especially the low tear volume or flow. Consequently, the results obtained by using these simple models might not reflect the release kinetics or biodegradation profile expected in the actual in vivo situation [18].

Millifluidic or microfluidic devices can potentially offer a more representative simulation environment of the eye by mimicking low tear volume and flow. These devices have been used in lab-on-a-chip and even organ-on-a-chip systems to emulate various human organs [19,20]. Notably, these technologies have already been implemented in drug-discovery and -delivery applications [21–24]. Beyond a more accurate biological simulation, these devices also significantly reduce reagent consumption while providing an increased assay throughput. The main barrier to adopting these devices for research has been their high cost. However, with the advancements in new fabrication technologies such as 3D printing and laser lithography, producing these devices, especially for customized chip and tailored assays, has become more cost effective [25,26].

Thus, the application of millifluidic and microfluidic devices could help develop a screening system to measure the degradation rate of biodegradable hydrogels and the subsequent drug or therapeutic release. Gelatin methacrylate (GelMA) was chosen as the biodegradable hydrogel in this study due to its broad applications in drug delivery [27,28]. Its biodegradation can be accelerated by matrix metalloproteinases (MMPs), the enzymes present in the tear film [29,30]. The degradation rate of GelMA can be controlled by modulating the levels of MMPs to which the gel is exposed. Polyvinyl alcohol (PVA) was selected as the model therapeutic agent contained within the biodegradable gel given its large molecular size, which ensures its entrapment within the gel matrix. Additionally, PVA is also used commonly as an ocular lubricant [31,32]. The aim of this study was to develop a screening platform by using a custom millifluidic device coupled with automated imaging analysis to simultaneously monitor both GelMA degradation and the subsequent release of PVA.

2. Materials and Methods

2.1. *Preparation of GelMA*

GelMA was prepared according to previously reported methods [33]. In brief, type A gelatin from porcine skin (10% *w*/*v*, Sigma-Aldrich, St. Louis, MO, USA) was reacted with methacrylic anhydride (1% *v*/*v*, Sigma-Aldrich, St. Louis, MO, USA) in a carbonate bicarbonate (CB) buffer (12.5 mM sodium bicarbonate, 87.5 mM sodium carbonate anhydrous, pH 9.4) at 50 °C for 1 h. This substitution reaction was stopped by adding acetic acid to a final concentration of 0.15% (*v*/*v*). The resulting product was dialyzed in 12–14 kDa dialysis tubes (Sigma-Aldrich, St. Louis, MO, USA) in deionized water for 24 h. Following the dialysis step, the solution was freeze-dried and then stored at −80 °C until use.

2.2. *Preparation of GelMA-PVA Hydrogels*

The freeze-dried GelMA was reconstituted in a solution of PBS to 10% *w*/*v* and then UV crosslinked by using a photoinitiator (lithium phenyl-2,4,6-trimethylbenzoylphosphinate

(LAP)). The GelMA hydrogels were cast into a disc shape with a radius of 2 mm and a thickness of 1 mm. A similar method was used to fabricate the GelMA-PVA hydrogels, which contained a 7.5% concentration of PVA. GelMA (20% *w*/*v*) was added to a LAP (1.2% *w*/*v*) solution prepared in PBS. A PVA (15% *w*/*v*) solution was prepared in PBS and heated for complete dissolution (~37 °C). The two solutions were added in equal amounts to make the GelMA/PVA prepolymer solution, which comprised GelMA (10%), PVA (7.5%) and LAP (0.6%). This prepolymer solution was then used to make polymer discs.

2.3. Biodegradation of GelMA with MMP9 by Mass Loss in a Vial

The GelMA hydrogel discs were dried by briefly dabbing the biomaterial with lens paper, and their initial weights were measured on a scale and recorded for t = 0. The hydrogel discs were then added to 1.7 mL microcentrifuge tubes which contained 1 mL of varying MMP9 (Gibco, Billings, MT, USA) concentrations (0, 25, 50, 100 and 200 µg/mL) in 1× phosphate buffered saline (PBS). The samples were incubated at 37 °C with gentle agitation. At t = 0, 4, 8, 12, 16 and 24 h, the samples were removed from the solution, dried and the dried weight was recorded.

2.4. Biodegradation of GelMA with MMP9 Using a Custom-Designed Millifluidic Device System

A custom-designed polydimethyl siloxane (PDMS) millifluidic device was provided by EyesoBio Inc. (Waterloo, ON, Canada). The device contains a series of microfluidic channels (2 mm width and 50 mm length) with a circular chamber (5 mm radius and 2 mm height) at the center for placing the samples (refer to Figure 1). Since GelMA is relatively transparent, the GelMA hydrogel discs were stained with a red dye solution (0.1% *v*/*v*, ClubHouse red food coloring, McCormick & Company, Baltimore, MD, USA) in 1× PBS to help visualize the degradation process. The entire device was connected by using Teflon tubing (1/16″ inner diameter × 1/32″ wall Tygon Tubing, Saint Gobain Performance Plastics, Courbevoie, France) with the inlet tubes connected to a 20 mL glass source-media reservoir (WHEATON® vials, Sigma-Aldrich DWK986541, St. Louis, MO, USA). The outlet tubes were connected to a peristaltic pump (Darwin Microfluidics BT100-1L, Paris, France). An overview of the experimental setup is shown in Figure 1.

Different concentrations of the MMP9 enzyme were prepared in 1× PBS (0, 50, 100 and 200 µg/mL) with 0.1% (*v*/*v*) red dye and were added to the source-media reservoirs. The entire experimental setup was placed inside a custom-designed acrylic chamber with temperature and humidity control equilibrated to 37 °C for 30 min prior to starting the biodegradation time course. Once equilibrated, the MMP9 solution flowed through the millifluidic device at 300 µL per minute. For comparison, using a different set of samples, the mass loss was also measured for the GelMA discs treated with the different concentrations of MMP9.

2.5. Image Analysis of Hydrogel Degradation

Images of the hydrogel biodegradation were obtained by using an iPhone 12 (Apple, Cupertino, CA, USA) running a time-lapse application (Life Lapse, Vancouver, BC, Canada), acquiring images every 60 s for the entirety of the time course (t = 20 h). Automated computational quantification of the hydrogel biodegradation was performed by using custom-written Python code (Python v3.11.3, https://www.python.org/ (accessed on 21 July 2023)). Images at each time frame were opened, and pixels in the entire image were scanned for a specific range of red color, corresponding to the hydrogel stained by the red dye. An image mask was created, such that those pixels identified as 'red' were assigned a value of 1, and all the others were assigned a value of 0. Next, the analysis pipeline distinguished between different hydrogel discs through grouping the image pixels that had a value of 1 and were near one another. Finally, the pipeline counted the number of pixels for each group (each hydrogel insert), and this was plotted over time. The values for the percentage (%) change in the GelMA hydrogel discs were calculated by dividing the surface area of the GelMA (in pixels) determined at each time point by the initial surface area at the start of the experiment. All the plots related to the time-lapse quantification of hydrogel biodegradation were generated by using Python and the Seaborn library to make statistical graphics in Python.

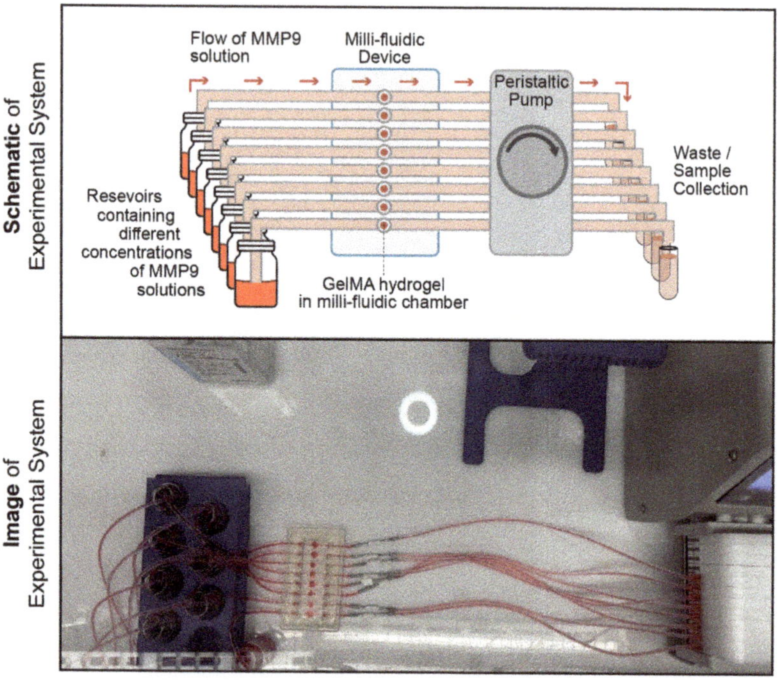

Figure 1. Setup of the millifluidic system for analyzing the biodegradation of GelMA hydrogels. A schematic diagram and photograph from a top-down view of the millifluidic system used in this study. The bottom photograph of the setup was acquired from the same fixed camera module used for all image-based biodegradation experiments. The depicted photo is thus representative of the quality (color accuracy and image resolution) of all time-lapse images in all biodegradation experiments.

2.6. Estimation of Average Biodegradation Rates

To estimate the average biodegradation rates of the hydrogel discs, the initial and final measurements of the hydrogel surface area (in counted pixels), or the time at which the insert fully degraded if the insert was no longer present by the end of the time course, was recorded. An assumption was made that the hydrogel degrades linearly to compare the approximated rates of degradation between different samples. The change in the surface area was normalized to the initial surface area of the hydrogel and divided by the time of the experiment, or the time to reach complete degradation, to obtain average rate measurements of the percent change in the hydrogel material per hour (%/h).

2.7. Release of PVA from Millifluidic Chip

All the GelMA-PVA hydrogel discs (10% GelMA, 7.5% PVA) analyzed in this study were prepared and used within 24 h. GelMA-PVA discs were placed in the circular chambers of the custom millifluidic device and treated with an MMP9 solution (0 and 200 μg/mL) using the same custom-designed experimental system described above. At t = 0, 1, 2, 3 and 17 h, 50 μL of the solution was removed from the glass reservoir and stored at 4 °C until the end of the experiment. Each sample was then used for the detection of PVA.

2.8. Detection of PVA

The detection of PVA was achieved by using previously published protocols [34,35]. In brief, a PVA-detection solution was formulated by using a solution of iodine (150 mM potassium iodide, 50 mM diiodine in deionized water, Sigma-Aldrich 221945 and 207772, St. Louis, MO, USA) and borate (64.7 mM boric acid in deionized water, Sigma-Aldrich B0394, St. Louis, MO, USA). To measure PVA in the solution, 150 µL of the PVA-detection solution was added to 50 µL of the sample in a 96-well plate and incubated at room temperature for 20 min with gentle shaking. The absorbance of the unknown samples, in addition to a set of standard samples of known PVA concentrations, prepared in PBS was then measured at 630 nm by using an Imaging Multimode Plate Reader (Cytation 5, Agilent BioTek Instruments, Winooski, VT, USA).

2.9. Quantification and Statistical Analysis

Statistical analyses were performed by using GraphPad Prism version 9.4.0 (GraphPad, La Jolla, CA, USA) and Python v3.11.3. To conduct significance tests for multiple comparisons of groups, a one-way analysis of variance (ANOVA) was used, as described in the figure legends. For linear correlations to compare the degradation profile between a conventional mass loss and the visual technique, the Pearson R correlation coefficient was used. Results with $p < 0.05$ were considered statistically significant: * $p < 0.05$, ** $p < 0.005$.

3. Results

3.1. Combined Millifluidics Imaging and Computational Analysis for Quantitative Characterization of GelMA Biodegradation

The work described here involves an experimental setup coupling a millifluidic device with a computational image-analysis pipeline that quantitatively measured the biodegradation of GelMA hydrogel discs continuously over the course of 20 h (Figure 2a). A series of time-lapse images of the GelMA biodegradation was acquired, and an image-analysis pipeline was applied (Figure 2b), which identified the image pixels that corresponded only to the GelMA material and recorded the change in the pixel area of the GelMA over time. As expected, the GelMA insert visibly degraded over time with MMP9 exposure, with complete biodegradation taking over 10 h when treated with 100 µg/mL MMP9, as seen in Figure 2c.

Two important observations were noted when utilizing the millifluidic chip. Firstly, the time to degrade GelMA was longer in these millifluidic devices compared to the GelMA degraded in a static 1 mL MMP9 solution (100 µg/mL) at the same concentration. The bulk degradation of GelMA in the static condition, with gentle agitation (50 rpm) at 37 °C, increased with greater concentrations of MMP9 and completely degraded around 8 h after treatment with the 100 µg/mL MMP9 solution (Figure 2d). In contrast, the complete degradation of the gels in the millifluidic chip took approximately 12 h in the 100 µg/mL MMP9 solution (Figure 2c). Secondly, the decrease in the GelMA disc dimensions during the hydrogel biodegradation within the device was more pronounced in the disc radius rather than the thickness (Figure 2e). This contrasts with the GelMA discs degraded by 100 µg/mL of MMP9 in a conventional microfuge tube, whereby the GelMA object is surrounded by the MMP9 solution, and an apparent reduction in the GelMA disc thickness can be observed in Figure 2f. It should be noted that the thickness of the discs within the device could not be observed during the course experiment, as images were acquired by using a top-down approach.

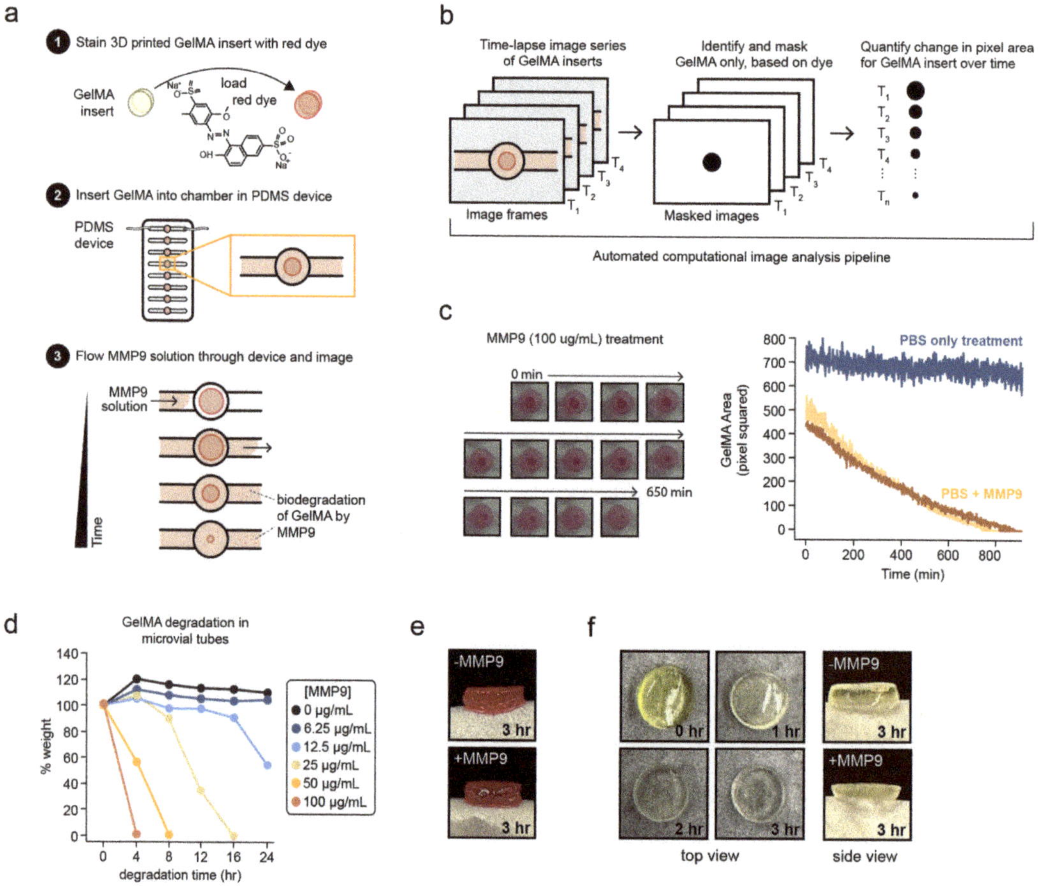

Figure 2. Time-lapse millifluidic imaging system with computational image-analysis capture kinetics of MMP9-dependent GelMA degradation. (**a**) Schematic diagram of the experimental approach to visually observe GelMA biodegradation. (**b**) Overview of the computational pipeline applied to all images acquired in the time-lapse experiments. (**c**) Representative images of stained GelMA discs within the millifluidic chamber over the course of 650 min of 100 µg/mL MMP9 treatment acquired via time-lapse imaging. Quantification of the change in GelMA disc size over time for discs with or without 100 µg/mL MMP9 in PBS (light and dark orange, and blue line traces, respectively, n = 2). (**d**) Percent of initial GelMA disc weight is plotted over time after exposure to the indicated concentrations of MMP9 in PBS. (**e**) Side view of a GelMA ocular disc after treatment with 100 µg/mL MMP9 in the millifluidic device. (**f**) Representative images (both top-down and side views) of GelMA ocular disc before and after treatment with 100 µg/mL MMP9 in a static vial.

Next, the ability of this system to accurately discern differences in the GelMA biodegradation rates was tested. The custom-designed millifluidic device could simultaneously accommodate eight samples; it provided a constant flow of seven different concentrations of the MMP9 solution and PBS as a control (Figure 3). The computational image-analysis pipeline was applied to these treated samples, and the change in the GelMA surface area over time was quantified (Figure 3a,b). There was a significant increase in the biodegradation rates with greater concentrations of MMP9 (Figure 3c–e). A similar trend was also observed when the mass-loss method was used to measure degradation for the GelMA discs in a static solution (Figure 2d).

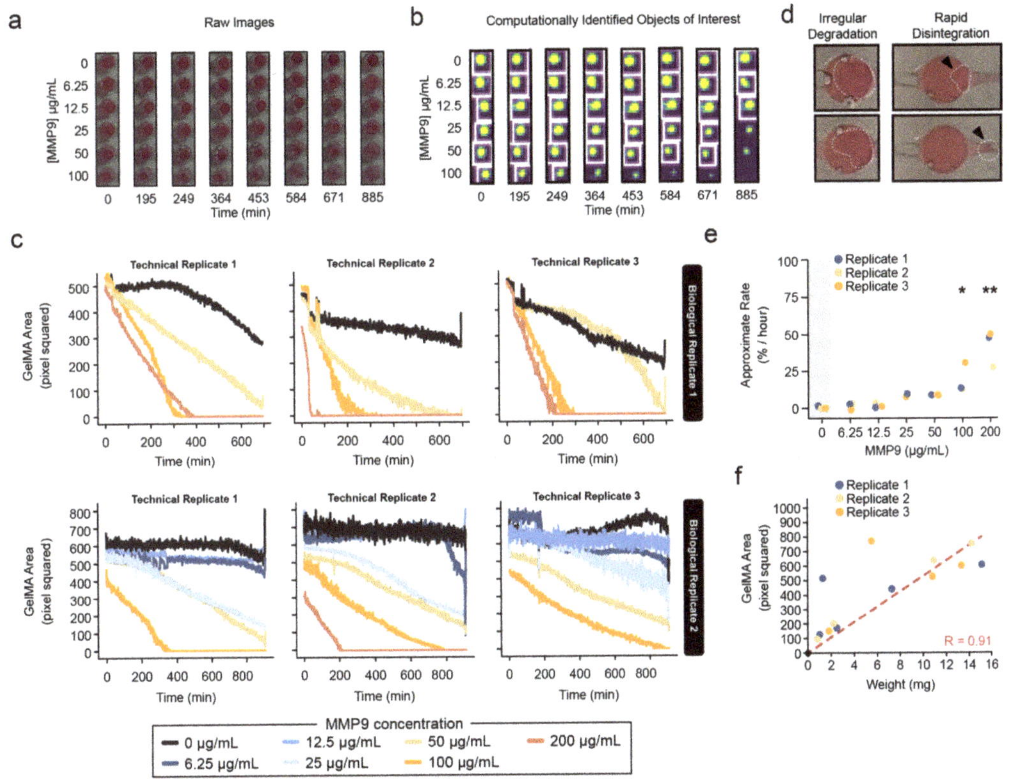

Figure 3. Computational image-analysis pipeline detects differences in GelMA biodegradation, which correlates well with conventional weight-based measurements of hydrogel biodegradation. (**a**) Representative images of GelMA inserts in custom-designed 8-chamber millifluidic devices during treatment with MMP9 over the course of 20 h. (**b**) Application of our automated custom image-analysis pipeline. Yellow indicates areas detected as stained GelMA inserts, and purple denotes areas not labeled as GelMA. (**c**) Quantification of two biological replicates (each with three technical replicates) of MMP9-dependent degradation of GelMA discs using our automated image pipeline. (**d**) Representative images of GelMA hydrogels undergoing irregular degradation or rapid disintegration during treatment with 200 µg/mL MMP9. White dotted outline indicates the location of the hydrogel, and black arrows indicate the location of GelMA biomaterial debris. (**e**) Pseudorates of GelMA biodegradation were calculated and plotted against MMP9 concentration (n = 3). Statistical significance determined by one-way ANOVA with Tukey multiple comparisons test: * $p < 0.05$, ** $p < 0.005$ (**f**) Linear correlation between the size of the GelMA discs and the weight of the same discs after being removed from the millifluidic device. Red dashed line represents the line of best fit with the Pearson correlation coefficient indicated (R).

It should be noted that very high MMP9 concentrations (>100 µg/mL) produced results with considerable variation between technical replicates (Figure 3c). In fact, at very high concentrations (200 µg/mL), the degradation was rapid and irregular. In some instances, a drastic decrease in the detectable material was observed for the GelMA, suggesting a sudden disintegration of the material rather than a gradual reduction in size that was observed in the GelMA hydrogel. Indeed, visible biodegradation debris could be seen flowing out of the device (Figure 3d). Despite these sources of variation, the overall average rates of GelMA degradation across the entire experiment generally agreed between biological replicates (Figure 3e). Most importantly, there was a very high positive agreement between the computationally measured sizes of the GelMA hydrogel samples as compared to their mass loss (R = 0.91, Figure 3f).

3.2. Release of Model Therapeutic PVA Can Be Quantified from the Millifluidic Device

Next, the simultaneous biodegradation and release of an encapsulated molecule were evaluated from the GelMA hydrogel discs. To this end, the release of PVA (as a model therapeutic) was quantified from the eluates from the millifluidic device, as illustrated in Figure 4. It was observed that the degradation of the GelMA-PVA hydrogel was substantially faster than that of the GelMA hydrogels alone (Figure 4a). Nevertheless, there was a detectable sustained release of PVA from the GelMA-PVA hydrogels over the 17 h of the MMP9 treatment (Figure 4b). Interestingly, PVA was detected even in the absence of MMP9, which suggests that some PVA can still be released from the hydrogel via passive diffusion. Indeed, a burst of PVA was detected at 1 hr of treatment in both enzyme and without-enzyme conditions. However, there was a greater increase in PVA detected over time in the eluates in the presence of MMP9 when compared with GelMA-PVA (Figure 4b). In addition to monitoring PVA release from the system, degraded GelMA was also quantified since it would also be present in the eluates. A high correlation (Pearson R = 0.97) was observed between the measured GelMA material in the eluates compared to the apparent hydrogel disc size quantified by the visual method (Figure 4c).

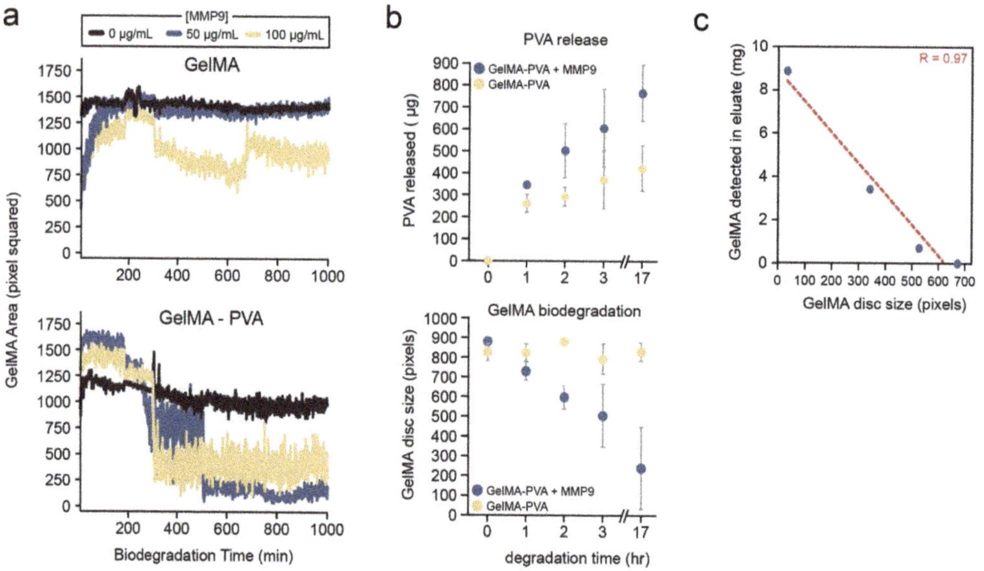

Figure 4. Simultaneous measurements of hydrogel degradation and concentrations of released compounds in device eluates. Computational quantification of the biodegradation of (**a**) GelMA and GelMA-PVA discs MMP9 at 0, 50 and 100 µg/mL. (**b**) Quantification of soluble PVA released from GelMA-PVA discs (top) and detection of degraded GelMA polymer (bottom) at the indicated times following MMP9 treatment. Error bars represent standard error of the mean. (**c**) Correlation between detected GelMA in the eluates and the size of the GelMA-PVA disc in the millifluidic device. Red dashed line represents the line of best fit with the Pearson correlation coefficient indicated (R).

4. Discussion

Quantifying hydrogel degradation is of significant interest in the drug-delivery field as the degradation profile of a biodegradable material can be leveraged for controlled drug delivery [10–12,36,37]. However, current methods to evaluate the biodegradation of biomaterials are extremely tedious and prone to significant experimental variability.

This is because the samples must be manually removed from the experimental system at each time point, dried and then measured. Consequently, researchers can choose only a feasible number of time points to capture snapshots of the degradation profile. However, for some material formulations, there are moments during degradation when the material can disintegrate rapidly over a short span (as this study noted), especially near the end of the degradation profile. Such crucial moments might be missed with just a snapshot of the degradation profile. Thus, novel in vitro assays to better characterize hydrogel and/or biomaterial degradation kinetics are required.

4.1. Novel Quantitative Millifluidic Imaging System to Quantify Hydrogel Biodegradation

This study aimed to develop a high-throughput screening methodology to continuously monitor the biodegradation of a GelMA hydrogel. The system employs a millifluidic chip to provide a steady flow, which can be adjusted as necessary to replicate physiological conditions or simulate accelerated degradation conditions. The system in this study was set up to run a total of 24 samples simultaneously, but this capacity can easily be expanded as required by either adding more sample channels to the device or connecting multiple devices in a series. The device also utilizes an automated imaging algorithm to acquire and analyze thousands of images of the degradation process over time without any need for manual measurements. Importantly, the computationally calculated degradation profile obtained by using our automated device and imaging platform correlated highly compared to the conventional mass-loss approach (Pearson R = 0.91). These results support the use of this visual-analysis method as an orthogonal approach to measure material degradation.

Despite the numerous advantages this automated system has over the more conventional mass-measurement approach, several considerations should be noted. Firstly, the current system only measures the surface area from a top view. Thus, thin samples, ideally in a disc shape, with a large front and back surface area, would be best suited for this analysis. Since this system does not measure material thickness, degradation measurements may deviate from the mass-loss method as the thickness of the material increases. Secondly, this method requires that the hydrogel exhibits a strong visual contrast against the background. This is unlikely for many hydrogels, such as GelMA, as they are transparent. Therefore, a hydrophilic red food dye was used to both stain the GelMA gels and was added to the MMP9 solution to outline the gel's overall shape as it degraded. The assumption is that the dye's absorption into the sample does not influence the sample's degradation rate. However, this assumption might not always be valid, as some chemical compounds can affect material properties [38,39]. Hence, it is important that the dye selected for this screening should have minimal impact on the properties of the hydrogel. Alternatively, if the material is fluorescent, then capturing images via fluorescence imaging is also possible with this approach. Nevertheless, the selection of an appropriately shaped biomaterial that can be stained with an inert dye would be highly suitable in this system.

One major advantage of this millifluidic system is that it allows for the collection of eluates for subsequent assays, enabling the simultaneous monitoring of biodegradation and the release of a therapeutic from the same sample. In this study, both the levels of GelMA and PVA present in the eluate were measured to (1) provide an additional method to monitor GelMA degradation and (2) evaluate the release of a loaded model therapeutic from a hydrogel. The degradation of GelMA was consistent over time and exhibited a strong linear correlation with the visual-analysis method (Pearson R= 0.97). Used in combination with the visual-analysis method, this assay aids in producing a reliable degradation profile. Furthermore, drugs that have been released from hydrogels may be used in conjunction with mathematical modeling to determine the type of release mechanisms that may be exhibited. In the conditions of this study, MMP9 likely acts by breaking down long polymeric chains of GelMA into smaller chains, causing the faster release of entrapped PVA from the inner core of the biomaterial. This mechanism could be described by Hopfenberg's model, but the true release kinetics will depend on the specific type of degradable polymer used, geometry and shape of the matrix and the presence of other chemical agents, among other factors [40]. In future studies, eluates from this system can be subjected to more sophisticated modeling of drug-release kinetic profiles as well as toxicity testing with cells. For example, eluted therapeutics with a well-defined release profile from this millifluidic system could be directly applied to human corneal epithelial cells exposed in a control and diseased state, such as hyperosmotic conditions to mimic dry eye syndrome. Cellular phenotypes, such as viability, the expression of proteins of interest and cellular morphological changes could be assessed through conventional means or through live-cell microscopy.

4.2. Potential for High-Throughput Screening of Hydrogels Used for Drug Delivery

One notable observation made in this study was that the addition of PVA into the GelMA disc could alter its biodegradation kinetics. Unsurprisingly, differences in the chemical composition of a hydrogel are one of many factors that can influence the material's physical and chemical properties, which ultimately influence the release kinetics of an encapsulated drug [41]. Other parameters that must be considered include the flow rates, volume, pH and temperature of the experimental system.

In the context of the ocular surface, there are other factors, such as blinking, that could affect the degradation rate. For instance, as the gel degrades, its internal structures may weaken, and even a small force from blinking could cause the gel to disintegrate instantly. For these reasons, a high-throughput and automated experimental system, such as the one presented in this study, would be beneficial for testing all these conditions and parameters simultaneously. Furthermore, recent technological advances have drastically increased the number of unique hydrogels that can be synthesized at one time [42,43]. One limiting factor could be the characterization of all these different formulations. The system developed in this study could significantly aid in the screening of these formulations. Finally, given that most degradation-time-course studies for polymers can span days, weeks or even months [44], an imaging system that allows researchers to quantitatively monitor the degradation remotely would reduce the time required to identify promising candidate materials. In the future, the goal is to also incorporate real-time analysis into this system as image data are gathered. Furthermore, it would be valuable to conduct in vitro–in vivo correlation studies in future studies to calibrate the system's parameters and generate representative physiological degradation profiles.

5. Conclusions

The developed screening platform was able to automatically monitor the degradation of a GelMA hydrogel by using a visual-imaging algorithm. The visual analysis showed a very strong positive correlation with the conventional mass-loss method used to measure material degradation. Furthermore, the developed system can also be used to measure the release of biodegraded material or a therapeutic from the same sample. In the future, this type of screening system could be adapted to measure the dissolution of various materials.

Author Contributions: Conceptualization, B.H., C.-M.P. and L.J.; methodology, B.H. and C.-M.P.; fabrication of GelMA ocular inserts, P.G. and P.S.; biodegradation of GelMA, B.H., P.G. and P.S.; millifluidic assays and experimentation, B.H.; mammalian cell cultures and assay, B.H., formal analysis and computational quantification, B.H.; writing—review and editing, B.H., P.G., P.S., C.-M.P. and L.J. All authors have read and agreed to the published version of the manuscript.

Funding: This project was supported and funded by Mitacs (through the Mitacs Accelerate program), InnoHK initiative and the Hong Kong Special Administrative Region Government, the Canadian Optometric Education Fund (COETF awarded to P.G.), NSERC CREATE Training in Global Biomedical Technology Research and Innovation, the Ontario Graduate Scholarship (OGS awarded to P.G.) and the Centre for Bioengineering and Biotechnology (CBB) at the University of Waterloo.

Institutional Review Board Statement: Not applicable.

Informed Consent Statement: Not applicable.

Data Availability Statement: The data can be shared upon request.

Acknowledgments: The University of Waterloo acknowledges that much of our work takes place on the traditional territory of the Neutral, Anishinaabeg and Haudenosaunee peoples. Our main campus is situated on the Haldimand Tract, the land granted to the Six Nations that includes six miles on each side of the Grand River. Our active work toward reconciliation takes place across our campuses through research, learning, teaching and community building, and is coordinated within the Office of Indigenous Relations.

Conflicts of Interest: Author B.H. was employed by the company EyesoBio Inc. C.M.P. and L.J. are advisors of EyesoBio Inc. The remaining authors declare that the research was conducted in the absence of any commercial or financial relationships that could be construed as a potential conflict of interest.

References

1. Lanier, O.L.; Manfre, M.G.; Bailey, C.; Liu, Z.; Sparks, Z.; Kulkarni, S.; Chauhan, A. Review of Approaches for Increasing Ophthalmic Bioavailability for Eye Drop Formulations. *AAPS PharmSciTech* **2021**, *22*, 107. [CrossRef] [PubMed]
2. Ahmed, S.; Amin, M.M.; Sayed, S. Ocular Drug Delivery: A Comprehensive Review. *AAPS PharmSciTech* **2023**, *24*, 66. [CrossRef] [PubMed]
3. Mofidfar, M.; Abdi, B.; Ahadian, S.; Mostafavi, E.; Desai, T.A.; Abbasi, F.; Sun, Y.; Manche, E.E.; Ta, C.N.; Flowers, C.W. Drug Delivery to the Anterior Segment of the Eye: A Review of Current and Future Treatment Strategies. *Int. J. Pharm.* **2021**, *607*, 120924. [CrossRef] [PubMed]
4. Han, H.; Li, S.; Xu, M.; Zhong, Y.; Fan, W.; Xu, J.; Zhou, T.; Ji, J.; Ye, J.; Yao, K. Polymer- and Lipid-Based Nanocarriers for Ocular Drug Delivery: Current Status and Future Perspectives. *Adv. Drug Deliv. Rev.* **2023**, *196*, 114770. [CrossRef]
5. Suri, R.; Beg, S.; Kohli, K. Target Strategies for Drug Delivery Bypassing Ocular Barriers. *J. Drug Deliv. Sci. Technol.* **2020**, *55*, 101389. [CrossRef]
6. Lynch, C.R.; Kondiah, P.P.D.; Choonara, Y.E.; du Toit, L.C.; Ally, N.; Pillay, V. Hydrogel Biomaterials for Application in Ocular Drug Delivery. *Front. Bioeng. Biotechnol.* **2020**, *8*, 228. [CrossRef]
7. Yang, C.; Yang, J.; Lu, A.; Gong, J.; Yang, Y.; Lin, X.; Li, M.; Xu, H. Nanoparticles in Ocular Applications and Their Potential Toxicity. *Front. Mol. Biosci.* **2022**, *9*, 931759. [CrossRef]
8. Jones, L.; Hui, A.; Phan, C.M.; Read, M.L.; Azar, D.; Buch, J.; Ciolino, J.B.; Naroo, S.A.; Pall, B.; Romond, K.; et al. CLEAR—Contact Lens Technologies of the Future. *Cont. Lens Anterior Eye* **2021**, *44*, 398–430. [CrossRef]
9. Kamaly, N.; Yameen, B.; Wu, J.; Farokhzad, O.C. Degradable Controlled-Release Polymers and Polymeric Nanoparticles: Mechanisms of Controlling Drug Release. *Chem. Rev.* **2016**, *116*, 2602. [CrossRef]
10. Senapati, S.; Mahanta, A.K.; Kumar, S.; Maiti, P. Controlled Drug Delivery Vehicles for Cancer Treatment and Their Performance. *Signal Transduct. Target. Ther.* **2018**, *3*, 7. [CrossRef]
11. Petersen, R.S.; Nielsen, L.H.; Rindzevicius, T.; Boisen, A.; Keller, S.S. Controlled Drug Release from Biodegradable Polymer Matrix Loaded in Microcontainers Using Hot Punching. *Pharmaceutics* **2020**, *12*, 1050. [CrossRef] [PubMed]
12. Benhabbour, S.R.; Kovarova, M.; Jones, C.; Copeland, D.J.; Shrivastava, R.; Swanson, M.D.; Sykes, C.; Ho, P.T.; Cottrell, M.L.; Sridharan, A.; et al. Ultra-Long-Acting Tunable Biodegradable and Removable Controlled Release Implants for Drug Delivery. *Nat. Commun.* **2019**, *10*, 4324. [CrossRef] [PubMed]
13. Welling, C.; Schwengler, H.; Strahl, B. In-Vitro Degradation Test for Screening of Biomaterials. In *Degradation Phenomena on Polymeric Biomaterials*; Springer: Berlin/Heidelberg, Germany, 1992; pp. 25–36. [CrossRef]
14. Hadavi, E.; de Vries, R.H.W.; Smink, A.M.; de Haan, B.; Leijten, J.; Schwab, L.W.; Karperien, M.H.B.J.; de Vos, P.; Dijkstra, P.J.; van Apeldoorn, A.A. In Vitro Degradation Profiles and In Vivo Biomaterial–Tissue Interactions of Microwell Array Delivery Devices. *J. Biomed. Mater. Res. B Appl. Biomater.* **2021**, *109*, 117–127. [CrossRef] [PubMed]
15. Azevedo, H.S.; Gama, F.M.; Reis, R.L. In Vitro Assessment of the Enzymatic Degradation of Several Starch Based Biomaterials. *Biomacromolecules* **2003**, *4*, 1703–1712. [CrossRef]
16. Phan, C.M.; Subbaraman, L.N.; Jones, L. In Vitro Drug Release of Natamycin from β-Cyclodextrin and 2-Hydroxypropyl-β-Cyclodextrin-Functionalized Contact Lens Materials. *J. Biomater. Sci. Polym. Ed.* **2014**, *25*, 1907–1919. [CrossRef]
17. Peng, C.C.; Kim, J.; Chauhan, A. Extended Delivery of Hydrophilic Drugs from Silicone-Hydrogel Contact Lenses Containing Vitamin E Diffusion Barriers. *Biomaterials* **2010**, *31*, 4032–4047. [CrossRef]
18. Pereira-da-Mota, A.F.; Vivero-Lopez, M.; Garg, P.; Phan, C.M.; Concheiro, A.; Jones, L.; Alvarez-Lorenzo, C. In Vitro–In Vivo Correlation of Drug Release Profiles from Medicated Contact Lenses Using an In Vitro Eye Blink Model. *Drug Deliv. Transl. Res.* **2023**, *13*, 1116–1127. [CrossRef]
19. Wu, Q.; Liu, J.; Wang, X.; Feng, L.; Wu, J.; Zhu, X.; Wen, W.; Gong, X. Organ-on-a-Chip: Recent Breakthroughs and Future Prospects. *Biomed. Eng. Online* **2020**, *19*, 9. [CrossRef]
20. Leung, C.M.; de Haan, P.; Ronaldson-Bouchard, K.; Kim, G.A.; Ko, J.; Rho, H.S.; Chen, Z.; Habibovic, P.; Jeon, N.L.; Takayama, S.; et al. A Guide to the Organ-on-a-Chip. *Nat. Rev. Methods Primers* **2022**, *2*, 33. [CrossRef]
21. Dittrich, P.S.; Manz, A. Lab-on-a-Chip: Microfluidics in Drug Discovery. *Nat. Rev. Drug Discov.* **2006**, *5*, 210–218. [CrossRef]

22. Liu, Y.; Sun, L.; Zhang, H.; Shang, L.; Zhao, Y. Microfluidics for Drug Development: From Synthesis to Evaluation. *Chem. Rev.* **2021**, *121*, 7468–7529. [CrossRef] [PubMed]
23. Staicu, C.E.; Jipa, F.; Axente, E.; Radu, M.; Radu, B.M.; Sima, F. Lab-on-a-Chip Platforms as Tools for Drug Screening in Neuropathologies Associated with Blood–Brain Barrier Alterations. *Biomolecules* **2021**, *11*, 916. [CrossRef] [PubMed]
24. Maurya, R.; Gohil, N.; Bhattacharjee, G.; Alzahrani, K.J.; Ramakrishna, S.; Singh, V. Microfluidics Device for Drug Discovery, Screening and Delivery. *Prog. Mol. Biol. Transl. Sci.* **2022**, *187*, 335–346. [CrossRef] [PubMed]
25. Ramasamy, M.; Ho, B.; Phan, C.M.; Qin, N.; Ren, C.L.; Jones, L. Inexpensive and Rapid Fabrication of PDMS Microfluidic Devices for Biological Testing Applications Using Low Cost Commercially Available 3D Printers. *J. Micromechanics Microengineering* **2023**, *33*, 105016. [CrossRef]
26. Bhattacharjee, N.; Urrios, A.; Kang, S.; Folch, A. The Upcoming 3D-Printing Revolution in Microfluidics. *Lab. Chip* **2016**, *16*, 1720. [CrossRef]
27. Bupphathong, S.; Quiroz, C.; Huang, W.; Chung, P.F.; Tao, H.Y.; Lin, C.H. Gelatin Methacrylate Hydrogel for Tissue Engineering Applications—A Review on Material Modifications. *Pharmaceuticals* **2022**, *15*, 171. [CrossRef]
28. Piao, Y.; You, H.; Xu, T.; Bei, H.P.; Piwko, I.Z.; Kwan, Y.Y.; Zhao, X. Biomedical Applications of Gelatin Methacryloyl Hydrogels. *Eng. Regen.* **2021**, *2*, 47–56. [CrossRef]
29. Akkurt Arslan, M.; Brignole-Baudouin, F.; Chardonnet, S.; Pionneau, C.; Blond, F.; Baudouin, C.; Kessal, K. Profiling Tear Film Enzymes Reveals Major Metabolic Pathways Involved in the Homeostasis of the Ocular Surface. *Sci. Rep.* **2023**, *13*, 15231. [CrossRef]
30. Smith, V.A.; Rishmawi, H.; Hussein, H.; Easty, D.L. Tear Film MMP Accumulation and Corneal Disease. *Br. J. Ophthalmol.* **2001**, *85*, 147–153. [CrossRef]
31. Teodorescu, M.; Bercea, M.; Morariu, S. Biomaterials of PVA and PVP in Medical and Pharmaceutical Applications: Perspectives and Challenges. *Biotechnol. Adv.* **2019**, *37*, 109–131. [CrossRef]
32. Allyn, M.M.; Luo, R.H.; Hellwarth, E.B.; Swindle-Reilly, K.E. Considerations for Polymers Used in Ocular Drug Delivery. *Front. Med.* **2021**, *8*, 787644. [CrossRef] [PubMed]
33. Rizwan, M.; Peh, G.S.L.; Ang, H.P.; Lwin, N.C.; Adnan, K.; Mehta, J.S.; Tan, W.S.; Yim, E.K.F. Sequentially-Crosslinked Bioactive Hydrogels as Nano-Patterned Substrates with Customizable Stiffness and Degradation for Corneal Tissue Engineering Applications. *Biomaterials* **2017**, *120*, 139–154. [CrossRef]
34. Procházková, L.; Rodríguez-Muñoz, Y.; Procházka, J.; Wanner, J. Simple Spectrophotometric Method for Determination of Polyvinylalcohol in Different Types of Wastewater. *Int. J. Environ. Anal. Chem.* **2014**, *94*, 399–410. [CrossRef]
35. Phan, C.M.; Walther, H.; Riederer, D.; Lau, C.; Lorenz, K.O.; Subbaraman, L.N.; Jones, L. Analysis of Polyvinyl Alcohol Release from Commercially Available Daily Disposable Contact Lenses Using an In Vitro Eye Model. *J. Biomed. Mater. Res. B Appl. Biomater.* **2019**, *107*, 1662. [CrossRef] [PubMed]
36. Kesharwani, P.; Bisht, A.; Alexander, A.; Dave, V.; Sharma, S. Biomedical Applications of Hydrogels in Drug Delivery System: An Update. *J. Drug Deliv. Sci. Technol.* **2021**, *66*, 102914. [CrossRef]
37. Buwalda, S.J.; Vermonden, T.; Hennink, W.E. Hydrogels for Therapeutic Delivery: Current Developments and Future Directions. *Biomacromolecules* **2017**, *18*, 316–330. [CrossRef] [PubMed]
38. Parhi, R. Cross-Linked Hydrogel for Pharmaceutical Applications: A Review. *Adv. Pharm. Bull.* **2017**, *7*, 515. [CrossRef]
39. Gastaldi, M.; Cardano, F.; Zanetti, M.; Viscardi, G.; Barolo, C.; Bordiga, S.; Magdassi, S.; Fin, A.; Roppolo, I. Functional Dyes in Polymeric 3D Printing: Applications and Perspectives. *ACS Mater. Lett.* **2021**, *3*, 1–17. [CrossRef]
40. Trucillo, P. Drug Carriers: A Review on the Most Used Mathematical Models for Drug Release. *Processes* **2022**, *10*, 1094. [CrossRef]
41. Hoare, T.R.; Kohane, D.S. Hydrogels in Drug Delivery: Progress and Challenges. *Polymer* **2008**, *49*, 1993–2007. [CrossRef]
42. Neto, A.I.; Demir, K.; Popova, A.A.; Oliveira, M.B.; Mano, J.F.; Levkin, P.A. Fabrication of Hydrogel Particles of Defined Shapes Using Superhydrophobic-Hydrophilic Micropatterns. *Adv. Mater.* **2016**, *28*, 7613–7619. [CrossRef] [PubMed]
43. Rosenfeld, A.; Oelschlaeger, C.; Thelen, R.; Heissler, S.; Levkin, P.A. Miniaturized High-Throughput Synthesis and Screening of Responsive Hydrogels Using Nanoliter Compartments. *Mater. Today Bio* **2020**, *6*, 100053. [CrossRef] [PubMed]
44. Resende, R.; Silva, A.; Marques, C.S.; Rodrigues Arruda, T.; Teixeira, S.C.; Veloso De Oliveira, T. Biodegradation of Polymers: Stages, Measurement, Standards and Prospects. *Macromol* **2023**, *3*, 371–399. [CrossRef]

pharmaceutics

Article

Development of ARPE-19-Equipped Ocular Cell Model for In Vitro Investigation on Ophthalmic Formulations

Simona Sapino [1,*], Giulia Chindamo [1], Elena Peira [1,*], Daniela Chirio [1], Federica Foglietta [1], Loredana Serpe [1], Barbara Vizio [2] and Marina Gallarate [1]

[1] Department of Drug Science and Technology, University of Turin, 10125 Turin, Italy; giulia.chindamo@unito.it (G.C.); daniela.chirio@unito.it (D.C.); federica.foglietta@unito.it (F.F.); loredana.serpe@unito.it (L.S.); marina.gallarate@unito.it (M.G.)
[2] Department of Medical Sciences, University of Turin, Via Genova 3, 10126 Turin, Italy; barbara.vizio@unito.it
* Correspondence: simona.sapino@unito.it (S.S.); elena.peira@unito.it (E.P.)

Abstract: Repeated intravitreal (IVT) injections in the treatment of retinal diseases can lead to severe complications. Developing innovative drug delivery systems for IVT administration is crucial to prevent adverse reactions, but requires extensive investigation including the use of different preclinical models (in vitro, ex vivo and in vivo). Our previous work described an in vitro tricompartmental ocular flow cell (TOFC) simulating the anterior and posterior cavities of the human eye. Based on promising preliminary results, in this study, a collagen scaffold enriched with human retinal pigmented epithelial cells (ARPE-19) was developed and introduced into the TOFC to partially mimic the human retina. Cells were cultured under dynamic flow conditions to emulate the posterior segment of the human eye. Bevacizumab was then injected into the central compartment of the TOFC to treat ARPE-19 cells and assess its effects. The results showed an absence of cytotoxic activity and a significant reduction in VEGF fluorescent signal, underscoring the potential of this in vitro model as a platform for researching new ophthalmic formulations addressing the posterior eye segment, eventually decreasing the need for animal testing.

Keywords: in vitro ocular flow cell; intravitreal injections; ARPE-19 scaffold; bevacizumab; drug delivery systems

Citation: Sapino, S.; Chindamo, G.; Peira, E.; Chirio, D.; Foglietta, F.; Serpe, L.; Vizio, B.; Gallarate, M. Development of ARPE-19-Equipped Ocular Cell Model for In Vitro Investigation on Ophthalmic Formulations. *Pharmaceutics* **2023**, *15*, 2472. https://doi.org/10.3390/pharmaceutics15102472

Academic Editor: Montse Mitjans Arnal

Received: 23 August 2023
Revised: 3 October 2023
Accepted: 13 October 2023
Published: 16 October 2023

1. Introduction

Treating retinal diseases with injections into the vitreous body is a common practice in the ophthalmic clinic. Repeated IVT administration is part of the treatment of certain diseases such as age-related macular degeneration (AMD) and diabetic macular edema (DME). However, in addition to being unpleasant and a reason for low patient compliance, IVT injections can lead to complications, such as retinal detachment, vitreous hemorrhage, and endophthalmitis [1].

The development of novel therapeutic systems that are able to release drugs in a delayed manner is therefore one of the most important goals in the field of ophthalmology. As a result of the increased permanence of the drugs in the posterior segment of the eye, fewer administrations would be required, making IVT therapies less invasive, more harmless, and more comfortable for the patients.

As with all new pharmaceutical preparations, the study of novel ophthalmic therapeutic systems involves the use of in vitro and in vivo experimental models in the preclinical phase [2]. In fact, once a candidate pharmaceutical formulation is identified, its development follows a detailed plan to ensure both safety and efficacy.

To date, preclinical studies for new preparations have been dominated by animal models. However, despite their importance, several efforts are underway at present to reduce the number of animals used in testing, both to comply with ethical concerns and to reduce costs. In addition, humans and animals differ in many ways, which is another concern with the employment of animal testing. This is especially true for experiments in ophthalmic research, in which animal models with intact vitreous humor are often used, which do not take into account structural changes induced by disease, age-related differences in vitreous humor, and interspecies variability (as an example, the volume of the rabbit vitreous is only around 1.5 mL, while it is 3–4 mL for humans).

The use of animals in medical and scientific research has recently been the subject of heated debate, and with recent changes to European legislation, specific funds have been allocated to research on alternative methods [3]. In this context, in vitro models as alternatives to animal testing become important, as they can speed up the course of medicinal product development and optimization while decreasing costs and reducing animal use [4,5]. Moreover, these alternative models can also decrease the huge gap between in vitro and in vivo studies, offering an alternative and/or support before moving to clinical trials [6,7]. Among alternative in vitro approaches, three-dimensional (3D) cell cultures recreate in vivo tissue microenvironments, and are able to increase cell–cell/matrix interactions, along with mechanical and chemical properties of tissue-like structures, compared to classic two-dimensional (2D) cell cultures [7,8]. Specifically, alternative models based on the seeding and culture of cells within porous 3D scaffolds composed of different materials with potentially tunable architectural complexity have also been recently described [8]. The current trend is to build bottom-up models that include anatomical and physiological factors, pharmacokinetic parameters, and consider physicochemical characteristics of drugs. These models are called pharmacokinetic models (PK models). Accordingly, some researchers have developed models to predict drug fate in the vitreous to accelerate the development and optimization of therapeutic dosage forms in the preclinical phase [9,10].

To quantify and predict the efficiency of drug delivery, it is essential to have in vitro models that mimic the human eye in terms of compartmentalization and mass transport processes that occur in vitreous humor. Indeed, some researchers [11] presented an experimental study of vitreous motion induced by saccadic eye movements, employing a model in which care was taken to correctly reproduce real saccadic eye movements.

Interestingly, an in vitro eye model (PK-EyeTM) has been developed to estimate human pharmacokinetics of IVT therapeutic compounds and formulations, which are cleared through the anterior route [12]. This model, designed with dimensions similar to the human eye, has proven to be highly effective in evaluating the clearance profiles of proteins like bevacizumab (BVZ) and ranibizumab, as well as poorly soluble drugs such as triamcinolone acetonide when administered as suspensions or formulated as IVT implants [13]. However, it does not provide insights into the tissue absorption and distribution of these injected formulations.

Another in vitro test described in the literature combines a vitreous model [14] and a simple system described by Loch and colleagues [15] in an attempt to create an in vitro system resembling the vitreous body and the applied forces that move the depot [16]. This model, called EyeMoS [17], is composed of a spherical eye chamber, obtained by 3D printing, housed on a rotating device and filled with gel of polyacrylamide, coated in turn with a thin layer of agarose gel. The chamber is provided with an inlet channel (for injection) and an outlet channel. However, this model presents a single chamber, and has no semi-permeable barriers or supports for line cells, limiting its use.

Some patented eyeball models are already available for ocular studies. This is the case for the "in vitro eyeball superfusion system" [18], which is a device able to preserve the normal morphology of an in vitro eyeball and maintain its ability to respond to stimuli. It comprises the in vitro eyeball storing unit and a thermostatic water feeding mechanism which drips a liquid with specific ion concentration on the surface of the isolated eyeball according to a certain speed to maintain the moisture state of a cornea.

An additional example is the "artificial eye assembly", which consists of layered components that offer pressurized multi-modular chambers. This assembly is valuable for investigating ocular pharmacokinetics while considering various ocular parameters and physiological conditions. Each chamber within the artificial eye can be pressurized at different levels, enabling the simulation of different wake and sleep cycles [19]. However, it should be noted that this artificial eye assembly does not include a compartment suitable for serving as a scaffold for retinal cell lines. Consequently, it is not suitable for conducting studies on the interaction between drugs and retinal cell lines.

Moreover, the "medical simulation human eye simulation module" [20] and "methods and devices for modeling the eye" have also been developed [21]. The former is a model for simulating the blinking and the pupil contracting mechanism, while the second is a biomimetic model of the eye comprising a convex scaffold, a fluidic device, and a fabricated eyelid coupled to a motor. In certain embodiments, the scaffold can be impregnated with one or more layers of keratocytes and epithelial cells. However, both of these models cannot be used for simulating IVT injections.

Starting from the above cited literature, particularly from the PK-EyeTM model [12], we designed and developed a Plexiglas tricompartmental eye flow cell (TOFC) that recreates the anterior and the posterior cavities of the human eye. As described in our previous paper [22], this artificial ocular model enables the simulation of IVT injections, the estimation of drug residence time in the posterior segment, and evaluation of its drainage through the anterior chamber of the eye. In the present paper, an evolution of such tricompartmental flow cells is presented, consisting of the insertion of a collagen scaffold enriched with human retinal cells mimicking the retina and allowing tests of cytotoxicity and efficacy.

For this purpose, a three-dimensional (3D) model of a human pigmented retinal (ARPE-19) cell seeded over a collagen porous scaffold has been introduced into the ocular cell and grown under a dynamic flow, in order to emulate the condition of the posterior segment of the human eye. The scaffold serves as a framework for the cells and emulates the natural extracellular matrix, allowing the assessment of interactions between the retinal cells and the drug being tested in a biologically relevant context.

The primary objective of this study is to evaluate the feasibility and practicality of this evolutionary approach. For these reasons, the viability of ARPE-19 cells over the 3D scaffold was initially evaluated under both dynamic and static conditions, the latter serving as a control. Subsequently, an analysis was conducted on a commercial solution of BVZ to examine its clearance profile and investigate its biological activity, particularly its anti-VEGF (vascular endothelial growth factor) properties. This comprehensive evaluation provides valuable insights into the behavior of retinal cells and the tested formulation, contributing to the overall understanding of the potential and applicability of this in vitro model.

2. Materials and Methods

2.1. Materials

Agar was from Alfa-Aesar (Ward Hill, MA, USA); hyaluronic acid sodium salt 1600 kDa (HA) was from Farmalabor (Barletta, Italy). Phosphate-buffered saline (PBS); Dulbecco's Modified Eagle Medium/Nutrient Mixture F-12 (DMEM-F12) fetal calf serum (FBS); sodium azide; L-glutamine; penicillin and streptomycin; MTT solution; and propidium iodide (PI) were from Sigma-Aldrich (St. Louis, MO, USA). Avastin® (Roche, Basilea, Switzerland) was kindly provided by Molinette Central Hospital (Turin, Italy). Tissue culture flasks and plates were from TPP, Trasadingen, Switzerland. Collagen porous scaffold was from Ultrafoam, Avitene; Davol Inc., Warwick, RI, USA. ARPE-19 cell line (ATCC-CRL-2302) was from ATCC® (Manassas, VA, USA). Collagenase IV was from Worthington Biochemical Corporation, Lakewood, NJ, USA. VEGF (JH121); sc-57496 was from Santacruz, DBA Italia SRL, Milan, Italy. Goat anti-mouse IgG H&L (Alexa Fluor® 647) ab150119 was from Abcam, Milan, Italy.

2.2. Methods

2.2.1. Samples Preparation

Avastin (25 mg/mL BVZ) was used undiluted for clearance study. However, for cytotoxicity experiments and anti-VEGF activity assessments, it was appropriately diluted in DMEM-F12 to achieve a concentration of 1 mg/mL BVZ.

An artificial fluid simulating the humor vitreous (HV) was prepared according to the literature [23]. Firstly, agar (0.4 g) was dissolved in 100 mL of pH 7.4 PBS or DMEM-F12 medium and then carefully vortexed using IKA T-25 Ultraturrax (IKA®-Werke GmbH, Staufen Germany). Separately, 1600 kDa hyaluronic acid sodium salt (HA) (0.5 g) was dispersed in 100 mL water. Equal volumes of both solutions were then mixed for 5 min using Ultraturrax to obtain a homogeneous medium to which a few drops of 0.02% *w/v* sodium azide were added. The mixture was cooled to room temperature (20 °C) until a gel-like consistency was reached.

The simulated HV prepared in DMEM-F12 medium was sterilized by autoclaving at 121 °C for 20 min, cooled down, and then enriched with fetal calf serum (10%, *v/v*), L-glutamine (2 mM), penicillin (100 units/mL), and streptomycin (100 μg/mL) before being used.

2.2.2. Clearance Study

To study the clearance profile of BVZ, the proposed Plexiglas model (TOFC) was set up without a scaffold, as previously described [22]. Figure 1 depicts the three compartments before assembly, with the anterior compartment containing a small cavity (0.25 mL) that mimics the anterior chamber of the eye, and the central compartment with a cavity volume of approximately 7.75 mL, which simulates the vitreous body. Additionally, two disks can be observed, highlighted in blue (anterior) and red (posterior), which simulate the physiological semipermeable barriers, namely the uveal trabecular and the retina, respectively. The anterior disk is designed with eight microholes (ID. 0.5 mm) distributed along the circumference to simulate the outflow pathway.

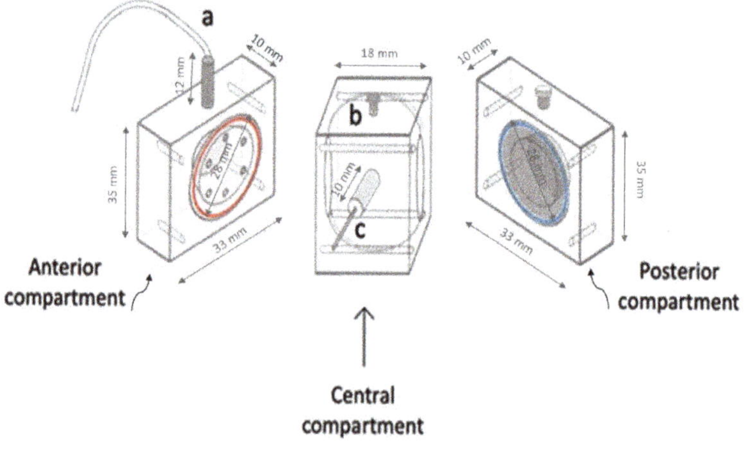

Figure 1. Schematic representation of the Plexiglas TOFC before assembly. The anterior compartment, on the left, features an outlet port located at the top (a) and a semipermeable disk (highlighted in red). The central compartment, in the middle, includes an injection port (b) and an inlet port (c). The posterior compartment, on the right, is equipped with a grid (highlighted in blue) that can be replaced with a retinal cell scaffold.

Before the experiment, the TOFC was filled with 8 mL of simulated HV. The central compartment of the cell was connected through the inlet port to the dispensing peristaltic pump (Minipuls®3, Gilson, Middleton, WI, USA) that provided a dynamic condition with a continuous aqueous flow of PBS (4.0 μL/min inflow). At starting time, an aliquot (200 μL) of BVZ 25 mg/mL was injected through the injection port at the bottom level in the simulated vitreous cavity of the cell. The injected dose of BVZ was about twice the standard clinical dose to account for the larger volume of this in vitro model. After the injection, at scheduled times up to 21 days, the aqueous fluid coming out from the TOFC via the outlet port of the anterior compartment was collected. Collected samples were stored at −20 °C prior to analysis for protein content by Bradford assay, a rapid and sensitive method used for measuring the concentrations of proteins. It is based on the shift in absorbance maximum of Coomassie brilliant blue G-250 dye from 465 to 595 nm following the binding to denatured proteins in the solution [24]. The experiment was repeated three times.

In a 96-well plate, 40 μL of each sample was mixed with 160 μL of Coomassie G-250 dye reagent solution diluted 1:4 with distilled water and incubated for 10 min at room temperature in the dark. Optical density was quantified at 595 nm in a plate reader. The readings were taken in triplicates and the mean and standard deviation were determined. The concentrations of unknown collected samples were estimated based on the standard curve derived from known concentrations of BVZ. Average measurements for blank (0 μg/mL of antibody) were subtracted from standards and unknown samples. Samples from each time point were evaluated in triplicate (n = 3) and the mean and standard deviation were determined.

2.2.3. Cell Line Culture

The human pigmented retinal (ARPE-19) cell line (ATCC-CRL-2302) was cultured as monolayers in a complete medium consisting of DMEM-F12 medium supplemented with fetal calf serum (10%, v/v), L-glutamine (2 mM), penicillin (100 units/mL), and streptomycin (100 μg/mL). Cells were maintained in culture at 37 °C in a humidified atmosphere containing 5% CO_2 in an incubator.

2.2.4. Generation of 3D Cultures and Development of ARPE-19 Scaffold

For standard 2D cell cultures, 75 cm^2 culture flasks were used. With the final aim of generating a 3D culture of ARPE-19, a commercial collagen porous scaffold of 12 mm diameter and 2 mm thickness was used. Each scaffold was first soaked overnight with a complete medium at 37 °C. Then, to understand the correct number of cells to seed over the scaffold, a first screening of different cell numbers for seeding was performed. Therefore, ARPE-19 cells in the exponential phase were detached using trypsin and counted, and different cell concentrations (2.5×10^5, 5×10^5, 1.0×10^6) were seeded over collagen scaffold and maintained in culture at 37 °C. To avoid cell attachment to the plastic surface of plates, each scaffold was therefore distributed into a 24-weel plate, previously coated with a 1.5% of sterilized agarose (Sigma-Aldrich); then, ARPE-19 cells were seeded over the scaffold. ARPE-19 cells were left to grow over the scaffold for 6 days and the medium was changed every other day. At the end, scaffolds enriched with cells were washed with PBS and incubated with MTT solution for 3 h at 37 °C in order to color cells and to monitor their distribution over the scaffold.

2.2.5. Setup of the TOFC Equipped with ARPE-19 Scaffold

ARPE-19 cells, grown in exponential phase in a plastic flask, were detached, counted, and 5×10^5 cells were then seeded over the collagen scaffold, as previously described. After six days of cell seeding, the ARPE-19 scaffold was placed on grids and properly introduced between the central and posterior compartment. The three compartments were then assembled using screws and filled with simulated HV. Next, the inlet port of TOFC was connected to a dispensing peristaltic pump (Minipuls® 3, Gilson, Middleton, WI, USA) via tubing (1.5 mm ID) to provide a continuous inflow (4.0 μL/min) of DMEM-F12, creating a dynamic condition referred to as d3D. To equilibrate the entire system, the ocular model equipped with ARPE-19 scaffold was left overnight in an incubator at 37 °C with 5% CO_2. The day following the equilibration, 200 μL of BVZ (1 mg/mL in DMEM-F12) was injected with a needle at the bottom of the central compartment containing 8 mL of simulated HV, in order to obtain a 25 μg/mL BVZ final concentration in the TCOF. This chosen dose was necessary to maintain a drug concentration within the TOFC that was compatible with ARPE-19 cells. The TOFC was then left for 48 h in an incubator at 37 °C with 5% CO_2 while being continuously perfused with DMEM-F12 at a 4.0 μL/min flow rate.

2.2.6. Incubation of ARPE-19 Scaffold in Static Condition

To compare the effects of BVZ on ARPE-19 cells treated in 3D condition (d3D) derived from the ocular cell setup, a static condition (s3D) was also established as a reference. Therefore, three scaffolds per experiment were incubated with BVZ (25 μg/mL) for 48 h in an incubator at 37 °C with 5% CO_2. Furthermore, the effect of BVZ treatment on scaffolds under s3D conditions was compared with that observed in untreated scaffolds under the same s3D conditions.

2.2.7. Flow Cytometry Analysis and Evaluation of Cell Viability

BVZ activity was monitored cytofluorimetrically by evaluating VEGF fluorescent signal over the cells. Scaffold from s3D or d3D models, treated with BVZ for 48 h, or untreated scaffolds, i.e., untreated s3D and untreated d3D, underwent collagenase IV treatment at 37 °C for 20 min. The cells were collected using centrifugation and stained with the primary antibody VEGF (JH121) (1:500) in PBS for 1 h at room temperature. At the end of incubation, the samples were washed with PBS and then incubated with the secondary antibody goat anti-mouse IgG H&L (Alexa Fluor® 647) and preabsorbed (1:2000) for 45 min at room temperature. At the end of the incubation, the cell pellet was washed with PBS and the sample was analyzed using a C6 flow cytometer (Accuri Cytometers, Milan, Italy). The analysis was performed by excluding cell debris based on forward scatter (FSC) and side scatter (SSC) parameters. VEGF fluorescent signal was then expressed as the integrated mean fluorescence intensity (iMFI), which represents the product of the frequency of VEGF positive cells and the mean fluorescence intensity of the cells. Moreover, to assess cell viability, digested cells from scaffolds, i.e., untreated s3D, s3D + BVZ, and untreated d3D and d3D + BVZ, were also incubated with propidium iodide (PI, 10 g/mL) for 20 min at 37 °C in PBS and then analyzed using a C6 flow cytometer. Three independent experiments were performed, with three replicates for each.

2.2.8. Statistical Analysis

Data are shown as mean values ± standard deviation of three independent experiments. Statistical analyses were performed using Prism 9.0 software (GraphPad, La Jolla, CA, USA). According to the design of the experiment under analysis, multiple *t*-tests, and one-way ANOVA and Bonferroni's tests were used to calculate the threshold of significance. The statistical significance threshold was set at $p < 0.05$.

3. Results

In the first part of the study, the in vitro ocular model (TOFC) was exploited to investigate the clearance profile of a monoclonal antibody, specifically BVZ, which is one of the most commonly used categories of IVT ophthalmic therapeutics.

Afterwards, the work proceeded with the setup of ARPE-19 scaffold and its insertion into the TOFC in order to carry out cell viability studies and to investigate the anti-VEGF efficacy of BVZ under dynamic conditions of continuous perfusion. For the sake of clarity, the sequence of experiments conducted in this study is represented in Figure 2.

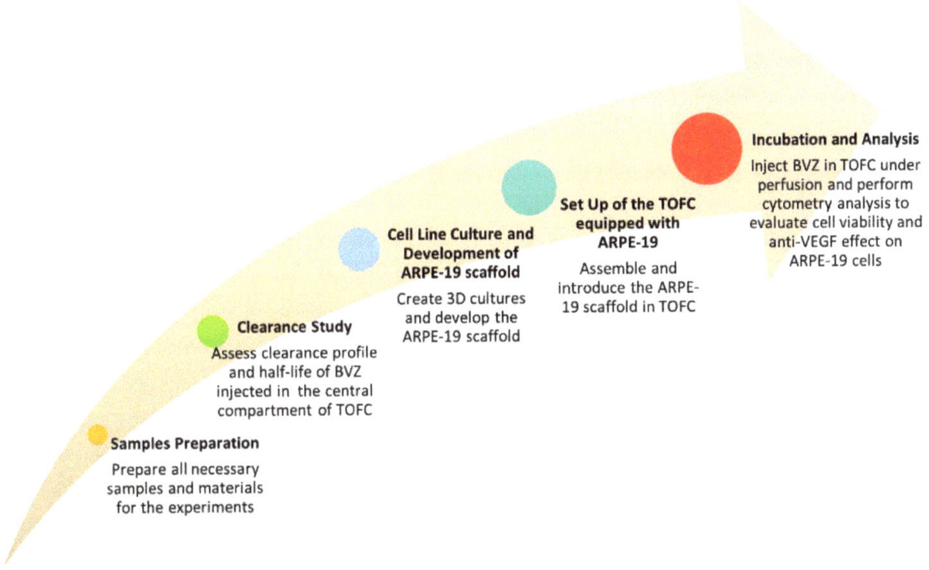

Figure 2. Flow chart representing the sequence of experiments performed to investigate the potential of TOFC equipped with ARPE-19 scaffold.

3.1. BVZ Clearance Study by TOFC

To estimate the BVZ clearance profile, the outflow from the TOFC was collected by the outlet port of the anterior compartment over a period of 21 days. A graphical representation of clearance and concentration profiles is provided in Figure 3a,b, respectively.

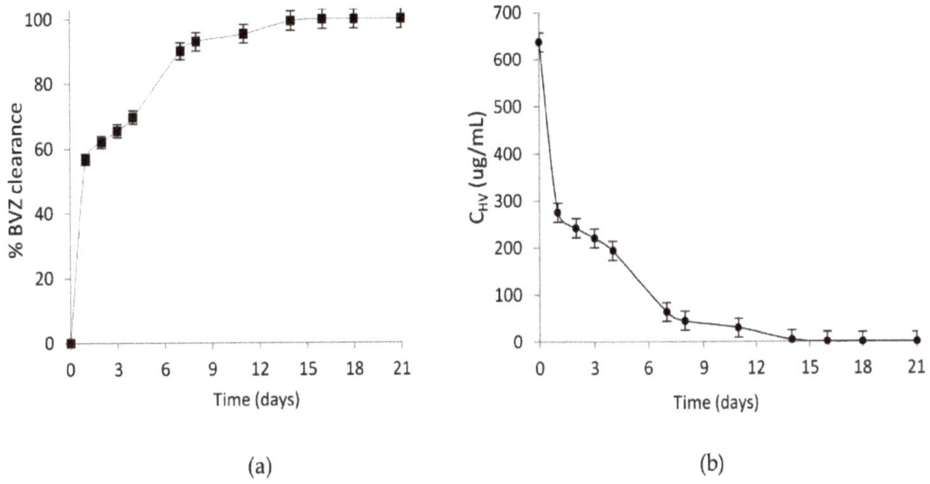

Figure 3. Graphical representation of BVZ (**a**) clearance profiles and (**b**) concentration in simulated HV after injection of BVZ (25 mg/mL) into the central compartment of the TOFC. Error bars in the graph represent the mean of three experiments.

The clearance profile, as depicted in Figure 3a, exhibited a first-order pattern characterized by a rapid initial increase followed by a more gradual upsurge. This behavior suggests a biphasic elimination process, possibly involving both saturable and non-saturable clearance mechanisms. These findings align with the known pharmacokinetic complexity of large molecular weight compounds.

In Figure 3b, the concentration profile shows a corresponding trend, indicating a decline in BVZ concentration in the HV over the observation period. Notably, the initial steep decline in concentration mirrored the rapid clearance phase observed in the clearance profile. The half-life of BVZ in TOFC was calculated to be 1.5 ± 0.4 days, underscoring the rapid elimination phase of the drug.

3.2. Development of ARPE-19 Scaffold and Equipping within TOFC

The correct distribution of cells inside the scaffold support represents a crucial aspect to determine the initial cellular setup required for each in vitro experiment. For this reason, at the end of 6 days of culture over the scaffold, the distribution of ARPE-19 cells in the scaffold was monitored using coloring cells with MTT solution (Figure 4). A homogeneous distribution and growth of the cells was observed in the scaffold with 5.0×10^5 cells seeded (Figure 4b), while, when 2.5×10^5 cells were seeded, just a peripheral distribution of the cells was observed (Figure 4a), like a 1.0×10^6 cell seeding condition (Figure 4c). Consequently, for further experiments, 5×10^5 was chosen as the starting seeding number of cells on the collagen scaffold.

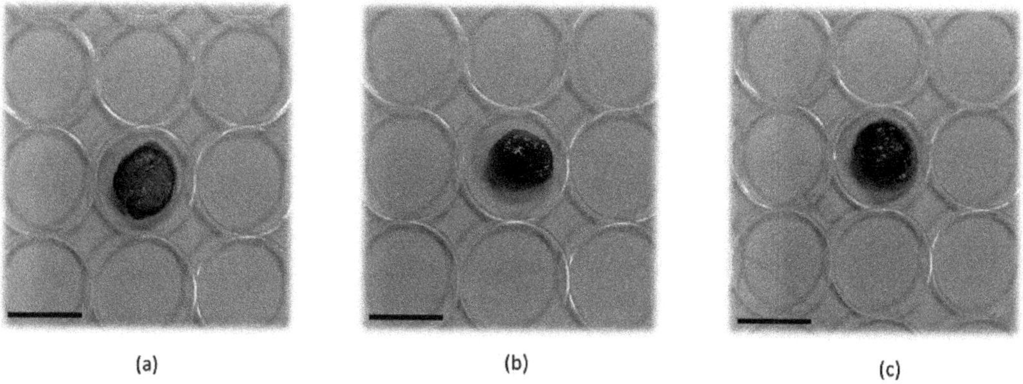

Figure 4. ARPE-19 cell distribution on collagen scaffold. ARPE-19 cells were grown over the collagen scaffold for 6 days and then scaffolds were incubated with MTT to stain cell distribution. Representative images of different cell seeding amounts: (**a**) 2.5×10^5; (**b**) 5.0×10^5; (**c**) 1.0×10^6. Scale bar: 10 mm.

Six days after the seeding, the ARPE-19 scaffold was vertically positioned between the central and the posterior compartment of the TOFC in order to simulate the retinal blood barrier. The three compartments were then assembled and connected to the peristaltic pump, as represented in Figure 5.

As shown in Figure 5, the developed ARPE-19 scaffold is placed between the central and posterior compartments and is supported by two grids to keep it in a vertical position. The inlet port is connected to a peristaltic pump via tubing (1.5 mm ID), providing continuous infusion of the completed cell culture medium (4.0 µL/min) to the area near the ARPE-19 scaffold. The aqueous outflow is collected from the anterior cavity via the outlet port, which is elevated to approximately 3.0 cm to maintain a full internal volume within the model by providing a small amount of back pressure. The overall size and volume of TOFC are approximately twice that of the human eye to facilitate analysis of drug distribution and pharmacokinetics in the ocular environment. Indeed, creating a model that is larger than the human eye allows for better visualization and analysis of drug behavior in the vitreous.

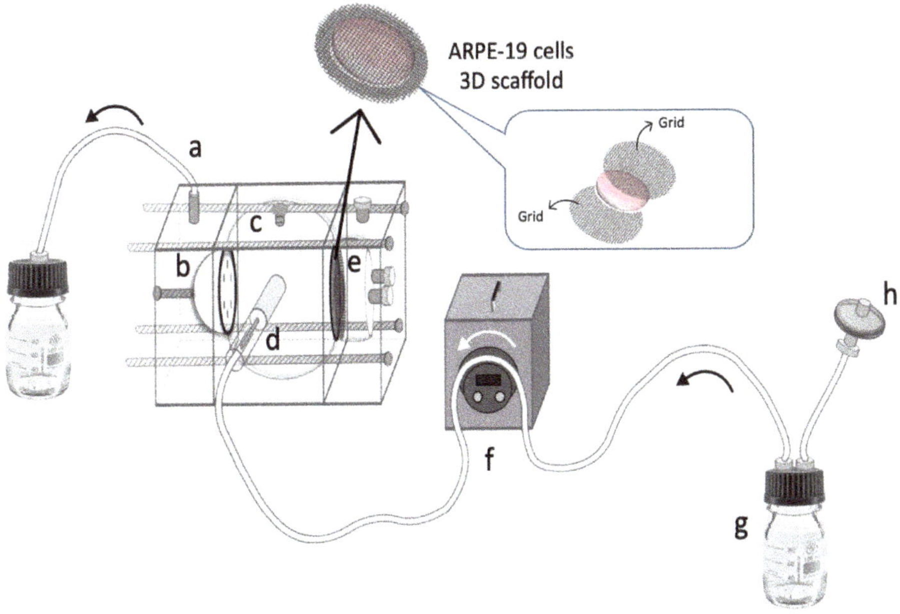

Figure 5. Schematic representation of the TOFC equipped with ARPE-19 scaffold. The model comprises: (a) an outlet port allowing outflow from the anterior compartment; (b) an 8-microhole perforated disk between the anterior and central compartment; (c) an injection port at the top of the central compartment; (d) an inlet port connected to a (f) peristaltic pump; (e) ARPE-19 scaffold vertically positioned between the central and the posterior compartment; (g) a reservoir of DMEM-F12 and (h) a sterile filter with 0.22 µm pore size.

3.3. Evaluation of Anti-VEGF Activity and Cell Viability

To assess the effectiveness of BVZ in inhibiting VEGF, ARPE-19 scaffold cultured under dynamic (d3D) conditions was analyzed 48 h after BVZ injection (0.2 mL, 1 mg/mL) in the central compartment of the TOFC. The results were further compared to both untreated d3D conditions and also versus ARPE-19 cell growth in an s3D condition or s3D incubated with BVZ at the same concentration (25 µg/mL).

This approach allowed for a comprehensive evaluation of BVZ activity and its impact on the ARPE-19 scaffold under different conditions. According to data obtained by flow cytometry, BVZ was able to reduce the VEGF fluorescent signal both in s3D and d3D (Figure 6a,b); it is the reduction that is only statistically significant ($p < 0.05$) in d3D conditions (Figure 6b) when compared to the respective untreated condition. Moreover, from the comparison of the VEGF fluorescence signal between s3D and d3D, it was discovered to be not statistically significant.

Moreover, the PI evaluation of the two considered scaffold conditions showed no statistically significant difference compared to the untreated scaffold conditions, showing that the BVZ concentration used did not affect cell viability over the scaffold (Figure 6e,f), as is also appreciated by the representative cytofluorimetric dot plots (Figure 6g,h).

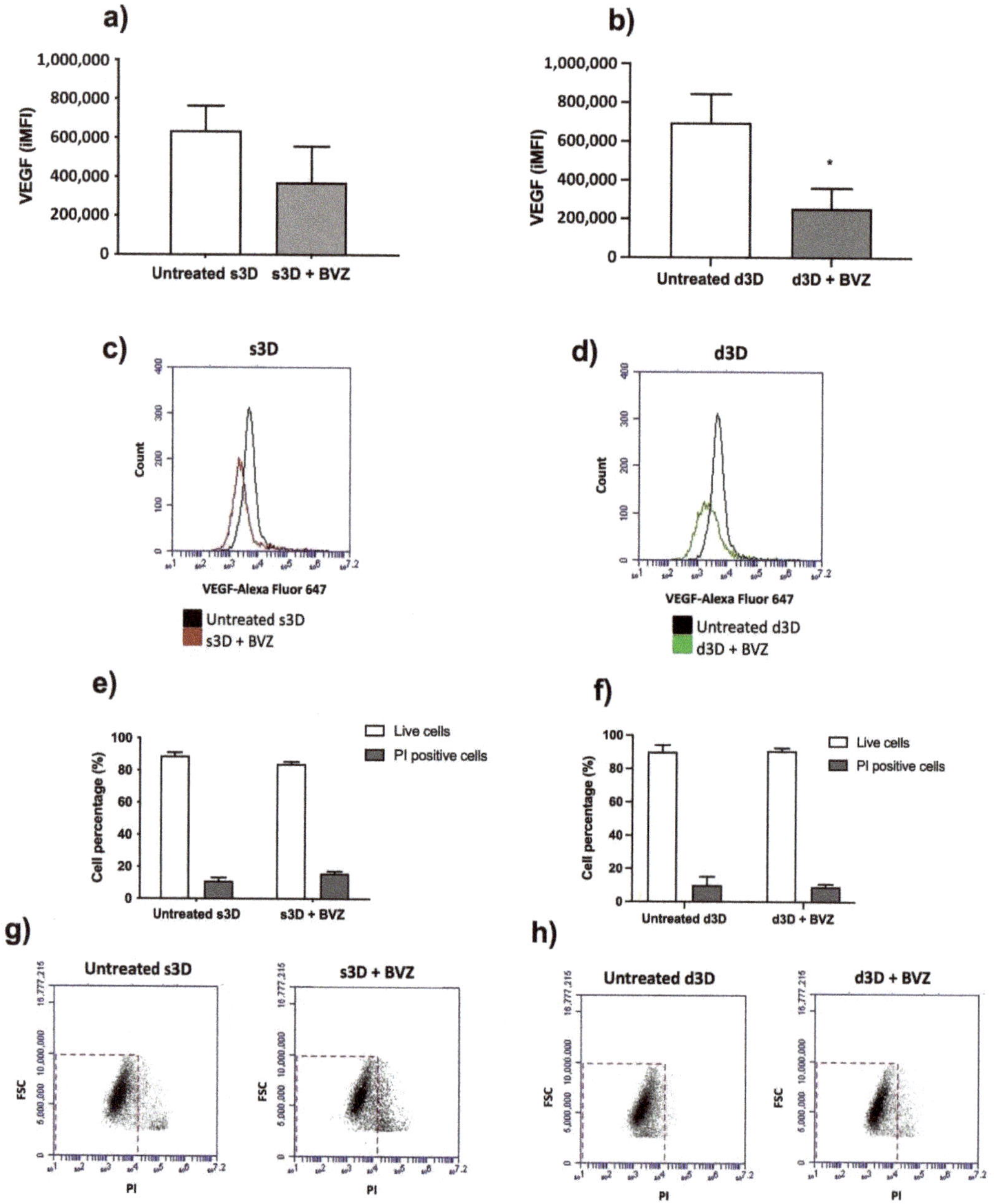

Figure 6. Evaluation of BVZ activity on VEGF. ARPE-19 cells grown under static (s3D; (**a**,**c**,**e**,**g**)) or dynamic condition (d3D; (**b**,**d**,**f**,**h**)) were left untreated or underwent BVZ treatment (25 µg/mL) for 48 h; then cytofluorimetric evaluation of VEGF on cells derived from scaffold was performed. VEGF fluorescent signal in ARPE-19 cells is shown as the integrated mean fluorescence (iMFI; (**a**,**b**)) along with representative flow cytometry plots (**c**,**d**). Statistically significant versus untreated condition d3D (Ctrl): * $p < 0.05$, $n = 3$). Propidium iodide (PI) staining is shown as positive cell percentage in s3D (**e**) or d3D (**f**) along with representative flow cytometry plots (**g**,**h**). Data are expressed as the percentage of cells ± standard deviation (no statistical significance of BVZ-treated scaffold versus untreated condition, $n = 3$).

4. Discussion

The development of a tricompartmental ocular flow model, namely the TOFC, arose from the need to find alternative models that enable the occurrence of pharmacokinetic and pharmacodynamic studies while limiting the use of animal experimentation during the initial development phase of new IVT ophthalmic therapies. After all, the search for alternative methods to animal experimentation is a topic of increasing interest that applies to the development of new therapeutic systems as a whole and arises from the need to respond to important ethical concerns. In vitro models have proven valuable for their ability to mimic physiological patterns, permitting the study of the safety and efficacy of potential therapeutics before they are tested in animal models or in human subjects [2].

In our previous research, TOFC was employed to assess the release profile and clearance of cefuroxime delivered within a nanoparticle system [22], whereas in this study, the same model was utilized to investigate the clearance of BVZ IVT administered as an anti-VEGF agent for a variety of ocular disorders.

The commercial solution of BVZ was injected without dilution at twice the standard clinical dose (5.0 mg BVZ; 0.2 mL) to account for the model's large volume. This dosage adjustment was necessary to ensure that the drug concentration inside the TCOF was comparable to that of the human eye and to enable the accurate analysis of drug distribution in the ocular environment and outflow.

The biphasic trend in the BVZ clearance profile observed in this study finds support in the literature. Ahn et al. compared the clearance of IVT-injected BVZ in vitrectomized versus non-vitrectomized control rabbit eyes. In both of the experimental groups, they observed a two-phase elimination pattern with a first fast distribution phase, followed by a second slow elimination phase [25].

The short half-life (1.5 ± 0.4 days) extrapolated by the clearance profile corresponds well with the steep initial decline in concentration observed in the concentration profile, providing a quantitative measure to the observed trend. This relatively short half-life suggests that a significant proportion of BVZ is cleared from the system within a short period after administration, necessitating the careful consideration of dosing frequency to maintain therapeutic efficacy.

Several in vivo studies analyzed the pharmacokinetic parameters of IVT-administered BVZ in different animal eye models, mainly rats, rabbits, or monkeys. It was encouraging that the BVZ half-life value found in this study is quite similar to that found by Gal-Or and colleagues [26], who investigated and characterized the presence of IVT-injected BVZ in the aqueous outflow channels of a rat model. According to their study, BVZ molecules passed through the aqueous outflow channels within 48 h following IVTl injection. In contrast, Nomoto et al. and Sinapis et al. [27,28] found the half-life of BVZ in the vitreous humor after IVT injection to be 6–6.61 days in rabbit eyes. In human eyes, at a similar dose, the half-life of BVZ is reported to be 4.9 days or 0.66 days in non-vitrectomized or vitrectomized eyes, respectively [29].

It is evident that the half-life of IVT-injected BVZ can vary significantly across different studies, mainly due to the specific experimental models employed and varying conditions such as vitrectomized versus non-vitrectomized eyes, and lentomized versus non-lentomized eyes. Therefore, given this variability, making direct comparisons among these studies may not be entirely appropriate.

Furthermore, it is important to emphasize that while in vitro experiments provide valuable insights, they cannot completely replace preclinical in vivo models. Instead, they should be considered as complementary tools, particularly useful for initial screening when selecting among various formulations those that warrant further investigation.

Beyond assessing the suitability of TOFC for studying IVT drug clearance, the primary emphasis of this study lies in introducing a novel element: a retinal cellular scaffold. Specifically, a scaffold of ARPE-19 cells that has been developed and positioned between the central and posterior compartments to partially simulate the retina. This allows for the creation of an artificial retina model that can be maintained in culture through the dynamic condition created by the peristaltic pump. Overall, the ocular flow cell equipped with the inserted ARPE-19 scaffold enables not only the assessment of resident time and drug clearance profile, but also the evaluation of the activity of drugs, whether they are free or entrapped in a drug delivery system.

Various in vitro models have been proposed in the literature to evaluate and describe drug distribution in the vitreous, but to the best of our knowledge, none of them have previously included a retinal cell culture scaffold in an assembled compartmentalized ocular model. Furthermore, most of the 3D models proposed take into consideration the realization of 3D models of the cornea, even if they are still far from the complex equipment of the eye, like for example, the lacrimal apparatus responsible for cleansing and supporting regeneration [30,31].

Recently, few works reported the use of alternative in vitro 3D models for ocular investigation. Auel and colleagues developed a technique to continuously observe the distribution of the drug in in vitro vitreous substitutes by using a 3D-printed device that allows the injection volume of 100 μL, which corresponds to a commonly therapeutically injected volume of IVT injection in vivo. This system therefore allows a reduction in the number of necessary animals in preclinical studies of new IVT dosage forms [32]. The use of 3D models in in vitro experimentations allows the recreation and maintenance of a suitable microenvironment to support cell growth and function, reducing the wide gap between in vitro and in vivo experimentations [7]. Among tissue engineering, porous 3D scaffolds are commonly used in several applications and can be made from various materials, according to the need and the type of pores required. In particular, porous scaffold networks that enable the transport of nutrients, removal of wastes, and facilitate the proliferation and migration of cells are essential. The porosity and pore size influences cell behavior and determines the final mechanical property of the scaffold [33].

Therefore, keeping these objectives in mind, the ARPE-19 scaffold was successfully developed and installed in the in vitro ocular model proposed in this study (Figure 5).

Several in vitro studies on ocular cells in culture, such as human retinal pigment epithelium, optic nerve head astrocytes, and human corneal cells, have been reported on the effect of BVZ [34,35]. BVZ has the main role to bind all circulating VEGF-A isoforms. By binding to VEGF-A, it prevents the interaction of VEGF-A with VEGFR and thereby inhibits the activation of VEGF signaling pathways that promote neovascularization [36]. Even though IVT injection uses minute amounts of the drug, the full-sized antibody, BVZ, has more potential to cause inflammatory and immune reactions over time. To avoid possibly severe systemic side effects, the treatment of ocular disease is usually limited to intraocular administration, in which case retinal toxicity is the primary concern [35]. Specifically, in the work of Kaempf and colleagues, neural retinal specimens were placed on nitrocellulose membranes and transferred to a sterile cell carrier under a perfusion system at 1 mL/h. The system was then treated with different concentrations of BVZ (0.25 mg/mL, 0.5 mg/mL, and 1.25 mg/mL). Authors underlined that in their model, BVZ was well tolerated by cells even if possible side effects on mature vessels had to be considered and may explain the higher risk for cardiovascular events in anti-VEGF treatments.

In support of our data, Chung and colleagues [37] developed an organotypic eye-on-a-chip model that mimics the retinal pigment epithelium (RPE)–choroid complex in vitro. This model consists of an RPE monolayer and adjacent perfusable blood vessel network, which supports the barrier function of the outer blood–retinal barrier. Treatment with BVZ caused a regression in the vessel network, demonstrating a significant antiangiogenic effect, confirming the main characteristic of the model to be used to evaluate not only the cytotoxic activity of a drug, but also to determine the appropriate drug dosage.

In the present study, a simplified prototype scaffold composed of a unique cell line (ARPE-19) was developed and employed. The selection of this specific cell line was based on the anatomical positioning of retinal pigment epithelium beneath neural cells within the retina, as well as its integral role as the initial component of the tri-layered structure constituting the blood–retinal barrier, which includes the retinal pigmented epithelium,

Bruch's membrane, and the vascular endothelium. Furthermore, the suitability of the ARPE-19 cell line for our investigations is underscored by its inherent ability to secrete vascular endothelial growth factor (VEGF) under normal physiological conditions [38]. This characteristic enabled us to assess the potential of this in vitro model for evaluating the anti-VEGF activity of BVZ.

Certainly, our study is not devoid of limitations. Firstly, like many other in vitro models designed to replicate the cellular and tissue environments of living organisms, our TOFC model should be interpreted with caution, as it inherently offers only a partial representation of real biological systems. Despite our efforts to faithfully recreate the ocular system and its existing barriers, our model does lack certain anatomical components, such as the lens. It is worth noting that the literature reports underscore the significant contribution of the lens to ocular pharmacokinetics, with one study indicating a substantial reduction in BVZ half-life in lensectomized eyes [39].

Another limitation that we aim to overcome in the future is related to the cellular scaffold. We are hopeful that in the near future we can develop a more realistic and representative model of the blood–retinal membrane by co-culturing retinal epithelial cells with retinal endothelial cells within the same 3D scaffold, as well as incorporating injury insults that induce retinal disease and loss of visual function. This approach should allow us to better mimic the complex interactions and barriers present in the ocular system, further improving the accuracy and applicability of our model for ocular pharmacokinetic studies.

In forthcoming research, in order to enhance our model, it will be imperative to consider the employment of alternative materials to Plexiglass and explore the potential utilization of 3D printing technology. 3D printing offers a more versatile and continually advancing technology within the biomedical field, which could provide us with a platform to construct more anatomically comprehensive and functionally representative ocular models.

5. Conclusions

In the present study, we demonstrated and confirmed that the TOFC is a new and promising in vitro ocular model with great potential. By developing a 3D ARPE-19 scaffold that partially mimics the presence of the retina, we were able to provide a more accurate representation of drug distribution in the vitreous cavity, as well as its biological activity. This information is crucial in the development of novel therapeutic strategies for posterior eye conditions.

As previously demonstrated [22], the TOFC proposed here has the capability of simulating the human eye environment, enabling the investigation of the clearance profile without the use of animal experimentation in the early stages of developing new ophthalmic therapeutics. This is important as it reduces the reliance on animal experimentation and can lead to faster and more ethical drug development.

Overall, the findings suggest that the ocular flow model equipped with ARPE-19 scaffold described in this study can be considered a promising platform for investigating pharmacokinetics and the activity of new ophthalmic formulations intended for the treatment of the posterior eye segment. Further studies are warranted to confirm these results and to explore the full potential of this in vitro model.

Author Contributions: Conceptualization, S.S. and E.P.; investigation and methodology, G.C. and D.C.; characterization analyses, E.P. and D.C.; in vitro methodology and analyses F.F., L.S. and B.V.; data curation, G.C and M.G.; writing and editing of the manuscript, S.S and F.F.; supervision, M.G. All authors have read and agreed to the published version of the manuscript.

Funding: This research received no external funding.

Institutional Review Board Statement: Not applicable.

Informed Consent Statement: Not applicable.

Data Availability Statement: Not applicable.

Acknowledgments: The authors are grateful to Vittorio Allocco of Alpeat s.a.s (Grugliasco, TO, Italy) for providing the technical support in realizing the TOFC.

Conflicts of Interest: The authors declare no conflict of interest.

References

1. Christensen, G.; Barut, L.; Urimi, D.; Schipper, N.; Paquet-durand, F. Investigating Ex Vivo Animal Models to Test the Performance of Intravitreal Liposomal Drug Delivery Systems. *Pharmaceutics* **2021**, *13*, 1013. [CrossRef] [PubMed]
2. Lehrmann, D.; Refaian, N.; Simon, M.; Rokohl, A.C.; Heind, L.M. Preclinical models in ophthalmic oncology—A narrative review. *Ann. Eye Sci.* **2022**, *7*, 14. [CrossRef]
3. 2021/2784(RSP). Available online: https://oeil.secure.europarl.europa.eu/oeil/popups/ficheprocedure.do?lang=en&reference=2021/2784 (accessed on 5 June 2023).
4. Gan, J.; Bolon, B.; Van Vleet, T.; Wood, C. Chapter 24—Alternative Models in Biomedical Research: In Silico, In Vitro, Ex Vivo, and Nontraditional In Vivo Approaches. In *Haschek and Rousseaux's Handbook of Toxicologic Pathology*, 4th ed.; Haschek, W.M., Rousseaux, C.G., Wallig, M.A., Bolon, B., Eds.; Academic Press: Cambridge, MA, USA, 2022; pp. 925–966. [CrossRef]
5. Verderio, P.; Lecchi, M.; Ciniselli, C.M.; Shishmani, B.; Apolone, G.; Manenti, G. 3Rs Principle and Legislative Decrees to Achieve High Standard of Animal Research. *Animals* **2023**, *13*, 277. [CrossRef] [PubMed]
6. Mengus, C.; Muraro, M.G.; Mele, V.; Amicarella, F.; Manfredonia, C.; Foglietta, F.; Muenst, S.; Soysal, S.D.; Iezzi, G.; Spagnoli, G.C. In Vitro Modeling of Tumor−Immune System Interaction. *ACS Biomater. Sci. Eng.* **2018**, *4*, 314–323. [CrossRef]
7. Foglietta, F.; Canaparo, R.; Muccioli, G.; Terreno, E.; Serpe, L. Methodological aspects and pharmacological applications of three-dimensional cancer cell cultures and organoids. *Life Sci.* **2020**, *254*, 117784–117785. [CrossRef]
8. Hirt, C.; Papadimitropoulos, A.; Muraro, M.G.; Mele, V.; Panopoulos, E.; Cremonesi, E.; Ivanek, R.; Schultz-Thater, E.; Droeser, R.A.; Mengus, C.; et al. Bioreactor-engineered cancer tissue-like structures mimic phenotypes, gene expression profiles and drug resistance patterns observed "in vivo". *Biomaterials* **2015**, *62*, 138–146. [CrossRef] [PubMed]
9. Fotaki, N. Flow-through cell apparatus (USP apparatus 4): Operation and features. *Dissolut. Technol.* **2011**, *18*, 46–49. [CrossRef]
10. Tojo, K. A pharmacokinetic model for ocular drug delivery. *Chem. Pharm. Bull.* **2004**, *52*, 1290–1294. [CrossRef]
11. Repetto, R.; Stocchino, A.; Cafferata, C. Experimental investigation of vitreous humour motion within a human eye model. *Phys. Med. Biol.* **2005**, *50*, 4729–4743. [CrossRef]
12. Awwad, S.; Lockwood, A.; Brocchini, S.; Khaw, P.T. The PK-Eye: A Novel in Vitro Ocular Flow Model for Use in Preclinical Drug Development. *J. Pharm. Sci.* **2015**, *104*, 3330–3342. [CrossRef]
13. Adrianto, M.F.; Annuryanti, F.; Wilson, C.G.; Sheshala, R.; Thakur, R.R. In vitro dissolution testing models of ocular implants for posterior segment drug delivery. *Drug Deliv. Transl. Res.* **2022**, *12*, 1355–1375. [CrossRef] [PubMed]
14. Loch, C.; Nagel, S.; Guthoff, R.; Seidlitz, A.; Weitschies, W. The Vitreous Model—A new in vitro test method simulating the vitreous body Model characterization. *Biomed. Eng. /Biomed. Tech.* **2012**, *57*, 281–284. [CrossRef]
15. Loch, C.; Bogdahn, M.; Stein, S.; Nagel, S.; Guthoff, R.; Weitschies, W.; Seidlitz, A. Simulation of Drug Distribution in the Vitreous Body After Local Drug Application into Intact Vitreous Body and in Progress of Posterior Vitreous Detachment. *J. Pharm. Sci.* **2014**, *103*, 517–526. [CrossRef]
16. Stein, S.; Auel, T.; Kempin, W.; Bogdahn, M.; Weitschies, W.; Seidlitz, A. Influence of the test method on in vitro drug release from intravitreal model implants containing dexamethasone or fluorescein sodium in poly (D,L-lactide-co-glycolide) or polycaprolactone. *Eur. J. Pharm. Biopharm.* **2018**, *127*, 270–278. [CrossRef] [PubMed]
17. Auel, T.; Großmann, L.; Schulig, L.; Weitschies, W.; Seidlitz, A. The EyeFlowCell: Development of a 3D-Printed Dissolution Test Setup for Intravitreal Dosage Forms. *Pharmaceutics* **2021**, *13*, 1394. [CrossRef]
18. Yang, X.; Guo, X.; Yang, Y.; Huang, J.; Xiong, X.; Xie, X.; Tan, X. In-Vitro Eyeball Superfusion System. Patent CN101406176A, 15 April 2009. Available online: https://worldwide.espacenet.com/patent/search?q=pn%3DCN101406176A (accessed on 6 May 2023).
19. Awwad, S.; Bouremel, Y.; Ibeanu, N.; Brocchini, S.J.; Khaw, P.T. Artificial Eye Assembly for Studying Ocular Pharmacokinetics. Patent WO2021186191A1, 31 August 2021. Available online: https://worldwide.espacenet.com/patent/search?q=pn%3DWO2021186191A1 (accessed on 6 May 2023).
20. Juhong, H.; Yambin, P. Medical Simulation Human Eye Simulation Module. Patent CN210378044U, 21 April 2020. Available online: https://worldwide.espacenet.com/patent/search?q=pn%3DCN210378044U (accessed on 21 June 2023).
21. Dongeun, H.; Jeongyun, S. Methods and Devices for Modelling the Eye. Patent US20170229043A1, 10 August 2017. Available online: https://worldwide.espacenet.com/patent/search?q=pn%3DUS2017229043A1 (accessed on 2 July 2023).
22. Sapino, S.; Peira, E.; Chirio, D.; Chindamo, G.; Guglielmo, S.; Oliaro-Bosso, S.; Barbero, R.; Vercelli, C.; Re, G.; Brunella, V.; et al. Thermosensitive nanocomposite hydrogels for intravitreal delivery of cefuroxime. *Nanomaterials* **2019**, *9*, 1461. [CrossRef]
23. Kummer, M.P.; Abbott, J.J.; Dinser, S.; Nelson, B.J. Artificial vitreous humor for in vitro experiments. In Proceedings of the Annual International Conference of the IEEE Engineering in Medicine and Biology, Lyon, France, 23–26 August 2007. [CrossRef]
24. Bradford, M.M. A rapid and sensitive method for the quantitation of microgram quantities of protein utilizing the principle of protein-dye binding. *Anal. Biochem.* **1976**, *72*, 248–254. [CrossRef]
25. Ahn, J.; Kim, H.; Woo, S.J.; Park, J.H.; Park, S.; Hwang, D.J.; Park, K.H. Pharmacokinetics of intravitreally injected bevacizumab in vitrectomized eyes. *J. Ocul. Pharmacol. Ther.* **2013**, *29*, 612–618. [CrossRef]

26. Gal-Or, O.; Dotan, A.; Dachbash, M.; Tal, K.; Nisgav, Y.; Weinberger, D.; Ehrlich, R.; Livnat, T. Bevacizumab clearance through the iridocorneal angle following intravitreal injection in a rat model. *Exp. Eye Res.* **2016**, *145*, 412–416. [CrossRef]
27. Nomoto, H.; Shiraga, F.; Kuno, N.; Kimura, E.; Fujii, S.; Shinomiya, K.; Nugent, A.K.; Hirooka, K.; Baba, T. Pharmacokinetics of Bevacizumab after Topical, Subconjunctival, and Intravitreal Administration in Rabbits. *Investig. Ophthalmol. Vis. Sci.* **2009**, *50*, 4807–4813. [CrossRef]
28. Sinapis, C.I.; Routsias, J.G.; Sinapis, A.I.; Sinapis, D.I.; Agrogiannis, G.D.; Pantopoulou, A.; Theocharis, S.E.; Baltatzis, S.; Patsouris, E.; Perrea, D. Pharmacokinetics of intravitreal bevacizumab (Avastin®) in rabbits. *Clin. Ophthalmol.* **2011**, *5*, 697–704. [CrossRef] [PubMed]
29. Moisseiev, E.; Waisbourd, M.; Ben-Artsi, E.; Levinger, E.; Barak, A.; Daniels, T.; Csaky, K.; Loewenstein, A.; Barequet, I.S. Pharmacokinetics of bevacizumab after topical and intravitreal administration in human eyes. *Graefes Arch. Clin. Exp. Ophthalmol.* **2014**, *252*, 331–337. [CrossRef] [PubMed]
30. Tegtmeyer, S.; Papantoniou, I.; Müller-Goymann, C.C. Reconstruction of an in vitro cornea and its use for drug permeation studies from different formulations containing pilocarpine hydrochloride. *Eur. J. Pharm. Biopharm.* **2001**, *51*, 119–125. [CrossRef] [PubMed]
31. Kutlehria, S.; Sachdeva, M.S. Role of In Vitro Models for Development of Ophthalmic Delivery Systems. *Crit. Rev. Ther. Drug Carrier Syst.* **2021**, *38*, 1–31. [CrossRef]
32. Auel, T.; Scherke, L.P.; Hadlich, S.; Mouchantat, S.; Grimm, M.; Weitschies, W.; Seidlitz, A. Ex Vivo Visualization of Distribution of Intravitreal Injections in the Porcine Vitreous and Hydrogels Simulating the Vitreous. *Pharmaceutics* **2023**, *15*, 786. [CrossRef]
33. Loh, Q.L.; Choong, C. Three-dimensional scaffolds for tissue engineering applications: Role of porosity and pore size. *Tissue Eng. Part B Rev.* **2013**, *19*, 485–502. [CrossRef] [PubMed]
34. Merz, P.R.; Röckel, N.; Ballikaya, S.; Auffarth, G.U.; Schmack, I. Effects of ranibizumab (Lucentis®) and bevacizumab (Avastin®) on human corneal endothelial cells. *BMC Ophthalmol.* **2018**, *18*, 316–323. [CrossRef]
35. Kaempf, S.; Johnen, S.; Salz, A.K.; Weinberger, A.; Walter, P.; Thumann, G. Effects of Bevacizumab (Avastin) on Retinal Cells in Organotypic Culture. *Investig. Ophthalmol. Vis. Sci.* **2008**, *49*, 3164–3171. [CrossRef]
36. Ferrara, N.; Hillan, K.J.; Gerber, H.P.; Novotny, W. Discovery and development of bevacizumab, an anti-VEGF antibody for treating cancer. *Nat. Rev. Drug Discov.* **2004**, *3*, 391–400. [CrossRef]
37. Chung, M.; Lee, S.; Lee, B.J.; Son, K.; Jeon, N.L.; Kim, J.H. Wet-AMD on a Chip: Modeling Outer Blood-Retinal Barrier In Vitro. *Adv. Healthc. Mater.* **2018**, *7*, 1700028–1700034. [CrossRef]
38. Ma, W.; Lee, S.E.; Guo, J.; Qu, W.; Hudson, B.I.; Schmidt, A.M.; Barile, G.R. RAGE ligand upregulation of VEGF secretion in ARPE-19 cells. *Investig. Ophthalmol. Vis. Sci.* **2007**, *48*, 1355–1361. [CrossRef] [PubMed]
39. Christoforidis, J.B.; Williams, M.M.; Wang, J.; Jiang, A.; Pratt, C.; Abdel-Rasoul, M.; Hinkle, G.H.; Knopp, M.V. Anatomic and pharmacokinetic properties of intravitreal bevacizumab and ranibizumab after vitrectomy and lensectomy. *Retina* **2013**, *33*, 946–952. [CrossRef] [PubMed]

pharmaceutics

MDPI

Article

Development and Bioactivity of Zinc Sulfate Cross-Linked Polysaccharide Delivery System of Dexamethasone Phosphate

Natallia V. Dubashynskaya [1,*], Anton N. Bokatyi [1], Andrey S. Trulioff [2], Artem A. Rubinstein [2], Igor V. Kudryavtsev [2] and Yury A. Skorik [1]

[1] Institute of Macromolecular Compounds of the Russian Academy of Sciences, Bolshoi VO 31, 199004 Saint Petersburg, Russia; qwezakura@yandex.ru (A.N.B.); yury_skorik@mail.ru (Y.A.S.)
[2] Institute of Experimental Medicine, Acad. Pavlov St. 12, 197376 Saint Petersburg, Russia; trulioff@gmail.com (A.S.T.); arrubin6@mail.ru (A.A.R.); igorek1981@yandex.ru (I.V.K.)
* Correspondence: dubashinskaya@gmail.com

Abstract: Improving the biopharmaceutical properties of glucocorticoids (increasing local bioavailability and reducing systemic toxicity) is an important challenge. The aim of this study was to develop a dexamethasone phosphate (DexP) delivery system based on hyaluronic acid (HA) and a water-soluble cationic chitosan derivative, diethylaminoethyl chitosan (DEAECS). The DexP delivery system was a polyelectrolyte complex (PEC) resulting from interpolymer interactions between the HA polyanion and the DEAECS polycation with simultaneous incorporation of zinc ions as a cross-linking agent into the complex. The developed PECs had a hydrodynamic diameter of 244 nm and a ζ-potential of +24.4 mV; the encapsulation efficiency and DexP content were 75.6% and 45.4 μg/mg, respectively. The designed DexP delivery systems were characterized by both excellent mucoadhesion and prolonged drug release (approximately 70% of DexP was released within 10 h). In vitro experiments showed that encapsulation of DexP in polysaccharide nanocarriers did not reduce its anti-inflammatory activity compared to free DexP.

Keywords: dexamethasone phosphate; zinc sulfate; polysaccharides; chitosan; hyaluronan; ocular delivery systems; mucoadhesion; anti-inflammatory activity

Citation: Dubashynskaya, N.V.; Bokatyi, A.N.; Trulioff, A.S.; Rubinstein, A.A.; Kudryavtsev, I.V.; Skorik, Y.A. Development and Bioactivity of Zinc Sulfate Cross-Linked Polysaccharide Delivery System of Dexamethasone Phosphate. *Pharmaceutics* **2023**, *15*, 2396. https://doi.org/10.3390/pharmaceutics15102396

Academic Editor: Sofia Lima

Received: 4 September 2023
Revised: 22 September 2023
Accepted: 25 September 2023
Published: 28 September 2023

1. Introduction

Various ocular pathologies of inflammatory genesis have a negative impact on the quality of life of patients and can lead to blindness [1]. Topical application of drugs is the preferred way to treat ocular diseases due to its non-invasiveness and safety [2]. Disadvantages of traditional ocular anti-inflammatory dosage forms (eye drops and ointments) are related to the rapid release of active pharmaceutical ingredients (APIs) and their subsequent rapid elimination from the site of administration due to the unique features of the anatomy and physiology of the eye (the tear film barrier, nasolacrimal duct drainage, constant rapid tear flow, and rapid precorneal clearance) [3–6], resulting in reduced bioavailability [7,8]. In addition, the anatomical corneal barrier and the low permeability of the cornea and sclera make topical application less effective for the treatment of posterior segment diseases [9]. The problem of rapid drug release from the dosage form can be solved by using polymeric solvents (e.g., cellulose derivatives, hyaluronic acid, etc.), which impart the necessary viscosity to the solution and thus modify the drug release [10,11]. However, these systems are not suitable for programmed and controlled drug release and corneal permeability improvement; in addition, they are not convenient to use because of the need for frequent application, resulting in low patient compliance [12].

One strategy to improve the biopharmaceutical properties of known drugs is the development of nanotechnology-based drug delivery systems, such as polymeric nano- and microparticles [1,10,13,14]. The particles in the form of interpolymer polyelectrolyte complexes (PECs) based on biopolymers (e.g., hyaluronic acid (HA), chitosan and its derivatives, etc.) are an attractive choice for the ocular delivery of anti-inflammatory drugs [15]. The incorporation of drug molecules into PECs of different structures allows the following: (i) to ensure selective targeting of the damaged tissues, (ii) to improve local bioavailability, (iii) to increase the residence time of the dosage form at the target site due to the mucoadhesive properties of biopolymers, (iv) to control the release rate from the polymer matrix, and (v) to reduce the degree and frequency of side effects [15–17]. In addition, the procedure for obtaining PECs is simple, convenient, and inexpensive and does not require the use of toxic reagents [1,18].

The physicochemical properties of polymeric particles, such as size, charge, and surface modification by targeting ligands (e.g., anti-VEGF antibodies [19], targeting peptide ICAM-1 [20], mannose [21], etc.), affect the efficiency of drug delivery and the efficacy of ocular disease treatment [22]. In this case, particles 50–400 nm in diameter are the preferred size for ophthalmic drug delivery because they provide more effective mucoadhesion and rapid penetration through the ocular barriers to the target site with less ocular irritation [10,23,24]. In addition, cationic nanocarriers have a longer residence time on the ocular mucosa due to their interaction with negatively charged mucus components, resulting in an enhanced ability to penetrate the drug into the eye [25,26]. On the other hand, the positive charge of the surface may prevent the particles from penetrating through the sclera and diffusing into the vitreous body due to their electrostatic binding with negatively charged components of these tissues [27]. By varying the conditions of PEC formation, it is possible to obtain polymeric carriers with desired physicochemical (size and surface charge) and pharmaceutical (rate and pattern of drug release) properties to improve ocular drug delivery, including anti-inflammatory agents of glucocorticoid nature, i.e., dexamethasone [28,29].

The disadvantages of biopolymer-based PECs are the relatively fast release of the drug (on average within 1–3 h) due to the disruption of ionic interactions between macromolecules under physiological conditions by the effect of pH and ionic strength [30]. This problem can be overcome by using different cross-linking agents such as metal ions (Zn^{2+}, Ca^{2+}, etc.) [31,32]. For instance, Tiyaboonchai et al. [33] used zinc sulfate to crosslink amphotericin B-containing nanoparticles based on polyethyleneimine and dextran. The introduction of zinc sulfate (25–50 mM) into the polyethyleneimine/dextran system in a 2:1 ratio resulted in a reduction in particle size from 800 nm to 300 nm and an increase in drug encapsulation efficiency from 70% to 80–90%. The Zn^{2+} ions can thus act as a reinforcing agent by cross-linking the polymer components. In addition, zinc-reinforced particles showed a drug release delay of up to 40% within 1 h.

Our previous studies have shown that polyanionic HA and polycationic diethylaminoethyl chitosan (DEAECS) with high degrees of substitution are promising for the formation of PECs [29]. In this case, stable complexes are formed whose size and charge depend on both the ratio of polymers and the order of mixing. The most stable PECs were obtained by mixing DEAEC and HA in ratios of 1:5 and 2:5. The hydrodynamic diameter of the obtained particles was 120–300 nm, and their surface charge ranged from −10 mV to −23 mV. In addition, according to our previous studies [30], the introduction of 20% DEAECS from the HA mass prolonged the release of colistin compared to the DEAECS-free complex by increasing the colloidal stability of the particles. In addition, both DEAECS and HA have attractive biomedical properties and are biodegradable, biocompatible, and non-toxic water-soluble polymers [34–37].

HA is a targeting ligand due to its high affinity for the CD44 and stabiliin-2 receptors, which are overexpressed at sites of inflammation and on the surface of immunocompetent cells (T and B lymphocytes and macrophages) [38–40], and chitosan and its cationic derivatives increase the permeability of drug molecules across the corneal surface due to their mucoadhesive properties and ability to open tight junctions [41]. For example, Mohamed et al. [42] developed chitosan nanoparticles loaded with the nonsteroidal anti-inflammatory drug meloxicam by electrostatic interaction between cationic chitosan and anionic drug using 0.25% sodium tripolyphosphate solution as a cross-linking agent. The resulting particles had a size of 200 to 600 nm, a ζ-potential of 25–54 mV, and an encapsulation efficiency of 70–90%. An in vitro study demonstrated sustained drug release within 72 h in PBS (pH 7.4). An ex vivo experiment demonstrated improved permeability of encapsulated meloxicam through both the cornea and sclera of rabbits compared to free drug. In in vivo studies, the dispersion of the obtained PECs showed enhanced anti-inflammatory activity and no ocular irritation compared to the solution of meloxicam eye drops. In another study [43], Ricci et al. developed mucoadhesive polyelectrolyte particles for ocular delivery of the nonsteroidal anti-inflammatory drug indomethacin based on chitosan and sulfobutyl ether-β-cyclodextrin with a diameter of 350 nm and a ζ-potential of +18 mV. The resulting particles were additionally coated with thiolated low-molecular-weight HA to reverse the surface charge to negative. The positively charged chitosan particles had excellent corneal permeability, making them attractive nanoplatforms for indomethacin delivery to the posterior segment of the eye. On the other hand, thiolated hyaluronic acid-coated particles showed prolonged residence time in the conjunctival sac, making them an optimal drug delivery system for the treatment of inflammatory diseases of the anterior segment of the eye.

The aim of the present work was to develop a suitable system to improve the local ocular delivery of glucocorticoids based on HA-DEAECS PECs with prolonged release and anti-inflammatory activity. Water-soluble dexamethasone phosphate (DexP) was chosen as a model glucocorticoid. DexP is one of the most effective drugs in the treatment of inflammatory diseases, but its high systemic toxicity, the need for long-term administration, and dose-dependent severe side effects limit its medical use [44]. The encapsulation of DexP in mucoadhesive polysaccharide-based PECs ensures its controlled release and targeted delivery and increases the residence time on the ocular mucosa, thereby reducing the dosage and frequency of side effects [45,46]. Furthermore, the use of zinc sulfate as a cross-linking agent can be beneficial not only for prolonging DexP release but also for potentiating/synergizing its pharmacological action through its own biological activity (including anti-inflammatory, antimicrobial, and wound healing) [28,47].

2. Materials and Methods

2.1. Materials and Reagents

Sodium hyaluronate with a viscosity average MW of 180,000 [48] was used in this work. DEAECS, with the values of degree of substitution 83% and degree of quaternization 14%, was previously synthesized and characterized [29]. The starting material for the synthesis of DEAECS was crab shell chitosan with an average MW of 37,000 and a degree of deacetylation (DDA) of 74% [49].

DexP, phosphate-buffered saline (PBS), zinc sulfate, mucin (type II), periodic acid, basic fuchsin, and sodium pyrosulfite were from Sigma-Aldrich (St. Louis, MI, USA), and the 1 M hydrochloric acid solution was from Acros Organics (Waltham, MA, USA).

2.2. General Methods

The hydrodynamic diameter (Dh) and the ζ-potential were determined by dynamic and electrophoretic light scattering (DLS and ELS), respectively, using a Compact-Z instrument (Photocor, Moscow, Russia) with a 659.7 nm He-Ne laser at 25 mV power and a detection angle of 90°. The polydispersity index (PDI) was determined by cumulants' analysis of the autocorrelation function using DynaLS software v. 2 (SoftScientific, Tirat Carmel, Israel, http://www.softscientific.com/science/downloads.html#evals (accessed on 3 September 2023)).

UV–VIS spectra were obtained with a UV-1700 PharmaSpec spectrophotometer (Shimadzu, Kyoto, Japan).

Quantification of zinc and phosphorus was performed by inductively coupled plasma atomic emission spectroscopy (ICP-AES) using a Shimadzu Icpe-9820 spectrometer (Shimadzu, Kyoto, Japan).

Particle morphology was examined by scanning electron microscopy (SEM) using a Tescan Mira 3 scanning electron microscope (Tescan, Brno, Czech Republic). The samples were placed on double-sided carbon tape and dried in a vacuum oven for 24 h. Images were acquired in the secondary electron mode at an accelerating voltage of 20 kV and an operating current of 543.3 pA. The distance between the sample and the detector was approximately 6 mm.

2.3. Preparation of PECs

Solutions of HA (10 mg/mL), DEAECS (10 mg/mL), $ZnSO_4$ (1 mg/mL), and DexP (1 mg/mL) were prepared in bi-distilled water. PECs were obtained by mixing the components according to the following procedures (Scheme 1):

(i) To the DexP solution, DEAECS solution was added, followed by the addition of HA solution (DexP-DEAECS-HA; Scheme 1a);
(ii) To the DexP solution, DEAECS solution was added, then zinc sulfate solution was added, followed by the addition of HA solution (DexP-DEAECS-Zn-HA; Scheme 1b);
(iii) To the DexP solution, HA solution was added, followed by the addition of DEAECS solution (DexP-HA-DEAECS; Scheme 1c);
(iv) To the DexP solution, HA solution was added, then zinc sulfate solution was added, followed by the addition of DEAECS solution (DexP-HA-Zn-DEAECS; Scheme 1d).

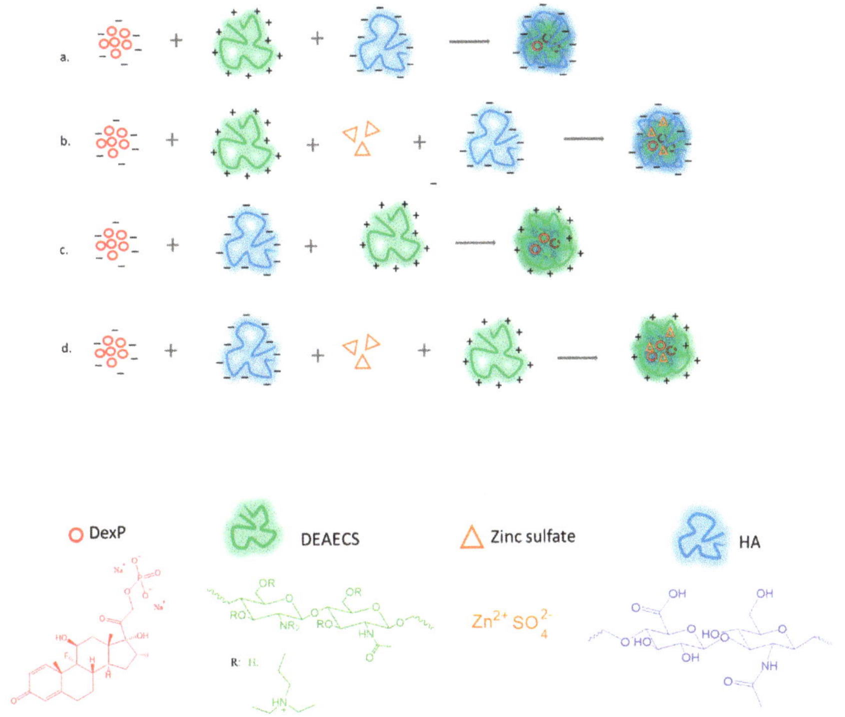

Scheme 1. Preparation of PECs: DexP-DEAECS-HA (**a**), DexP-DEAECS-Zn-HA (**b**), DexP-HA-DEAECS (**c**), and DexP-HA-Zn-DEAECS (**d**).

All solutions were added dropwise with a 23G needle under ultrasound treatment conditions (at 20 W, pulse-on 3 s and pulse-off 7 s, total 180 s) using a Bandelin Sonopuls mini 20 probe ultrasonicator (Bandelin Electronics, Berlin, Germany). The resulting systems were concentrated by ultrafiltration at 4500 rpm using a Vivaspin® Turbo 4 centrifugal concentrator with a pore size of 10,000 MWCO (Sartorius AG, Göttingen, Germany) to separate the non-encapsulated components (DexP and $ZnSO_4$). Various PEC formation parameters are shown in Table 1. The formed PECs were freeze-dried using a 10 N freeze dryer (Fanbolun Ltd., Guangzhou, China).

Table 1. Formation conditions and properties of the PECs (mean ± standard deviation, n = 3).

Formulation and Mass Ratio of Initial Components	Scheme	Dh (nm)	PDI	ζ-Potential (mV)	EE (%)	DexP Content (μg/mg)	Zn^{2+} Content (%)
DexP-DEAECS 1:5	1a	710 ± 318	0.7	+17.9 ± 0.7	77.8	-	-
DexP-DEAECS-HA 1:5:10	1a	518 ± 124 514 ± 136 *	0.5 0.5 *	−17.8 ± 0.2 −18.1 ± 0.3 *	37.8	24.6	-
DexP-DEAECS-Zn 1:5:1	1b	604 ± 162	0.3	+18.1 ± 0.5	86.7	-	-
DexP-DEAECS-Zn-HA 1:5:1:10	1b	702 ± 158 714 ± 142 *	0.3 0.3 *	−17.0 ± 0.2 −17.2 ± 0.4 *	58.5	35.7	2.2 ± 0.7
DexP-HA-DEAECS 1:5:10	1c	154 ± 28 155 ± 34 *	0.2 0.2 *	+26.8 ± 0.5 +26.1 ± 0.7 *	10.5	7.0	-
DexP-HA-Zn 1:5:1	1d	950 ± 253	0.6	−21.4 ± 0.6	30.3	-	-
DexP-HA-Zn-DEAECS 1:5:1:10	1d	244 ± 56 256 ± 61 *	0.1 0.1 *	+24.4 ± 0.3 +25.3 ± 0.2 *	75.6	45.4	2.3 ± 0.8

* Particle parameters after storage for 24 h as an aqueous dispersion at room temperature.

2.4. Encapsulation Efficiencies and DexP Content

Encapsulation efficiency (EE) and DexP content (μg/mg) were determined by measuring the concentration of unloaded DexP (indirect method). The PEC suspension was concentrated by ultrafiltration (see Section 2.3). The amount of encapsulated DexP in the PEC was calculated from the difference between the total amount of DexP used to prepare the PECs and the amount of DexP in the filtrate. The concentration of DexP in the filtrate was determined spectrophotometrically at a wavelength of 242 nm using a calibration curve (10 mm quartz cuvette, UV-visible spectrophotometer Shimadzu UV-1700 Pharma Spec, Japan). The results were calculated according to the following equations:

$$\text{EE }(\%) = \frac{(\text{DexP mass total} - \text{DexP mass in the filtrate}) \times 100}{\text{DexP mass total}} \quad (1)$$

$$\text{DexP content }(\mu\text{g/mg}) = \frac{(\text{Dex mass total} - \text{Dex mass in the filtrate}) \times 1000}{\text{PEC mass}} \quad (2)$$

2.5. In Vitro DexP Release

The release test conditions were selected based on the FDA recommendation for dissolution methods for topical ophthalmic dosage forms [13]. A 10 mg sample was dispersed in PBS (2 mL, pH 7.4) and incubated at 32 °C. At specified time intervals, the nanosuspension was ultracentrifuged at 4500 rpm using a 10,000 MWCO Vivaspin®Turbo4 centrifugal concentrator, and the volume of dissolution medium was replenished with fresh PBS. The amount of DexP released was determined spectrophotometrically.

2.6. Mucoadhesion

The mucin binding efficiency was evaluated by mucin adsorption using the two-step periodic acid/Schiff colorimetric method [50,51]. Periodic acid was prepared as follows: 10 μL of 50% periodic acid was added to 7 mL of 7% acetic acid. Schiff's reagent was prepared as follows: 100 mL of 1% aqueous basic fuchsin was added to 20 mL of 1 M HCl; the resulting mixture was decolorized twice for 5 min with 300 mg activated charcoal.

Sodium pyrosulfite (0.1 g per 6 mL of Schiff's reagent) was added just before use, and the resulting solution was incubated at 37 °C until it became colorless or pale yellow (about 90–100 min).

The calibration curve was constructed as follows: 200 μL of freshly prepared periodic acid was added to 2 mL of standard mucin solutions (0.02–0.08 mg/mL). The resulting solutions were incubated at 37 °C for 120 min to complete the periodate oxidation; then, colorless Schiff reagent (200 μL) was added and allowed to stand for 30 min at room temperature (the solution turned pink). The absorbance of the standards was measured at 565 nm.

Mucin solution (0.5 mg/mL; 1 mL) was added to the DexP-DEAECS-Zn-HA and DexP-HA-Zn-DEAECS (0.5 mg/mL; 10 mL) with magnetic stirring at 500 rpm, and the mixture was incubated at 37 °C for 60 min. The resulting mixture was centrifuged at 4500 rpm for 60 min, and the supernatant was used to measure the free mucin concentration using the calibration curve. A solution containing all the components of the analyzed solution, except for the analyte, was used as a reference solution. Mucoadhesiveness (mucin binding efficiency) was calculated using the following equation:

$$\text{Mucoadhesiveness}\ (\%) = \frac{(m_o - m_s) \times 100}{m_o} \quad (3)$$

where m_o is the initial mucin mass and m_s is the mucin mass in the supernatant.

2.7. *Anti-Inflammatory Activity*

Human monocytic leukemia cells (THP-1 cells) were used to study the in vitro effects of DexP and DexP-containing PECs. Cell line THP-1 was obtained from the Collection of Vertebrate Cell Cultures maintained by the Institute of Cytology of the Russian Academy of Sciences. THP-1 cells were cultured at 37 °C in a humidified atmosphere with 5% CO_2 in RPMI-1640 medium (Biolot, St. Petersburg, Russia) supplemented with 10% (*v*/*v*) heat-inactivated fetal calf serum (FBS, Gibco Inc., Grand Island, NY, USA), 2 mM L-glutamine (Biolot, St. Petersburg, Russia), and 50 μg/mL gentamicin (Biolot, St. Petersburg, Russia), as previously described [13]. Primarily, we investigated the effects of DexP on cell viability, and flow cytometry based on YO-PRO-1/PI staining was performed to detect viable and apoptotic cells. YO-PRO-1 iodide (Molecular Probes, Eugene, OR, USA) was used at a final concentration of 250 nM, and propidium iodide (PI, Merck KGaA, Darmstadt, Germany) was used at a final concentration of 1 μM. Method principles and "gating strategy" were described previously [52]. A minimum of 10,000 THP-1 cells were analyzed per sample. Flow cytometry data were obtained using a Navios™ flow cytometer (Beckman Coulter, Beckman Coulter Inc., Indianapolis, IN, USA) equipped with 405, 488, and 638 nm lasers and analyzed using Navios software v.1.2 and Kaluza™ software v.2.0 (Beckman Coulter, Beckman Coulter Inc., Indianapolis, IN, USA). Data were presented as median and interquartile range, Me (Q25; Q75). Differences between groups were analyzed using a non-parametric Mann–Whitney U test with a value of $p < 0.05$.

Next, we investigated the ability of DexP, $ZnSO_4$, and DexP/Zn^{2+}-containing PECs to suppress in vitro activation of THP-1 cells. We activated THP-1 cells in vitro by adding recombinant human tumor necrosis factor-α protein (final concentration 2 ng/mL, BioLegend Inc., San Diego, CA, USA), while untreated THP-1 cells were used as a negative control. The test compounds (DexP, $ZnSO_4$, DexP-HA-DEAECS, DexP-HA-Zn-DEAECS, DexP-DEAECS-HA, DexP-DEAECS-Zn-HA, and HA-DEAECS) were added to 200 μL THP-1 cell suspension (200 μL cell culture medium containing 1 × 105 cells in suspension) and incubated for 24 h in 96-well flat-bottom culture plates (Sarstedt, Germany). The concentrations of the compounds tested were equivalent to a DexP concentration of 0.1 μg/mL. The cells were then transferred to 75 mm × 12 mm flow cytometry tubes (Sarstedt, Germany) and washed with 4 mL sterile PBS (centrifugation at 300× *g* for 5 min). The resulting cell sediments were resuspended in 100 μL fresh sterile PBS and stained with mouse anti-human CD54-PE antibody (clone HA58, isotype—mouse IgG1, κ; BioLegend Inc., San Diego, CA,

USA) for 15 min in the dark as described previously [14]. Finally, THP-1 cell samples were washed again and stained with DAPI (final concentration 1 µg/mL; BioLegend Inc., San Diego, CA, USA) to distinguish between live and dead cells. A minimum of 10,000 single THP-1 cells were collected per sample. Flow cytometry data were obtained using a Navios™ flow cytometer (Beckman Coulter Inc., CA, USA) equipped with 405, 488, and 638 nm lasers and analyzed using Navios software v.1.2 and Kaluza™ software v.2.0 (Beckman Coulter Inc., CA, USA). The intensity of CD54 expression was finally measured as mean fluorescence intensity (MFI) on the cell surface of viable THP-1 cells. Data were presented as median and interquartile range, Me (Q25; Q75). Differences between groups were analyzed using a non-parametric Mann–Whitney U test with a value of $p < 0.05$.

3. Results and Discussion

3.1. Preparation and Characterization of the PECs

DEAECS is an alkylated derivative of chitosan with a high positive charge density. Typically, the substitution reaction proceeds through both amine and hydroxyl groups, and 0–15% of the diethylaminoethyl groups are alkylated to form quaternary ammonium groups [29]. The first step of our study was to investigate the interaction of the water-soluble cationic polymer DEAECS with negatively charged DexP molecules using spectrophotometry [53]. Titration of the DexP solution (0.025 mg/mL) with the DEAECS solution (0.3 mg/mL) showed a change in the shape of the DexP absorption spectrum and a decrease in absorption intensity with increasing polymer content (hypochromic effect), indicating that these components interact with each other (Figure 1).

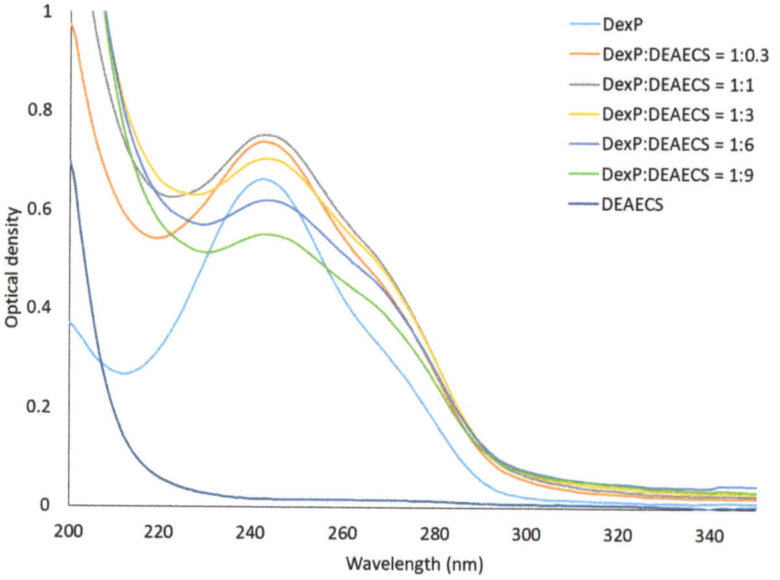

Figure 1. UV–VIS absorption spectra of mixtures of DEAECS and DexP at different ratios in water.

In the second step, it was of interest to investigate the tri-component systems DexP-DEAECS-HA and DexP-HA-DEAECS by DLS. Furthermore, zinc sulfate solution was added to the tri-component systems (DexP-DEAECS-Zn-HA and DexP-HA-Zn-DEAECS) to better control the strength of the formed PECs, their size, and their surface charge. DEAECS is capable of chelating Zn^{2+} cations via amino and hydroxyl groups. The deprotonated amino groups are responsible for the complexing properties, while the protonated amino groups provide electrostatic interactions with both DexP anions and carboxylate groups of HA [32]. In addition, Zn^{2+} cations also bind to the phosphate group of DexP and the carboxylate group of HA [31]. Thus, particle formation is the result of complex interactions (Figure 2). The data obtained by the DLS method are shown in Table 1.

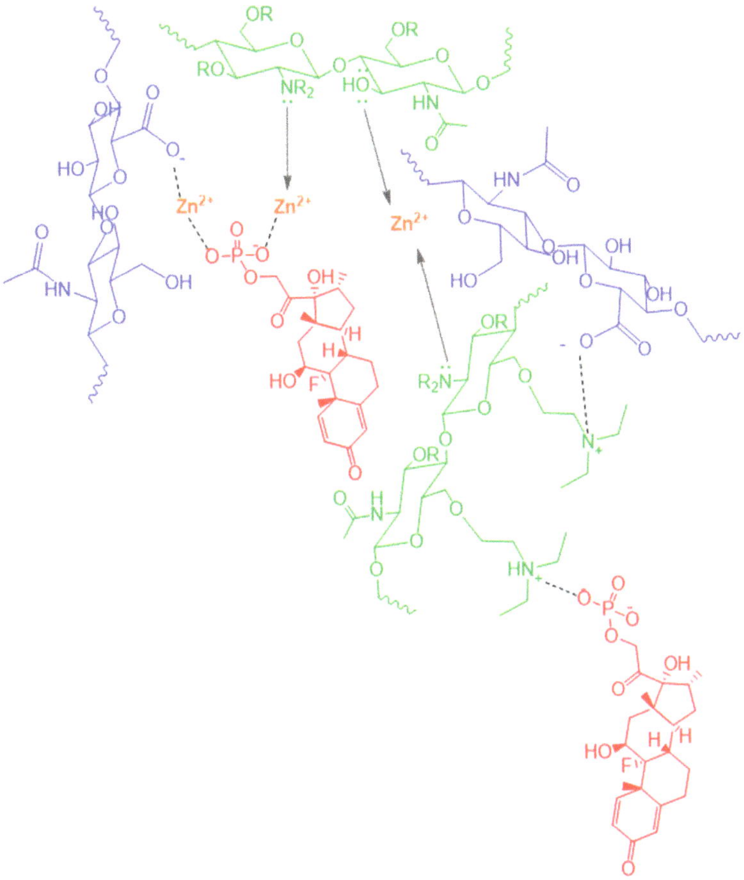

Figure 2. Some possible interactions in a system consisting of DexP, Zn^{2+}, and polymers (DEAECS and HA).

The order of polyelectrolyte mixing influenced both particle size and particle size distribution (PDI). The addition of zinc ions contributed to a decrease in particle size and an increase in particle size uniformity due to the cross-linking effect. Thus, the interaction of DexP with DEAECS resulted in the formation of large polymeric particles (DexP-DEAECS) with a size of 710 nm, a positive surface charge (ζ-potential of +17.9 mV), and a high PDI of 0.7. After the addition of HA (DexP-DEAECS-HA, Scheme 1a) to this system, the particle size was reduced to 518 nm, and PECs with a negative ζ-potential (−17.8 mV) were formed (Table 1). The introduction of zinc ions into the DexP-DEAECS system reduced both the particle size (to 604 nm) and the PDI to a value of 0.3 (DexP-DEAECS-Zn). The addition of HA to this system resulted in the formation of negatively charged (ζ-potential of −17 mV) PECs sized at 702 nm (DexP-DEAECS-Zn-HA, Scheme 1b).

By changing the mixing order of DEAECS and HA, we were able to obtain PECs with acceptable size (154 nm) and PDI (0.2), as well as a high ζ-potential of +26.8 mV (DexP-HA-DEAECS, Scheme 1c). The introduction of zinc ions into the mixture of DexP and HA resulted in the formation of large polydisperse particles (950 nm, PDI 0.6). Further treatment of the resulting system with DEAECS resulted in PECs with the desired size (244 nm) and narrow size distribution (PDI 0.1), as well as a suitable ζ-potential (24.4) to ensure colloidal stability of the system (DexP-HA-Zn-DEAECS, Scheme 1d). It should be noted that PDI values of 0.2 and below are generally considered acceptable for polymeric drug delivery systems [54]. The obtained particles retained their parameters, including size, ζ-potential, and PDI, for at least 24 h (Table 1).

The EE is an important parameter that determines the suitability of the process for PEC formation. As shown in Table 1, the order of mixing the components and the addition of zinc ions (cross-linking agent) affected the EE of DexP. DEAECS efficiently bound DexP (DexP-DEAECS, EE 77.8%), but when HA was added, some DexP was displaced, and the EE decreased to 37.8% (DexP-DEAECS-HA). In contrast, the addition of Zn^{2+} promoted an increase in EE to 86.7% due to additional binding of DexP molecules (DexP-DEAECS-Zn), which also led to an increase in EE to 58.5% when HA was added to the system (DexP-DEAECS-Zn-HA).

When DEAECS was added to the mixture of DexP and HA, the EE was only 10.5% (DexP-HA-DEAECS), apparently indicating a primary interaction between the polyelectrolytes. However, the introduction of the zinc ions increased the EE to 30.3% and 75.6% (DexP-HA-Zn and DexP-HA-Zn-DEAECS, respectively).

UV–VIS spectra of three- and four-component systems show the interaction of DexP with DEAECS and a stepwise increase in the turbidity (baseline enhancement due to light scattering) of the PEC nanosuspension due to the formation of insoluble polymeric particles DexP-DEAECS-Zn-HA (Figure 3a) as well as DexP-HA-Zn-DEAECS (Figure 3b).

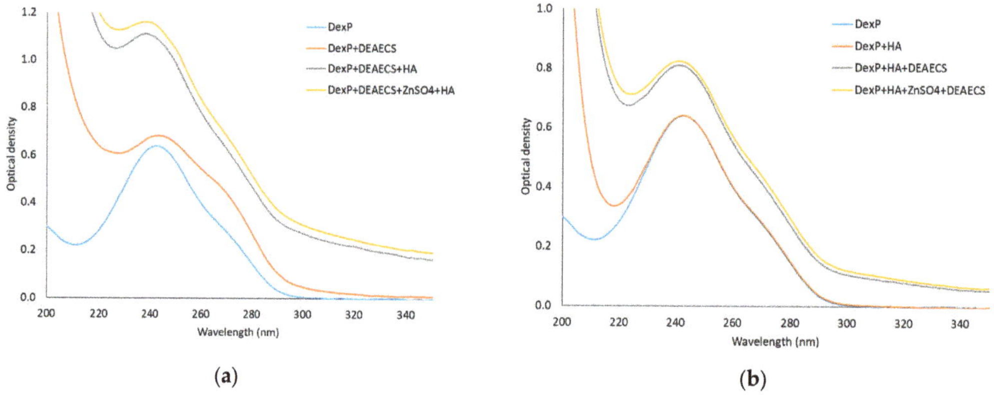

Figure 3. UV–VIS absorption spectra upon stepwise formation of DexP-DEAECS-Zn-HA (**a**) and DexP-HA-Zn-DEAECS (**b**).

SEM images of DexP-DEAECS-Zn-HA (Figure 4a) and DexP-HA-Zn-DEAECS (Figure 4b) showed the presence of spherical particles; the sizes of the PECs obtained in the solid state correspond to their hydrodynamic diameters, which is an indirect marker of the stiffness of zinc-containing PECs [48].

3.2. *In Vitro DexP Release Kinetics from the PECs*

DexP in water interacts with polycationic DEAECS to form PECs as a result of the subsequent addition of polyanionic HA; the resulting PECs are further strengthened and stabilized by the introduction of zinc ions due to their cross-linking effect. However, under physiological conditions, due to the influence of pH and ionic strength, the bonds between the components are weakened, diffusion is increased, and drug molecules are released [30]. The in vitro kinetics of DexP release in PBS at 32 °C is shown in Figure 5.

DexP release from zinc-free PECs (DexP-DEAECS-HA and DexP-HA-DEAECS) was rapid within 2–4 h. In contrast, Zn^{2+}-containing particles were characterized by delayed release, with a total of 98 and 70% DexP release in 10 h from DexP-DEAECS-Zn-HA and DexP-HA-Zn-DEAECS, respectively. The presence of DEAECS on the surface of polymeric particles prolonged drug release both by increasing the colloidal stability of PECs and by limiting diffusion due to ionic interactions of the polycationic polymer with the DexP anion. Thus, both the presence of zinc ions and an increase in the content of polycationic DEAECS in the system modified the release of DexP from the corresponding PECs. DexP-containing polymeric nanocarriers with these release profiles are attractive topical glucocorticoid delivery systems.

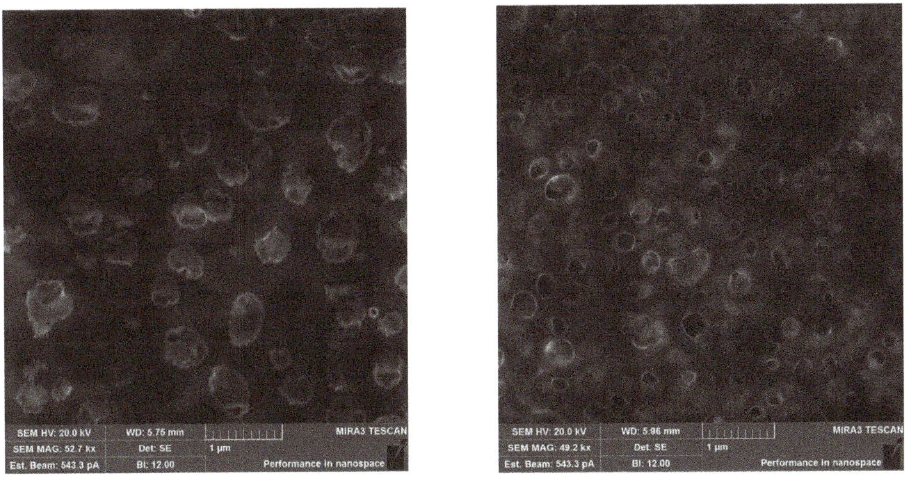

(**a**) (**b**)

Figure 4. SEM images of DexP-DEAECS-Zn-HA (**a**) and DexP-HA-Zn-DEAECS (**b**).

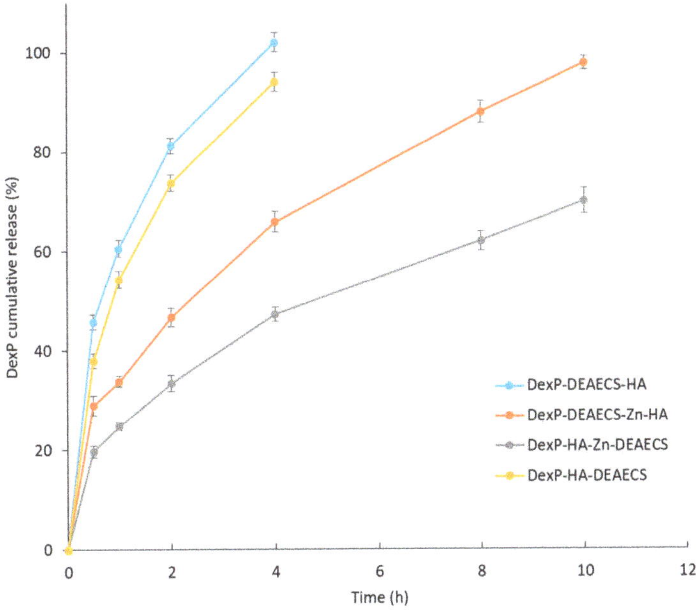

Figure 5. Release of DexP from the PECs in PBS at 32 °C. Data are presented as mean ± standard deviation (n = 3).

Assuming diffusion-controlled release, the cumulative DexP release curves were linearized according to the Higuchi and Korsmeyer–Peppas kinetic models [55,56]. The fitting parameters are shown in Table 2.

Table 2. Fitting parameters of the kinetic models of DexP release.

Formulation	Kinetic Model *				
	Higuchi $Q = K_H t^{0.5}$ (4)		Korsmeyer-Peppas $Q = K_{KP} t^n$ (5)		
	K_H	R^2	K_{KP}	n	R^2
DexP-DEAECS-HA	54.9	0.9743	65.0	0.50	0.9986
DexP-DEAECS-Zn-HA	31.9	0.9906	37.1	0.40	0.9966
DexP-HA-DEAECS	49.8	0.9865	51.0	0.50	0.9943
DexP-HA-Zn-DEAECS	22.6	0.9915	25.5	0.43	0.9993

* Q is the cumulative DexP release (%); K_H is the Higuchi constant; K_{KP} is the release rate constant; n is the release exponent, t is the time.

The kinetics of DexP release were in good agreement with both the Higuchi (4) and Korsmeyer–Peppas (5) models. The values of the release exponent ($n \leq 0.5$) characterize the drug release mechanism as a Fickian diffusion (Case I transport) and diffusion-controlled process, which is typical for this type of polymeric particle [57].

3.3. *Mucoadhesion of the PECs*

Mucoadhesive ocular drug delivery systems adhere to the corneal mucosa, thereby increasing drug residence time and local bioavailability [58]. Both DEAECS and HA are capable of intermolecular interaction with various functional groups of mucin through hydrogen bonding and entanglement of polymer chains, as well as electrostatic bonding and hydrophobic interaction [58,59]. The mucoadhesion of DexP-DEAECS-Zn-HA and DexP-HA-Zn-DEAECS was tested as they were the most promising nanocarriers in terms of DexP release profile. The mucoadhesive properties were evaluated by the ability of the particles to bind mucin in aqueous solution. The amount of mucin adsorbed was measured by the change in free mucin concentration in the supernatant according to Equation (3). It was shown (Figure 6) that both DexP-DEAECS-Zn-HA and DexP-HA-Zn-DEAECS effectively bound mucin (mucoadhesive capacity was approximately 40 and 59%, respectively); however, the use of DEAECS-coated PECs with a positive surface charge increased the mucoadhesive capacity of the particles 1.5-fold. Thus, because of their ability to bind to mucin, zinc-containing PECs can prevent the rapid clearance of DexP from the corneal surface, indicating their promise in the treatment of inflammatory eye diseases.

3.4. *Anti-Inflammatory Activity of the PECs*

Our results showed that DexP, $ZnSO_4$, HA-DEAECS, and DexP/Zn^{2+}-containing PECs had no significant cytotoxic effect on TNFa-untreated THP-1 cells (Table 3). We also found that the combination treatment of THP-1 cells with TNFa and DexP, $ZnSO_4$, HA-DEAECS, and DexP/Zn^{2+}-containing PECs also had no significant effect on the viability of THP-1 cells. These results indicated that DexP, $ZnSO_4$, HA-DEAECS, and DexP/Zn^{2+}-containing PECs had no cytotoxic effects on THP-1 cells.

We then examined the effects of DexP, $ZnSO_4$, HA-DEAECS, and DexP/ Zn^{2+}-containing PECs on TNFa-induced cell surface CD54 expression by THP-1 cells (Table 4). The results confirmed that our TNFa stimulation effectively increased cell surface CD54 expression on THP-1 cells (4.61 (3.77; 5.55) MFI in negative controls vs. 0.77 (0.60; 0.86) MFI after 24 h in vitro co-culture with 2 ng/mL TNFa, $p < 0.001$). Interestingly, we found that two types of DexP-containing systems (DexP-HA-DEAECS and DexP-HA-Zn-DEAECS) increased CD54 expression on THP-1 cells without TNFa stimulation. Finally, we found that all DexP/ Zn^{2+}-containing PECs significantly downregulated CD54 expression on TNFa-treated THP-1 cells, whereas $ZnSO_4$ solution had no effect on CD54 expression. Taken together, our results indicate that DexP/Zn-containing PECs were effective in suppressing TNFa-induced THP-1 cell activation and exhibited anti-inflammatory activity in vitro.

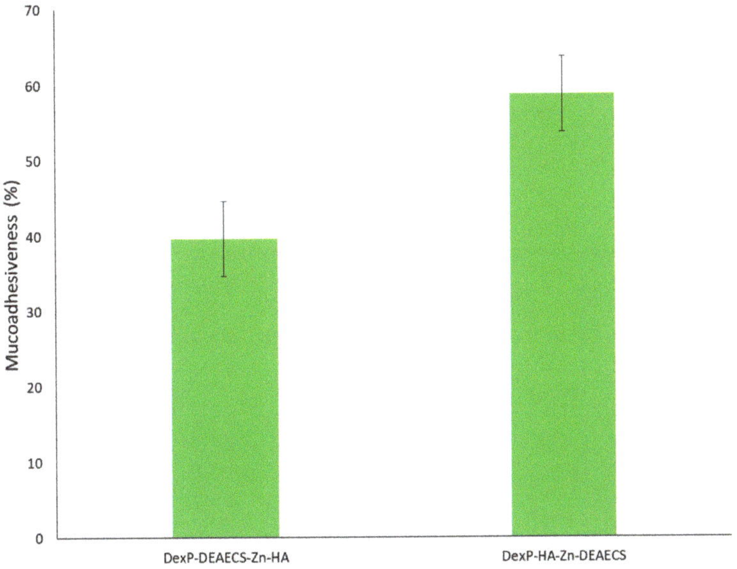

Figure 6. Mucoadhesiveness of DexP-DEAECS-Zn-HA and DexP-HA-Zn-DEAECS. Data are presented as mean ± standard deviation (n = 3).

Table 3. Cell viability (the corresponding numbers of live YO-PRO-1negPIneg cells) staining of THP-1 cells treated with DexP, $ZnSO_4$, HA-DEAECS, and DexP/ Zn^{2+}-containing PECs for 24 h as detected by YO-PRO-1/PI staining (n = 9). Data are presented as median and interquartile range, Me (Q25; Q75).

Sample	no TNFa Added	2 ng/mL TNFa
Negative control	95.94 (95.63; 96.30)	96.08 (95.65; 96.28)
DexP-HA-DEAECS	96.44 (96.10; 96.63)	96.20 (95.70; 96.31)
DexP-DEAECS-Zn-HA	96.32 (96.21; 96.63)	96.17 (95.93; 96.34)
HA-DEAECS	96.07 (95.61; 96.34)	96.06 (95.84; 96.25)
$ZnSO_4$	96.60 (96.23; 96.75)	96.09 (95.83; 96.40)
DexP-HA-Zn-DEAECS	96.25 (96.03; 96.49)	96.09 (95.95; 96.27)
DexP	96.46 (96.18; 96.48)	95.74 (95.50; 96.13)
DexP-DEAECS-HA	96.20 (96.06; 96.39)	96.22 (96.01; 96.35)

Table 4. CD54 expression by THP-1 cells in vitro treated with DexP, $ZnSO_4$, HA-DEAECS, and DexP/ Zn^{2+}-containing PECs. Data are presented as median and interquartile range, Me (Q25; Q75) (n = 6); data are presented as CD54 MFI.

Sample	no TNFa Added	2 ng/mL TNFa
Negative control	0,77 (0,60; 0,86)	4,61 (3,77; 5,55)
DexP-HA-DEAECS	1.01 (0.81; 1.03) **	2.24 (2.15; 2.41) **
DexP-DEAECS-Zn-HA	0.80 (0.65; 1.17)	1.90 (1.84; 2.37) **
HA-DEAECS	0.66 (0.61; 0.68)	2.63 (2.47; 3.63) *
$ZnSO_4$	0.64 (0.61; 0.64)	3.84 (3.40; 4.06)
DexP-HA-Zn-DEAECS	0.95 (0.89; 1.36) *	2.71 (2.44; 3.05) **
DexP	0.62 (0.59; 0.67)	1.26 (1.09; 1.63) **
DexP-DEAECS-HA	0.80 (0.74; 0.87)	1.93 (1.78; 2.00) **

* and **—the differences from the negative control (THP-1 cells without addition of DexP, $ZnSO_4$, and DexP/ Zn^{2+}-containing PECs) were significant at $p < 0.05$ and $p < 0.01$, respectively, according to the non-parametric Mann–Whitney U test.

4. Conclusions

We have developed a simple and convenient technique for obtaining DEAECS- and HA-based PECs with pronounced anti-inflammatory activity. The advantages of this technique are (i) easy preparation and mild preparation conditions, (ii) use of aqueous solutions, (iii) use of biocompatible and biodegradable polysaccharides, (iv) the possibility to control the size and surface charge of the formed PECs, (v) high EE, (vi) prolonged drug release within 10 h, and (vii) effective mucoadhesion.

It can be concluded that the key factor for the formation of stable particles of 200–300 nm size is the polyelectrolyte interaction between oppositely charged polymers upon the addition of DEAECS to HA. However, the obtained PECs have a low EE (10.5%) and a fast DexP release (within 2 h). The use of zinc ions as a cross-linking agent increased the EE to 75.6% and prolonged the drug release to 10 h.

The results indicate that the developed PECs are promising nanocarriers with desirable properties (including size, charge, EE, drug release profile, and mucoadhesion). Based on these data, we plan to extend our research to in vivo experiments with the goal of creating a topical DexP delivery system with enhanced bioavailability and improved therapeutic properties.

Author Contributions: Conceptualization, N.V.D. and Y.A.S.; methodology, N.V.D., A.N.B., A.S.T., I.V.K. and Y.A.S.; investigation, N.V.D., A.N.B., A.S.T. and A.A.R.; writing—original draft preparation, N.V.D. and I.V.K.; writing—review and editing, Y.A.S.; supervision, Y.A.S.; project administration Y.A.S.; funding acquisition, N.V.D. All authors have read and agreed to the published version of the manuscript.

Funding: This study was financially supported by the Russian Science Foundation (project 23-23-00148).

Institutional Review Board Statement: Not applicable.

Informed Consent Statement: Not applicable.

Data Availability Statement: The data are contained within the article.

Conflicts of Interest: The authors declare no conflict of interest. The funders had no role in the design of the study, in the collection, analyses, or interpretation of data, in the writing of the manuscript, or in the decision to publish the results.

References

1. Han, H.; Li, S.; Xu, M.; Zhong, Y.; Fan, W.; Xu, J.; Zhou, T.; Ji, J.; Ye, J.; Yao, K. Polymer-and lipid-based nanocarriers for ocular drug delivery: Current status and future perspectives. *Adv. Drug Deliv. Rev.* **2023**, *196*, 114770. [CrossRef] [PubMed]
2. Steinmetz, J.D.; Bourne, R.R.; Briant, P.S.; Flaxman, S.R.; Taylor, H.R.; Jonas, J.B.; Abdoli, A.A.; Abrha, W.A.; Abualhasan, A.; Abu-Gharbieh, E.G. Causes of blindness and vision impairment in 2020 and trends over 30 years, and prevalence of avoidable blindness in relation to VISION 2020: The Right to Sight: An analysis for the Global Burden of Disease Study. *Lancet Glob. Health* **2021**, *9*, e144–e160. [CrossRef] [PubMed]
3. Cone, R.A. Barrier properties of mucus. *Adv. Drug Deliv. Rev.* **2009**, *61*, 75–85. [CrossRef]
4. Alshaikh, R.A.; Waeber, C.; Ryan, K.B. Polymer based sustained drug delivery to the ocular posterior segment: Barriers and future opportunities for the treatment of neovascular pathologies. *Adv. Drug Deliv. Rev.* **2022**, *187*, 114342. [CrossRef] [PubMed]
5. Mofidfar, M.; Abdi, B.; Ahadian, S.; Mostafavi, E.; Desai, T.A.; Abbasi, F.; Sun, Y.; Manche, E.E.; Ta, C.N.; Flowers, C.W. Drug delivery to the anterior segment of the eye: A review of current and future treatment strategies. *Int. J. Pharm.* **2021**, *607*, 120924. [CrossRef]
6. Sun, S.; Li, J.; Li, X.; Lan, B.; Zhou, S.; Meng, Y.; Cheng, L. Episcleral drug film for better-targeted ocular drug delivery and controlled release using multilayered poly-ε-caprolactone (PCL). *Acta Biomater.* **2016**, *37*, 143–154. [CrossRef]
7. Billowria, K.; Sandhu, N.K.; Singh, B. Topical Advances in Mucoadhesive Ocular Drug Delivery System. *Curr. Drug Deliv.* **2023**, *20*, 1127–1140. [CrossRef]
8. Subrizi, A.; Del Amo, E.M.; Korzhikov-Vlakh, V.; Tennikova, T.; Ruponen, M.; Urtti, A. Design principles of ocular drug delivery systems: Importance of drug payload, release rate, and material properties. *Drug Discov. Today* **2019**, *24*, 1446–1457. [CrossRef]
9. Baudouin, C.; Labbé, A.; Liang, H.; Pauly, A.; Brignole-Baudouin, F. Retinal and eye research. *Prog. Retin. Eye Res.* **2010**, *29*, 312e334.
10. Dubashynskaya, N.; Poshina, D.; Raik, S.; Urtti, A.; Skorik, Y.A. Polysaccharides in ocular drug delivery. *Pharmaceutics* **2019**, *12*, 22. [CrossRef]

11. Urtti, A. Challenges and obstacles of ocular pharmacokinetics and drug delivery. *Adv. Drug Deliv. Rev.* **2006**, *58*, 1131–1135. [CrossRef] [PubMed]
12. Almeida, H.; Amaral, M.H.; Lobão, P.; Sousa Lobo, J.M. Applications of poloxamers in ophthalmic pharmaceutical formulations: An overview. *Expert Opin. Drug Deliv.* **2013**, *10*, 1223–1237. [CrossRef] [PubMed]
13. Dubashynskaya, N.V.; Golovkin, A.S.; Kudryavtsev, I.V.; Prikhodko, S.S.; Trulioff, A.S.; Bokatyi, A.N.; Poshina, D.N.; Raik, S.V.; Skorik, Y.A. Mucoadhesive cholesterol-chitosan self-assembled particles for topical ocular delivery of dexamethasone. *Int. J. Biol. Macromol.* **2020**, *158*, 811–818. [CrossRef] [PubMed]
14. Dubashynskaya, N.V.; Bokatyi, A.N.; Golovkin, A.S.; Kudryavtsev, I.V.; Serebryakova, M.K.; Trulioff, A.S.; Dubrovskii, Y.A.; Skorik, Y.A. Synthesis and characterization of novel succinyl chitosan-dexamethasone conjugates for potential intravitreal dexamethasone delivery. *Int. J. Mol. Sci.* **2021**, *22*, 10960. [CrossRef]
15. Tsai, C.-H.; Wang, P.-Y.; Lin, I.-C.; Huang, H.; Liu, G.-S.; Tseng, C.-L. Ocular drug delivery: Role of degradable polymeric nanocarriers for ophthalmic application. *Int. J. Mol. Sci.* **2018**, *19*, 2830. [CrossRef]
16. Wang, C.; Pang, Y. Nano-based eye drop: Topical and noninvasive therapy for ocular diseases. *Adv. Drug Deliv. Rev.* **2023**, *194*, 114721. [CrossRef]
17. Liu, Y.-C.; Lin, M.T.-Y.; Ng, A.H.C.; Wong, T.T.; Mehta, J.S. Nanotechnology for the treatment of allergic conjunctival diseases. *Pharmaceuticals* **2020**, *13*, 351. [CrossRef]
18. Mitchell, M.; Billingsley, M.; Haley, R.; Marissa, E.; Nicholas, A. Langer Robert. Engineering precision nanoparticles for drug delivery. *Nat. Rev. Drug Discov.* **2021**, *20*, 101–124. [CrossRef]
19. Zhao, X.; Seah, I.; Xue, K.; Wong, W.; Tan, Q.S.W.; Ma, X.; Lin, Q.; Lim, J.Y.; Liu, Z.; Parikh, B.H. Antiangiogenic nanomicelles for the topical delivery of aflibercept to treat retinal neovascular disease. *Adv. Mater.* **2022**, *34*, 2108360. [CrossRef]
20. Hsueh, P.-Y.; Ju, Y.; Vega, A.; Edman, M.C.; MacKay, J.A.; Hamm-Alvarez, S.F. A multivalent ICAM-1 binding nanoparticle which inhibits ICAM-1 and LFA-1 interaction represents a new tool for the investigation of autoimmune-mediated dry eye. *Int. J. Mol. Sci.* **2020**, *21*, 2758. [CrossRef]
21. Torretta, S.; Scagliola, A.; Ricci, L.; Mainini, F.; Di Marco, S.; Cuccovillo, I.; Kajaste-Rudnitski, A.; Sumpton, D.; Ryan, K.M.; Cardaci, S. D-mannose suppresses macrophage IL-1β production. *Nat. Commun.* **2020**, *11*, 6343. [CrossRef]
22. Weng, Y.; Liu, J.; Jin, S.; Guo, W.; Liang, X.; Hu, Z. Nanotechnology-based strategies for treatment of ocular disease. *Acta Pharm. Sin. B* **2017**, *7*, 281–291. [CrossRef]
23. Liu, D.; Lian, Y.; Fang, Q.; Liu, L.; Zhang, J.; Li, J. Hyaluronic-acid-modified lipid-polymer hybrid nanoparticles as an efficient ocular delivery platform for moxifloxacin hydrochloride. *Int. J. Biol. Macromol.* **2018**, *116*, 1026–1036. [CrossRef]
24. Almeida, H.; Amaral, M.H.; Lobão, P.; Silva, A.C.; Loboa, J.M.S. Applications of polymeric and lipid nanoparticles in ophthalmic pharmaceutical formulations: Present and future considerations. *J. Pharm. Pharm. Sci.* **2014**, *17*, 278–293. [CrossRef] [PubMed]
25. Imperiale, J.C.; Acosta, G.B.; Sosnik, A. Polymer-based carriers for ophthalmic drug delivery. *J. Control. Release* **2018**, *285*, 106–141. [CrossRef]
26. Martens, T.F.; Remaut, K.; Deschout, H.; Engbersen, J.F.; Hennink, W.E.; Van Steenbergen, M.J.; Demeester, J.; De Smedt, S.C.; Braeckmans, K. Coating nanocarriers with hyaluronic acid facilitates intravitreal drug delivery for retinal gene therapy. *J. Control. Release* **2015**, *202*, 83–92. [CrossRef]
27. Radhakrishnan, K.; Sonali, N.; Moreno, M.; Nirmal, J.; Fernandez, A.A.; Venkatraman, S.; Agrawal, R. Protein delivery to the back of the eye: Barriers, carriers and stability of anti-VEGF proteins. *Drug Discov. Today* **2017**, *22*, 416–423. [CrossRef]
28. Fang, L.; Liu, J.; Liu, Z.; Zhou, H. Immune modulating nanoparticles for the treatment of ocular diseases. *J. Nanobiotechnol.* **2022**, *20*, 496. [CrossRef] [PubMed]
29. Raik, S.V.; Gasilova, E.R.; Dubashynskaya, N.V.; Dobrodumov, A.V.; Skorik, Y.A. Diethylaminoethyl chitosan–hyaluronic acid polyelectrolyte complexes. *Int. J. Biol. Macromol.* **2020**, *146*, 1161–1168. [CrossRef] [PubMed]
30. Dubashynskaya, N.V.; Raik, S.V.; Dubrovskii, Y.A.; Demyanova, E.V.; Shcherbakova, E.S.; Poshina, D.N.; Shasherina, A.Y.; Anufrikov, Y.A.; Skorik, Y.A. Hyaluronan/diethylaminoethyl chitosan polyelectrolyte complexes as carriers for improved colistin delivery. *Int. J. Mol. Sci.* **2021**, *22*, 8381. [CrossRef]
31. Cao, J.; Naeem, M.; Noh, J.-K.; Lee, E.H.; Yoo, J.-W. Dexamethasone phosphate-loaded folate-conjugated polymeric nanoparticles for selective delivery to activated macrophages and suppression of inflammatory responses. *Macromol. Res.* **2015**, *23*, 485–492. [CrossRef]
32. Sun, S.; Wang, A. Adsorption properties and mechanism of cross-linked carboxymethyl-chitosan resin with Zn (II) as template ion. *React. Funct. Polym.* **2006**, *66*, 819–826. [CrossRef]
33. Tiyaboonchai, W.; Woiszwillo, J.; Middaugh, C.R. Formulation and characterization of amphotericin B–polyethylenimine–dextran sulfate nanoparticles. *J. Pharm. Sci.* **2001**, *90*, 902–914. [CrossRef] [PubMed]
34. Chen, L.; Zheng, Y.; Feng, L.; Liu, Z.; Guo, R.; Zhang, Y. Novel hyaluronic acid coated hydrophobically modified chitosan polyelectrolyte complex for the delivery of doxorubicin. *Int. J. Biol. Macromol.* **2019**, *126*, 254–261. [CrossRef]
35. Tripodo, G.; Trapani, A.; Torre, M.L.; Giammona, G.; Trapani, G.; Mandracchia, D. Hyaluronic acid and its derivatives in drug delivery and imaging: Recent advances and challenges. *Eur. J. Pharm. Biopharm.* **2015**, *97*, 400–416. [CrossRef]
36. Sionkowska, A.; Gadomska, M.; Musiał, K.; Piątek, J. Hyaluronic acid as a component of natural polymer blends for biomedical applications: A review. *Molecules* **2020**, *25*, 4035. [CrossRef]

37. Raik, S.V.; Andranovitš, S.; Petrova, V.A.; Xu, Y.; Lam, J.K.-W.; Morris, G.A.; Brodskaia, A.V.; Casettari, L.; Kritchenkov, A.S.; Skorik, Y.A. Comparative study of diethylaminoethyl-chitosan and methylglycol-chitosan as potential non-viral vectors for gene therapy. *Polymers* **2018**, *10*, 442. [CrossRef]
38. Lee, G.Y.; Kim, J.-H.; Choi, K.Y.; Yoon, H.Y.; Kim, K.; Kwon, I.C.; Choi, K.; Lee, B.-H.; Park, J.H.; Kim, I.-S. Hyaluronic acid nanoparticles for active targeting atherosclerosis. *Biomaterials* **2015**, *53*, 341–348. [CrossRef]
39. Burdick, J.A.; Prestwich, G.D. Hyaluronic acid hydrogels for biomedical applications. *Adv. Mater.* **2011**, *23*, H41–H56. [CrossRef]
40. Teder, P.; Vandivier, R.W.; Jiang, D.; Liang, J.; Cohn, L.; Puré, E.; Henson, P.M.; Noble, P.W. Resolution of lung inflammation by CD44. *Science* **2002**, *296*, 155–158. [CrossRef]
41. Nagpal, K.; Singh, S.K.; Mishra, D.N. Chitosan nanoparticles: A promising system in novel drug delivery. *Chem. Pharm. Bull.* **2010**, *58*, 1423–1430. [CrossRef] [PubMed]
42. Mohamed, H.; Shafie, A.M.A.; Mekkawy, A.I. Chitosan Nanoparticles for Meloxicam Ocular Delivery: Development, Vitro Characterization, and In Vivo Evaluation in a Rabbit Eye Model. *Pharmaceutics* **2022**, *14*, 893. [CrossRef] [PubMed]
43. Ricci, F.; Racaniello, G.F.; Lopedota, A.; Laquintana, V.; Arduino, I.; Lopalco, A.; Cutrignelli, A.; Franco, M.; Sigurdsson, H.H.; Denora, N. Chitosan/sulfobutylether-β-cyclodextrin based nanoparticles coated with thiolated hyaluronic acid for indomethacin ophthalmic delivery. *Int. J. Pharm.* **2022**, *622*, 121905. [CrossRef] [PubMed]
44. Dubashynskaya, N.V.; Bokatyi, A.N.; Skorik, Y.A. Dexamethasone conjugates: Synthetic approaches and medical prospects. *Biomedicines* **2021**, *9*, 341. [CrossRef] [PubMed]
45. Dubey, V.; Mohan, P.; Dangi, J.S.; Kesavan, K. Brinzolamide loaded chitosan-pectin mucoadhesive nanocapsules for management of glaucoma: Formulation, characterization and pharmacodynamic study. *Int. J. Biol. Macromol.* **2020**, *152*, 1224–1232. [CrossRef]
46. Lynch, C.; Kondiah, P.P.; Choonara, Y.E.; du Toit, L.C.; Ally, N.; Pillay, V. Advances in biodegradable nano-sized polymer-based ocular drug delivery. *Polymers* **2019**, *11*, 1371. [CrossRef]
47. Wu, G.; Ma, F.; Xue, Y.; Peng, Y.; Hu, L.; Kang, X.; Sun, Q.; Ouyang, D.F.; Tang, B.; Lin, L. Chondroitin sulfate zinc with antibacterial properties and anti-inflammatory effects for skin wound healing. *Carbohydr. Polym.* **2022**, *278*, 118996. [CrossRef]
48. Dubashynskaya, N.V.; Bokatyi, A.N.; Gasilova, E.R.; Dobrodumov, A.V.; Dubrovskii, Y.A.; Knyazeva, E.S.; Nashchekina, Y.A.; Demyanova, E.V.; Skorik, Y.A. Hyaluronan-colistin conjugates: Synthesis, characterization, and prospects for medical applications. *Int. J. Biol. Macromol.* **2022**, *215*, 243–252. [CrossRef]
49. Raik, S.V.; Poshina, D.N.; Lyalina, T.A.; Polyakov, D.S.; Vasilyev, V.B.; Kritchenkov, A.S.; Skorik, Y.A. N-[4-(N, N, N-trimethylammonium) benzyl] chitosan chloride: Synthesis, interaction with DNA and evaluation of transfection efficiency. *Carbohydr. Polym.* **2018**, *181*, 693–700. [CrossRef]
50. Hejjaji, E.M.; Smith, A.M.; Morris, G.A. Evaluation of the mucoadhesive properties of chitosan nanoparticles prepared using different chitosan to tripolyphosphate (CS: TPP) ratios. *Int. J. Biol. Macromol.* **2018**, *120*, 1610–1617. [CrossRef]
51. Yamabayashi, S. Periodic acid—Schiff—Alcian Blue: A method for the differential staining of glycoproteins. *Histochem. J.* **1987**, *19*, 565–571. [CrossRef]
52. Mindukshev, I.V.; Kudryavtsev, I.V.; Serebriakova, M.K.; Trulioff, A.S.; Gambaryan, S.P.; Sudnitsyna, J.S.; Avdonin, P.V.; Jenkins, R.O.; Goncharov, N.V. Chapter 26—Flow cytometry and light-scattering techniques in evaluation of nutraceuticals. In *Nutraceuticals*, 2nd ed.; Gupta, R.C., Lall, R., Srivastava, A., Eds.; Academic Press: Cambridge, MA, USA, 2021; pp. 379–393. [CrossRef]
53. Nazarova, A.; Khannanov, A.; Boldyrev, A.; Yakimova, L.; Stoikov, I. Self-assembling systems based on pillar [5] arenes and surfactants for encapsulation of diagnostic dye dapi. *Int. J. Mol. Sci.* **2021**, *22*, 6038. [CrossRef]
54. Danaei, M.; Dehghankhold, M.; Ataei, S.; Hasanzadeh Davarani, F.; Javanmard, R.; Dokhani, A.; Khorasani, S.; Mozafari, M. Impact of particle size and polydispersity index on the clinical applications of lipidic nanocarrier systems. *Pharmaceutics* **2018**, *10*, 57. [CrossRef]
55. Siepmann, J.; Peppas, N.A. Higuchi equation: Derivation, applications, use and misuse. *Int. J. Pharm.* **2011**, *418*, 6–12. [CrossRef]
56. Korsmeyer, R.W.; Gurny, R.; Doelker, E.; Buri, P.; Peppas, N.A. Mechanisms of solute release from porous hydrophilic polymers. *Int. J. Pharm.* **1983**, *15*, 25–35. [CrossRef]
57. Zhang, Z.; Zhang, R.; Chen, L.; Tong, Q.; McClements, D.J. Designing hydrogel particles for controlled or targeted release of lipophilic bioactive agents in the gastrointestinal tract. *Eur. Polym. J.* **2015**, *72*, 698–716. [CrossRef]
58. Graça, A.; Gonçalves, L.M.; Raposo, S.; Ribeiro, H.M.; Marto, J. Useful in vitro techniques to evaluate the mucoadhesive properties of hyaluronic acid-based ocular delivery systems. *Pharmaceutics* **2018**, *10*, 110. [CrossRef]
59. Menchicchi, B.; Fuenzalida, J.; Bobbili, K.B.; Hensel, A.; Swamy, M.J.; Goycoolea, F. Structure of chitosan determines its interactions with mucin. *Biomacromolecules* **2014**, *15*, 3550–3558. [CrossRef]

pharmaceuticals

MDPI

Article

Development of Osthole-Loaded Microemulsions as a Prospective Ocular Delivery System for the Treatment of Corneal Neovascularization: In Vitro and In Vivo Assessments

Yali Zhang [1], Jingjing Yang [2], Yinjian Ji [1], Zhen Liang [2], Yuwei Wang [1,*] and Junjie Zhang [2,*]

1 The First of Clinical Medicine, Henan University of Chinese Medicine, Zhengzhou 450046, China; zyl1638905393@163.com (Y.Z.); jyj17856819199@126.com (Y.J.)

2 Ophthalmology Department, Henan Provincial People's Hospital, Henan Eye Hospital, Zhengzhou University People's Hospital, Zhengzhou 450003, China; yangjj9089@163.com (J.Y.); liangzhenxh@126.com (Z.L.)

* Correspondence: wangyuwei612@163.com (Y.W.); zhangjunjie@zzu.edu.cn (J.Z.)

Abstract: Osthole (OST), a natural coumarin compound, has shown a significant inhibitory effect on corneal neovascularization (CNV). But, its effect on treating CNV is restricted by its water insolubility. To overcome this limitation, an OST-loaded microemulsion (OST-ME) was created to improve the drug's therapeutic effect on CNV after topical administration. The OST-ME formulation comprised Capryol-90 (CP-90), Cremophor® EL (EL-35), Transcutol-P (TSP) and water, and sodium hyaluronate (SH) was also included to increase viscosity. The OST-ME had a droplet size of 16.18 ± 0.02 nm and a low polydispersity index (0.09 ± 0.00). In vitro drug release from OST-ME fitted well to the Higuchi release kinetics model. Cytotoxicity assays demonstrated that OST-ME was not notably toxic to human corneal epithelial cells (HCECs), and the formulation had no irritation to rabbit eyes. Ocular pharmacokinetics studies showed that the areas under the concentration–time curves (AUC_{0-t}) in the cornea and conjunctiva were 19.74 and 63.96 μg/g*min after the administration of OST-ME, both of which were 28.2- and 102.34-fold higher than those after the administration of OST suspension (OST-Susp). Moreover, OST-ME (0.1%) presented a similar therapeutic effect to commercially available dexamethasone eye drops (0.025%) on CNV in mouse models. In conclusion, the optimized OST-ME exhibited good tolerance and enhanced 28.2- and 102.34-fold bioavailability in the cornea and conjunctiva tissues compared with suspensions in rabbit eyes. The OST-ME is a potential ocular drug delivery for anti-CNV.

Keywords: osthole; microemulsion; ocular drug delivery system; pharmacokinetic; corneal neovascularization

Citation: Zhang, Y.; Yang, J.; Ji, Y.; Liang, Z.; Wang, Y.; Zhang, J. Development of Osthole-Loaded Microemulsions as a Prospective Ocular Delivery System for the Treatment of Corneal Neovascularization: In Vitro and In Vivo Assessments. *Pharmaceuticals* **2023**, *16*, 1342. https://doi.org/10.3390/ph16101342

Academic Editors: Rosario Pignatello, Hugo Almeida, Carmelo Puglia and Debora Santonocito

Received: 15 August 2023
Revised: 13 September 2023
Accepted: 19 September 2023
Published: 22 September 2023

1. Introduction

The cornea is highly specialized avascular tissue [1], a feature that is required for optical performance. After corneal injury or infection, the new vessels might develop from the corneal limbus, and corneal transparency changes. Thus, loss of vision is the general reason for blindness worldwide. Although transplant operations can improve eyesight, they often fail when neovascularization occurs and result in immune rejection [2]. It has been reported that about 1.4 million people develop corneal neovascularization (CNV) in America, accounting for 4.14% of ocular diseases [3]. The avascularity of the cornea is dependent on the two counterbalancing systems of proangiogenic factors and antiangiogenic factors [4,5]. However, inflammation, chemical burns, infections, nutrition status and other damage factors disrupt the balance of the two systems. Many cytokines, such as vascular endothelial growth factor (VEGF) and matrix metalloproteinase (MMP), have great effects during the formation of CNV. Current clinical pharmacological therapeutics for CNV include anti-inflammatory and immunosuppressive agents and VEGF inhibitors [6]. Among them, topically administered steroids are still a first choice for anti-CNV [7]. However, the frequent application of steroids will lead to some adverse reactions, such as corneal infection, cataracts or glaucoma [8], which makes it urgent to look for a better method to cure CNV.

Osthole (OST) is obtained from many medicinal plants such as *Cnidium monnieri* (L.) Cusson and has been verified to have potential therapeutic applications due to its multiple significant pharmacological activities, including anticancer, antiosteoporotic and antiproliferative effects. Previous studies have also shown that OST not only reduces intraocular pressure [9], but also inhibits CNV [10]. However, its water insolubility (0.63 μg/mL) and low bioavailability significantly restrict its eye applications [11]. Therefore, it is very vital to exploit suitable dosage forms for OST.

In recent years, the OST-loaded drug delivery systems have been extensively studied to enhance their solubility and bioavailability, including injections, inclusion compounds, solid dispersions, gels and other dosage forms, which aimed for systemic administration [12]. However, the limitation of OST was still unaddressed. Recently, an OST-loaded drug delivery system was improved by nano-emulsions and liposomes to promote the therapy of Alzheimer's disease [13,14]. However, OST-loaded nanocarriers for ocular drug delivery (ODD) have not yet been reported, and some important properties, such as the stability and efficacy of topical ocular administration, remain unresolved in research. Moreover, the eyes are a very complicated tissue, and their unique anatomy restricts the absorption and permeation of most active agents [15]. Thus, ODD remains a challenging task for researchers. The major challenges in ODDs for topical administration are poor corneal permeability and a short residence time on the ocular mucosa [16]. In recent years, lipid-based nanocarrier systems have obtained great attention for ODD systems in ocular diseases and shown numerous benefits, such as enhancing the bioavailability of water insoluble drugs, increasing permeability across ocular tissues, providing sustained drug release and reducing some side effects [16,17]. Microemulsions (MEs) are particularly suitable for ODD, as they overcome many problems, including enhancing residence time and promoting penetration in the corneal. Furthermore, MEs are simple, cheap, easy to produce and sterilize and thermodynamically stable.

The goal of the study was to prepare OST-loaded microemulsion (OST-ME) to treat CNV. The OST-ME was optimized using the experimental statistical design technique (central composite design response surface methodology, CCD-RSM). The OST-ME was characterized by some important parameters, such as droplet size (DS), polydispersity index (PDI), morphology, drug entrapment efficiency (EE) and drug loading (DL). The in vitro drug release from the OST-ME was evaluated. The cytotoxicity of OST-ME was assessed in human corneal epithelial cells (HCECs). Furthermore, we evaluated the therapeutic effect of OST-ME as topical eye drops for anti-CNV in a mouse model, and irritation and the pharmacokinetic profiles in rabbit eyes were also investigated.

2. Results

2.1. Solubility Study

The solubilities of OST in each vehicle are shown in Figure 1. The solubility of OST in Capryol-90 (CP-90, 145.67 ± 10.63 mg/g) was the highest among the oil solvents and that in Transcutol P (TSP, 398.42 ± 6.56 mg/g) as the cosurfactant was much higher than that with the cosurfactant in Polyethylene glycol (PEG400). Thus, CP-90 was chosen as the oil phase, while TSP was chosen as the cosurfactant in the OST-ME formulation. However, the solubilities of OST in Cremophor® EL-35 (EL-35) and Tween-80 (TW-80) were 143.31 ± 3.69 mg/g and 157.90 ± 14.96 mg/g, with no significant difference, so the emulsifying abilities of EL-35 and TW-80 had to be further tested to select a suitable surfactant.

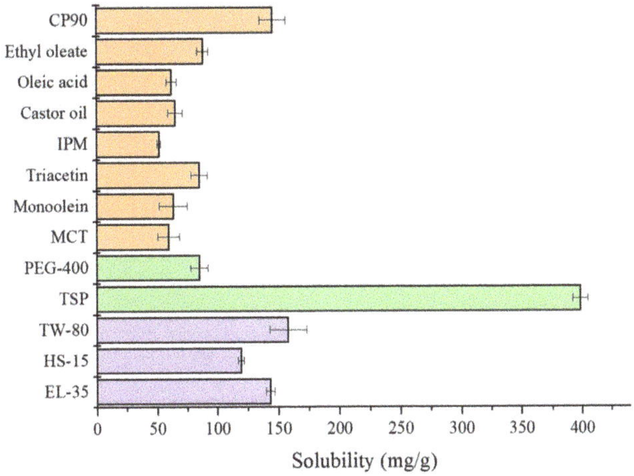

Figure 1. The screen data of OST in oils, surfactants and cosurfactants.

2.2. Screening the Emulsification Abilities of TW-80 and EL-35

The transmittance values of the emulsions prepared by emulsifying CP-90 with TW-80 and EL-35 were 90.76 ± 3.76% and 99.23 ± 0.39%, respectively, as shown in Figure 2. The transmittance of the emulsion consisting of CP-90 and EL-35 was higher than that of the emulsion consisting of CP-90 and TW-80, which demonstrated that EL-35 had a better ability to emulsify CP-90. Thus, EL-35 was selected as the surfactant.

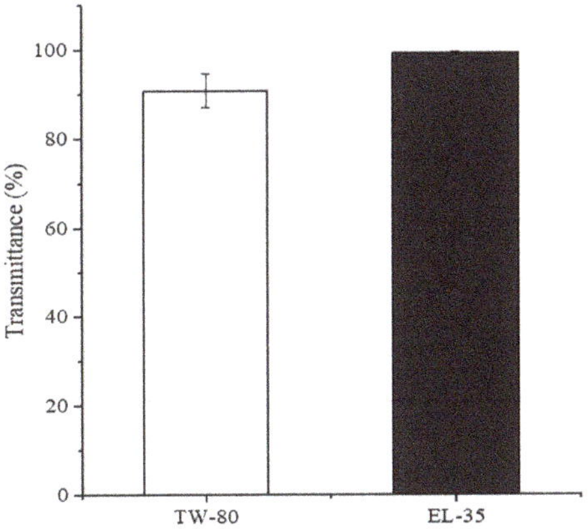

Figure 2. Transmittance of the emulsion consisting of CP-90 and surfactant.

2.3. Construction of Pseudoternary Phase Diagrams

Pseudo-ternary phase diagrams (PTPDs) were constructed to determine the optimal range of ingredient concentrations. The PTPDs with EL-35 and TSP of different Km values are shown in Figure 3. The MEs' regions were at a maximum when the Km values were between 2–4. Thus, the range of Km values was 2–4, and the oil concentration was 2–5% in further studies.

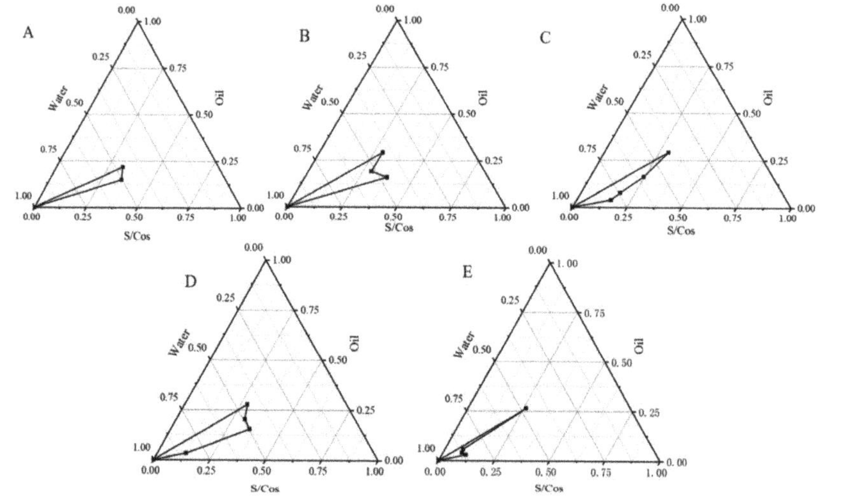

Figure 3. PTPDs of systems with different Km: (**A**) Km = 1:1; (**B**) Km = 2:1; (**C**) Km = 3:1; (**D**) Km = 4:1; (**E**) Km = 5:1.

2.4. Central Composite Design Response Surface Methodology

The independent variables, oil concentration (X_1) and Km (X_2), had a significant effect on the response variables, including DS (Y_1) and PDI (Y_2). The DS and PDI values from the thirteen runs showed variations from 14.51 nm to 34.67 nm and 0.08 to 0.40, respectively (Table 1). The equations generated for each response are as follows:

$$Y_1 = 20.81 - 5.24\,X_1 + 7.03\,X_2 - 0.3475\,X_1X_2 + 3.23\,X_1^2 + 1.83\,X_2^2 - 0.1461\,X_1^2X_2 + 7.22\,X_1X_2^2\ (R^2 = 0.9961) \quad (1)$$

$$Y_2 = 0.1340 - 0.1096\,X_1 + 0.0707\,X_2 - 0.0300\,X_1X_2 + 0.0536\,X_1^2 + 0.0811\,X_2^2 + 0.0393\,X_1^2X_2 + 0.1546\,X_1X_2^2\ (R^2 = 0.9977) \quad (2)$$

Mathematical Equations (1) and (2) describe the relationship between DS (Y_1) or PDI (Y_2) and the independent variables oil concentration and Km, respectively. The coefficients (R^2) were 0.9961 and 0.9977, respectively, which means that there is a good fit between the independent variables and the DS and PDI. The effect of these independent variables on the DS and PDI of the OST-ME are shown in Figure 4, and the predicted and actual values of DS and PDI are shown in Figure 5.

Table 1. The factors and levels of CCD-RSM (X_1: oil concentration; X_2: Km; Y_1: DS; Y_2: PDI).

Independent Variables			Value of Response			
			Actual Value		Predicted Value	
Formulation	X_1(%)	X_2	Y_1 (nm)	Y_2	Y_1 (nm)	Y_2
1	2	3	14.51	0.194	14.31	0.199
2	4.56066	3.70711	34.39	0.397	34.92	0.397
3	4.56066	2.29289	31.14	0.369	31.93	0.362
4	3.5	3	22.07	0.142	21.97	0.148
5	3.5	3	20.30	0.134	20.07	0.131
6	3.5	3	20.36	0.139	20.01	0.135
7	2.43934	2.29289	16.68	0.093	17.22	0.095
8	3.5	2	34.67	0.387	34.85	0.392
9	5	3	34.39	0.384	34.46	0.388
10	3.5	4	19.84	0.083	19.88	0.087
11	3.5	3	20.28	0.139	20.07	0.148
12	3.5	3	21.02	0.131	21.01	0.137
13	2.43934	3.70711	21.32	0.237	20.93	0.244

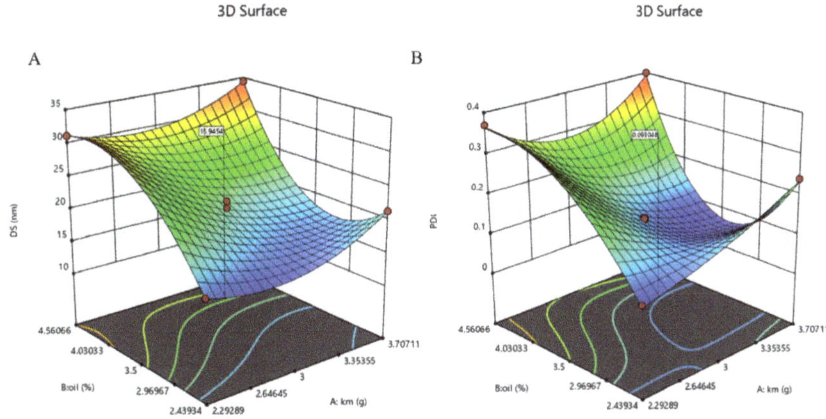

Figure 4. 3D response surface plot showing the effect of independent variables on (**A**) DS and (**B**) PDI.

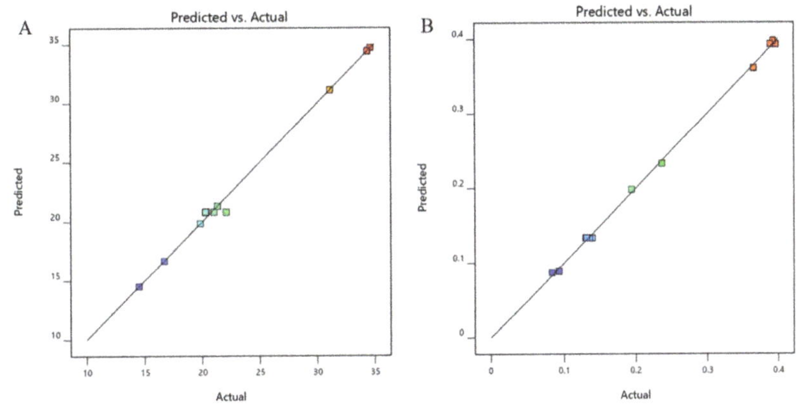

Figure 5. The predicted and actual values of (**A**) DS and (**B**) PDI.

2.5. Preparation and Characterization of the OST-ME

According to the abovementioned optimization experiments, the optimized OST-ME formulation contained 2.44% CP-90, 5.35% EL-35 and 2.21% TSP. Three OST-ME samples were made according to the optimal formulation; they were colorless and had good physical stability. A TEM image, DS (16.18 ± 0.02 nm) and PDI (0.09 ± 0.00) of OST-ME are shown in Figure 6, and other characterization results are listed in Table 2. The EE% and DL% were 99.15 ± 0.66% and 3.70 ± 0.53%, respectively. The osmolarity value was 298.89 ± 1.54 mOsm/kg and the pH value was 6.61 ± 0.99, both of which meet the requirements of eye drops.

Table 2. Characterization of optimized OST-ME.

DS (nm)	PDI	pH	Osmolarity (mOsm/kg)	EE (%)	DL (%)	ZP (mv)
16.18 ± 0.02	0.09 ± 0.00	6.61 ± 0.99	298.89 ± 1.54	99.15 ± 0.66	3.70 ± 0.53	−1.18 ± 0.97

Note: DS, droplet size; PDI, polydispersity index; EE, entrapment efficiency; DL, drug loading; ZP, zeta potential.

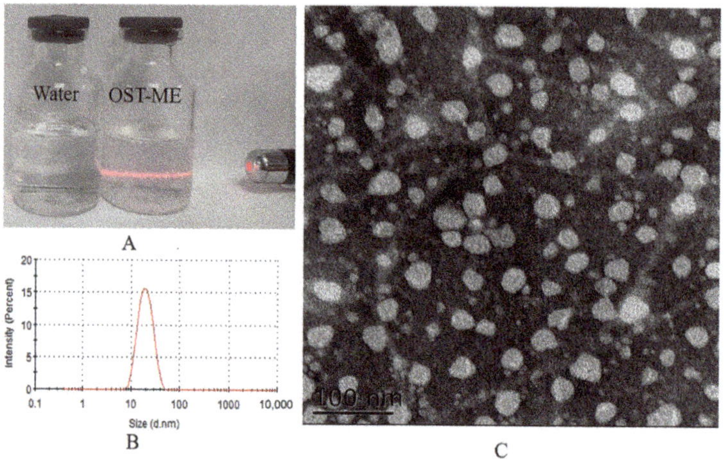

Figure 6. The appearance (**A**), the DS distribution (**B**) and the TEM image (**C**) of the OST-ME (scale bar = 100 nm).

2.6. Fourier Transform Infrared Spectroscopy Analyses

An Fourier Transform Infrared (FTIR) spectroscopy examination was tested to identify probable interactions between OST and the other excipients during preparation of the ME. The FT-IR spectra of OST, blank ME, OST-ME and the blank ME/OST PM are displayed in Figure 7. The FT-IR spectrum of pure OST has characteristic peaks at 1750 cm^{-1} for C=O stretching, C-H stretching in the range of 2900–3100 cm^{-1}, C=C stretching in the 1500–1650 cm^{-1} range and C-O stretching at 1640–1750 cm^{-1}. The results are similar to those reported in a previous paper [18]. The FTIR spectrum of the PM showed a combination of the OST and blank-ME individual spectra, but some of the characteristic peaks of OST still existed, indicating that no interaction happened between the pure OST and blank-ME. OST-ME and blank-ME had similar spectra, and no new peaks were observed. The characteristic peak of the pure drug did not appear in the OST-ME spectrum, suggesting that the pure drug was completely dissolved by CP-90 (oil phase). Previous similar results have been reported in the research on luliconazole-loaded nanoemulsions and tacrolimus-loaded microemulsions [19,20].

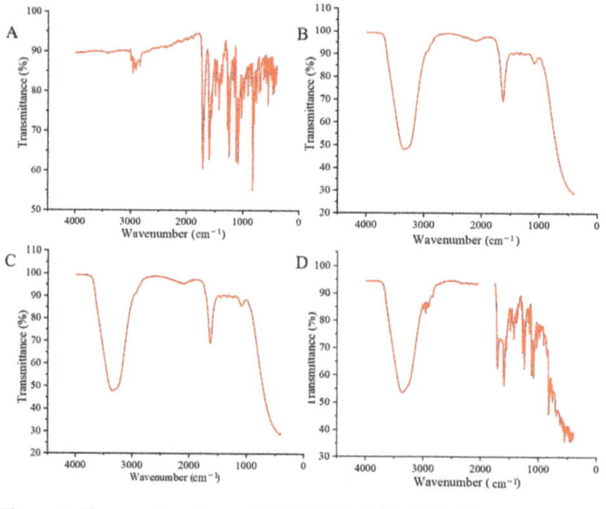

Figure 7. The spectra of pure OST (**A**), blank-ME (**B**), OST-ME (**C**) and PM (**D**).

2.7. Short-Term Stability

The results of the stability investigation are shown in Figure 8. The appearance of the OST-ME was transparent and colorless, which showed that OST was stable in the ME system during the test period. No significant changes in the chemical or physical characteristics (EE, PS, PDI and pH) were observed at 4 °C. However, at 25 °C, both the DS and the PDI showed a slow upward trend; the DS changed from 15.99 ± 0.22 nm to 18.98 ± 0.27 nm, and the PDI increased from 0.10 ± 0.02 to 0.27 ± 0.02. The EE% and pH showed decreasing trends: the EE% decreased from 97.97 ± 0.17% to 94.86 ± 0.09% and the pH value deceased from 6.65 ± 0.13 to 6.05 ± 0.17. Thus, OST-ME could be stable at 4 °C.

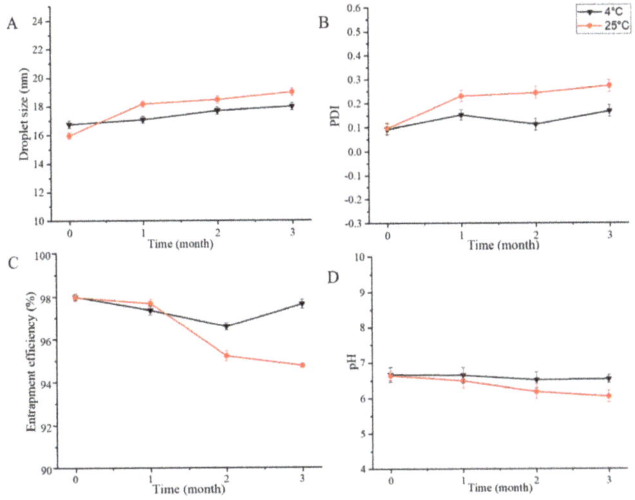

Figure 8. Stability study of OST-ME (**A**) DS, (**B**) PDI, (**C**) EE, (**D**) pH.

2.8. *In Vitro* Drug Release Study

The drug release profiles of OST-ME and OST suspension (OST-Susp) in simulated tear fluid (STF, pH 7.4) are shown in Figure 9. The OST-ME had a better sustained release, which was observed at 48 h of dialysis. It is evident that the cumulative release rate of OST-ME was much higher than the OST-Susp ($p < 0.01$). The result shows that the microemulsion-based formulation shows increased OST release compared to the suspensions. The cumulative release percentage of OST-ME is initially rapid, with over 20.01% of the loaded drug being released in the first 10 h. After this phase, there is a steady gradual increase over the next 38 h. The release data were fitted to different dissolution models, including the zero-order, first-order, Higuchi and Korsmeyer–Peppas models, and the Higuchi equation fitted the curve well for the OST-ME (R^2 = 0.99). While the release percentage of OST-Susp is initially rapid with over 14.12% of the loaded drug being released in the first 4 h, then there is a slight increase over the next 44 h. The Korsmeyer–Peppas equation fitted the curve well for the OST-ME (R^2 = 0.93). All equation fitting and correlation coefficient results are listed in Table 3.

Table 3. The different mathematical models' fitting for OST-ME and OST-Susp.

	Mathematical Models								
Formulation	Zero-order		First-order		Higuchi		Korsmeyer–Peppas		
	K(h)	R^2	K(h)	R^2	K($h^{1/2}$)	R^2	K(h)	n	R^2
OST-ME	0.77	0.92	0.25	0.86	5.42	0.99	7.62	0.42	0.98
OST-Susp	0.09	0.13	0.51	0.94	1.23	0.38	10.14	0.16	0.14

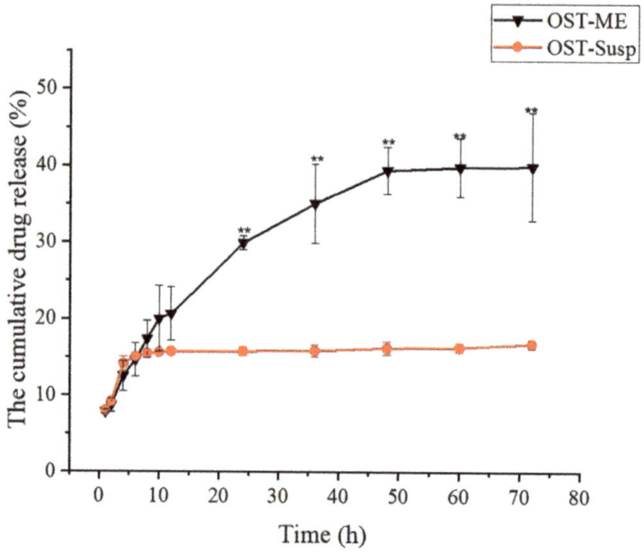

Figure 9. In vitro drug release profiles of OST-ME and OST-Susp. Data represented as mean ± SD, n = 3 (** $p < 0.01$ vs. OST-Susp. Independent samples *t*-test).

2.9. *In vitro Cell Viability Study*

The cell toxicity of OST-ME was evaluated by the CCK-8 assay. The cytotoxicity profiles of the OST-ME and blank-ME after incubation at different time points are shown in Figure 10A–D, respectively. The figure demonstrates that OST-ME is safe for HCECs after different durations of incubation, as indicated by the high cell viability percentage (>80%).

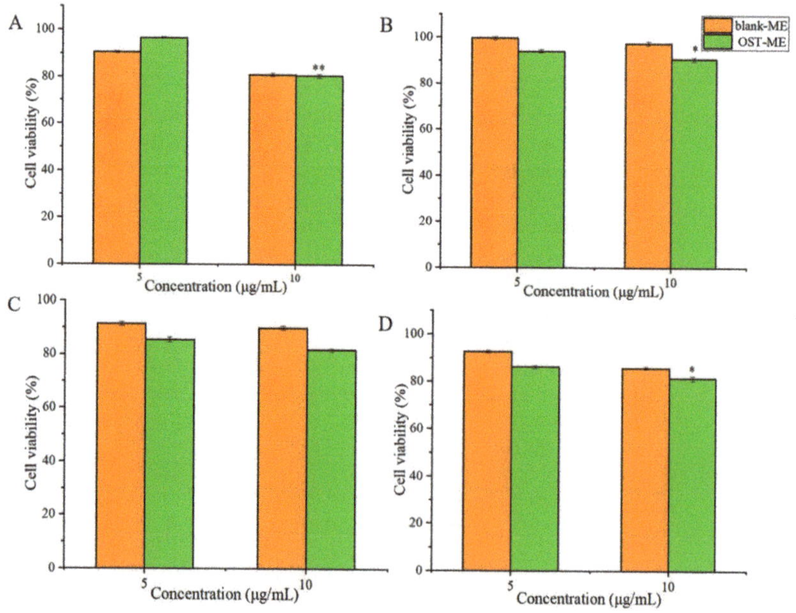

Figure 10. Histogram of the percentage cell viability of OST-ME. Results of CCK-8 assay at incubation times of (**A**) 0.25 h, (**B**) 1 h, (**C**) 2 h and (**D**) 4 h with blank-ME and OST-ME (5 μg/mL, 10 μg/mL). * $p < 0.05$, ** $p < 0.01$ vs. 5 μg/mL OST-ME. Independent samples *t*-test.

2.10. The Ocular Irritation Test

The study was tested with rabbits according to the modified Draize test. No obvious ocular irritancy symptoms were detected in the test or control eyes. The scores in terms of the cornea, conjunctiva, redness, discharge and iris alterations were 0 in all rabbits. Moreover, the image of the irritation result was photographed by the sodium fluorescein (Figure 11A) [21]. Hematoxylin and eosin (H&E) stained tissue sections were used to assess cell structure and tissue integrity. Representative micrographs of three types of tissues (cornea, conjunctiva and iris) treated with OST-ME and saline are shown in Figure 11B. The figure of the cornea, conjunctiva and iris showed smooth and clear tissue structures in the experiment group and control group. These results illustrate that OST-ME meets the needs of safety and is nonirritating, which suggests suitability for ocular drug delivery.

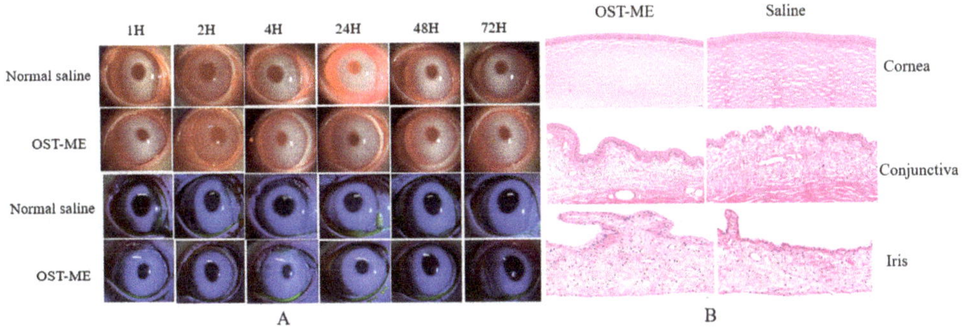

Figure 11. Ocular irritation result (**A**) and histopathological analysis of cornea, iris and conjunctiva (**B**).

2.11. Ocular Pharmacokinetics Study

The distributions of OST in the corneal and conjunctival tissue are shown in Figure 12, and the ocular pharmacokinetics parameters are shown in Table 4. The OST concentrations in the corneal and conjunctival tissue were much greater in the OST-ME group than in the OST-Susp group after a single administration. Moreover, the levels of OST in the OST-Susp group declined to below the limit of quantitation (LOQ, 0.025 μg/mL) 10 min and 15 min after administration. The AUC_{0-t} value of the corneal and conjunctival tissue in the OST-ME group were 19.74 and 63.96 μg/g·min, respectively. Therefore, the ME displayed a notable advantage over OST suspension in increasing the permeability of OST across the cornea and conjunctiva.

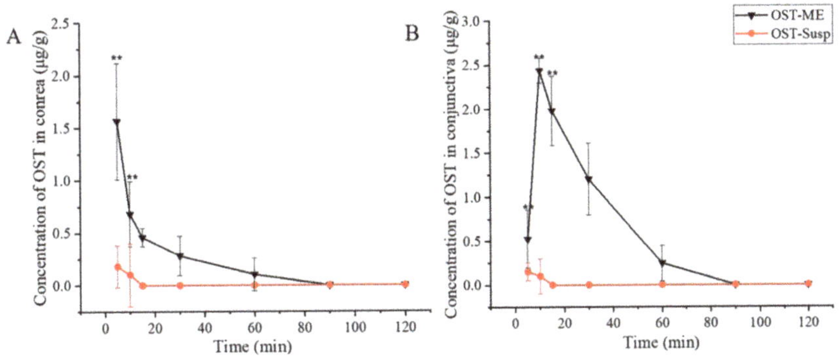

Figure 12. Concentration-time curves of OST in rabbit cornea (**A**) and conjunctiva (**B**) (** $p < 0.01$ vs. OST-Susp).

Table 4. The results of pharmacokinetic parameters.

Tissue	Pharmacokinetic Parameters	Unit	OST-ME	OST-Susp
Cornea	C_{max}	μg/g	1.56 ± 0.55	0.18 ± 0.21
	T_{max}	min	5	5
	$T_{1/2}$	min	28	/
	$AUC_{0\text{-}t}$	μg/g·min	19.74	0.7
Conjunctiva	C_{max}	μg/g	2.44 ± 0.14	0.15 ± 0.11
	T_{max}	min	10	5
	$T_{1/2}$	min	25	/
	$AUC_{0\text{-}t}$	μg/g·min	63.96	0.625

Note: AUC, area under curve.

2.12. *In Vivo Anti-CNV Efficacy in Mice*

The Image and Area of CNV

The anti-CNV effect of OST-ME was evaluated. As shown in Figure 13A, the burn areas of the epitheliums were similar among the groups, and there was no significant difference. To observe whether OST-ME can restrain CNV, the images (Figure 13B) were taken by microscope camera system. After treatment on day 1, CNV had already grown from the corneal limbus in all groups. The CNV showed an increasing trend on days 3 and 7 (Figure 13B) in the saline treatment group. On day 3 after treatment, although CNV had continued the growth trend, CNV in the 0.1% OST-ME (M), 0.2% OST-ME (H) and Dexamethasone (DEX) groups had shorter and thinner new vessels than that in the 0.05% OST-ME (L) and saline groups. On day 7 after treatment, the CNV of the M (0.1% OST-ME) and H (0.2% OST-ME) groups was reduced (Figure 14A). The areas of the saline group were significantly higher than other groups ($p < 0.05$) (Figure 14B), but there was no significant difference between group M and H ($p > 0.05$). These results demonstrated the OST-ME can restrain CNV.

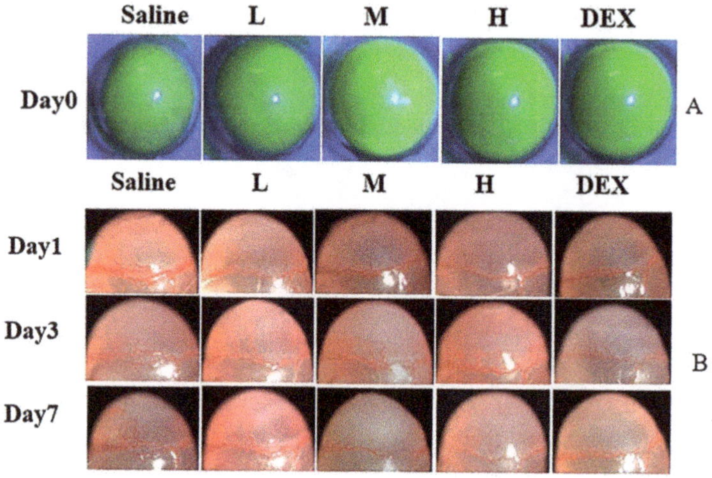

Figure 13. The fluorescein sodium images after modeling on day 0 (**A**) and slit lamp images of CNV in different groups on days 1, 3 and 7 (**B**).

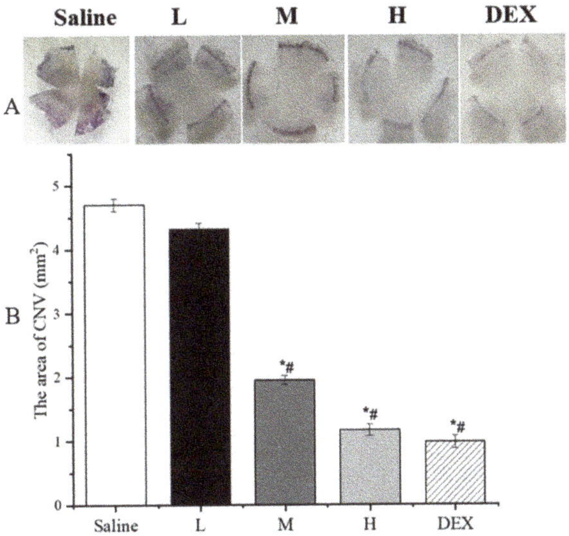

Figure 14. (**A**) Hematoxylin staining images of different groups on day 7. (**B**) The area of CNV 7 days after alkali burn (* $p < 0.05$ vs. saline group; # $p < 0.05$ vs. L group).

2.13. Histopathological Examination

The H&E section was used to evaluate the structural difference among every group. As illustrated in Figure 15A, the normal cornea showed orderly arranged epithelial cells and no structural or pathological changes in the vasculature. In Figure 15B, the epithelial cells in the saline group were arranged in an orderly manner, but irregular collagen fibers and an enlarged fiber space in the stroma were observed, and new vasculature existed in the corneal structure. Compared with the normal group (Figure 15B), the pathological conditions between the L and M groups (Figure 15C,D) were notably improved to some extent. The epithelial cells and collagen fibers in the stroma between the H and DEX groups were more remarkably improved, and angiogenesis was notably reduced (Figure 15E,F). The result illustrated that the M and H doses of OST-ME can restrain CNV.

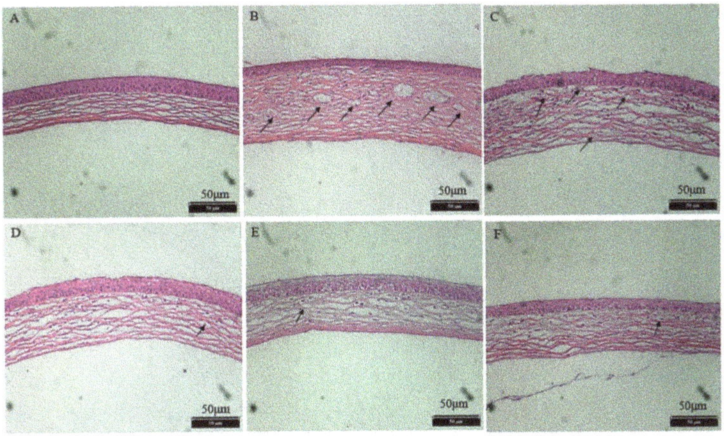

Figure 15. H&E staining of cornea (x 200): (**A**) the normal group; (**B**) the saline group; (**C**) the 0.05% OST-ME group; (**D**) the 0.1% OST-ME group; (**E**) the 0.2% OST-ME group; (**F**) the DEX group. The black arrow indicates cornea neovascularization.

2.14. Enzyme Linked Immunosorbent Assay

To investigate the effect of OST-ME on protein expression in CNV, the concentrations of VEGF-A and MMP-9 among total protein were assessed by ELISA. On days 3 and 7, the levels of VEGF-A and MMP-9 in group M, H and DEX were notable lower than those in the saline group ($p < 0.05$) after administration of the corresponding drug. The result illustrated that OST-ME could restrain the level of VEGF-A and MMP-9 in the CNV model (Figure 16).

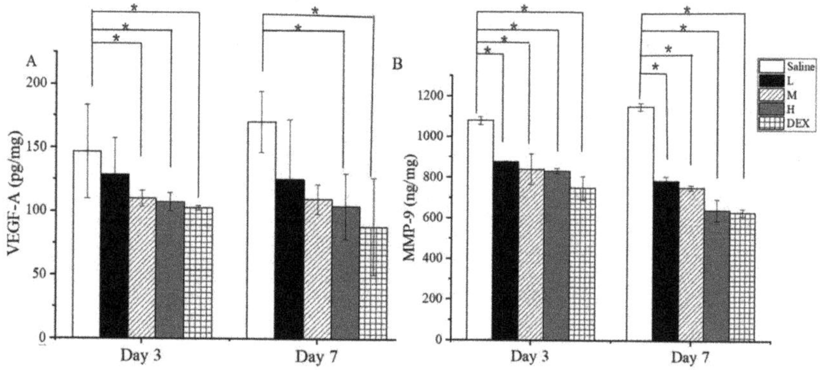

Figure 16. The concentration of VEGF-A (**A**) and MMP-9 (**B**) in corneal tissues at day 3 and day 7 (* $p < 0.05$ vs. saline group).

3. Discussion

Previous studies have shown that some pro-angiogenic cytokines, such as VEGF and MMP, would increase in animal models of CNV [22–24]. It has been reported that OST, a new antiangiogenic drug, could inhibit the overexpression of VEGF and MMP [25,26], and topical administration of OST could inhibit CNV established by alkali burns in mice [10]. However, the poor water solubility of OST (0.63 μg/mL) limits its clinical application in ophthalmology [11]. MEs, as one of the most prospective forms of nano-carriers for drug delivery systems, have shown some advantages over traditional eye drops for ocular applications [27]. It has been reported that using MEs as vehicles results in good store stability, good corneal permeation, sustained drug release and ultimately increased drug bioavailability in the eye [28,29]. In the present investigation, an oil-in-water (O/W) ME loaded with OST was successfully produced and showed good in vitro and in vivo characteristics.

All inactive ingredients selected for use in the OST-ME formulations, such as CP-90, EL-35, TSP and SH, were included in the FDA Inactive Ingredients Database, and no organic solvents were used in the preparation process, which could avoid potential toxicity due to organic residue. The three excipients are safe and harmless and have already been approved in Europe for topical applications [30], and were thus selected for use in ophthalmic preparation in this study. CP-90 and TSP were selected as the oil phase and cosurfactant because of the high solubility of OST in these solvents. EL-35 was selected as the surfactant, as it had a stronger ability to emulsify the oil phase than TW-80. Moreover, EL-35 and TSP are less affected by pH changes and have been widely applied to improve the bioavailability of insoluble drugs [31].

The PTPDs provided useful information on various ME compositions. The larger the regional area of the ME in the PTPDs, the stronger the ability to form ME [32]. The formulation was optimized based on the PTPDs and CCD-RSM. The response surface plot relationship of the independent variable to DS and PDI is shown in Figure 4. A nonlinear mathematical model was used to fit the result by CCD-RSM. The optimized OST-ME with a small DS was obtained. Figure 4A shows that the DS decreased as the amount of oil and Km decreased. Figure 4B shows that the PDI also decreased as the amount of oil and Km decreased.

In vitro drug release has a significant effect on predicting and understanding the nature of a formulation. The drug release curve of the OST-ME and OST-Susp were better fitted to the Higuchi and first-order equations, and the R^2 values are 0.99 and 0.94, respectively. The cumulative drug release of the OST-ME was higher than the OST-Susp over 96 h. These data illustrated that the ME has a better ability to release drugs. These results also gave a value of n of 0.42 ($n < 0.43$), which illustrated that OST release from OST-ME was dependent on Fickian diffusion [33]. Although in vitro drug release experiments provide important information for in vivo experiments, they cannot replace data obtained from in vivo studies.

When ophthalmic drug delivery systems for topical application are developed, ocular safety is always a critical issue. The Draize eye test is a commonly used way to assess the irritation of eye drops and it was used to assess the irritation caused by OST-ME in this study [34]. Here, the eye irritation scores were both 0 in the experiment group and control group, indicating no eye irritation and suggesting good biocompatibility and tolerance. In this study, HCECs were also used to evaluate cell toxicity, and the results illustrated that the OST-ME has good cytocompatibility at proper concentrations.

The pharmacokinetic study was conducted in rabbit eyes. This study had strengths and weaknesses and could directly evaluate the drug concentration in the corneal and conjunctiva tissue. However, since cornea and conjunctiva tissue are not consecutively sampled, it is impossible to harvest tissues from the same animal at every time point. So, the drug level will be impacted by individual absorption and metabolism to some extent [35]. Compared to OST-Susp, OST-ME rapidly penetrated the cornea and conjunctiva due to its ultrasmall particle size, which allowed the material to penetrate into the tissue via the transcellular pathway. It has been reported that ex vivo silicate nanoparticles with a particle size of 40 nm can penetrate bovine corneas [36]. Moreover, some surfactants could also decrease interfacial surface tension and increase the drug permeability across epithelial cells [37]. The conjunctival tissue is more permeable to drugs than the corneal tissue [38], and the drug level in the corneal and conjunctival is affected by individual metabolism [35]. Nevertheless, conjunctival drug absorption was deemed useless due to its distribution by the capillaries and lymphatics into systemic circulation [39]. Correspondingly, in our investigation, OST was undetected in the aqueous humor. The charge and size of a drug and many other factors could influence its permeation across eye barriers [38]. Therefore, the corneal penetration mechanism still needs to be further studied.

Various causes can result in CNV, but chemical injury is clinically one of the most common. In this experiment, an alkali burn injury model was used to induce corneal angiogenesis and evaluate the treatment effect of OST-ME. The results demonstrated that the OST-ME (H) treatment could significantly inhibit CNV when the eye drop was instilled four times a day. The antiangiogenic effects of OST-ME were verified by evaluating the area of CNV (Figure 14B) and H&E-stained sections at each time point (Figure 15). Additionally, 0.1% OST-ME can restrain the level of VEGF-A and MMP-9 in the cornea total protein concentration. It has also been reported that MMP-9 and MMP-2 could play a very important role in CNV [40]. Our results indicated that OST-ME could significantly inhibit the expression of MMP-9. Other researchers have also shown that CNV can be effectively inhibited by topically administering OST suspensions in a carboxymethylcellulose sodium (CMC-Na) solution [10]. The test group, which was treated with a high concentration of the OST-ME, produced results that were not different from those in the DEX group in our investigation, suggesting that OST is a potential alternative to DEX for an anti-CNV drug.

4. Materials and Methods

4.1. Materials

Osthole (OST), isopropyl myristate (IPM), and monoolein were provided by Macklin Biochemical Co., Ltd. (Shanghai, China). Medium-chain triglycerides (MCTs) were purchased from Yunhong Chemical Preparation Excipients Technology Co., Ltd. (Shanghai, China). Ethyl oleate and triacetin were obtained from J&K Scientific Technology Co., Ltd. (Beijing, China). Oleic acid was provided by Tokyo Chemical Industries Co., Ltd. (Tokyo, Japan). Propylene glycol dicaprylate (PGD) and castor oil were provided by Hunan Er-Kang Pharmaceutical Co., Ltd. (Changsha, China). PEG400 was obtained from Solarbio Life Science (Beijing, China). EL-35 was obtained from Shanghai Puzhen Biotechnology Co., Ltd. (Shanghai, China). Kolliphor HS-15 (HS-15) was obtained from BASF SE (Ludwigshafen, Germany). Tween-80 (TW-80) was obtained from Sichuan Jinshan Pharmaceutical Co., Ltd. (Guangyuan, China). TSP and CP-90 were acquired from Gattefosse (Saint-Priest, France). Glycerin was provided by Huikang Pharmaceutical Co., Ltd. (Lishui, Zhejiang, China). Sodium hyaluronate (SH) was obtained from Furuida Biochemical Co., Ltd. (Qingdao, Shandong, China). A Cell Counting Kit-8 (CCK-8) was acquired from APExBIO (Houston, TX, USA). Mice MMP-9 and VEGF-A enzyme linked immunosorbent assay (ELISA) kits were acquired from Elabscience Biotechnology (Wuhan, China). Dexamethasone (DEX) sodium phosphate solution were provided by Huaqing Pharmaceutical Co., Ltd. (Xinxiang, China).

4.2. Animals

New Zealand white rabbits (2.0–2.5 kg) and male BALB/c mice (6–8 weeks old, 20 ± 2 g) were obtained from Huaxing Experimental Animal Breeding Co. (Zhengzhou, China). All rabbits and mice were provided a standard daily diet and water and placed in lab that was kept at 23 °C ± 2 °C with a 12 h light/12 h dark cycle. Every animal was experimented on according to the principle of the Association for Research in Vision and Ophthalmology (ARVO) declaration.

4.3. OST Assay by High Performance Liquid Chromatography

The OST concentration was measured by the high performance liquid chromatography (HPLC) method according to a previous report [41,42]. Briefly, the HPLC system (Milford, MA, USA) was equipped with a Waters Symmetry® C18 column (4.6 × 250 mm, 5μm), and the column temperature was set at 40 °C. The mobile phase was made up of methanol–water (85:15, *v*/*v*) under an isocratic conditions flow rate of 1.0 mL/min and the injection volume was 10 μL. The ultraviolet (UV) detector wavelength was 322 nm. The OST concentration was determined from the standard curve.

4.4. Solubility Study

To obtain suitable ingredients for the preparation of OST-MEs, the solubilities of OST in different oils (CP-90, ethyl oleate, oleic acid, castor oil, IPM, triacetin, monoolein and MCTs), surfactants (EL-35, TW-80 and HS-15) and cosurfactants (PEG400 and TSP) were investigated according to a previous report [43,44]. All undissolved drugs were removed from the samples, and the samples were diluted with methanol and assayed using a UV-visible spectrophotometer (UV1800SPC, Shanghai, China) at 322 nm [45]. Each experiment was prepared in triplicate.

4.5. Emulsification Ability

The ability of the selected surfactant to emulsify the oil phase was assessed according to a previous report [46]. Emulsions transmittance was tested at 650 nm using a UV, taking purified water as a blank control group. Each sample was determined in triplicate.

4.6. Pseudo-Ternary Phase Diagrams

The aforementioned three ingredients (oil phase, surfactant and cosurfactant) were chosen to constitute the PTPDs by the water titration phase inversion emulsification (PIE) method according to a previous report [47]. The area had a low viscosity and the transparency appearance was deemed as the ME. The weight percents of the oil, S/Cos and water were recorded and calculated. Then, PTPD was prepared by Origin software (Version 8.0, Northampton, MA, USA).

4.7. Optimization of the OST-ME Formulation

The OST-ME formulation was optimized by the experimental statistical design technique with the Design Expert® software (V 12.0.1.0, Minneapolis, MN, USA). CCD-RSM was applied to investigate the effects of independent variables (X_1: oil concentration, %; and X_2: Km range) and their interaction over the dependent variables (Y_1: DS; and Y_2: PDI) [48,49]. The two-variable relations are shown in Table 5.

Table 5. The OST-ME was optimized by CCD-RSM.

	Levels				
Factors (independent variables)	−1.414	−1	0	1	1.414
X_1 (oil concentration, %)	2	2.44	3.5	4.56	5
X_2 (Km range)	2	2.29	3	3.71	4
Responses (dependent variables)			Desirability constraints		
Y_1: DS (nm)			Minimize		
Y_2: PDI			Minimize		

Note: DS, droplet size; PDI, polydispersity index.

4.8. Preparation of the OST-ME

The optimal OST-ME formulation could be obtained from the CCD-RSM optimization results and was prepared using the PIE method. Briefly, three selected ingredients were weighed and homogenously mixed at 37 °C. Then, OST was added in the homogenous mixture and dissolved under magnetic stirring. Then, distilled water was added in the mixture until the transparent light blue solution was obtained. Lastly, 10 mL of 0.2% (*w*/*v*) SH solution was added to the OST-ME solution, and the total volume of the mixed solution was 20 mL. The OST-ME was filtered using a 0.22 μm filter. Each sample was prepared in triplicate.

4.9. Characterization of the OST-ME

4.9.1. Determination of Droplet Size, Zeta Potential and Polydispersity Index

The average DS, ZP and PDI values of the OST-ME were tested by dynamic light scattering (Zetasizer, NanoZS90, Worcestershire, UK). All samples were diluted (1:20, *v*/*v*) with purified water, and each experiment was performed in triplicate.

4.9.2. Assessment of Entrapment Efficiency and Drug Loading

To calculate the EE% and DL% of OST-ME, 3 mL of OST-ME was added to centrifugal filter tubes (Amicon Ultra4, Ireland Regenerated Celluloses, MWCO: 10 kD) to separate the free OST from the OST-ME by centrifuge (Centrifuge 5810 R, Eppendorf, Germany). All samples were assayed by the aforementioned HPLC method. The value was calculated by the following equations:

$$EE\% = \frac{W_t - W_f}{W_t} \times 100 \quad (3)$$

$$DL\% = \frac{\text{Weight of the drug in the ME}}{\text{Weight of the drug and nanocarrier}} \times 100 \quad (4)$$

where W_t is the weight of the OST in the ME and W_f is the weight of the free drug in the ME.

4.10. Morphological Observations of the OST-ME

The morphology of the optimized OST-ME was observed by transmission electron microscopy (TEM) (Philips Company, Holland Tecnai 12, Eindhoven, The Netherlands). Briefly, OST-ME was diluted 50-fold with purified water before the TEM study. Then, the diluted OST-ME was applied to a carbon-coated copper grid. After drying, OST-ME samples were observed and photographed by TEM at 25 °C.

4.11. pH and Osmotic Pressure

The pH and osmolality of the OST-ME were tested by pH meter and freezing point osmometer (STY-A, Tianjin, China). Each experiment was conducted in triplicate.

4.12. Fourier Transform Infrared Spectroscopy Analyses

In this study, the OST, Blank-ME, OST-ME and the physical mixture (PM) of 20 mL of Blank-ME/OST (each experimental sample contained 20 mg of OST) were characterized by an AVATAR 370 FTIR instrument (Alpha II, Bruker, Germany). All samples were measured at 25 °C in the range of 4000–400 cm^{-1} [50].

4.13. Short-Term Stability

The stability of the optimized OST-ME was assessed for three months. Briefly, the OST-ME was prepared by filtration sterilization, and five milliliters of the sample was loaded in sterilized polypropylene eye drop bottles, sealed with a cover under a cleaning bench and then placed at 4 °C and 25 °C. Both the physical and chemical stabilities of OST-ME formulations were evaluated. All tests were performed on day 0 and at 1, 2 and 3 months, and samples were analyzed in triplicate.

4.14. In vitro Drug Release

The drug release of OST was conducted via dialysis in simulated tear fluid (STF, pH 7.4), containing 0.1% TW-80 as the solubilizer, which served as the release medium. The release of OST was analyzed by HPLC, and the cumulative release percentage (Q) of OST was calculated at relevant time points (according to Equation (3)). The Q was fitted to the zero-order kinetics, first-order kinetics, Higuchi and Korsmeyer–Peppas models, and the release curves were drawn using Origin software (Version 8.0, Northampton, MA, USA). The OST-Susp was chosen as the control.

$$Q\% = \frac{C_n V + V_i \sum_{i=0}^{i=n} C_i}{W_0} \times 100 \quad (5)$$

Here, W_0 is the total weight of the OST in the OST-ME, C_n is the OST concentration in STF at t_n, V is the total volume of STF, V_i and C_i are the sample volume and concentration at t_i, respectively, and t_n is the nth sampling time [51].

4.15. Cytotoxicity

The toxicity of OST-ME to HCECs was evaluated with CCK-8 assays. HCECs at a density of 1×10^4 cells per well were exposed to different concentrations of OST-ME (5 μg/mL and 10 μg/mL) and corresponding concentrations of blank-ME, which were cultured for 0.25, 1, 2 and 4 h. Then, 10% CCK-8 (100 μL) was added to every well and cultured for 4 h, and the optical density (OD) of all samples was tested at 450 nm with a microplate reader (PerkinElmer 2104 Multilabel Reader, Shanghai, China). All results were calculated by Equation (4) [52].

$$\text{Cell viability\%} = \frac{OD_{Sample} - OD_{blank}}{OD_{control} - OD_{blank}} \times 100 \quad (6)$$

4.16. Ocular Irritation Test

The irritation of the OST-ME was measured by six white rabbits according to the Draize eye test [53,54]. None of the eyes of any rabbits had eye disease. A quantity of 100 μL of the OST-ME was instilled into the right eye, while the contralateral eye used 0.9% saline solution as a control. Both eyes of all rabbits were examined, scored and recorded for signs of ocular irritation after administration of 1, 2, 4, 24, 48 and 72 h. The results were recorded according to the Draize technique [34]. Furthermore, the rabbits were euthanized via an injection of 4% pentobarbital sodium solution through the ear vein 72 h after exposure. The eyeballs were dissected and fixed with FAS, and after staining with

H&E, histopathological observation of the corneal, conjunctival and iris was performed using an optical microscope (Nikon 80i, Nikon Corporation, Tokyo, Japan) [55].

4.17. *Ocular Pharmacokinetics*

4.17.1. Grouping and Dosing

Forty-two healthy rabbits were randomly divided into two groups (test group and control group, 21 rabbits in each group), which were randomly divided into seven subgroups (n = 3), respectively. Both eyes of each animal were instilled with 50 μL of 0.1% OST-ME in the test group and the OST-Susp in the control group. The animals were euthanized by an injection of 4% phenobarbital sodium solution at scheduled time points. The corneal and conjunctival tissues were collected. Then, the tissues were weighed and stored at −80 °C for HPLC analysis. The drug in the tissue samples was extracted according to a previous report [56].

4.17.2. Analysis of Ocular Tissues

A validated method reported in a previous study was revised to gain OST from corneal and conjunctival tissue [57]. Briefly, the harvested conjunctiva and cornea samples were cut into pieces and soaked in methanol (0.4 mL) and then stored at 4 °C for 24 h. All samples were centrifuged (12,000 rpm, 10 min) and the supernatant was drawn and determined by the abovementioned HPLC method. Corneal and conjunctival tissue working solutions were acquired by diluting the standard solutions with corresponding blank rabbit tissues in order to prepare the rabbit tissue calibration curves. The pharmacokinetic parameters were obtained using DAS2.1.1 software (Anhui Provincial Center for Drug Clinical Evaluation, Wuhu, China).

4.18. *Anti-CNV Study*

Establishment of CNV Model

The CNV mouse model was established using the alkali burn method described in a previous report [58]. After one day, CNV was imaged by slit lamp microscope. Then, eighty mice were randomly divided into five groups (n = 16). Every mouse in each group was instilled with 5 μL of saline (saline group) or the same volume OST-ME (L, 0.05%, *w*/*v*), OST-ME (M, 0.1%, *w*/*v*), OST-ME (H, 0.2%, *w*/*v*) or dexamethasone (DEX, 0.025%, *w*/*v*). Each group was treated four times a day for a total of 7 days.

4.19. *Assessment and Quantification of CNV Area*

After treatment days 1, 3 and 7, CNV images of all animals were taken by microscope [58]. To quantitatively analyze the CNV area, a corneal flat mount method was used. On day 7, aortic perfusion was performed on three mice in each group. Then, the right eye of each mouse was enucleated and fixed in FAS at 4 °C, after which the corneal tissue was dissected and flattened for taking imaging. The area was calculated with the following Equation (5) [59,60].

$$A = C/12 \times 3.1416 \times \left[r^2 - (r - L)^2\right] \tag{7}$$

Here, A is the area, C is the number of clock hours of CNV that were involved, L is the length of the new blood vessel and r is the corneal radius [61].

4.20. *Histopathological Examination*

After day 7, three mice were sacrificed and the whole eyeball was enucleated from each. The corneas were separated and fixed in FAS trimming for hematoxylin-eosin (H&E) staining and histopathological observations.

4.21. *Enzyme Linked Immunosorbent Assay*

The expression levels of VEGF-A and MMP-9 in the corneas were measured. After days 3 and 7, five mice were sacrificed in each group, and the corneal samples were dissected and saved at −80 °C until analysis. The corneal samples were rewarmed at 4 °C for half an hour before analysis. The samples were treated according to the previous method [58]. The concentration of VEGF-A and MMP-9 in the corneas was measured according to the manufacturers' instructions. All samples of the OD were tested by a microplate reader at 450 nm.

4.22. Statistical Analysis

All results were analyzed by SPSS software (SPSS version 21, Chicago, IL, USA). Fisher's least significant difference (LSD) test was recorded to compare the differences between every group; $p < 0.05$ was considered as statistical significance. All data were recorded as the mean ± standard deviation (SD).

5. Conclusions

In this study, an optimized OST-ME formulation was successfully generated and characterized. The formulation showed good tolerance. Moreover, the formulation had good storage stability at 4 °C. In vitro drug release studies illustrated that OST-ME had a better sustained drug release rate than OST-Susp. In vivo pharmacokinetic studies illustrated that OST-ME had better bioavailability than OST-Susp and that the retention time of OST-ME on the cornea was prolonged. In addition, OST-ME effectively inhibited CNV and decreased VEGF-A and MMP-9 protein expression. In summary, OST-ME could be a potential drug for anti-CNV.

Author Contributions: All authors contributed to the study's conception and design; study design, Y.Z., Y.W. and J.Z.; validation, J.Y.; formal analysis, Y.Z. and J.Y.; investigation, Z.L. and Y.J.; data curation, Y.Z. and J.Y.; writing original draft preparation, Y.Z. and J.Y.; writing—review and editing, Y.Z. and J.Y.; project administration, Y.J. All authors have read and agreed to the published version of the manuscript.

Funding: This work was supported by scientific research of traditional Chinese medicine in Henan province (2023ZY2045). This research was funded by the Henan Eye Hospital Basic Science Research Program, grant number 22JCQN008.

Institutional Review Board Statement: All institutional and national guidelines for the care and use of laboratory animals were followed. The animal study protocol was approved by the Ethical Committee of Experimental Animal Care of the Henan Eye Institute (protocol code HNEECA-2022-09 and HNEECA-2022-10; approved by May 2022).

Informed Consent Statement: Not applicable.

Data Availability Statement: Data is contained within the article.

Acknowledgments: The authors are grateful to the Henan Provincial Institute of Food for the animal housing. The authors are grateful for the funding provided by scientific research of traditional Chinese medicine in Henan province (2023ZY2045) and the Henan Eye Hospital Basic Science Research Program, grant number 22JCQN008.

Conflicts of Interest: The authors have no relevant financial or non-financial interests to disclose.

References

1. Mukwaya, A.; Peebo, B.; Xeroudaki, M.; Ali, Z.; Lennikov, A.; Jensen, L.; Lagali, N. Factors regulating capillary remodeling in a reversible model of inflammatory corneal angiogenesis. *Sci. Rep.* **2016**, *6*, 32137. [CrossRef] [PubMed]
2. Skobe, M.; Dana, R. Blocking the path of lymphatic vessels. *Nat. Med.* **2009**, *15*, 993–994. [CrossRef] [PubMed]
3. Lee, P.; Wang, C.C.; Adamis, A.P. Ocular Neovascularization: An Epidemiologic Review. *Surv. Ophthalmol.* **1998**, *43*, 245–269. [CrossRef]
4. Senturk, B.; Cubuk, M.O.; Ozmen, M.C.; Aydin, B.; Guler, M.O.; Tekinay, A.B. Inhibition of VEGF mediated corneal neovascularization by anti-angiogenic peptide nanofibers. *Biomaterials* **2016**, *107*, 124–132. [CrossRef] [PubMed]
5. Wang, Z.; Liu, C.-H.; Huang, S.; Chen, J. Wnt Signaling in vascular eye diseases. *Prog. Retin. Eye Res.* **2019**, *70*, 110–133. [CrossRef] [PubMed]
6. Zhang, C.; Yin, Y.; Zhao, J.; Li, Y.; Wang, Y.; Zhang, Z.; Niu, L.; Zheng, Y. An Update on Novel Ocular Nanosystems with Possible Benefits in the Treatment of Corneal Neovascularization. *Int. J. Nanomed.* **2022**, *17*, 4911–4931. [CrossRef] [PubMed]

7. Liarakos, V.S.; Papaconstantinou, D.; Vergados, I.; Douvali, M.; Theodossiadis, P.G. The Effect of Subconjunctival Ranibizumab on Corneal and Anterior Segment Neovascularization: Study on an Animal Model. *Eur. J. Ophthalmol.* **2014**, *24*, 299–308. [CrossRef] [PubMed]
8. Comstock, T.L.; Holland, E.J. Loteprednol and tobramycin in combination: A review of their impact on current treatment regimens. *Expert Opin. Pharmacother.* **2010**, *11*, 843–852. [CrossRef]
9. Fan, Y.; Wei, J.; Guo, L.; Zhao, S.; Xu, C.; Sun, H.; Guo, T. Osthole Reduces Mouse IOP Associated with Ameliorating Extracellular Matrix Expression of Trabecular Meshwork Cell. *Investig. Opthalmol. Vis. Sci.* **2020**, *61*, 38. [CrossRef]
10. Zhang, Q.-Y.; Tao, S.-Y.; Lu, C.; Li, J.-J.; Li, X.-M.; Jiang, Q.; Yan, B. Osthole: A Traditional Chinese Medicine for Ocular Anti-Angiogenic Therapy. *Ophthalm. Res.* **2020**, *63*, 483–490. [CrossRef]
11. Sun, C.; Gui, Y.; Hu, R.; Chen, J.; Wang, B.; Guo, Y.; Lu, W.; Nie, X.; Shen, Q.; Gao, S.; et al. Preparation and Pharmacokinetics Evaluation of Solid Self-Microemulsifying Drug Delivery System (S-SMEDDS) of Osthole. *AAPS PharmSciTech* **2018**, *19*, 2301–2310. [CrossRef] [PubMed]
12. Zheng, L.; Shen, L.; Li, Z.; Zhang, X.; Wu, M.; Zhang, Y.; Liu, J. Design, Preparation, and Evaluation of Osthol Poly-Butyl-Cyanoacrylate Nanoparticles with Improved In Vitro Anticancer Activity in Neuroblastoma Treatment. *Molecules* **2022**, *27*, 6908. [CrossRef]
13. Song, Y.; Wang, X.; Wang, X.; Wang, J.; Hao, Q.; Hao, J.; Hou, X. Osthole-Loaded Nanoemulsion Enhances Brain Target in the Treatment of Alzheimer's Disease via Intranasal Administration. *Oxid. Med. Cell. Longev.* **2021**, *2021*, 8844455. [CrossRef] [PubMed]
14. Kong, L.; Li, X.-T.; Ni, Y.-N.; Xiao, H.-H.; Yao, Y.-J.; Wang, Y.-Y.; Ju, R.-J.; Li, H.-Y.; Liu, J.-J.; Fu, M.; et al. Transferrin-Modified Osthole PEGylated Liposomes Travel the Blood-Brain Barrier and Mitigate Alzheimer's Disease-Related Pathology in APP/PS-1 Mice. *Int. J. Nanomed.* **2020**, *15*, 2841–2858. [CrossRef] [PubMed]
15. Bachu, R.D.; Chowdhury, P.; Al-Saedi, Z.H.F.; Karla, P.K.; Boddu, S.H.S. Ocular Drug Delivery Barriers—Role of Nanocarriers in the Treatment of Anterior Segment Ocular Diseases. *Pharmaceutics* **2018**, *10*, 28. [CrossRef] [PubMed]
16. Gautam, N.; Kesavan, K. Development of microemulsions for ocular delivery. *Ther. Deliv.* **2017**, *8*, 313–330. [CrossRef] [PubMed]
17. Jacob, S.; Nair, A.B.; Shah, J.; Gupta, S.; Boddu, S.H.S.; Sreeharsha, N.; Joseph, A.; Shinu, P.; Morsy, M.A. Lipid Nanoparticles as a Promising Drug Delivery Carrier for Topical Ocular Therapy—An Overview on Recent Advances. *Pharmaceutics* **2022**, *14*, 533. [CrossRef]
18. Yun, F.; Kang, A.; Shan, J.; Zhao, X.; Bi, X.; Li, J.; Di, L. Preparation of osthole-polymer solid dispersions by hot-melt extrusion for dissolution and bioavailability enhancement. *Int. J. Pharm.* **2014**, *465*, 436–443. [CrossRef]
19. Yang, J.; Liang, Z.; Lu, P.; Song, F.; Zhang, Z.; Zhou, T.; Li, J.; Zhang, J. Development of a Luliconazole Nanoemulsion as a Prospective Ophthalmic Delivery System for the Treatment of Fungal Keratitis: In Vitro and In Vivo Evaluation. *Pharmaceutics* **2022**, *14*, 2052. [CrossRef]
20. Wan, T.; Pan, J.; Long, Y.; Yu, K.; Wang, Y.; Pan, W.; Ruan, W.; Qin, M.; Wu, C.; Xu, Y. Dual roles of TPGS based microemulsion for tacrolimus: Enhancing the percutaneous delivery and anti-psoriatic efficacy. *Int. J. Pharm.* **2017**, *528*, 511–523. [CrossRef]
21. Li, Z.; Liu, R.; Guo, Z.; Chu, D.; Zhu, L.; Zhang, J.; Shuai, X.; Li, J. Celastrol-based nanomedicine promotes corneal allograft survival. *J. Nanobiotechnol.* **2021**, *19*, 341. [CrossRef] [PubMed]
22. Giannaccare, G.; Pellegrini, M.; Bovone, C.; Spena, R.; Senni, C.; Scorcia, V.; Busin, M. Anti-VEGF Treatment in Corneal Diseases. *Curr. Drug Targets* **2020**, *21*, 1159–1180. [CrossRef] [PubMed]
23. Voiculescu, O.B.; Voinea, L.M.; Alexandrescu, C. Corneal neovascularization and biological therapy. *J. Med. Life* **2015**, *8*, 444–448. [PubMed]
24. Torrecilla, J.; Gómez-Aguado, I.; Vicente-Pascual, M.; del Pozo-Rodríguez, A.; Solinís, M.Á.; Rodríguez-Gascón, A. MMP-9 Downregulation with Lipid Nanoparticles for Inhibiting Corneal Neovascularization by Gene Silencing. *Nanomaterials* **2019**, *9*, 631. [CrossRef]
25. Yao, F.; Zhang, L.; Jiang, G.; Liu, M.; Liang, G.; Yuan, Q. Osthole attenuates angiogenesis in an orthotopic mouse model of hepatocellular carcinoma via the downregulation of nuclear factor-κB and vascular endothelial growth factor. *Oncol. Lett.* **2018**, *16*, 4471–4479. [CrossRef] [PubMed]
26. Yin, S.; Liu, H.; Wang, J.; Feng, S.; Chen, Y.; Shang, Y.; Su, X.; Si, F. Osthole Induces Apoptosis and Inhibits Proliferation, Invasion, and Migration of Human Cervical Carcinoma HeLa Cells. *Evid.-Based Complement. Altern. Med. eCAM* **2021**, *2021*, 8885093. [CrossRef] [PubMed]
27. Ustundag Okur, N.; Çağlar, E.Ş.; Siafaka, P.I. Novel Ocular Drug Delivery Systems: An Update on Microemulsions. *J. Ocul. Pharmacol. Ther.* **2020**, *36*, 342–354. [CrossRef]
28. Kalam, M.A.; Alshamsan, A.; Aljuffali, I.A.; Mishra, A.K.; Sultana, Y. Delivery of gatifloxacin using microemulsion as vehicle: Formulation, evaluation, transcorneal permeation and aqueous humor drug determination. *Drug Deliv.* **2016**, *23*, 886–897. [CrossRef]
29. Gupta, A.; Nayak, K.; Misra, M. Cow ghee fortified ocular topical microemulsion; in vitro, ex vivo, and in vivo evaluation. *J. Microencapsul.* **2019**, *36*, 603–621. [CrossRef]
30. Sánchez-López, E.; Espina, M.; Doktorovova, S.; Souto, E.; García, M. Lipid nanoparticles (SLN, NLC): Overcoming the anatomical and physiological barriers of the eye—Part II—Ocular drug-loaded lipid nanoparticles. *Eur. J. Pharm. Biopharm.* **2017**, *110*, 58–69. [CrossRef]

31. Xi, J.; Chang, Q.; Chan, C.K.; Meng, Z.Y.; Wang, G.N.; Sun, J.B.; Wang, Y.T.; Tong, H.H.Y.; Zheng, Y. Formulation Development and Bioavailability Evaluation of a Self-Nanoemulsified Drug Delivery System of Oleanolic Acid. *AAPS PharmSciTech* **2009**, *10*, 172–182. [CrossRef] [PubMed]
32. Zakkula, A.; Gabani, B.B.; Jairam, R.K.; Kiran, V.; Todmal, U.; Mullangi, R. Preparation and optimization of nilotinib self-micro-emulsifying drug delivery systems to enhance oral bioavailability. *Drug Dev. Ind. Pharm.* **2020**, *46*, 498–504. [CrossRef]
33. Liang, Z.Z.Z.; Zhang, Z.; Yang, J.; Lu, P.; Zhou, T.; Li, J.; Zhang, J. Assessment to the Antifungal Effects in vitro and the Ocular Pharmacokinetics of Solid-Lipid Nanoparticle in Rabbits. *Int. J. Nanomed.* **2021**, *16*, 7847–7857. [CrossRef] [PubMed]
34. Wilhelmus, K.R. The Draize Eye Test. *Surv. Ophthalmol.* **2001**, *45*, 493–515. [CrossRef] [PubMed]
35. Zhou, T.; Miao, Y.; Li, Z.; Lu, P.; Liang, Z.; Yang, J.; He, J.; Xia, H.; Zhang, Z.; Zhang, J. A Comparative Ocular Pharmacokinetics Study of Preservative-Free Latanoprost Unit-Dose Eye Drops and a Benzalkonium Chloride-Preserved Branded Product Following Topical Application to Rabbits. *J. Ocul. Pharmacol. Ther.* **2020**, *36*, 522–528. [CrossRef] [PubMed]
36. Mohammadpour, M.; Hashemi, H.; Jabbarvand, M.; Delrish, E.M. Penetration of Silicate Nanoparticles into the Corneal Stroma and Intraocular Fluids. *Cornea* **2014**, *33*, 738–743. [CrossRef]
37. Rahman, M.A.; Hussain, A.; Hussain, S.; Mirza, M.A.; Iqbal, Z. Role of excipients in successful development of self-emulsifying/microemulsifying drug delivery system (SEDDS/SMEDDS). *Drug Dev. Ind. Pharm.* **2013**, *39*, 1–19. [CrossRef]
38. Moiseev, R.V.; Morrison, P.W.J.; Steele, F.; Khutoryanskiy, V.V. Penetration Enhancers in Ocular Drug Delivery. *Pharmaceutics* **2019**, *11*, 321. [CrossRef]
39. Liu, D.; Li, J.; Cheng, B.; Wu, Q.; Pan, H. Ex Vivo and in Vivo Evaluation of the Effect of Coating a Coumarin-6-Labeled Nanostructured Lipid Carrier with Chitosan-*N*-acetylcysteine on Rabbit Ocular Distribution. *Mol. Pharm.* **2017**, *14*, 2639–2648. [CrossRef]
40. Zhang, J.; Wang, S.; He, Y.; Yao, B.; Zhang, Y. Regulation of matrix metalloproteinases 2 and 9 in corneal neovascularization. *Chem. Biol. Drug Des.* **2020**, *95*, 485–492. [CrossRef]
41. An, F.; Wang, S.H.; Zhang, D.S.; Zhang, L.; Mu, J.X. Pharmacokinetics of osthole in rabbits. *Yao Xue Xue Bao Acta Pharm. Sin.* **2003**, *38*, 571–573.
42. Li, Y.; Meng, F.; Xiong, Z.; Liu, H.; Li, F. HPLC Determination and Pharmacokinetics of Osthole in Rat Plasma after Oral Administration of Fructus Cnidii Extract. *J. Chromatogr. Sci.* **2005**, *43*, 426–429. [CrossRef] [PubMed]
43. Kesharwani, P.; Jain, A.; Srivastava, A.K.; Keshari, M.K. Systematic development and characterization of curcumin-loaded nanogel for topical application. *Drug Dev. Ind. Pharm.* **2020**, *46*, 1443–1457. [CrossRef] [PubMed]
44. Zhang, R.; Yang, J.; Luo, Q.; Shi, J.; Xu, H.; Zhang, J. Preparation and in vitro and in vivo evaluation of an isoliquiritigenin-loaded ophthalmic nanoemulsion for the treatment of corneal neovascularization. *Drug Deliv.* **2022**, *29*, 2217–2233. [CrossRef] [PubMed]
45. Shao, B.; Sun, L.; Xu, N.; Gu, H.; Ji, H.; Wu, L. Development and Evaluation of Topical Delivery of Microemulsions Containing Adapalene (MEs-Ap) for Acne. *AAPS PharmSciTech* **2021**, *22*, 125. [CrossRef] [PubMed]
46. Farghaly, D.A.; Aboelwafa, A.A.; Hamza, M.Y.; Mohamed, M.I. Microemulsion for topical delivery of fenoprofen calcium: In vitro and in vivo evaluation. *J. Liposome Res.* **2018**, *28*, 126–136. [CrossRef] [PubMed]
47. Wang, L.; Yan, W.; Tian, Y.; Xue, H.; Tang, J.; Zhang, L. Self-Microemulsifying Drug Delivery System of Phillygenin: Formulation Development, Characterization and Pharmacokinetic Evaluation. *Pharmaceutics* **2020**, *12*, 130. [CrossRef]
48. Tang, S.Y.; Manickam, S.; Wei, T.K.; Nashiru, B. Formulation development and optimization of a novel Cremophore EL-based nanoemulsion using ultrasound cavitation. *Ultrason. Sonochem.* **2012**, *19*, 330–345. [CrossRef]
49. Galooyak, S.S.; Dabir, B. Three-factor response surface optimization of nano-emulsion formation using a microfluidizer. *J. Food Sci. Technol.* **2015**, *52*, 2558–2571. [CrossRef]
50. Li, Y.-H.; Wang, Y.-S.; Zhao, J.-S.; Li, Z.-Y.; Chen, H.-H. A pH-sensitive curcumin loaded microemulsion-filled alginate and porous starch composite gels: Characterization, in vitro release kinetics and biological activity. *Int. J. Biol. Macromol.* **2021**, *182*, 1863–1873. [CrossRef]
51. Yang, W.; Li, H.; Pan, T.; Cui, Y.; Li, X.; Gao, J.; Shen, S. Improved oral bioavailability of poorly water-soluble glimepiride by utilizing microemulsion technique. *Int. J. Nanomed.* **2016**, *11*, 3777–3788. [CrossRef] [PubMed]
52. Yang, J.; Yan, J.; Zhou, Z.; Amsden, B.G. Dithiol-PEG-PDLLA Micelles: Preparation and Evaluation as Potential Topical Ocular Delivery Vehicle. *Biomacromolecules* **2014**, *15*, 1346–1354. [CrossRef] [PubMed]
53. Rasoanirina, B.N.V.; Lassoued, M.A.; Miladi, K.; Razafindrakoto, Z.; Chaâbane-Banaoues, R.; Ramanitrahasimbola, D.; Cornet, M.; Sfar, S. Self-nanoemulsifying drug delivery system to improve transcorneal permeability of voriconazole: In-vivo studies. *J. Pharm. Pharmacol.* **2020**, *72*, 889–896. [CrossRef] [PubMed]
54. Teba, H.E.; Khalil, I.A.; El Sorogy, H.M. Novel cubosome based system for ocular delivery of acetazolamide. *Drug Deliv.* **2021**, *28*, 2177–2186. [CrossRef] [PubMed]
55. Huang, Y.; Tao, Q.; Hou, D.; Hu, S.; Tian, S.; Chen, Y.; Gui, R.; Yang, L.; Wang, Y. A novel ion-exchange carrier based upon liposome-encapsulated montmorillonite for ophthalmic delivery of betaxolol hydrochloride. *Int. J. Nanomed.* **2017**, *12*, 1731–1745. [CrossRef] [PubMed]
56. Yang, J.; Ma, Y.; Luo, Q.; Liang, Z.; Lu, P.; Song, F.; Zhang, Z.; Zhou, T.; Zhang, J. Improving the solubility of vorinostat using cyclodextrin inclusion complexes: The physicochemical characteristics, corneal permeability and ocular pharmacokinetics of the drug after topical application. *Eur. J. Pharm. Sci.* **2022**, *168*, 106078. [CrossRef] [PubMed]

57. Li, J.; Ma, B.; Zhang, Q.; Yang, X.; Sun, J.; Tang, B.; Cui, G.; Yao, D.; Liu, L.; Gu, G.; et al. Simultaneous determination of osthole, bergapten and isopimpinellin in rat plasma and tissues by liquid chromatography–tandem mass spectrometry. *J. Chromatogr. B* **2014**, *970*, 77–85. [CrossRef] [PubMed]
58. Luo, Q.; Yang, J.; Xu, H.; Shi, J.; Liang, Z.; Zhang, R.; Lu, P.; Pu, G.; Zhao, N.; Zhang, J. Sorafenib-loaded nanostructured lipid carriers for topical ocular therapy of corneal neovascularization: Development, in-vitro and in vivo study. *Drug Deliv.* **2022**, *29*, 837–855. [CrossRef]
59. Irani, Y.D.; Scotney, P.D.; Klebe, S.; Mortimer, L.A.; Nash, A.D.; Williams, K.A. An Anti–VEGF-B Antibody Fragment Induces Regression of Pre-Existing Blood Vessels in the Rat Cornea. *Investig. Opthalmol. Vis. Sci.* **2017**, *58*, 3404–3413. [CrossRef]
60. Li, Z.; Li, J.; Zhu, L.; Zhang, Y.; Zhang, J.; Yao, L.; Liang, D.; Wang, L. Celastrol nanomicelles attenuate cytokine secretion in macrophages and inhibit macrophage-induced corneal neovascularization in rats. *Int. J. Nanomed.* **2016**, *11*, 6135–6148. [CrossRef]
61. Huang, X.; Han, Y.; Shao, Y.; Yi, J.-L. Efficacy of the nucleotide-binding oligomerzation domain 1 inhibitor Nodinhibit-1 on corneal alkali burns in rats. *Int. J. Ophthalmol.* **2015**, *8*, 860–865. [CrossRef]

pharmaceutics

MDPI

Article

Discovery and Potential Utility of a Novel Non-Invasive Ocular Delivery Platform

Weizhen (Jenny) Wang * and Nonna Snider

Department of R&D, JeniVision Inc., Irvine, CA 92617, USA
* Correspondence: wangjenny@jenivision.com

Abstract: To this day, the use of oily eye drops and non-invasive retinal delivery remain a major challenge. Oily eye drops usually cause ocular irritation and interfere with the normal functioning of the eye, while ocular injections for retinal drug delivery cause significant adverse effects and a high burden on the healthcare system. Here, the authors report a novel topical non-invasive ocular delivery platform (NIODP) through the periorbital skin for high-efficiency anterior and posterior ocular delivery in a non-human primate model (NHP). A single dose of about 7 mg JV-MD2 (omega 3 DHA) was delivered via the NIODP and reached the retina at a Cmax of 111 μg/g and the cornea at a Cmax of 66 μg/g. The NIODP also delivered JV-DE1, an anti-inflammatory agent in development for dry eye diseases, as efficiently as eye drops did to the anterior segments of the NHP. The topical NIODP seems to transport drug candidates through the corneal pathway to the anterior and via the conjunctiva/sclera pathway to the posterior segments of the eye. The novel NIODP method has the potential to reshape the landscape of ocular drug delivery. This is especially the case for oily eye drops and retinal delivery, where the success of the treatment lies in the ocular tolerability and bioavailability of drugs in the target tissue.

Keywords: AMD; cornea; docosahexaenoic acid (DHA); drug delivery; non-invasive ocular delivery platform (NIODP); ocular disease; oily eye drops; omega 3; retina; retinal delivery; retinal diseases

Citation: Wang, W.; Snider, N. Discovery and Potential Utility of a Novel Non-Invasive Ocular Delivery Platform. *Pharmaceutics* **2023**, *15*, 2344. https://doi.org/10.3390/pharmaceutics15092344

Academic Editors: Francisco Javier Otero-Espinar and Kevin Ita

Received: 11 August 2023
Revised: 31 August 2023
Accepted: 13 September 2023
Published: 19 September 2023

1. Introduction

Tolerability and suitability issues can limit the use of various materials or delivery routes for ocular drug administration, particularly for oily eye drops and retinal drugs. While eye drops are very often used to treat ocular surface diseases, intravitreal injections or implants are mainly used to treat posterior ocular diseases. Since Vitravene® (fomivirsen sodium) became the first FDA-approved intravitreally injected therapeutic agent in 1998, the ophthalmic pharmaceutical industry has been in urgent need of a breakthrough in ocular drug delivery.

Topical eye drop administration is well known for its capacity to provide necessary and efficient pharmaceutically effective doses to most anterior ocular tissues, usually with higher local drug levels than oral administration and minimal systemic exposure and side effects [1,2]. While most active pharmaceutical ingredients (APIs) are lipophilic, commercialized eye drops are often used in a more ocularly tolerable aqueous formulation that may be subjected to fast elimination by tears compared to an oily formulation. Eye drops containing castor oil as a vehicle have been found to cause corneal toxicity. This is not observed with the use of Aleurites, camelina, maize, and olive oils, suggesting that oil formulations may still be useful as ophthalmic solutions [2]. Although oily eye drop formulations may increase the solubility and pharmacologic effects of the drug, they often cause ocular discomfort, such as vision blurring and foreign body sensations, due to the high viscosity and refractive index of oily contents [2,3]. This is the main limiting factor for their use as eye drop formulations.

Posterior ocular drug delivery is a major challenge due to the complex anatomy and the dynamic physiological barrier of the eye, which significantly affect the availability of treatments. The physicochemical properties of drugs, formulations, delivery systems, and routes of administration are major factors affecting intraocular bioavailability; they have been explored to enable effective ocular drug delivery [4]. Oral administration and eye drops are the two currently available non-invasive routes of delivery used to treat ocular diseases. Due to the blood–retina barrier, the retinal bioavailability of drugs via oral administration is extremely low and comes with very high unnecessary systemic exposure. In individual baboon neonates, it was demonstrated that the absorption of DHA to the retina from blood circulation reached a plateau when DHA in plasma or red blood cells (RBCs) was approximately 6% of the weight of total fatty acids in the diet [5], meaning that DHA in dietary supplements beyond a certain limit may not be absorbed into the retina. Additionally, the delivery efficiency of DHA from the diet to RBCs in baboon neonates was mostly between 0.013% and 0.04% of the DHA dose, while the correlated diet-to-retina DHA delivery efficiency was calculated to be in the range of 0.0003% to 0.001% [6]. Topical eye drops, a more direct route with lower systemic exposure, have also been shown to be very inefficient for posterior segment delivery. Only <3% of the dosed drug amount in eye drop formulations reached the aqueous humor, and 0.001% or less reached the retina [7,8]. Thus, for the retinal delivery of DHA, the oral route requires megadose systemic exposure, and oily eye drops cause intolerable adverse ocular effects, meaning that both methods are highly inefficient.

While orally administered drugs reach the retina through the blood circulation, the use of topical eye drops is believed to channel drugs to the posterior ocular segments via two possible routes: (1) the corneal route, where the drug penetrates the corneal surface and continues to diffuse through anterior ocular tissues (aqueous humor, lens/iris/ciliary body) to the vitreous humor and may then reach the retina; and (2) the conjunctiva/scleral route, where a drug diffuses from the conjunctiva of the ocular surface through the scleral water channels/pores to reach the retina [7,9]. The concentration gradient of dissolved drugs is the driving force for molecules to permeate through the lipophilic membrane barriers of the eye (i.e., the conjunctiva and/or cornea) along the corneal and scleral pathways [7,10]. For a drug with favorable physicochemical properties (e.g., molecular weight, radius, charge, and lipophilicity), the scleral pathway provides a bypass around the anterior segment barriers (the lens, iris, and ciliary body), allowing drug permeation to the back of the eye [11,12].

Although many rabbit and rodent studies claim to have achieved successful retinal delivery by applying high doses of small molecules or proteins in eyedrop formulations, successful translation to larger species or clinical success has not yet been achieved, and topical eye drops remain highly inefficient for posterior segment delivery [13–15]. In these rabbit and rodent studies, the amount of therapeutic agents reaching the retina was mostly in the range of a 0.01 to 0.1 μg/g concentration after a typical eye drop regimen [13,16–19]. In such circumstances, retinal delivery due to systemic exposure cannot be ruled out because of the small body volume of these animal models. Therefore, rabbit and rodent models may not be appropriate for studies of posterior segment drug delivery [13].

The current standard of care for retinal drug delivery is intravitreal injection or implant [20], and the efforts to improve retinal drug delivery are heavily focused on two aspects. The first is slow-release, long-acting ocular drug formulations/implants for macromolecules (such as anti-VEGF (vascular endothelial growth factor)) or steroids that increase the duration of action or reduce the frequency of injection. Recently, a second aspect has emerged that concentrates on more targeted routes of delivery, such as subconjunctival, suprachoroidal, subretinal, and trans-scleral injections. These new delivery techniques, although potentially less invasive, still require repeated injections into the eye. In addition, ocular injections are usually not suitable for the delivery of small molecules as they tend to have short half-lives (usually less than 10 h) of bioavailability in the target tissues [9,14,21]. Other than in steroid treatments, such as dexamethasone intravitreal implants and triamcinolone intravitreal injections [22,23], there are currently no non-steroidal small molecules approved for use to treat retinal diseases. This is not because small molecules cannot treat such diseases, but rather due to the hindered capacity of the currently available delivery methods. As a matter of fact, small molecules, such as VEGF receptor inhibitors, platelet-derived growth factor receptor inhibitors, tyrosine kinase inhibitors, and complement inhibitors, have been presented in scientific publications and listed in ongoing pipelines as potential treatments of dry/wet age-related macular degeneration (AMD) and other retinal diseases [24–27]. The route of delivery is often through slow-release invasive implants or oral administration with systemic exposure.

Here, we describe the discovery of a novel non-invasive ocular delivery platform (NIODP) that successfully delivered drug candidates with high bioavailability and high efficiency not only to the front, but also to the back of the nonhuman primate (NHP) eye through topical administration to the periorbital skin.

2. Materials and Methods

2.1. Compounds

The chemical structure of JV-DE1 and JV-MD2 (two small molecules currently under development in the JeniVision pipeline) are presented in Figure 1. JV-DE1 (also known as JV-DE1, RO1138452, CAY10441) was custom synthesized at Raybow Pharmaceutical Science and Technology Co., Ltd., Hangzhou, China. JV-MD2 (DHA free acid) and compound X (described in Sections 2.2 and 2.6) were purchased from Sigma-Aldrich, St. Louis, MO, USA. These compounds also served as internal standards (IS) for the relative analytical assays.

(a) JV-DE1

(b) JV-MD2

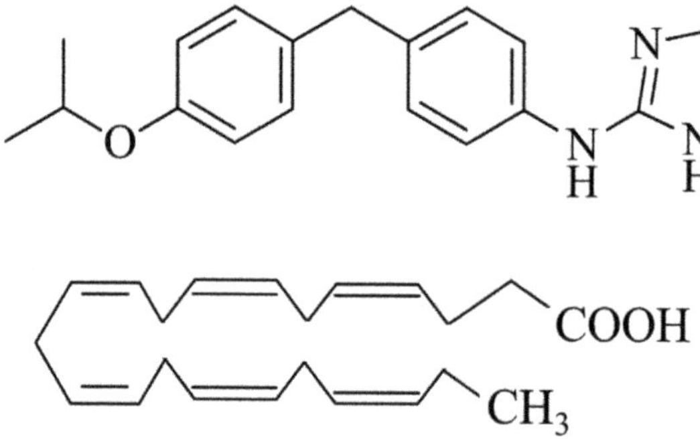

Figure 1. Chemical structures of (**a**) JV-DE1 (RO1138452, CAY10441), 4,5-dihydro-N-[4-[[4-(1-methylethoxy)phenyl]methyl]phenyl]-1H-imadazol-2-amine, formula weight 309.4; and (**b**) JV-MD2 (DHA), cis-4,7,10,13,16,19-docosahexaenoic acid, formula weight 328.49.

2.2. Formulations

JV-DE1 eye drop formulation: JV-DE1 was dissolved in 2.4% polyoxyl 35 castor oil and 0.2% glycerol in pH7.6 Tris-buffered saline to 2.4 mg/mL (0.24% *w*/*v*).

Formulations for NIODP application: JV-DE1 was dissolved in medium-chain triglyceride oil to 5.3 mg/g (0.53% *w*/*w*). The original JV-MD2 stock of 98% was diluted in linoleic acid oil pre-dissolved with compound X. The final concentration of JV-MD2 was 215.21 mg/g (21.5% *w*/*w*) and compound X was 16.14 mg/g. A pen brush with a 3-mL reservoir was used as the applicator for each formulation.

2.3. Non-Invasive Ocular Delivery Platform (NIODP)

NIODP is a JeniVision proprietary topical ocular drug delivery route via the periorbital skin, i.e., the skin area around the eye orbit, which was first used for glaucoma drug delivery to the anterior chamber of the eye [28]; here, it was discovered to be a novel route for ocular drug delivery, particularly for retinal drugs, as depicted in Figure 2.

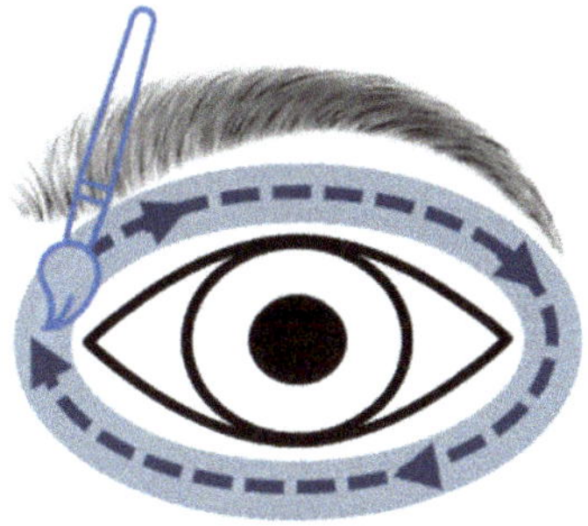

Figure 2. Non-invasive ocular delivery platform (NIODP). A novel drug delivery method to the front and back of the eye via periorbital skin application.

2.4. Choice of Animals for Eye Drop and NIODP Ocular Biodisposition Studies

A pilot ocular biodisposition study is often utilized in the research and discovery phase, prior to Good Laboratory Practices (GLP) pharmacokinetic studies, to assess the feasibility of the delivery route and reliability of the animal model, as well as to minimize the unnecessary use of animals to be sacrificed, especially in studies of higher species such as non-human primates (NHPs). The biodisposition describes a drug's distribution ("where") at a certain time point ("when"). As long as an ocular biodisposition study is designed so that it can answer the questions of "when" and "where" in a generally consistent trend, ideally at multiple time points, such a study design has been accepted by the FDA and for peer-reviewed publications, especially when higher species are used in the studies [6,28–31].

Rabbits are an ideal model to study topical eye drop formulation delivery, especially to the anterior chamber of the eye. Compared to rodents, rabbits share more common anatomical and biochemical features with humans, such as a larger eye size [32]. Monkeys were chosen for the initial NIODP concept validation as the most suitable animal model due to their hairless periorbital skin, the size of their eyeballs, and the fact that they have a similar ocular anatomy to humans, in order to maximize the usually low animal-to-human translational success rate in non-invasive retinal delivery. Non-naïve NHPs washed out from previously unrelated studies were used for the experiment. For analytical method development and validation, ocular blank matrixes were harvested from animals of a control group after unrelated terminal studies.

2.5. Biodisposition of JV-DE1 Eye Drops in New Zealand Rabbits

Five male New Zealand rabbits aged 4–7 months were used in this study. The animals were housed individually in polypropylene cages (530 mm × 630 mm × 320 mm) and in an environmentally monitored, well-ventilated conventional room maintained at a temperature of 18–26 °C and a relative humidity of 40–70%. A certified rabbit diet was provided ad libitum daily during the quarantine and study periods. The nutritional ingredients and designated chemicals of the diet were analyzed by a qualified institute once quarterly.

The in-life procedures and sample collections were performed at Joinn Laboratory Inc. (Suzhou, China). A single dose of 50 μL (120 μg) per eye of the 0.24% JV-DE1 eye drops was applied to both eyes of the animals at time 0 using a pipet. This dose was chosen based on the maximum amount deliverable as an eye drop. Blood samples were collected from all five study animals at 0 h pre-dosing. For every time point of 0.5, 2, 4, 8, and 24 h post-dose, one animal was euthanized and the ocular tissues (anterior sclera, aqueous humor, bulbar conjunctiva, ciliary body, cornea, iris, posterior sclera, and retina) of both eyes were collected. Plasma samples were collected before each euthanization.

Sample preparation and bioanalysis were performed at Medicilon Preclinical Research LLC (Shanghai, China). Solid ocular tissues were homogenized with 9- to 49-fold (1 g tissue in 9 mL to 49 mL, *w*/*v*) of cold homogenization buffer (50% methanol/H_2O). Aliquots of plasma or aqueous humor, as well as the homogenized tissue samples, were mixed with 8-fold volumes of 200 ng/mL warfarin in a methanol solution. After vortexing and centrifuging, an aliquot of supernatants was transferred to a 96-well plate for LC-MS/MS analysis. JV-DE1 is a synthesized new chemical entity (NCE). The absence of the endogenous compound was verified by JeniVision with a battery of pre-clinical GLP and non-GLP studies, including analytical studies in monkey, dog, and rabbit tissues.

2.6. Biodisposition of JV-DE1 and JV-MD2 Delivered via NIODP in Non-Human Primates

Four female cynomolgus non-naïve monkeys aged 3–4 years used for unrelated projects were washed out prior to this study. The monkey maintenance pelleted feed was purchased from Beijing HFK Bioscience Co. Ltd. (Beijing, China) or other qualified sources and was provided ad libitum throughout the in-life portion of the study. During the acclimation period and the experiment, the animals were housed individually (1 monkey/cage) in stainless-steel wire-mesh-type cages in a group housing.

All experiments were performed at Medicilon. A single dose of about 31.2 mg of the 5.3 μg/mg JV-DE1 formulation, i.e., 165.3 ± 4.6 μg (mean ± SEM) per eye of JV-DE1, was applied to the right eye (OD); and a single dose of about 31.48 ± 0.43 mg of the 215.2 μg/mg JV-MD2 formulation, i.e., 6775 ± 92 μg (mean ± SEM) per eye, was applied to the left eye (OS) of each animal at time 0 via NIODP (this formulation also contained 16.14 μg/mg of compound X (mean 508 μg per OS)), which did not diffuse beyond the periorbital skin. A pen brush was used to dose each formulation with three to four circular motions for even distribution. The doses of the test articles were selected based on their solubility/concentration with the maximum deliverable volume on the periorbital skin of the animals. The administered dose was calculated by the weight difference of the pen brush before and after administration. Animals were restrained from eye rubbing in restraint chairs for 2 h after dosing, with access to food and drink. A blood sample was collected from one of the study animals at pre-dosing. For every time point of 0.5, 3, 6, and 24 h post-dose, one animal was euthanized and the ocular tissues (upper eyelid, cornea, retina, and vitreous humor) of both eyes were collected. Plasma samples were collected before each euthanization.

For the convenience of tissue processing and sample extraction, only upper eyelids were collected to represent the entirety of the periorbital tissue. Ocular tissues were homogenized by adding a 9-fold volume of 50% methanol/H_2O per gram of tissue. For the LC-MS/MS sample preparation, a 50 μL aliquot of plasma, aqueous humor, vitreous humor, or tissue homogenate was thoroughly mixed with a 250 μL extraction solution of CHCl3/EtOH (1:1); then, a 210 μL supernatant of the samples was transferred to a 96-well plate after centrifugation. The samples were evaporated in nitrogen gas (N2) until dried. Each sample was redissolved in 200 μL MeOH, of which 2 μL was injected for the LC-MS/MS analysis.

2.7. LC-MS/MS Methods for JV-DE1 in Rabbit Plasma and Ocular Tissues

The liquid chromatography (LC) system comprised a Waters (Waters Corporation, Milford, CT, USA) Ultra Performance Liquid Chromatography (UPLC) equipped with an ACQUITY UPLC binary solvent manager, an ACQUITY UPLC sample manager, an ACQUTIY UPLC sample organizer, and an ACQUITY UPLC column heater HT. The mass spectrometric (MS) analysis was performed using a Triple Quad 6500+ (Applied Biosystems/MDS Sciex, Concord, ON, Canada) with an ESI ion source. The data acquisition and control system were created using Analyst 1.6.3 and 1.7.1 Software from Applied Biosystems/MDS Sciex. The LC/MS conditions for JV-DE1 are described in Supplementary Table S1a–c.

2.8. LC-MS/MS Methods for JV-DE1 and JV-MD2 in Monkey Plasma and Ocular Tissues

The LC system was the same as that described in Section 2. The MS analysis was performed using a Triple Quad 5500 with an ESI ion source, and the data acquisition and control system were Analyst 1.6.3 software from Applied Biosystems/MDS Sciex.

The LC/MS conditions for JV-DE1 are described in Supplementary Table S2. The LC conditions were as follows: ACQUITY UPLC ® BEH C18 1.7 μm, 2.1 mm × 50 mm; the mobile phase Column A, 0.1% formic acid in water; and Column B, 0.1% formic acid in acetonitrile. The flow rate was 0.6 ml/min, the column temperature was 50 °C, and the injection volume was 2 μL. The MS conditions were as follows: scan type, positive MRM; ion source, turbo spray; ionization model, ESI; nebulizer gas 1, 55 psi; gas 2, 55 psi; curtain gas, 40 psi; CAD, 10; ionspray voltage, 5500 V; and temperature, 550 °C.

The LC/MS conditions for JV-MD2 (DHA) are described in Supplementary Table S3. The LC conditions were as follows: ACQUITY UPLC® BEH C18 1.7 μm, 2.1 mm × 50 mm; the mobile phase Column A, 10 mm NH_4AC in H_2O; and Column B, CAN. The flow rate was 0.5 mL/min, the column temperature was 40 °C, and the injection volume was 4 μL. The MS conditions were as follows: scan type, negative MRM; ion source, turbo spray; ionization model, ESI; nebulizer gas 1, 55 psi; gas 2, 55 psi; curtain gas, 40 psi; CAD, 9; ionspray voltage, 5500 V; and temperature, 550 °C.

3. Results

3.1. JV-DE1 Ocular and Plasma Bioavailability Delivered by Eye Drops in New Zealand Rabbits: The Evolution of Eye Drop Administration to Glaucoma Drug Periorbital Skin Delivery, to the Discovery of the Non-Invasive Ocular Delivery Platform (NIODP)

The topical periorbital skin route (i.e., via the skin area around the eye orbit) for ocular drug delivery was first used to deliver JV-GL1, a prostanoid EP_2 receptor agonist, to treat glaucoma, with successful intraocular-pressure-lowering effects in normotensive cynomolgus monkeys [28] and in open-angle glaucoma or ocular hypertension patients in a Phase 1b/2a clinical trial (NCT04761705). Prior to the discovery of the novel topical periorbital skin route, JV-GL1 demonstrated highly effective and long-duration anti-glaucoma effects as eye drops in ocular normotensive monkeys [28].

JV-DE1 (RO1138452) is an anti-inflammatory dual antagonist of the prostanoid IP receptor and PAF receptor, with a pKi of 9.3 (ki = 0.5 nM) for human IP receptor and 7.9 (Ki = 1.3 nM) for human PAF receptor [33]. It is in development at JeniVision for the treatment of dry eye disease. When a 50 μL JV-DE1 eye drop formulation was administered by pipetting to the right eye (OD) at 120 μg/eye to New Zealand rabbits (Table 1), it accumulated at high concentrations in the ocular surface tissues of the bulbar conjunctiva (Cmax ~16 μg/g) and cornea (Cmax ~12 μg/g) as expected, followed by the anterior sclera (Cmax 1.7856 μg/g), ciliary body/iris (Cmax 0.3049 μg/g), and posterior sclera (Cmax 0.2395 μg/g). The JV-DE1 also reached the retina at a Cmax of 0.0920 μg/g, which is much higher than the 0.0026 μg/g Cmax in vitreous humor. The JV-DE1 eye drop concentration gradient in ocular tissues (Figure 3) was consistent with its maximum ocular delivery efficiency (presented as % administered dose), which was conjunctiva (1.3929%) > cornea (0.8622%) > anterior sclera (0.2982%) > posterior sclera (0.0197%) > ciliary body/iris (0.0174%) > retina (0.0047%) > vitreous humor (0.0023%). There was no significant systemic exposure of JV-DE1 when applied via eye drops, as the drug concentration was no more than 0.001 μg/mL in the plasma throughout the 0.5, 3, and 6 h post-dose time points, with a 24 h clearance.

Table 1. JV-DE1 in New Zealand rabbits following the administration of a single eye drop in the right eye.

Test Article		**JV-DE1 (0.24% *w/v*)**				
Dosing site		Topical eye drop (OD)				
Rabbit ID		All	2036281	2036282	2036283	2036284
Time (h)		0	0.5	3	6	24
Dose level (μg/eye)		0	120	120	120	120
Drug in plasma (μg/mL)		BLQ	0.0010	0.0003	0.0001	BLQ
Drug in vitreous humor (μg/mL)		NF *	0.0026	0.0017	0.0012	0.0004
Drug in OD Tissues (μg/g)	Conjunctiva	NF *	16.4919	5.1781	0.5660	0.9937
	Cornea	NF *	12.1249	5.9526	5.1255	0.5422
	Anterior sclera	NF *	1.7856	0.9263	1.4785	0.0932
	Ciliary body/iris	NF *	0.1054	0.3049	0.2314	0.0289
	Posterior sclera	NF *	0.2090	0.2395	0.1512	0.0645
	Retina	NF *	0.0920	0.0491	0.0589	0.0068
	Vitreous humor (μg/mL)	NF *	0.0026	0.0017	0.0012	0.0004
% Administered Dose	Conjunctiva		1.3929	0.4477	0.1288	0.1467
	Cornea		0.8622	0.4239	0.3709	0.0254
	Anterior sclera		0.2982	0.1068	0.2139	0.0127
	Ciliary body/iris		0.0084	0.0174	0.0137	0.0021
	Posterior sclera		0.0153	0.0323	0.0197	0.0088
	Retina		0.0047	0.0036	0.0037	0.0004
	Vitreous humor		0.0023	0.0012	0.0007	0.0004

OD: right eye; BLQ: below the limit of quantification, given a value of 0 in the relevant calculations; LLOQ: lower limit of quantitation, equal to 0.0001 μg/mL, given a value of 0 in the relevant calculations thereafter. Delivery efficiency = % of administered dose = 100X (drug content in tissue (μg))/dose level (μg/eye). NF *: not found in undosed animals of various preclinical species, as JV-DE1 is a synthetic novel chemical entity.

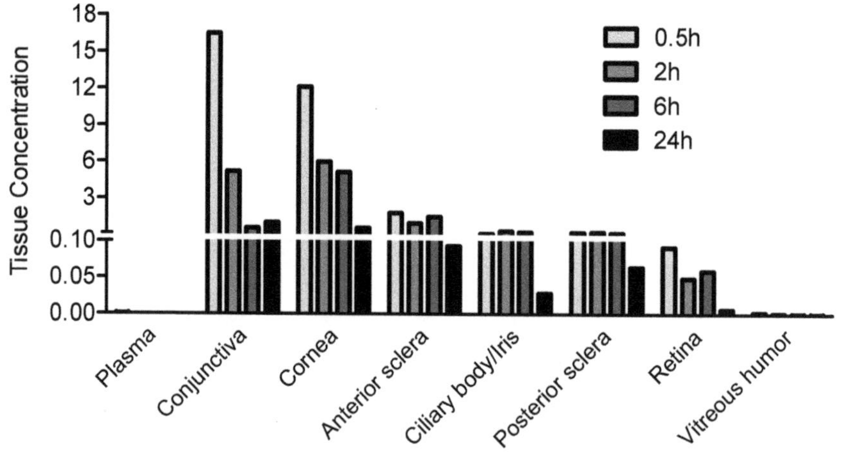

Figure 3. JV-DE1 bioavailability in New Zealand rabbit plasma and ocular tissues when administered as eye drops. A single dose of JV-DE1 (120 μg/eye) was delivered to the right eyes (OD). *N* = four animals in study. The JV-DE1 level is presented as μg/g of solid tissues or μg/mL of aqueous tissues.

Although the 0.0047% retinal delivery efficiency of JV-DE1 eye drops in rabbits was about five times higher compared to the maximum of 0.001% efficiency usually seen in most eye drops dosed to lower animal species, a 10- to 100-fold increase in retinal delivery efficiency demonstrated in a large animal species is desirable to ensure clinical success. Since a substantial increase in the drug load is hard to achieve as an eye drop formulation due to limitations related to drug solubility, ocular tolerability, and suitability, the follow-up studies (as described in Sections 3.2 and 3.3) on ocular drug delivery via the periorbital skin route were undertaken in the hope of achieving pharmaceutically effective retinal doses in larger animal species.

3.2. *JV-DE1 Ocular and Plasma Bioavailability after a Single-Dose NIODP Application in Non-Human Primates*

JV-DE1 was topically applied on the periorbital skin at about 165.3 μg/eye to the right eye (OD) of four cynomolgus monkeys (Table 2). A substantial quantity of the drug was found in the eyelid/periorbital skin (Cmax 26.54 μg/g) and cornea (Cmax 9.30 μg/g). On the other hand, the retina (Cmax 0.0455 μg/g) and vitreous humor (Cmax 0.0190 μg/g) exhibited the lowest drug levels. Therefore, the concentration gradient remained similar to the eye drop application, where the dosing site of NIODP (eyelid/periorbital skin) > cornea > retina > vitreous humor (Figure 4). The plasma concentrations remained ≤ 0.0003 μg/mL, near the lower limit of quantitation (LLOQ, 0.0001 μg/mL), showing no significant systemic exposure of JV-DE1 in the current study via NIODP application, similar to the eye drop administration.

Table 2. JV-DE1 in cynomolgus monkeys following a single-dose administration via NIODP.

Test Article		JV-DE1 (0.53% *w/w*)				
Dosing site		Periorbital skin (OD)				
Animal no.		101	101	102	103	104
Time (h)		0	0.5	3	6	24
Dose level (μg/eye)		0	179.1	160.6	162.2	159.3
Drug in plasma (μg/mL)		BLQ	0.0001	0.0002	0.0003	BLQ
Drug in OD Tissues (μg/g)	Eyelid/periorbital skin	NF *	26.5354	32.4547	7.9456	11.5978
	Cornea	NF *	9.2993	16.6887	23.9295	1.6213
	Retina	NF *	0.0396	0.0279	0.0455	0.0055
	Vitreous humor (μg/mL)	NF *	0.0152	0.0079	0.0039	0.0190
% Administered Dose	Eyelid/periorbital skin		0.6370	1.4956	0.3477	0.7501
	Cornea		0.1921	0.3430	0.5900	0.0326
	Retina		0.0004	0.0004	0.0005	0.0002
	Vitreous humor		0.0047	0.0029	0.0031	0.0018

OD: right eye; BLQ: below the limit of quantification, given a value of 0 in the relevant calculations. LLOQ: lower limit of quantitation, equal to 0.0001 μg/mL, given a value of 0 in the relevant calculations thereafter. Delivery efficiency = % of administered dose = 100X (drug content in tissue (μg))/dose level (μg/eye). NF *: not found in undosed animals of various preclinical species, as JV-DE1 is a synthetic novel chemical entity.

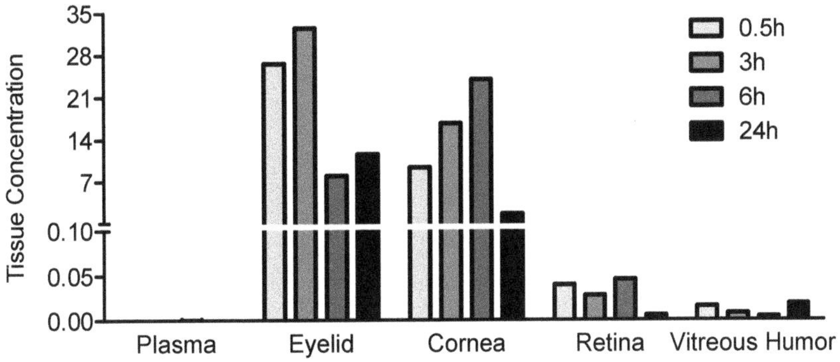

Figure 4. JV-DE1 bioavailability in monkey plasma and ocular tissues delivered via NIODP. A single dose of JV-DE1 was administered to the right eye (OD) at 165.4 μg/eye (mean). Eyelid/periorbital skin is collectively labeled as "Eyelid". *N* = four animals in the study. The JV-DE1 level is presented as μg/g of solid tissue or μg/mL of fluid samples.

3.3. *JV-MD2 Ocular and Plasma Bioavailability via NIODP in Non-Human Primates*

JV-MD2 (DHA omega 3 free acid) was administered via NIODP at approximately 6775 µg/eye to the left eye (OS) of four cynomolgus monkeys. The endogenous levels of DHA in the ocular tissues were determined during method validation from the mean of a double-blank matrix measured during method validation, where BLQ is below the limit of quantification, with a lower limit of quantitation (LLOQ) = 0.5 µg/mL. Substantial quantities of JV-MD2 remained in the eyelid/periorbital skin (11–420 µg/g vs. the BLQ baseline), cornea (22–66 µg/g vs. the BLQ baseline), and retina (47–111 µg/g vs. the 17 µg/g baseline), at all post-dose time points of 0.5, 3, 6, and 24 h (Table 3). It is notable that JV-MD2 rapidly reached its Cmax of 111 µg/g in the retina within 0.5 h post-dosage from the endogenous level of 17 µg/g. In the vitreous humor, JV-MD2 remained below BLQ at all timepoints except for at 24 h post-dose (2 µg/mL). The JV-MD2 concentration gradient was as follows: the dosing site of NIODP (eyelid/periorbital skin) > retina > cornea >> vitreous humor. This is generally concordant with the maximum percentage of the administered dose achieved within 30 min of dosing, which was eyelid/periorbital skin (0.4288%) > retina (0.0343%) > cornea (0.0283%) >> vitreous humor. The post-dose plasma levels of JV-MD2 showed a range of 1–3 µg/mL, with no significant fluctuation around the 2 µg/mL pre-dosing baseline.

Table 3. JV-MD2 in cynomolgus monkeys after a single-dose administration via NIODP.

Test Article		**JV-MD2 (DHA (21.5% *w/w*)**				
Dosing site		Periorbital skin (OS)				
Animal no.		101	101	102	103	104
Time (h)		0	0.5	3	6	24
Dose level (µg/eye)		0	6568	6768	7018	6747
Drug in plasma (µg/mL)		2	2	3	2	1
Drug in OS Tissues (µg/g)	Eyelid/periorbital skin	BLQ *	381	420	11	16
	Cornea	BLQ *	66	22	22	26
	Retina	17 *	111	67	79	47
	Vitreous humor	BLQ *	0	0	0	2
% Administered Dose	Eyelid/periorbital skin		0.4288	0.3844	0.0149	0.0197
	Cornea		0.0283	0.0109	0.0149	0.0173
	Retina **		0.0343	0.0264	0.0228	0.0175
	Vitreous humor		0.0000	0.0000	0.0000	0.0236

OS: left eye; BLQ: below the limit of quantification, given a value of 0 in relevant calculations. LLOQ: lower limit of quantitation, equal to 0.5 µg/mL, and given a value of 0 in relevant calculations thereafter. Delivery efficiency = % of administered dose = 100X (drug content in tissue (µg))/dose level (µg/eye). * Mean of calculated endogenous DHA from the double-blank matrix measured during method validation. ** Endogenous DHA was subtracted when calculating % administered dose in the retina.

4. Discussion

According to the tissue concentration gradient (Figure 3) and the % of the administered dose in ocular tissues (Table 1) derived from the rabbit eye drop biodisposition study, most of the JV-DE1 followed a typical "corneal route" of cornea → anterior tissues (ciliary body/iris) → vitreous humor where JV-DE1 lost the driving force to reach the retina; in the meantime, a small portion of the JV-DE1 may also have taken the "conjunctiva–sclera route", i.e., conjunctiva → sclera → retina. Changing the site of delivery from the ocular surface to the application of eye drops to the periorbital skin around the eye via NIODP did not improve retinal delivery of JV-DE1. Rather, the maximum delivery efficiency in the retina was about 10-fold lower, dropping from 0.0047% via eye drop application to 0.0005% via NIODP, albeit not in a head-to-head comparison, as the studies were conducted in different species. Nonetheless, the tissue concentration gradient again indicated that the JV-DE1 levels achieved in the retina were mainly through the same conjunctiva–sclera pathway as the eye drops. JV-DE1 seems to bypass the vitreous humor to reach the retina, since, in both delivery routes, the retinal bioavailability seems to be higher than that of the vitreous humor. The retinal Cmax of JV-DE1 (RO1138452) was 0.0920 µg/g (297 nM) for eye drop administration in rabbits and 0.0455 µg/g (147 nM) for NIODP in monkeys. This Cmax value is at least 100-fold higher than the Ki on the human receptors of prostanoid IP (ki = 0.5 nM) and PAF (Ki = 1.3 nM) and may be sufficient to treat retinal diseases if the same delivery efficiency is translatable from rabbits to humans as eye drops or from monkeys to humans via NIODP. However, while it may be tolerable to apply the 0.53% (*w*/*w*) oily formulation once daily via NIODP, the 0.24% (*w*/*v*) aqueous eye drop formulation may cause eye irritation in humans.

Although both molecules are amphipathic, JV-DE1 can form an aqueous formulation, while JV-MD2 (DHA) is a fatty acid with much lower water solubility. This difference in physicochemical properties makes it easier for DHA to penetrate cell membranes and diffuse through biological tissues to achieve efficient transcellular and intracellular distributions. We have discovered a novel non-invasive ocular delivery platform, and demonstrated that the application of less than 7 mg of JV-MD2 (DHA) via NIODP can reach a Cmax of 66µg/g in the cornea and 111 µg/g in the retina, where the delivery efficiencies were 0.01–0.42% in the eyelid/periorbital skin (site of application), 0.01–0.03% in the cornea, and 0.01–0.04% in the retina of NHPs. Like JV-DE1 (administered either as eye drops or via NIODP), JV-MD2 seems to reach the retina via the conjunctiva–sclera pathway when administered via NIODP, with a preferred distribution in the retina over the cornea (Figure 5). Interestingly, the biodistribution of JV-MD2 only appeared in the vitreous humor at 24 h post-dose but not at any earlier time points of 0.5, 3, or 6 h post-dose; moreover, there was no endogenous DHA detected in the blank matrix. Thus, excess JV-MD2 may diffuse from the retina to vitreous humor over time if other reasons, such as animal-to-animal variation, can be ruled out.

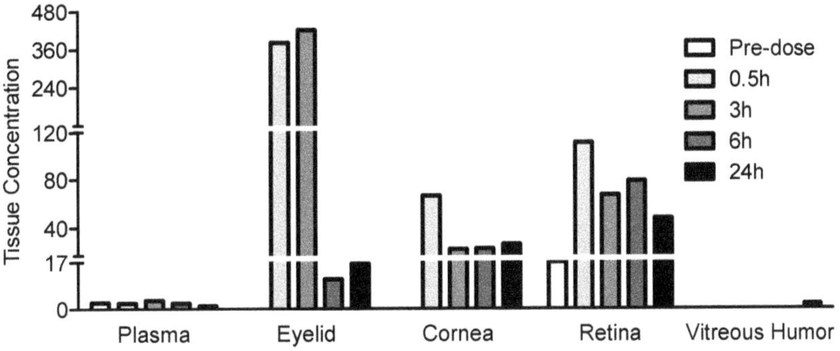

Figure 5. JV-MD2 bioavailability in monkey plasma and ocular tissues delivered via NIODP. A single dose of JV-MD2 was administered at 6775 µg/eye (mean) to the left eye (OS). Eyelid/periorbital skin is collectively labeled as "eyelid". *N* = four animals in the study. The JV-MD2 level is presented as µg/g of solid tissue or µg/mL of fluid sample.

In contrast to traditional eye drop administration, which targets the cornea mostly for anterior ocular drug delivery, the conjunctival–scleral pathway has not previously been considered a major drug delivery route, although ocular drug penetration may occur via this pathway. The conjunctival–scleral pathway may provide a much larger surface area for drug absorption than the cornea [34]. Compared to the cornea, the relatively leaky and hydrophilic conjunctival tissue can provide approximately 230-fold larger intercellular spaces that are more permeable even to macromolecules, such as proteins and peptides [3]. Connected to the conjunctiva is the sclera, a network of collagen fibers, proteoglycans, and glycoproteins in an aqueous medium forming scleral water channels 30–350 nm in size [9,12], spacious enough for the passage of macromolecules. The suprachoroid is located between the sclera and the choroid. Since the choroid bleeds into the suprachoroid space

(SCS), the exchange of biomolecules between the choroid, SCS, and sclera is barrier-free. Because of this permeability, as well as being less invasive and having higher bioavailability than intravitreal injection, suprachoroidal injection has been under investigation since 2013 for retinal delivery [35–37]. The fenestrated capillaries in the choroid are highly permeable and allow for high concentrations and the rapid diffusion of nutrients in the extra-vascular space of the choroid [38]. Bruch's membrane (BrM) is a thin layer of extracellular matrix, which is a selectively permeable membrane between the retina and choroid and regulates the exchange of nutrients, oxygen, minerals, and by-products of the visual cycle through passive diffusion, influenced by the weight, size, and shape of the diffusing molecule. While some complement proteins, such as FHL-1, factor D, and C5a, are allowed to diffuse through, most complement proteins (including the low-molecular-weight C3a) are unable to do so [39,40]. Finally, before any drug reaches the retina, it must pass the retinal pigment epithelium (RPE), which also forms the outer blood–retina barrier (BRB), regulating drug permeability via physicochemical properties, such as molecular weight, lipophilicity, protein binding, and concentration gradient [12].

Age-related macular degeneration (AMD) in the elderly is the leading cause of irreversible vision loss. Early or intermediate stages of AMD (dry AMD) are defined by the formation of lipid-rich deposits of drusen between the RPE and the BrM, as well as the accumulation of choroidal macrophages. Geographic atrophy (GA), one of the advanced stages of AMD, is characterized by the confluent deterioration of the RPE and photoreceptor and choroidal neovascularization. Wet (or neovascular) AMD, another advanced stage of AMD, is characterized by invasive choroidal neovascularization (CNV) with accompanying macrophage accumulation in the retina, which breaks from the BrM and can lead to retinopathy [41]. Genetic variations in the innate immune system and poor diet are the two main factors contributing to drusen genesis and disease progression in AMD [42]. The mechanistic target of rapamycin (mTOR), a sensor of nutrient availability and growth factors, has been implicated in multiple diseases like cancer, diabetes, and neurodegenerative diseases; they are characterized by inflammation, as well as aging, referred to as "inflammaging" [43–45]. The activation of mTORC1 has been associated with the formation of drusen-like deposits in photoreceptors; dietary supplementation with DHA alleviated most pathologies in a mouse model with advanced AMD pathologies [42]. The once-daily intragastric administration of DHA effectively inhibited laser-induced CNV formation in mice, which was associated with the suppressed protein expression of NF-κB, VGFER2, and VEGF, major players in the angiogenic pathway in cancer and advanced stages of AMD [46]. Upon the induction of pathological stimuli, activated macrophages were recruited to the affected site, i.e., the back of the eye in the case of AMD, to secrete proinflammatory cytokines, recruit more macrophages, and accelerate disease progression. Omega 3 fatty acids provoke major alterations in gene expression in macrophages to decrease cytokine production while increasing phagocytosis to eliminate pathogens. It is worth noting that the anti-inflammatory effect mediated by DHA was more potent than that of EPA; the only cytokine secretion increased by the omega 3 fatty acid treatment was the anti-inflammatory cytokine IL-10, while many other cytokines, such as IL-1β, TNF-α, and IL-6, were found to be decreased in omega-3-fatty-acid-treated macrophages [47]. Therefore, the mechanism of action of DHA in early and intermediate dry AMD treatments is thought to involve the suppression of drusen genesis via mTORC inhibition, the alteration of the function of macrophages toward an anti-inflammation phenotype by inhibiting proinflammatory cytokine production, and the mediation of anti-neovascularization effects by inhibiting the effects of VEGF in the choroid and retina. Given the success in treating early- or intermediate-stage dry AMD by DHA, it is logical to anticipate the prevention of late-stage AMD, wet AMD, and geographic atrophy, which have prevalence levels of approximately 10% of all individuals with AMD [48,49] (Figure 6a).

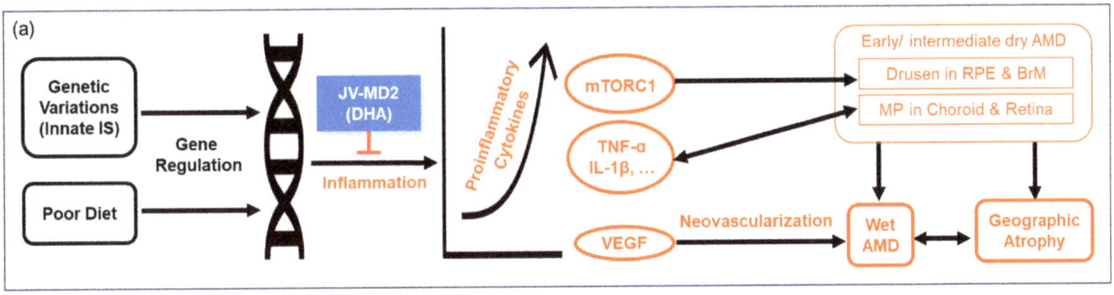

(b)

- DHA molecular target and potency: RXRα receptor EC50 5~10μM; PPARγ receptor EC50 > 10μM (Oxidized DHA EC50 0.4~3.7μM); COX-2 IC50 18 μM; Kinases: PKC, PKA, MAPK, CaMKII, IC50 34~36 μM.
- JV-MD2 via NIODP retinal delivery: about 7mg/eye → retinal Cmax 338 μM
- Retinal delivery efficiency: NIODP (0.04%) > Eye drops (0.001% or less) ≥ Oral (0.001% or less)

Figure 6. MOA and pharmacological effects of DHA on AMD. (**a**) The anti-inflammatory effects of DHA on drusen genesis, proinflammatory cytokine secretion, and macrophage accumulation in the choroid and retina. (**b**) DHA molecular target, potency, and retinal delivery efficiency via various routes. IS, immune system; RPE, retinal pigment epithelium; BrM, Bruch's membrane; MP, macrophages.

Regarding human clinical trials for dry AMD treatment, in 2015, Georgiou and Prokopiou reported preliminary but promising therapeutic results of taking 5 g/day omega 3 in patients with mild-to-moderate visual impairment of dry AMD [50]. Then, in 2022, in an ARVO annual meeting abstract, the same group reported that 3.7 g daily oral administration of omega 3 fatty acids improved objective and subjective vision in patients with dry AMD and SD [51]. A peer-reviewed article has not yet been published. In a three-year randomized clinical study of patients with early lesions of AMD, the omega-3-supplemented (840 mg/day DHA and 270 mg/day EPA) patients who had high red blood cell membrane EPA and DHA levels were significantly protected against choroidal neovascularization of AMD compared with those in the olive oil placebo group [52]. Additionally, the preventative effect of omega 3 in AMD has clearly been demonstrated in a large number of epidemiological studies, using different methodologies, populations, and geographical sites with a high degree of consistency [53]. However, no interventive treatment effect from omega 3 consumption was found in patients with advanced AMD [54]. This may be due to two reasons: (a) the poor absorption and poor retinal delivery efficiency of orally administered omega 3, even with mega dosage [7,53,55]; and (b) the pharmaceutically effective doses for disease treatment are usually expected to be at least a few times higher than the doses for disease prevention, where normal physiological levels are good enough for maintaining health. For example, the European Food Safety Authority (EFSA) suggested that the amount of EPA+DHA required to lower triglyceride is 2–4 g/day and 3 g/day to lower blood pressure, which are, respectively, about 4- to 13-fold higher than the daily consumption recommended to stay healthy according to the World Health Organization (WHO) [56].

A healthy retina contains a high concentration of DHA (the active ingredient of JV-MD2), which is not only important in the maintenance of normal retinal integrity and visual function, but also plays anti-inflammatory, anti-apoptotic, and neuroprotective roles [56,57]. DHA analogs may act as anti-inflammatory lipid mediators to activate peroxisome-proliferator-activated receptors (PPARs) and retinoid X receptors (RXRs). As a natural ligand, DHA induced a protective effect in rat retinal neuronal cultures to promote the survival and differentiation of photoreceptors by activating RXRs and the downstream signaling pathways [58]. The EC_{50} of DHA was about 5–10 μM for human RXRα receptor, and an oxidized form of DHA can be as potent as an EC_{50} of 0.4 μM for human

PPARγ [59,60]. It was suggested that DHA and its more potent metabolites compete with the more biologically potent arachidonic acid on the COX-2 (IC_{50} 18 μM) signaling cascade and can shift the proinflammatory state to a more anti-inflammatory one [61,62]. DHA was able to suppress inflammation through reducing IL-1β production with a potency of IC_{50} = 4.6 μM in the human THP-1 macrophage cell line [63]. DHA was also found to reduce the activity of protein kinase C (PKC), cAMP-dependent protein kinase A (PKA), mitogen-activated protein kinase (MAPK), and Ca21/calmodulin-dependent protein kinase II (CaMKII) at an IC_{50} of 34–36 μM in in vitro functional assays [64]. For retinal disease treatments, a local drug concentration 3- to 10-fold higher than EC_{50} or IC_{50} is desirable, which may be readily achieved in the retina utilizing the NIODP, as demonstrated in our current study, where the application of just 7 mg/eye of DHA in NHP yielded a retina DHA Cmax of 111 μg/g (about 338 μM) (Figure 6b). This JV-MD2 retinal Cmax is at least 10-fold higher than the EC_{50} or IC_{50} of most mediators in the omega 3 DHA signaling cascade. Such concentration is believed to be enough to treat retinal diseases because the success of drug treatments lies in the effective drug concentration deliverable to the target tissue [65]. Moreover, we believe that much higher DHA retinal concentrations can be achieved via NIODP using formulations with a higher concentration and more frequent dosing, if necessary.

Because of the "500 Dalton rule" for passive skin penetration [66], small molecules are the best candidates for NIODP delivery. However, liposomes up to 600 nm in diameter have been reported to penetrate the skin through intercellular lipids of the stratum corneum [67,68]. Liposomes with an average size of 300 nm in diameter were reported to penetrate deeper into skin layers, and those with a 70 nm diameter showed the best dermal delivery performance [69,70]. For reference, the average molecular widths are 2.5 nm for DNA, 10 nm for proteins, 100 nm for a typical virus, and 1000 nm for a bacterium [71]. A previous publication indicated that liposomes can deliver macromolecules through the skin [72]. In posterior ocular delivery, nanocarriers have been reported to overcome the ocular barriers, as nanoparticles <250 nm were usually easily taken up by retinal cells via endocytosis [9,73]. Therefore, it is possible that NIODP may have the potential to be utilized for macromolecular therapeutics packed in liposomes for retinal delivery. More vigorous research is necessary.

The NIODP via periorbital skin application is also a novel route for anterior ocular drug delivery. It has successfully delivered JV-GL1, a prostaglandin EP2 receptor agonist, for glaucoma treatment in a phase 1b/2a clinical trial with satisfactory efficacy, while avoiding ocular adverse effects commonly associated with prostaglandin eye drops directly applied to the ocular surface. It is important to note that, for issues of solubility or ocular tolerability, most hydrophobic vitamins and supplements, including omega 3, cannot be conveniently used as high-dose eye drops. The NIODP makes it possible to deliver these molecules for the potential treatment of anterior ocular diseases, such as dry eye disease, uveitis, etc., with minimum irritation or interference with normal ocular functions. A summary of the therapeutic agents (JV-GL1, JV-DE1, and JV-MD2) that were successfully delivered through periorbital skin administration to the targeted tissues is shown in Figure 7.

Notably, like most eye drops used in a range of reasonable ocular doses (0.01–0.5%), the systemic exposure of JV-DE1 was very low when using both eye drops and NIODP as delivery routes with a 24 h clearance. Additionally, when delivered as a single dose at about 7 mg per eye via NIODP, JV-MD2 also did not significantly change the baseline omega 3 levels in the plasma. Therefore, while achieving breakthrough retinal delivery efficiency, the systemic exposure via NIODP application may not pose a great concern; this may also be determined by the physicochemical properties and biosafety profile of the drug.

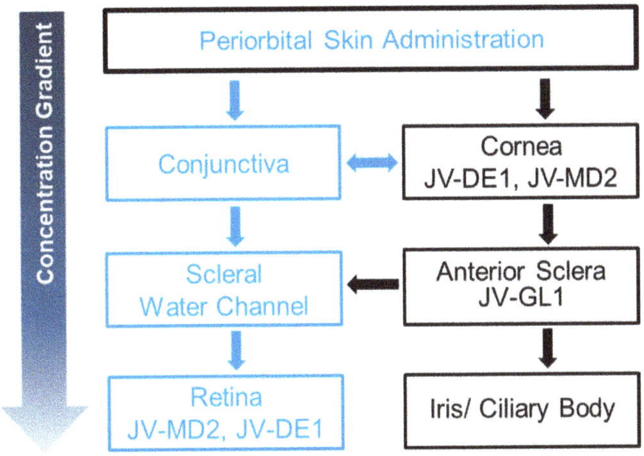

Figure 7. Proposed concentration gradient of drug distribution administered through NIODP and drug candidates found in the targeted tissue. The JV-GL1 biodistribution is unpublished (JeniVision data).

Similar to JV-DE1 applied via eye drops, both JV-DE1 and JV-MD2 applied via NIODP seem to reach the retina via the conjunctiva–sclera pathway (Figure 7). The potential advantages of NIODP include (a) a breakthrough in non-invasive, high-efficiency retinal delivery; (b) a much more ocularly tolerable delivery method than eye drops for therapeutic agents known to cause ocular adverse effects or interfere with normal functioning of the eye, such as drug ingredients that cause eye irritation due to ocularly intolerable drug property or concentration, or oily formulations causing vision blurriness and eye stress; and (c) another topical ocular delivery route without significant systemic exposure, just like the traditional eye drop administration, but potentially more convenient for self-administration or administration by a care-giver.

Like any other delivery route (oral, intravenous injection, eye drop, or intravitreal injection), NIODP delivery has its prerequisite conditions of use. However, such limitations do not discount its value as a novel non-invasive ocular delivery platform, which is not just specific to DHA or JV-DE1. A successful NIODP delivery is determined by the physicochemical properties of the drug; it must (a) have permeability through the periorbital skin, which is determined by its molecular weight, lipophilicity, and solubility; (b) have good solubility/concentration to establish a sufficient concentration gradient to drive efficient, high-bioavailability diffusion from the anterior to posterior ocular tissues; and (c) be compatible with the local tissue, such as the sclera water channel, in order to travel through and reach the retina.

In summary, any drug that can penetrate the periorbital skin and can diffuse through ocular tissues may be deliverable by NIODP, which is presented in this report as a novel general delivery platform for ocular delivery to both the anterior and posterior segments of the eye. The site of periorbital skin application enables the utilization of the conjunctiva–sclera pathway for a much higher retinal delivery efficiency using NIODP compared to eye drop delivery. Good bioavailability is driven by the concentration gradient of ocular tissues, where the drug solubility plays an important role when the delivery volume is fixed. Due to the "500 Dalton rule" for passive skin penetration, small molecules are the best candidates for NIODP delivery. With more thorough research, it may be possible to utilize NIODP for the retinal delivery of macromolecular therapeutics packed in liposomes or other nanocarriers. Nonetheless, our studies demonstrated the potential of NIODP for use in the high-efficiency drug delivery of small molecules for the treatment of various ocular disorders, particularly for retinal diseases.

5. Conclusions

The discovery of a novel non-invasive ocular delivery platform has opened up new possibilities for the effective topical delivery of molecules that are currently difficult to deliver to both the front and back of the eye. The NIODP is a combination of periorbital skin administration with topical drug formulation for ocular, particularly retinal, delivery. JV-MD2 (DHA) has been successfully delivered by NIODP with a high efficiency and high bioavailability to the retina. When the essential fatty acid DHA, with a multi-anti-inflammatory mechanism of action, reaches the retina at a concentration up to 10-fold higher than the normal EC_{50} or IC_{50} of its molecular targets, a better therapeutic efficacy can be anticipated for retinal diseases (such as early or intermediate AMD, thus preventing late-stage AMD) and avoiding or minimizing the frequency of invasive ocular injections. With further study and more experimental evidence, the NIODP could provide significant opportunities to address the serious medical need in drug delivery for the treatment of eye diseases without irritation or injection, transforming the retinal health landscape.

6. Patents

Patent (pending) resulting from the work reported in this manuscript: Delivery methods for Treating Eye Diseases, by W.W., D.W., and N.S.

Supplementary Materials: The following supporting information can be downloaded at: https://www.mdpi.com/article/10.3390/pharmaceutics15092344/s1, Table S1a: LC conditions for JV-DE1 in rabbit plasma samples. Table S1b: LC conditions for JV-DE1 in rabbit ocular tissues. Table S1c: MS conditions for JV-DE1 in rabbit plasma and ocular tissues. Table S2: LC/MS process conditions for JV-DE1 in monkey plasma and ocular tissues. Table S3: LC/MS process conditions for JV-MD2 (DHA) in monkey plasma and ocular tissues.

Author Contributions: Conceptualization and methodology, W.W.; data analysis, W.W.; interpretation and investigation, W.W. and N.S.; writing—original draft preparation, W.W.; writing—review and editing, W.W. and N.S.; visualization, W.W. and N.S.; supervision, project administration, and resources, W.W. All authors have read and agreed to the published version of the manuscript.

Funding: This research received no external funding.

Institutional Review Board Statement: All experiments were conducted in accordance with the ARVO Statement on the Use of Animals in Ophthalmic and Vision Research. All experimental procedures followed protocols approved by the committees on animal research and ethics of the contracted research organizations: Joinn Laboratory Inc. (Suzhou, China) for rabbit studies and Medicilon Preclinical Research LLC (Shanghai, China) for monkey studies.

Informed Consent Statement: Informed consent was obtained from all subjects enrolled in the clinical study.

Data Availability Statement: Data are available on request due to restrictions related to privacy and confidentiality.

Conflicts of Interest: W.W. is one of the major shareholders of JeniVision. N.S. declares no conflict of interest. For JeniVision, the company had no role in tissue sample analysis, collection and calculation of the data in the study report provided by the contract research organizations (Joinn and Medicilon).

References

1. Mosteller, M.W.; Gebhardt, B.M.; Hamilton, A.M.; Kaufman, H.E. Penetration of topical cyclosporine into the rabbit cornea, aqueous humor, and serum. *Arch. Ophthalmol.* **1985**, *103*, 101–102. [CrossRef] [PubMed]
2. Said, T.; Dutot, M.; Christon, R.; Beaudeux, J.L.; Martin, C.; Warnet, J.M.; Rat, P. Benefits and side effects of different vegetable oil vectors on apoptosis, oxidative stress, and P2X7 cell death receptor activation. *Investig. Ophthalmol. Vis. Sci.* **2007**, *48*, 5000–5006. [CrossRef] [PubMed]
3. Agarwal, P.; Craig, J.P.; Rupenthal, I.D. Formulation Considerations for the Management of Dry Eye Disease. *Pharmaceutics* **2021**, *13*, 207. [CrossRef] [PubMed]
4. Agrahari, V.; Mandal, A.; Agrahari, V.; Trinh, H.M.; Joseph, M.; Ray, A.; Hadji, H.; Mitra, R.; Pal, D.; Mitra, A.K. A comprehensive insight on ocular pharmacokinetics. *Drug Deliv. Transl. Res.* **2016**, *6*, 735–754. [CrossRef] [PubMed]

5. Sarkadi-Nagy, E.; Wijendran, V.; Diau, G.Y.; Chao, A.C.; Hsieh, A.T.; Turpeinen, A.; Nathanielsz, P.W.; Brenna, J.T. The influence of prematurity and long chain polyunsaturate supplementation in 4-week adjusted age baboon neonate brain and related tissues. *Pediatr. Res.* **2003**, *54*, 244–252. [CrossRef]
6. Sarkadi-Nagy, E.; Wijendran, V.; Diau, G.Y.; Chao, A.C.; Hsieh, A.T.; Turpeinen, A.; Lawrence, P.; Nathanielsz, P.W.; Brenna, J.T. Formula feeding potentiates docosahexaenoic and arachidonic acid biosynthesis in term and preterm baboon neonates. *J. Lipid Res.* **2004**, *45*, 71–80. [CrossRef]
7. Sripetch, S.; Loftsson, T. Topical drug delivery to the posterior segment of the eye: Thermodynamic considerations. *Int. J. Pharm.* **2021**, *597*, 120332. [CrossRef]
8. Hughes, P.M.; Olejnik, O.; Chang-Lin, J.E.; Wilson, C.G. Topical and systemic drug delivery to the posterior segments. *Adv. Drug Deliv. Rev.* **2005**, *57*, 2010–2032. [CrossRef]
9. Tsai, C.H.; Wang, P.Y.; Lin, I.C.; Huang, H.; Liu, G.S.; Tseng, C.L. Ocular Drug Delivery: Role of Degradable Polymeric Nanocarriers for Ophthalmic Application. *Int. J. Mol. Sci.* **2018**, *19*, 2830. [CrossRef]
10. Lakhani, P.; Patil, A.; Majumdar, S. Recent advances in topical nano drug-delivery systems for the anterior ocular segment. *Ther. Deliv.* **2018**, *9*, 137–153. [CrossRef]
11. Molokhia, S.A.; Thomas, S.C.; Garff, K.J.; Mandell, K.J.; Wirostko, B.M. Anterior eye segment drug delivery systems: Current treatments and future challenges. *J. Ocul. Pharm. Ther.* **2013**, *29*, 92–105. [CrossRef] [PubMed]
12. Varela-Fernandez, R.; Diaz-Tome, V.; Luaces-Rodriguez, A.; Conde-Penedo, A.; Garcia-Otero, X.; Luzardo-Alvarez, A.; Fernandez-Ferreiro, A.; Otero-Espinar, F.J. Drug Delivery to the Posterior Segment of the Eye: Biopharmaceutic and Pharmacokinetic Considerations. *Pharmaceutics* **2020**, *12*, 269. [CrossRef] [PubMed]
13. Rodrigues, G.A.; Lutz, D.; Shen, J.; Yuan, X.; Shen, H.; Cunningham, J.; Rivers, H.M. Topical Drug Delivery to the Posterior Segment of the Eye: Addressing the Challenge of Preclinical to Clinical Translation. *Pharm. Res.* **2018**, *35*, 245. [CrossRef] [PubMed]
14. Kim, H.M.; Woo, S.J. Ocular Drug Delivery to the Retina: Current Innovations and Future Perspectives. *Pharmaceutics* **2021**, *13*, 108. [CrossRef]
15. Gote, V.; Sikder, S.; Sicotte, J.; Pal, D. Ocular Drug Delivery: Present Innovations and Future Challenges. *J. Pharm. Exp. Ther.* **2019**, *370*, 602–624. [CrossRef] [PubMed]
16. Nomoto, H.; Shiraga, F.; Kuno, N.; Kimura, E.; Fujii, S.; Shinomiya, K.; Nugent, A.K.; Hirooka, K.; Baba, T. Pharmacokinetics of bevacizumab after topical, subconjunctival, and intravitreal administration in rabbits. *Invest. Ophthalmol. Vis. Sci.* **2009**, *50*, 4807–4813. [CrossRef]
17. Davis, B.M.; Normando, E.M.; Guo, L.; Turner, L.A.; Nizari, S.; O'Shea, P.; Moss, S.E.; Somavarapu, S.; Cordeiro, M.F. Topical delivery of Avastin to the posterior segment of the eye in vivo using annexin A5-associated liposomes. *Small* **2014**, *10*, 1575–1584. [CrossRef]
18. De Cogan, F.; Hill, L.J.; Lynch, A.; Morgan-Warren, P.J.; Lechner, J.; Berwick, M.R.; Peacock, A.F.A.; Chen, M.; Scott, R.A.H.; Xu, H.; et al. Topical Delivery of Anti-VEGF Drugs to the Ocular Posterior Segment Using Cell-Penetrating Peptides. *Investig. Ophthalmol. Vis. Sci.* **2017**, *58*, 2578–2590. [CrossRef]
19. Sigurdsson, H.H.; Konraethsdottir, F.; Loftsson, T.; Stefansson, E. Topical and systemic absorption in delivery of dexamethasone to the anterior and posterior segments of the eye. *Acta Ophthalmol. Scand.* **2007**, *85*, 598–602. [CrossRef]
20. Hartman, R.R.; Kompella, U.B. Intravitreal, Subretinal, and Suprachoroidal Injections: Evolution of Microneedles for Drug Delivery. *J. Ocul. Pharm. Ther.* **2018**, *34*, 141–153. [CrossRef]
21. Del Amo, E.M.; Rimpela, A.K.; Heikkinen, E.; Kari, O.K.; Ramsay, E.; Lajunen, T.; Schmitt, M.; Pelkonen, L.; Bhattacharya, M.; Richardson, D.; et al. Pharmacokinetic aspects of retinal drug delivery. *Prog. Retin. Eye Res.* **2017**, *57*, 134–185. [CrossRef] [PubMed]
22. Karti, O.; Saatci, A.O. Intravitreal Dexamethasone Implant in the Treatment of Non-Infectious Uveitic Macular Edema. *Med. Hypothesis Discov. Innov. Ophthalmol.* **2018**, *7*, 169–175. [PubMed]
23. Villegas, V.M.; Gold, A.S.; Wildner, A.; Latiff, A.; Murray, T.G. Intravitreal triamcinolone acetonide: A "real world" analysis of visual acuity, pressure and outcomes. *Int. J. Ophthalmol.* **2016**, *9*, 789–791. [PubMed]
24. Cao, L.; Weetall, M.; Bombard, J.; Qi, H.; Arasu, T.; Lennox, W.; Hedrick, J.; Sheedy, J.; Risher, N.; Brooks, P.C.; et al. Discovery of Novel Small Molecule Inhibitors of VEGF Expression in Tumor Cells Using a Cell-Based High Throughput Screening Platform. *PLoS ONE* **2016**, *11*, e0168366. [CrossRef]
25. Roskoski, R., Jr. The role of small molecule platelet-derived growth factor receptor (PDGFR) inhibitors in the treatment of neoplastic disorders. *Pharm. Res.* **2018**, *129*, 65–83. [CrossRef]
26. Kaiser, P.K. Retina Pipeline 2021 Ongoing Innovation Wet AMD. Available online: https://retinatoday.com/images/retina-pipeline/retina-pipeline-2021/pdfs-for-download/Wet-AMD-Retina-Pipeline-Poster.pdf (accessed on 20 January 2022).
27. Kaiser, P.K. Retina Pipeline 2021 Ongoing Innovation Dry AMD. Available online: https://retinatoday.com/images/retina-pipeline/retina-pipeline-2021/pdfs-for-download/Dry-AMD-Retina-Pipeline-Poster.pdf (accessed on 20 January 2022).
28. Woodward, D.F.; Wang, J.W.; Coleman, R.A.; Woodrooffe, A.J.; Clark, K.L.; Stamer, W.D.; Tao, G.; Fan, S.; Toris, C.B. A Highly Effective and Ultra-Long-Acting Anti-Glaucoma Drug, with a Novel Periorbital Delivery Method. *J. Ocul. Pharm. Ther.* **2019**, *35*, 265–277. [CrossRef]

29. Dilbeck, M.D.; Spahr, Z.R.; Nanjappa, R.; Economides, J.R.; Horton, J.C. Columnar and Laminar Segregation of Retinal Input to the Primate Superior Colliculus Revealed by Anterograde Tracer Injection Into Each Eye. *Investig. Ophthalmol. Vis. Sci.* **2022**, *63*, 9. [CrossRef]
30. Zarbin, M.A.; Novack, G. N-of-1 Clinical Trials: A Scientific Approach to Personalized Medicine for Patients with Rare Retinal Diseases Such as Retinitis Pigmentosa. *J. Ocul. Pharm. Ther.* **2021**, *37*, 495–501. [CrossRef]
31. Woodward, D.F.; Wenthur, S.L.; Rudebush, T.L.; Fan, S.; Toris, C.B. Prostanoid Receptor Antagonist Effects on Intraocular Pressure, Supported by Ocular Biodisposition Experiments. *J. Ocul. Pharm. Ther.* **2016**, *32*, 606–622. [CrossRef]
32. Zernii, E.Y.; Baksheeva, V.E.; Iomdina, E.N.; Averina, O.A.; Permyakov, S.E.; Philippov, P.P.; Zamyatnin, A.A.; Senin, I.I. Rabbit Models of Ocular Diseases: New Relevance for Classical Approaches. *CNS Neurol. Disord. Drug Targets* **2016**, *15*, 267–291. [CrossRef]
33. Bley, K.R.; Bhattacharya, A.; Daniels, D.V.; Gever, J.; Jahangir, A.; O'Yang, C.; Smith, S.; Srinivasan, D.; Ford, A.P.; Jett, M.F. RO1138452 and RO3244794: Characterization of structurally distinct, potent and selective IP (prostacyclin) receptor antagonists. *Br. J. Pharm.* **2006**, *147*, 335–345. [CrossRef] [PubMed]
34. Watsky, M.A.; Jablonski, M.M.; Edelhauser, H.F. Comparison of conjunctival and corneal surface areas in rabbit and human. *Curr. Eye Res.* **1988**, *7*, 483–486. [CrossRef] [PubMed]
35. Chiang, B.; Jung, J.H.; Prausnitz, M.R. The suprachoroidal space as a route of administration to the posterior segment of the eye. *Adv. Drug Deliv. Rev.* **2018**, *126*, 58–66. [CrossRef] [PubMed]
36. Tyagi, P.; Kadam, R.S.; Kompella, U.B. Comparison of suprachoroidal drug delivery with subconjunctival and intravitreal routes using noninvasive fluorophotometry. *PLoS ONE* **2012**, *7*, e48188. [CrossRef]
37. Scheive, M.; Yazdani, S.; Hajrasouliha, A.R. The utility and risks of therapeutic nanotechnology in the retina. *Ther. Adv. Ophthalmol.* **2021**, *13*, 25158414211003381. [CrossRef]
38. Tornquist, P.; Alm, A.; Bill, A. Permeability of ocular vessels and transport across the blood-retinal-barrier. *Eye* **1990**, *4*, 303–309. [CrossRef]
39. Hammadi, S.; Tzoumas, N.; Ferrara, M.; Meschede, I.P.; Lo, K.; Harris, C.; Lako, M.; Steel, D.H. Bruch's Membrane: A Key Consideration with Complement-Based Therapies for Age-Related Macular Degeneration. *J. Clin. Med.* **2023**, *12*, 2870. [CrossRef]
40. Clark, S.J.; McHarg, S.; Tilakaratna, V.; Brace, N.; Bishop, P.N. Bruch's Membrane Compartmentalizes Complement Regulation in the Eye with Implications for Therapeutic Design in Age-Related Macular Degeneration. *Front. Immunol.* **2017**, *8*, 1778. [CrossRef]
41. Ambati, J.; Atkinson, J.P.; Gelfand, B.D. Immunology of age-related macular degeneration. *Nat. Rev. Immunol.* **2013**, *13*, 438–451. [CrossRef]
42. Cheng, S.Y.; Cipi, J.; Ma, S.; Hafler, B.P.; Kanadia, R.N.; Brush, R.S.; Agbaga, M.P.; Punzo, C. Altered photoreceptor metabolism in mouse causes late stage age-related macular degeneration-like pathologies. *Proc. Natl. Acad. Sci. USA* **2020**, *117*, 13094–13104. [CrossRef]
43. Casciano, F.; Zauli, E.; Rimondi, E.; Mura, M.; Previati, M.; Busin, M.; Zauli, G. The role of the mTOR pathway in diabetic retinopathy. *Front. Med.* **2022**, *9*, 973856. [CrossRef] [PubMed]
44. Leonardi, G.C.; Accardi, G.; Monastero, R.; Nicoletti, F.; Libra, M. Ageing: From inflammation to cancer. *Immun. Ageing* **2018**, *15*, 1. [CrossRef] [PubMed]
45. Zou, Z.; Tao, T.; Li, H.; Zhu, X. mTOR signaling pathway and mTOR inhibitors in cancer: Progress and challenges. *Cell Biosci.* **2020**, *10*, 31. [CrossRef] [PubMed]
46. Li, X.; Gao, S.; Zhang, Y.; Xin, M.; Zuo, C.; Yan, N.; Xia, Q.; Zhang, M. Dihydroartemisinin Inhibits Laser-Induced Choroidal Neovascularization in a Mouse Model of Neovascular AMD. *Front. Pharm.* **2022**, *13*, 838263. [CrossRef]
47. Gutierrez, S.; Svahn, S.L.; Johansson, M.E. Effects of Omega-3 Fatty Acids on Immune Cells. *Int. J. Mol. Sci.* **2019**, *20*, 5028. [CrossRef]
48. Department of Ophthalmology, H.M.S. AMD Treatment Guidelines. Available online: https://eye.hms.harvard.edu/eyeinsights/2015-january/age-related-macular-degeneration-amd#:~:text=Ninety%20percent%20of%20all%20people,legal%20blindness%20from%20the%20disease (accessed on 27 July 2023).
49. Nielsen, M.K. Geographic Atrophy. Available online: https://eyewiki.aao.org/Geographic_Atrophy#:~:text=It%20starts%20typically%20in%20the,of%20all%20individuals%20with%20AMD (accessed on 27 July 2023).
50. Georgiou, T.; Prokopiou, E. The New Era of Omega-3 Fatty Acids Supplementation: Therapeutic Effects on Dry Age-Related Macular Degeneration. *J. Stem Cells* **2015**, *10*, 205–215.
51. Prokopiou, K.; Kolovos, P.; Tsangari, H.; Bandello, F.; Rossetti, L.M.; Mastropasqua, L.; Mohand-Said, S.; Georgiou, T. A prospective, multicentre, randomised, double-blind study designed to assess the potential effects of omega-3 fatty acids supplementation in dry age-related macular degeneration or Stargardt disease. *Investig. Ophthalmol. Vis. Sci.* **2022**, *63*, 377-F0208.
52. Souied, E.H.; Delcourt, C.; Querques, G.; Bassols, A.; Merle, B.; Zourdani, A.; Smith, T.; Benlian, P.; Nutritional, A.M.D.T.S.G. Oral docosahexaenoic acid in the prevention of exudative age-related macular degeneration: The Nutritional AMD Treatment 2 study. *Ophthalmology* **2013**, *120*, 1619–1631. [CrossRef]
53. Souied, E.H.; Aslam, T.; Garcia-Layana, A.; Holz, F.G.; Leys, A.; Silva, R.; Delcourt, C. Omega-3 Fatty Acids and Age-Related Macular Degeneration. *Ophthalmic Res.* **2015**, *55*, 62–69. [CrossRef]

54. Edelhauser, H.F.; Rowe-Rendleman, C.L.; Robinson, M.R.; Dawson, D.G.; Chader, G.J.; Grossniklaus, H.E.; Rittenhouse, K.D.; Wilson, C.G.; Weber, D.A.; Kuppermann, B.D.; et al. Ophthalmic drug delivery systems for the treatment of retinal diseases: Basic research to clinical applications. *Investig. Ophthalmol. Vis. Sci.* **2010**, *51*, 5403–5420. [CrossRef]
55. Khoo, H.E.; Ng, H.S.; Yap, W.S.; Goh, H.J.H.; Yim, H.S. Nutrients for Prevention of Macular Degeneration and Eye-Related Diseases. *Antioxidants* **2019**, *8*, 85. [CrossRef]
56. Querques, G.; Forte, R.; Souied, E.H. Retina and omega-3. *J. Nutr. Metab.* **2011**, *2011*, 748361. [CrossRef]
57. Calder, P.C. Omega-3 fatty acids and inflammatory processes. *Nutrients* **2010**, *2*, 355–374. [CrossRef]
58. German, O.L.; Monaco, S.; Agnolazza, D.L.; Rotstein, N.P.; Politi, L.E. Retinoid X receptor activation is essential for docosahexaenoic acid protection of retina photoreceptors. *J. Lipid Res.* **2013**, *54*, 2236–2246. [CrossRef]
59. Lengqvist, J.; Mata De Urquiza, A.; Bergman, A.C.; Willson, T.M.; Sjovall, J.; Perlmann, T.; Griffiths, W.J. Polyunsaturated fatty acids including docosahexaenoic and arachidonic acid bind to the retinoid X receptor alpha ligand-binding domain. *Mol. Cell Proteom.* **2004**, *3*, 692–703. [CrossRef]
60. Itoh, T.; Yamamoto, K. Peroxisome proliferator activated receptor gamma and oxidized docosahexaenoic acids as new class of ligand. *Naunyn Schmiedebergs Arch. Pharm.* **2008**, *377*, 541–547. [CrossRef]
61. Calder, P.C. Omega-3 polyunsaturated fatty acids and inflammatory processes: Nutrition or pharmacology? *Br. J. Clin. Pharm.* **2013**, *75*, 645–662. [CrossRef]
62. Li, X.; Yu, Y.; Funk, C.D. Cyclooxygenase-2 induction in macrophages is modulated by docosahexaenoic acid via interactions with free fatty acid receptor 4 (FFA4). *FASEB J.* **2013**, *27*, 4987–4997. [CrossRef]
63. Iverson, C.; Bacong, A.; Liu, S.; Baumgartner, S.; Lundstrom, T.; Oscarsson, J.; Miner, J.N. Omega-3-carboxylic acids provide efficacious anti-inflammatory activity in models of crystal-mediated inflammation. *Sci. Rep.* **2018**, *8*, 1217. [CrossRef]
64. Mirnikjoo, B.; Brown, S.E.; Kim, H.F.; Marangell, L.B.; Sweatt, J.D.; Weeber, E.J. Protein kinase inhibition by omega-3 fatty acids. *J. Biol. Chem.* **2001**, *276*, 10888–10896. [CrossRef]
65. Djebli, N.; Khier, S.; Griguer, F.; Coutant, A.L.; Tavernier, A.; Fabre, G.; Leriche, C.; Fabre, D. Ocular Drug Distribution After Topical Administration: Population Pharmacokinetic Model in Rabbits. *Eur. J. Drug Metab. Pharmacokinet.* **2017**, *42*, 59–68. [CrossRef]
66. Bos, J.D.; Meinardi, M.M. The 500 Dalton rule for the skin penetration of chemical compounds and drugs. *Exp. Dermatol.* **2000**, *9*, 165–169. [CrossRef]
67. Schramlova, J.; Blazek, K.; Bartackova, M.; Otova, B.; Mardesicova, L.; Zizkovsky, V.; Hulinska, D. Electron microscopic demonstration of the penetration of liposomes through skin. *Folia Biol.* **1997**, *43*, 165–169.
68. Souto, E.B.; Macedo, A.S.; Dias-Ferreira, J.; Cano, A.; Zielinska, A.; Matos, C.M. Elastic and Ultradeformable Liposomes for Transdermal Delivery of Active Pharmaceutical Ingredients (APIs). *Int. J. Mol. Sci.* **2021**, *22*, 9743. [CrossRef]
69. Bisht, R.; Mandal, A.; Jaiswal, J.K.; Rupenthal, I.D. Nanocarrier mediated retinal drug delivery: Overcoming ocular barriers to treat posterior eye diseases. *Wiley Interdiscip. Rev. Nanomed. Nanobiotechnol.* **2018**, *10*, e1473. [CrossRef]
70. Ghasemiyeh, P.; Mohammadi-Samani, S. Potential of Nanoparticles as Permeation Enhancers and Targeted Delivery Options for Skin: Advantages and Disadvantages. *Drug Des. Dev. Ther.* **2020**, *14*, 3271–3289. [CrossRef]
71. Shah, S.M.; Ashtikar, M.; Jain, A.S.; Makhija, D.T.; Nikam, Y.; Gude, R.P.; Steiniger, F.; Jagtap, A.A.; Nagarsenker, M.S.; Fahr, A. LeciPlex, invasomes, and liposomes: A skin penetration study. *Int. J. Pharm.* **2015**, *490*, 391–403. [CrossRef]
72. NanoSense Lesson 2: Scale of Objects, Student Materials. Available online: https://nanosense.sri.com/activities/sizematters/sizeandscale/SM_Lesson2Student.pdf (accessed on 27 July 2023).
73. Duangjit, S.; Opanasopit, P.; Rojanarata, T.; Ngawhirunpat, T. Characterization and In Vitro Skin Permeation of Meloxicam-Loaded Liposomes versus Transfersomes. *J. Drug Deliv.* **2011**, *2011*, 418316. [CrossRef]

pharmaceutics

MDPI

Article

Travoprost Liquid Nanocrystals: An Innovative Armamentarium for Effective Glaucoma Therapy

Mohamed A. El-Gendy [1], Mai Mansour [2], Mona I. A. El-Assal [1], Rania A. H. Ishak [2,*] and Nahed D. Mortada [2]

[1] Department of Pharmaceutics and Pharmaceutical Technology, Faculty of Pharmacy, Future University in Egypt, Cairo 11835, Egypt
[2] Department of Pharmaceutics and Industrial Pharmacy, Faculty of Pharmacy, Ain Shams University, Cairo 11566, Egypt
* Correspondence: raniaaziz@pharma.asu.edu.eg

Abstract: To date, the ophthalmic application of liquid crystalline nanostructures (LCNs) has not been thoroughly reconnoitered, yet they have been extensively used. LCNs are primarily made up of glyceryl monooleate (GMO) or phytantriol as a lipid, a stabilizing agent, and a penetration enhancer (PE). For optimization, the D-optimal design was exploited. A characterization using TEM and XRPD was conducted. Optimized LCNs were loaded with the anti-glaucoma drug Travoprost (TRAVO). Ex vivo permeation across the cornea, in vivo pharmacokinetics, and pharmacodynamic studies were performed along with ocular tolerability examinations. Optimized LCNs are constituted of GMO, Tween® 80 as a stabilizer, and either oleic acid or Captex® 8000 as PE at 25 mg each. TRAVO-LNCs, F-1-L and F-3-L, showed particle sizes of 216.20 ± 6.12 and 129.40 ± 11.73 nm, with EE% of 85.30 ± 4.29 and 82.54 ± 7.65%, respectively, revealing the highest drug permeation parameters. The bioavailability of both attained 106.1% and 322.82%, respectively, relative to the market product TRAVATAN®. They exhibited respective intraocular pressure reductions lasting for 48 and 72 h, compared to 36 h for TRAVATAN®. All LCNs exhibited no evidence of ocular injury in comparison to the control eye. The findings revealed the competence of TRAVO-tailored LCNs in glaucoma treatment and suggested the potential application of a novel platform in ocular delivery.

Keywords: ocular delivery; liquid crystalline nanostructures; glaucoma; Travoprost; D-optimal design; ex vivo permeation; pharmacokinetics; pharmacodynamics

Citation: El-Gendy, M.A.; Mansour, M.; El-Assal, M.I.A.; Ishak, R.A.H.; Mortada, N.D. Travoprost Liquid Nanocrystals: An Innovative Armamentarium for Effective Glaucoma Therapy. *Pharmaceutics* **2023**, *15*, 954. https://doi.org/10.3390/pharmaceutics15030954

Academic Editors: Rosario Pignatello, Francisco Javier Otero-Espinar, Hugo Almeida, Carmelo Puglia and Debora Santonocito

Received: 5 December 2022
Revised: 9 March 2023
Accepted: 13 March 2023
Published: 15 March 2023

1. Introduction

Since their discovery, liquid crystalline nanostructures (LCNs) have gained esteem as nanoparticle systems for drug delivery. LCNs are typically composed of amphiphilic lipids such as monoolein (MO), additionally well-known as glycerol monooleate (GMO), and phytantriol (PYT), along with stabilizers such as Poloxamer 407. As a result, they make tremendous self-assembling entities for encapsulating both lipophilic and hydrophilic substances [1]. LCNs can be beneficial for ophthalmic drug delivery, where the high surface area of LCNs could endorse adhesion and hence drug penetration through the corneal epithelium, allowing for greater bioavailability. However, and to our best knowledge, LCNs are scarcely exploited for ocular administration [2–15]. Moreover, the integration of new stabilizers other than P407 is still limited in research.

Glaucoma is a set of progressive eye illnesses due to the rise of intraocular pressure (IOP), which ranges from 10 to 24 mmHg in a healthy human eye [16]. Elevated intraocular pressure (IOP) can lead to many eye complications. This elevation may produce plodding harm to the optic nerve, where the continuous long-term injury may result in a failure of communications between the retina and the brain and finally a loss of vision. Glaucoma is the second-leading cause of visual loss after cataracts. Different measures, such as laser treatment, surgery, and pharmacological treatment, can reduce IOP. Medicines such as adrenergic agonists, inhibitors of carbonic anhydrase, beta-blockers, analogs of prostaglandin, and hyperosmotic and myotic medicines are encompassed in the medicinal treatment of glaucoma. These medication types either increase the fluid flow from the eye or reduce the eye fluid generation. The foremost line of treatment for glaucoma in most countries is prostaglandin analogs; Latanoprost (Xalatan®), Travoprost (Travatan®), and Bimatoprost (Careprost®) are examples [17]. The prostaglandin analogs thereby reduce the IOP in the eye by increasing the draining of the aqueous humor.

Travoprost (TRAVO) differs from the other marketed prostaglandin analogs in being a full agonist at the prostaglandin F receptor (FP receptor), whereas the others are partial agonists with lower efficacy [18]. TRAVO is an isopropyl ester prodrug [17] hydrolyzed to the biologically active free acid by corneal esterases upon absorption into the eye after topical ocular administration. Despite its efficacy, Travoprost suffers from several major drawbacks as it is extremely hydrophobic with a log P of 4.6, has poor aqueous solubility of 7.59×10^{-3} g/L, and has a rapid terminal elimination half-life of approximately 45 min, thus affecting its ocular bioavailability [3,19].

In the literature, TRAVO has been loaded into a number of nanocarriers aiming to improve its corneal penetrability, ocular bioavailability, and hence its therapeutic efficacy. TRAVO-loaded nanoemulsion prepared by Ismail et al., 2020, showed an enhancement in the drug absorption better than that of the commercially available product Travatan®, as demonstrated by better bioavailability in terms of Cmax and AUC, and it also sustained the IOP lowering period. Moreover, the nanoemulsion formulation has been proven to be safe and nonirritant to ocular surfaces [3]. Self-assembled lipid DNA nanoparticles (NPs) were prepared by Schnichels et al. (2020) and loaded with TRAVO for glaucoma treatment. After eye drop instillation, TRAVO-NPs showed a prolonged adherence time to the eye that extended to one hour. Furthermore, the pharmacokinetic results disclosed that TRAVO-NPs delivered at least twice the drug quantity that was delivered by the free drug [20]. Additionally, Lambert et al. (2015) prepared a nano-sponge (NS) and examined the efficacy after intravitreal administration with the aim to lower the IOP in mice. The NS were loaded either with Brimonidine (an alpha-adrenergic agonist) or TRAVO, then their efficacy was compared. NS loaded with Brimonidine lowered IOP up to 30% for a duration of 6 days, whereas TRAVO-NS lowered IOP by about 19% to 29% for 4 days when compared to saline solution injection [21].

Yet, neither the ocular application of LCNs nor the impact of incorporating penetration enhancers (PEs) has been well reconnoitered. In addition, mounting the bioavailability of TRAVO with long-lasting effects was one of the challenges to be overcome. Hence, the present work focused on LCNs preparation and statistical optimization with the inclusion of new stabilizers and penetration enhancers. The optimized formulas were then chosen for the loading of the anti-glaucomic drug, Travoprost (TRAVO). Morphological examination, thermal behavior, and crystallinity studies were conducted. An ex vivo study was performed across the excised cornea of rabbits to assess the permeability of TRAVO-loaded LCNs. The selected medicated formulas were then exposed to in vivo pharmacodynamic and pharmacokinetic studies in comparison to Travatan®, which is the market product.

2. Materials and Methods

2.1. Materials

Glyceryl monooleate was generously provided by Danisco, Grindsted, Denmark. Poloxamer 407 (P407), Tween® 80, Kolliphor® HS 15 (formely regarded as Solutol® HS), Cholesterol, Brij® 52, Myrj® S40, Acetonitrile, Phosphoric acid, Methanol (HPLC grade), Betamethasone, Dapoxetine, Tertiary butyl-methyl ether (TBME), Acetonitrile, Formic acid, Glacial acetic acid, Formalin, Ethyl alcohol, Xylol, Hematoxylin and Eosin (H & E) stain were purchased from Sigma Aldrich, St. Louis, Missouri, USA. Oleic acid was bought from Loba Chemie, Mumbai, India. Triglycerides of caprylic acid (Captex® 8000) and mono/diglycerides of caprylic acid (Capmul® MCM C8 EP/NF) were provided by the ABITEC Corporation, Columbus, OH, USA. El-Nasr Pharmaceuticals, Al Qalyubia, Egypt, supplied the sodium dihydrogen phosphate and sodium hydrogen phosphate. Lecithin® (L-α-Phosphatidylcholine, egg about 72%) was procured from Fisher Scientific (Leicestershire, UK). Phytantriol (PYT) was kindly obtained from EVA Pharma, Giza, Egypt. Tocopherol polyethylene glycol 1000 succinate (TPGS) was kindly supplied by Isochem (Vert-Le-Petit, France). Travoprost (TRAVO) was kindly gifted from Orchidia Pharmaceutical Industries, Dakahlia, Egypt. Travatan® eye drops (Novartis Pharmaceuticals UK Ltd., London, UK) were purchased from a community pharmacy. Fully-grown male New Zealand white rabbits, weighing 2.5 kg ± 0.5 kg, were granted from the Ophthalmology Research Institute, Giza, Egypt.

2.2. Preparation of Plain and TRAVO-Loaded LCNs

GMO, stabilizer, and penetration enhancer (PE) were melted in a beaker on a hot plate set to 60 °C to make plain LCNs. Then, using a heated plate with a magnetic stirrer (MS-300HS, Misung Scientific Co., Gyeonggi-do, Korea), the aqueous phase was poured into the lipid phase while being agitated at 500 rpm for 2 h. After that, a homogenizer was used to homogenize the dispersions for 1 min at 15,000 rpm (Silent Heidolph Crusher, Schwabach, Germany). The dispersion prepared was left at room temperature to be cooled down till it congealed, then kept at 5 ± 3 °C in a refrigerator, producing plain LCNs. For loaded LCNs, a calculated amount of TRAVO was weighed using an analytical balance (Sartorius CPA 225D, Gottingen, Germany) and added to the lipid phase, and the emulsification with the aqueous phase was then performed [22], producing TRAVO-LCNs with a concentration of 40 µg/mL equivalent to that of the marketed product Travatan®.

2.3. Experimental Design

Based on the results obtained from a preliminary study, the LCNs were prepared and optimized using a D-optimal experimental design, which allows a statistical evaluation of three independent variables, including the stabilizer amount (A) and the types of both PE (B) and stabilizer (C). GMO was the lipid of choice; in addition, three different stabilizer types were investigated: P407, Tween 80, and TPGS, all ranging in amounts from 1.25 to 25 mg, with or without the presence of a penetration enhancer (PE). Oleic acid, Captex® 8000, and Capmul® MCM were the PEs explored. Twenty formulations were prepared with different levels of variables as presented in Table 1. The dependent variables studied were the particle size (Y1), polydispersity index (Y2), and zeta potential (Y3) of the made LCNs.

Table 1. The results of dependent variables of the prepared liquid crystalline nanostructures formulae based on the D-optimal design.

Formula Code	Factor A	Factor B	Factor C	Responses * ± SD		
	Stabilizer Amount (mg)	PE Type	Stabilizer Type	Y1: PS (nm)	Y2: PDI	Y3: ZP (mV)
F1	1.25	Capmul® MCM	TPGS	346.45 ± 30.05	0.40 ± 0.04	−40.80 ± 5.05
F2	1.25	None	Tween 80	666.35 ± 60.83	0.50 ± 0.05	−41.15 ± 2.34
F3	21.4375	Captex® 8000	Tween 80	182.53 ± 24.43	0.43 ± 0.09	−36.58 ± 1.13
F4	25	Oleic acid	TPGS	232.55 ± 38.41	0.46 ± 0.01	−74.75 ± 7.34
F5	25	None	Tween 80	260.80 ± 57.46	0.42 ± 0.08	−31.50 ± 0.42
F6	11.9375	Captex® 8000	TPGS	205.05 ± 9.57	0.38 ± 0.02	−36.98 ± 1.50
F7	4.8125	Captex® 8000	P407	160.38 ± 5.05	0.15 ± 0.04	−20.58 ± 0.46
F8	25	None	TPGS	109.08 ± 6.53	0.36 ± 0.06	−26.20 ± 2.51
F9	20.25	Capmul® MCM	P407	150.70 ± 7.51	0.32 ± 0.07	−17.85 ± 1.16

Table 1. *Cont.*

Formula Code	Factor A	Factor B	Factor C	Responses * ± SD		
	Stabilizer Amount (mg)	PE Type	Stabilizer Type	Y1: PS (nm)	Y2: PDI	Y3: ZP (mV)
F10	1.25	Oleic acid	P407	160.63 ± 10.95	0.32 ± 0.04	−66.65 ± 5.72
F11	1.25	Captex® 8000	Tween 80	561.25 ± 66.22	0.57 ± 0.05	−52.78 ± 9.94
F12	1.25	Oleic acid	Tween 80	176.03 ± 5.91	0.37 ± 016	−72.70 ± 6.88
F13	17.875	None	P407	307.35 ± 36.12	0.61 ± 0.07	−19.28 ± 1.84
F14	4.8125	Oleic acid	TPGS	226.80 ± 22.52	0.42 ± 0.04	−81.03 ± 7.71
F15	21.675	Oleic acid	P407	333.83 ± 51.39	0.47 ± 0.03	−37.18 ± 2.88
F16	4.21875	Capmul® MCM	Tween 80	579.53 ± 229.65	0.58 ± 0.17	−41.53 ± 3.81
F17	25	Captex® 8000	P407	147.78 ± 11.14	0.32 ± 0.05	−15.18 ± 0.95
F18	25	Capmul® MCM	Tween 80	418.25 ± 117.58	0.39 ± 0.07	−26.40 ± 1.27
F19	8.375	None	TPGS	180.75 ± 29.95	0.33 ± 0.05	−29.48 ± 1.91
F20	21.4375	Capmul® MCM	TPGS	195.28 ± 17.76	0.41 ± 0.04	−32.93 ± 1.54

* All data are mean of triplicates ± SD. SD—standard deviation; PS—particle size; PDI—polydispersity index; ZP—zeta potential; PE—penetration enhancer.

2.4. *Quantitative Analysis of TRAVO Using High-Performance Liquid Chromatography (HPLC)*

TRAVO was quantitatively analyzed using HPLC (LC-20AT, Shimadzu, Japan) with the assay method implemented by the USP (USP 40, Travoprost Ophthalmic Solution Monograph). The mobile phase comprises a filtered and degassed mixture of deionized water, adjusted to pH 3 using phosphoric acid, and acetonitrile at a volume ratio of 35:65. The flow rate was adjusted to 1 mL/min, and the column temperature was set at 25°C. Under these chromatographic conditions, TRAVO was analyzed in the injected samples of 10 µL volume, detected at a UV wavelength of 220 nm, and eluted at a retention time of 3.5 min. According to ICH guidelines, the assay method's linearity, accuracy, precision, limit of detection (LOD), and limit of quantitation (LOQ) were all verified.

2.5. *Characterization of the Fabricated Travoprost Loaded LCNs*

2.5.1. Particle Size (PS), Polydispersity Index (PDI), and Zeta Potential (ZP)

The Malvern Zetasizer Nano Series (Malvern, Worcestershire, UK) was used to perform dynamic light scattering (DLS) on all prepared dispersions in order to obtain the average PS and PDI. The same device was used to measure the ZP values using the Laser Doppler Anemometry (LDA) technique. At 25 °C, measurements were carried out in triplicate. The samples' counts ranged from 200 to 500 Kcps by dilution with deionized water [23].

2.5.2. Determination of TRAVO Entrapment Efficiency (EE%)

Briefly, 500 µL of TRAVO-LCNs were loaded into the upper chamber of a Nano-sep® (centrifuge tubes, Pall Life Sciences, Arizona, USA) and then centrifuged at 7000 rpm for 30 min using a cooling micro-centrifuge (Labogene-Scan speed 1524, GryozenCo., Ltd., Yuseoung-gu, Daejeon 305-301, Korea) adjusted at 4 °C. The concentration of free TRAVO in the supernatant collected in the lower chamber was determined quantitatively using the HPLC instrument, as previously described, using the following equation:

$$EE\% = \frac{A - B}{A} \times 100 \quad (1)$$

where A is the initial amount of the drug added and B is the amount that remained free in the supernatant.

2.5.3. LCNs Morphology Investigation Using High-Performance Transmission Electron Microscopy (TEM)

F-1-L, F-3-L, F-4-L, and F-5-L optimum TRAVO-LCNs were chosen to investigate their morphological structures using HR-TEM. Imaging samples were obtained by adding 0.005 mL of the formula to a 300-mesh copper grid that was carbon-coated and placed on filter paper. The grid was given 3–5 min to dry at room temperature after the extra droplets were wiped away. Using an HR-TEM and a digital camera, the samples were photographed while remaining unstained and mounted on a holder.

2.5.4. Crystallinity Study Using X-ray Powder Diffraction (XRPD)

For studying the crystallinity of the dried samples, the representative formulae were lyophilized by a freezer dryer (Christ, Alpha2-4LD Plus, Harz, Germany), which are plain GMO-based formulae (F-1-O, F-3-O, F-4-O, and F-5-O), with F-1-O composed of oleic acid as PE and Tween 80 as a stabilizer, while F-3-O, F-4-O, and F-5-O composed of Captex® 8000 as PE and Tween 80, TPGS, and P407 as the stabilizer, respectively, were subjected to XRPD. The four formulae were compared to a dried PE-free formula composed of GMO and P407 as the lipid and stabilizer, respectively, which are the components of a typical cubic LCN. Cu-ka radiation, a voltage of 40 kV, and a current of 40 mA were used in an X-ray powder diffractometer (Philips, PW 3710, Caerphilly, United Kingdom). From 5° to 50° at 2θ, all measures were implemented at a scan rate of 2°/min.

2.6. *Ex Vivo Study for Corneal Permeation of TRAVO-Loaded LCNs*

The ex vivo corneal penetration study was conducted on the eight optimized TRAVO-loaded LCN formulae (F-1-L to F-8-L) in comparison to drug solution (DS) using a customized Franz diffusion cell with an area of diffusion of 0.28 cm^2 across excised rabbit corneas. The Research Ethics Committee of the Faculty of Pharmacy at Ain Shams University approved all animal procedures (acceptance number: REC-ASU 54).

Rabbits with average weights of 2.5 ± 0.5 kg were euthanized by urethane injection in the marginal ear vein. The oculomotor muscles, palpebral conjunctivas, and optic nerve plexus were trimmed by trained personnel using ophthalmic scissors, then the eyeballs were removed, and the corneas were excised after being cleaned. They were gently rinsed with simulated tear fluid (STF), composed of 6.7 g NaCl, 2.0 g $NaHCO_3$, and 0.08 g $CaCl_2$ in 1 L of deionized water, pre-adjusted to a temperature of 34 °C. The fresh corneas were clamped between the two compartments of the Franz diffusion cell. A calculated volume of each formula, equivalent to 40 µg of TRAVO, was added to the donor compartment. Aliquots of 20 mL of STF were placed into the receptor compartment, and magnetic stirring at 50 rpm was allowed throughout the entire experiment. A sample of 300 µL was taken from each chamber at 0.5, 1, 2, 4, 6, and 8 h and replenished with fresh STF. The amount of drug permeated across the cornea was assayed by the validated method previously described using HPLC [7]. The cumulative amounts of TRAVO permeated per unit corneal area (µg/cm2) were measured and plotted against time.

Different corneal permeability parameters were measured from the permeation results, including steady-state flux (Jss) and permeability coefficient (Kp). The corneal permeation rate at steady state (Jss, µg/cm^2/h) was determined from the slope of the linear part of the permeation curve. The apparent permeability coefficient (Kp) was calculated by the following equation:

$$Kp = Jss/Co$$

where Jss is the steady state flux and Co is the original concentration of the drug in the donor compartment [24].

2.7. *Stability Study of the Selected TRAVO-Loaded LCNs*

The physical stability of the selected TRAVO-LCNs (F-1-L and F-3-L) was evaluated by keeping them under refrigeration (5 ± 3 °C) for 90 days. The PS, PDI, ZP, and EE% were all evaluated before and after 30 and 90 days of storage, respectively.

2.8. Sterilization of TRAVO Loaded LCNs by Gamma Irradiation

The chosen TRAVO-LCNs (F-1-L and F-3-L) were exposed to gamma radiation using a ^{60}Co radiation source at room temperature at a dosage rate of 5 kGy/h. The doses of radiation were 5, 10, 15, and 25 kGy. After being exposed to gamma rays, the physicochemical characteristics of the chosen formulae were evaluated, and their differences from non-irradiated samples were statistically compared [25].

The sterilization efficacy of the different gamma radiation doses applied to F-1-L and F-3-L was evaluated by a sterility test. The amounts of surviving bacteria and fungi were totaled to determine the suitable dose of gamma irradiation for sterilization. Sterility testing was carried out under aseptic conditions using fluid thioglycolate media, which is primarily intended for the culture of anaerobic bacteria but can also detect aerobic bacteria and soybean casein digest media, which are suitable for both fungi and aerobic bacteria. Each tested formula had two sterility test tubes, one as a negative control to check the sterility of the media used and the other as a positive control containing the tested formula itself. After a 14-day incubation period, the media was macroscopically examined for visual microbial growth and turbidity [25].

2.9. In Vivo Ocular Evaluation of the Selected TRAVO-Loaded LCNs

The optimized medicated formulae (F-1-L and F-3-L) were selected for in vivo evaluation as they showed the highest ocular flux and permeation.

2.9.1. Pharmacodynamic Study in Rabbits Using Steroid-Induced Ocular Hypertension Model

The pharmacodynamic investigation included nine New Zealand white rabbits weighing approximately 2.5 kg $\pm$ 0.5 kg (3 rabbits per group) [26]. Throughout the test, the rabbits were maintained in isolated cages and supplied a conventional meal and water [26]. The rabbits were categorized randomly into three groups (G-I, G-II, and G-III). The left eyes served for induction and treatments, while the right ones served as negative controls (non-induced and non-treated). A corticosteroid injection was used to cause ocular hypertension (glaucoma). For 3 weeks, the rabbits in each group were given a 0.7 mL sub-conjunctival suspension of 0.1% betamethasone in the left eye [27]. When all rabbits' intraocular pressure (IOP) was raised to the glaucomatous level (IOP > 24 mmHg) [3], 100 µL of either F-1-L or F-3-L was instilled once in the left eyes of G-I and G-II rabbits, respectively, and 100 µL of the marketed product Travatan® eye drops was instilled once in the left eyes of G-III rabbits. A tonometer (Schiötz tonometer, Rudolf Riester GmbH, Germany) with a 10 g plunger load was used to measure IOP in the three groups. The plunger of the tonometer was pressed against the center of the cornea, and the reading was then taken once the disc was carefully lowered to the corneal surfaces [28]. The measurements were performed initially and at time intervals of 0.5, 1, 2, 4, 6, 8, 10, 12, 24, 36, 48, 60, and 72 h after the initial dose instillation, and the IOP values were recorded. Calculation of the percent of IOP reduction took place at each time interval (t) for each treatment group based on the initial IOP value (after induction) using the following equation:

$$\%\text{IOP Reduction} = \frac{\text{IOP(initial)} - \text{IOP(t)}}{\text{IOP(initial)}} \times 100 \quad (2)$$

2.9.2. Pharmacokinetic Study in Rabbits

A tiny needle was placed across the cornea, right above the corneoscleral limbus in the anterior chamber of the eye, to extract drug-free aqueous humor from healthy rabbits. The samples were frozen in vials at −20 °C for later analysis and then thawed at room temperature for LC-MS/MS calibration curve construction. After administration of 100 µL of F-1-L, F-3-L, and Travatan® to groups G-I, G-II, and G-III, respectively, samples of aqueous humor (50 µL) were withdrawn from the rabbits' eyes at intervals of 0.5, 1, 2, 4, 6, 8, 12, 24, and 48 h. Samples were collected by a small needle inserted into the anterior chamber and stored at −20 °C for LC-MS/MS quantification of the drug. The pharmacokinetic parameters calculated were the maximum concentration of the drug in the aqueous humor (Cmax), the time needed to reach the maximum concentration (Tmax), the mean residence time (MRT), and the area under the concentration–time curve ($AUC_{0\text{-}48}$ and AUC_{inf}). The relative bioavailability (F%) was also calculated for each LCN formulation with respect to Travatan® by the following equation:

$$\text{Relative Bioavailability}(F\%) = \frac{\text{AUC(inf) of LCN formula}}{\text{AUC(inf) of Travatan}^{\circledR}} \tag{3}$$

Quantitative Determination of TRAVO Using LC-MS/MS

Samples of the aqueous humor with a volume of 0.5 mL were placed in tubes made of glass with a volume of 7 mL. Internal standard (IS) solution (100 ng/mL Dapoxetine) was added at a volume of 50 µL. The vortex took place for 1 min for the samples. The rocker-mixer Reax II was used to mix the extraction solvent made of (4 mL tertiary butyl-methyl ether (TBME)) with the samples for a 10 min duration. Samples were centrifuged at 1790 *g* for 10 min at 4 °C, and the upper organic layer was moved into fresh tubes and evaporation took place using a vacuum concentrator until dry. A specific volume of mobile phase was added to the formed dry residues, then the reconstituted samples were mixed in a vortex for a minute and finally analyzed using LC-MS/MS (4500 LC-MS/MS MASS SPECTROMETER, AB SCIEX INSTRUMENTS, Concord, Ontario, L4K, 4V8, Canada). A sample volume of 10 µL was injected into an LC system using a C18 column. The isocratic mobile phase, composed of 80% acetonitrile and 20% water containing 0.1% formic acid, was delivered at a flow rate of 1.0 mL/min into the mass spectrometer's electrospray ionization chamber. MS/MS detection in positive ion mode was used to analyze TRAVO and Dapoxetine (IS) by operating a mass spectrometer furnished with a Turbo Ion Spray Interface with a voltage set at 5500 V at 500 °C. The ions were identified using the multiple reactions monitoring (MRM) mode. Analyst software (version 1.4.2) was used to process the analytical data [29].

2.9.3. Ocular Tolerability

The Draize test was implemented to compare the ocular safety of the chosen TRAVO-LCN formulations to the commercially available eye product (Travatan®). This was achieved by assessing the administered preparation's potential irritating effects. After the solution was delivered into the rabbit's eye, the potential for corneal, iridial, and conjunctival injury was evaluated. The glaucomatous eyes of rabbits treated with the tested formulations were examined for symptoms of redness, swelling, ulceration, or blindness using the three groups from the prior pharmacodynamic investigation [28,30]. The animals' right eyes served as negative controls in all three groups. After the initial dose, rabbits were examined at predetermined time intervals of 1 h, 24 h, 72 h, and 14 days. Conjunctival redness or chemosis, iris inflammation, and corneal opacity were graded on a scale of 0–4, 0–2, 0–3, and 0–4. The lower the score, the less harmful the formulation [31].

2.9.4. Histopathological Examinations

The safety of the specified TRAVO-LCN formulas on ocular tissues was confirmed through histopathological testing in comparison to the positive glaucomatous control eye. After euthanasia, tissue samples from the rabbits' eyes were obtained. After that, they were fixed with Davidson's Solution, which was made up of 300 mL 95% ethyl alcohol, 100 mL glacial acetic acid, 200 mL 10% neutral buffered formalin, and finally 300 mL distilled water [32]. After enucleation and trimming, the eyes were immediately placed in the solution. To keep the eye immersed, a gauze pad was employed. The globe was kept in the solution for 24 h before being removed and placed in 10% formalin. Trimmed tissue samples were cleaned and dehydrated in alcohol. After that, the dehydrated samples were cleaned in xylene, fixed in paraffin blocks, and sectioned at a thickness of 4–6 µm. For histological analysis, under a light optical microscope (Olympus Venox-S, AH-2, Tokyo, Japan), the acquired tissue sections were deparaffinized with xylol, and staining with H&E took place [33].

2.10. Statistical Analysis

All results were expressed as mean ± standard deviation (SD). All experimental data were statistically evaluated and optimized based on a D-optimal design using software named Design-Expert® (Version 7, Stat-Ease Inc., Minneapolis, Minnesota, USA). The generated equation models were checked for validation by comparing the experimental results with the predicted ones. The following equation was used for the calculation of the prediction error:

$$\text{Prediction error} = \frac{\text{Predicted} - \text{Experimental}}{\text{Experimental}} \times 100 \tag{4}$$

Statistical analysis of the results was performed for all pharmacokinetic parameters by employing one-way analysis of variance (ANOVA) in SPSS software (IBM 20).

3. Results and Discussion

3.1. Experimental Design

Considering the preliminary study's findings (Tables S1–S3, Supplementary Data), a D-optimal design was implemented, and twenty LCN formulas were prepared by varying the stabilizer amounts ranging from 1.25 to 25 mg (Factor A), in the absence or presence of various PEs (Factor B: None, oleic acid, Captex® 8000, Capmul® MCM), and different types of stabilizers (Factor C: P407, Tween 80, TPGS), aiming to select the optimized LCN formulations in terms of PS, PDI, and ZP for further drug loading. The average values of the measured responses (PS (Y1), PDI (Y2), and ZP (Y3)) for the prepared LCN formulations according to the experimental design are presented in Table 1.

The data revealed that nano-sized particles were formed with PS varying between 109.08 ± 6.53 and 666.35 ± 60.83 nm, where the lowest PS value was obtained by F8 containing the highest amount of TPGS (25 mg) as a stabilizer without any PE, while the highest one was obtained by F2 containing the lowest amount (1.25 mg) of Tween 80 and no PE as well. It can be noticed that PS of TPGS-stabilized formulae were rather comparable to those of P407-LCNs, where their respective sizes ranged between 109.08 ± 6.53 and 346.45 ± 30.05 nm, 147.78 ± 11.14, and 333.83 ± 51.39 nm, while those containing Tween exhibited higher PS ranging from 176.03 ± 5.91 to 666.35 ± 100.83 nm. In addition, it is obvious that the inclusion of a higher or lower amount of stabilizer revealed inconsistent results, which depended on the type of stabilizer and/or PE used.

The obtained PDI values varied from 0.15 ± 0.04 to 0.61 ± 0.07, indicating good PS distribution. It can be noticed that the respective PDI data of Tween, TPGS, and P407-stabilized LCN formulae ranged between 0.37 ± 016 and 0.58 ± 0.17, 0.33 ± 0.05 and 0.46 ± 0.01, and 0.15 ± 0.04 and 0.61 ± 0.07, noting the large variability in size distributions, particularly in the case of formulations prepared with P407.

Finally, the ZP results of all prepared LCN formulae showed high negative magnitudes ranging from −15.18 ± 0.95 to −81.03 ± 7.71 mV, indicating a high electrostatic stabilization. The obtained data revealed higher negativity values and hence better particle-particle repulsion and stability for both Tween 80 and TPGS-based formulations than those prepared using P407, as the respective ZP values ranged between −26.40 ± 1.27 and −72.70 ± 6.88 mV, −26.20 ± 2.51 and −81.03 ± 7.71 mV, and −15.18 ± 0.95 and −66.65 ± 5.72 mV.

3.1.1. Data Analysis

PS Response

In influencing the effectiveness of cellular absorption and the biodistribution of the nanocarriers, PS is one of the most important parameters [34,35]. In general, small-sized monodispersed nanosystems are preferred over large ones, as the latter may result in ocular irritation and discomfort [36]. PS is an important feature for ocular delivery as it affects intraocular penetration. Membrane permeability decreased with the increase in PS, where particles < 400 nm showed greater penetration through the corneal mucosa [8].

The ANOVA results (Table 2) of the PS response showed that both the stabilizer amount (A) and type (C) significantly affected the sizes of the formed LCNs ($p < 0.05$), while the type of PE (B) revealed a non-significant effect on PS ($p > 0.05$). The main effect plots illustrated in Figure 1 showed that upon increasing the amount of stabilizer from 1.25 to 25 mg, the average PS of the produced LCNs decreased significantly ($p < 0.05$), irrespective of the type of stabilizer. This is ascribed to the fact that the stabilizer acts as a size-controlling agent, which prevents the growth and coalescence of nanoparticles. The obtained result is in agreement with the findings of Das et al. [37], who formulated silver nanoparticles using different stabilizer concentrations. The results revealed that the particles prepared without using any stabilizer are coarser in size than those prepared using a stabilizer. Ishak et al., 2017, also found that the higher amount of Tween 80 led to a significant decrease in the PS of the prepared nanocarriers [38]. Mansour et al., 2017 [39] also noticed that the PS was significantly increased ($p < 0.05$) by increasing the amount of lipid while keeping the amount of P407 constant, or, in other words, the PS decreased as the lipid: P407 weight ratio decreased, as described by Nakano et al., 2001 [40]. This may be explained by the fact that the stabilizers utilized are hydrophilic polymers or surfactants, which improve the positive curvature of cubosomes while decreasing their negative curvature when compared to hydrophobic substances such as lipids [39]. According to the nucleation and growth model described by Lamer and Dinegar, a low stabilizer concentration might reduce the nucleation and lower the formation of an enormous number of nuclei and henceforward aid the growth of larger nanoparticles [41].

Table 2. ANOVA test results of all responses studied, according to the D-optimal design.

Terms	Responses					
	PS		PDI		ZP	
	F-Value	*p*-Value	*F*-Value	*p*-Value	*F*-Value	*p*-Value
Model	24.88 *	0.0393	30.8 *	0.0319	27.57 *	<0.0001
A	35.36 *	0.0271	0.0143 ^{NS}	0.9156	11.32 *	0.0051
B	7.19 ^{NS}	0.1245	10.81 ^{NS}	0.0859	36.7 *	<0.0001
C	58.43 *	0.0168	51.71 *	0.019	16.79 *	0.0002
AB	15.64 ^{NS}	0.0607	2.67 ^{NS}	0.2846	-	-
AC	16.62 ^{NS}	0.0567	46.22 *	0.0212	-	-
BC	16.1 ^{NS}	0.0596	42.95 *	0.0229	-	-

A—stabilizer amount; B—PE type; C—stabilizer type; PS—particle size; PDI—polydispersity index; ZP—zeta potential. * Significant at 5% probability ($p < 0.05$). ^{NS} non-significant.

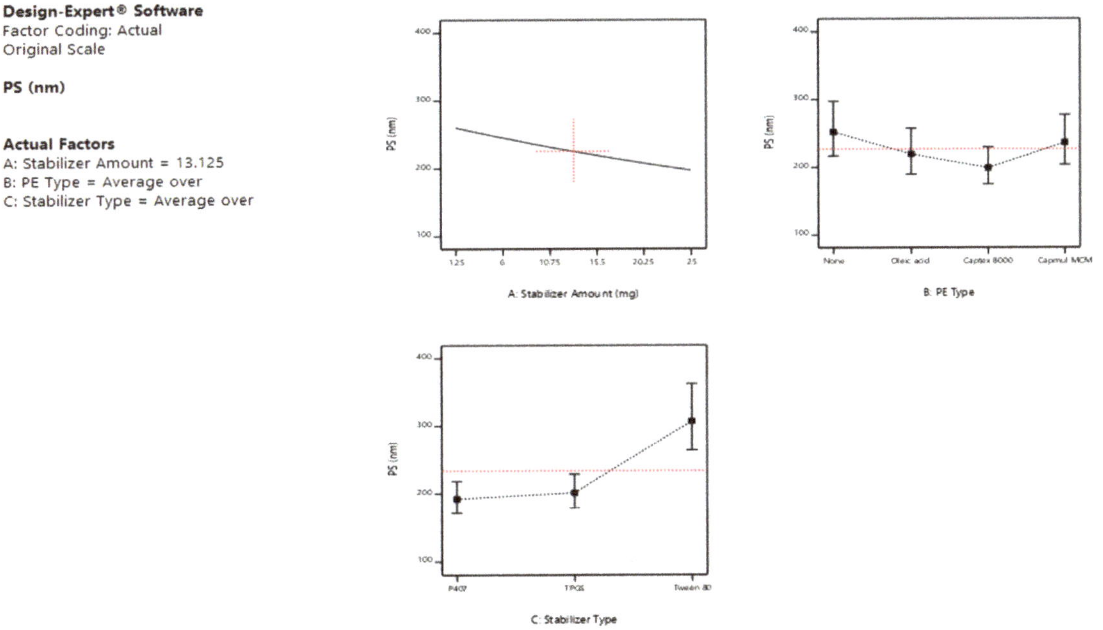

Figure 1. Main effect plots showing the effect of the independent variables; (**A**) stabilizer amount, (**B**) penetration enhancer type, and (**C**) stabilizer type on the particle size of the prepared LCNs.

Further inspection of the main effect plot Figure 1 revealed that the stabilizer type exhibited a substantial impact on the average PS of the prepared LCNs ($p < 0.05$). Changing the stabilizer type was associated with variable effects, as the addition of Tween 80 caused a buildup in LCN size when compared to P407 and TPGS, which showed comparable smaller PS under the same formulation conditions. These results are consistent with Dibaei et al. (2019) [42], who revealed that using TPGS as a stabilizer in curcumin-loaded nanosuspensions produced NPs exhibiting the lowest PS among all the prepared NPs. Since P407 has a longer hydrophobic alky chain length than Tween 80, they showed smaller PS as the emulsifying effect was positively correlated to the emulsifier's alkyl carbon chain length. In other words, the longer the alkyl carbon chain, the better the emulsifying effect [43].

In addition, the plots of Figure 1 demonstrated that the absence/presence of PE, as well as the type of PE, used did not have a significant impact on the mean sizes of the produced LCNs confirming the results of the ANOVA test.

All the two-way interactions, AC, BC, and AB exhibited no significant influences on the PS of LCNs with p values >0.05.

PDI Response

Based on the ANOVA results (Table 2), it was obvious that the PDI was significantly affected only by the stabilizer type (C) ($p < 0.05$), with no significant effect of both A and B factors ($p > 0.05$), i.e., the stabilizer amount and the type of PE. The 2-FI interactions AC and BC revealed significant effects on the size distributions of the formed LCNs ($p < 0.05$), while AB was not significant as the p-value exceeded 0.05.

Low PDI values indicate monodispersed nanoparticles, while higher ones [32] indicate polydispersed ones [39]. As obvious from the main effect plots presented in Figure 2, Tween 80-stabilized LCNs showed higher PDI values than those prepared with P407 and TPGS, confirming the significant effect of the stabilizer type on PDI. The increase in particle heterogeneity upon using Tween 80 could be attributed to the agglomerates or micelles composed of free stabilizers that did not share in the formation of cubosomes and hence decreased the homogeneity of the nano-dispersion [44]. Low PDI values were obtained using P407, indicating a uniform size and a good distribution of particles, which is in agreement with those obtained by Patil et al., 2019, who used P407 as a stabilizer while preparing cubosomes with GMO as a lipid [45].

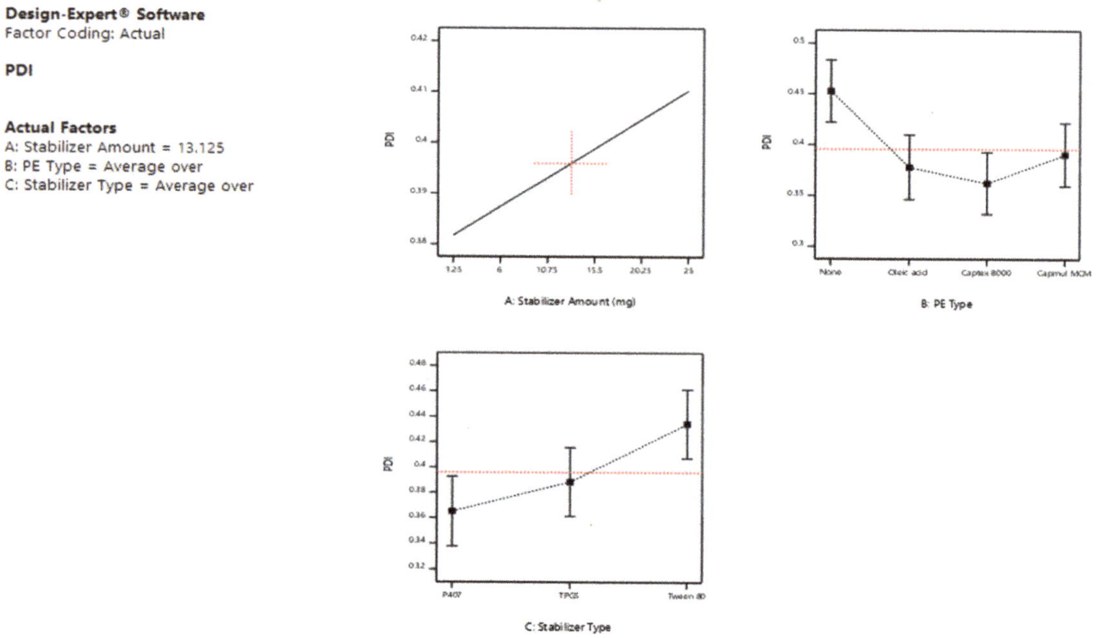

Figure 2. Main effect plots showing the effect of the independent variables; (**A**) stabilizer amount, (**B**) penetration enhancer type, and (**C**) stabilizer type on the PDI of the prepared LCNs.

Zeta Potential Response

The surface charge of LCNs is a crucial parameter for ensuring the stability of the generated nano-dispersions. The need for a reasonably stable formulation is highlighted by the reported fabrication of a physically stable LCN with a ZP value of at least −30 mV or −20 mV to be electrostatically stabilized or sterically stabilized systems, respectively [42,46]. The ANOVA results (Table 2) revealed that all three ZP model terms, A, B, and C, were significantly affecting the ZP values with p values < 0.05.

By observing Figure 3, a positive correlation occurs between the amount of the stabilizer and the corresponding ZP values, which is to say that increasing stabilizer content from 1.25 to 25 mg caused an increase in ZP values, which is to say a decrease in the ZP negative magnitudes. Our data are in agreement with earlier studies by Sun et al., 2004, who coated model nanoparticles with Tween 80 as a tool for delivering drugs to the brain. This may be because the adsorbed surface layer of non-ionic surfactant is probably masking the surface charge of the LCNs, as the more the adsorbed non-ionic surfactant is, the thicker the adsorbed layer and the more positive shift in ZP values [47].

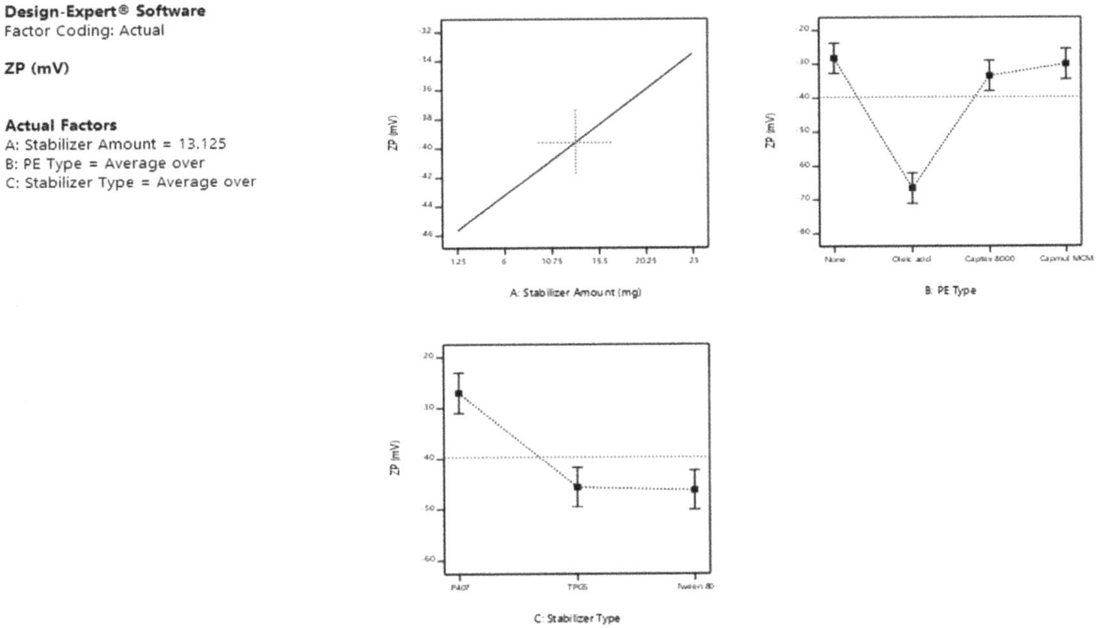

Figure 3. Main effect plots showing the effect of the independent variables; (**A**) stabilizer amount, (**B**) PE type, and (**C**) stabilizer type on the ZP of the prepared LCNs.

Regarding the type of stabilizer, Tween 80 and TPGS showed higher negative magnitudes of ZP values compared to P407; this could refer to the capability of the latter to cover efficiently the surface of the formed particles owing to its high molecular weight (12,600 g/mol) compared to those of TPGS (1542 g/mol) and Tween 80 (1310 g/mol) [34]. The decline in ZP magnitudes suggests the formation of a stabilized polymer layer [48].

As for the PE type, the negativity of ZP values of oleic acid-based LCNs was significantly higher than both Captex® 8000 and Capmul® MCM-LCNs. This increase is brought on by the oleic acid molecules' free carboxylic groups, which have negative charges [39]. The amphiphilic nature of these glycerides, which tend to be adsorbed onto the LCN surfaces, displaying a shielding effect, was also linked to the decreased ZP values of Captex 8000 and Capmul MCM [49].

3.1.2. Model Validation and Optimization

For model validation and optimization, the optimized formulations were chosen according to the numerical optimization generated from the Design Expert® software. This optimization process was conducted to optimize the LCN formulations based on formulation constraints: factor A: at the lowest and highest stabilizer amounts; factor B: at each PE type; and factor C: the stabilizer type in range. The target goals were adjusted as follows: (1) minimize PS, (2) minimize PDI, and (3) ZP <-25 mV. Eight formulae were then selected based on the highest desirability function (D) approaching unity. The optimized formulation compositions are presented in Table 3. The collected experimental findings were contrasted with those predicted, and the prediction error (% bias) for each response model was then determined. The experimental and predicted data and the calculated prediction errors are collected in Table 3. As shown, the results of the prediction error are all below 20%, confirming the validity and prediction capability of the three response models [50].

Table 3. Compositions, experimental and predicted data, and prediction error (%) of PS, PDI, and ZP responses of the optimized liquid crystalline nanostructures.

Formula Code	A: Stabilizer Amount (mg)	B: PE Type	C: Stabilizer Type	Experimental Results * ± SD			Predicted Results			Prediction Error (%)		
				PS (nm)	PDI	ZP (mV)	PS (nm)	PDI	ZP (mV)	PS	PDI	ZP
F-1-O	25	Oleic acid	Tween 80	238.11 ± 17.21	0.26 ± 0.01	−67.30 ± 2.81	207.32	0.22	−67.11	14.85	19.09	0.28
F-2-O	1.25	Oleic acid	P407	160.63 ± 8.80	0.32 ± 0.02	−66.65 ± 6.91	155.98	0.31	−60.07	2.98	1.29	10.96
F-3-O	25	Captex® 8000	Tween 80	159.10 ± 10.98	0.39 ± 0.01	−32.40 ± 5.17	167.59	0.41	−34.02	5.07	3.67	4.75
F-4-O	25	Captex® 8000	TPGS	143.05 ± 12.67	0.47 ± 0.04	−26.89 ± 2.10	119.54	0.40	−33.42	19.62	17.20	19.54
F-5-O	4.252	Captex® 8000	P407	176.10 ± 9.74	0.17 ± 0.02	−21.30 ± 3.29	167.75	0.15	−25.44	4.98	18.49	16.27
F-6-O	1.25	Captex® 8000	P407	205.50 ± 13.45	0.14 ± 0.03	−24.20 ± 2.12	171.77	0.12	−26.97	19.63	14.75	10.28
F-7-O	1.25	Capmul® MCM	TPGS	346.45 ± 18.21	0.40 ± 0.02	−40.80 ± 1.17	336.90	0.41	−42.12	2.84	1.59	3.13
F-8-O	25	Capmul® MCM	TPGS	167.03 ± 10.90	0.33 ± 0.04	−29.10 ± 3.22	187.60	0.40	−29.98	10.97	17.66	2.93

* All experimental data are mean of triplicates ± SD. SD—standard deviation; PS—particle size; PDI—polydispersity index; ZP—zeta potential; PE—penetration enhancer.

3.2. Preparation of TRAVO-Loaded LCNs

Based on the optimization results obtained from the D-optimal design, the eight optimized formulae were selected for drug loading. These formulations were loaded with TRAVO at a concentration of 40 μg/mL mimicking that of the marketed product Travatan®, and then coded F-1-L, F-2-L, F-3-L, F-4-L, F-5-L, F-6-L, F-7-L, and F-8-L. They were prepared by the addition of calculated drug amount to the melted lipid using the hot melt emulsification technique previously described. The prepared TAVO-loaded LCN formulations were then subjected to in vitro and ex vivo characterization.

3.3. Characterization of TRAVO-Loaded LCNs

3.3.1. PS, PDI, and ZP

It can be noticed from Table 4 that all the loaded LCN formulae (F-1-L–F-8-L) showed a nano-sized range from 129.40 ± 11.73 to 361.57 ± 29.21 nm. The PDI values were within the acceptable range (< 0.5), indicating the size uniformity of the prepared formulations. Both formulations (F-1-L and F-3-L) containing Tween 80 as a stabilizer, although used at its highest amount (25 mg), showed variable PS; 216.20 ± 6.12 and 129.40 ± 11.73 nm, respectively. This is mostly due to the discrepancy in the PE used as oleic acid and Captex® 8000, respectively. This may be attributed to the effect of Captex® 8000, which acts as a surface-active agent due to its amphiphilic property, as it supports lowering the tension at the particle-water interface and hence reducing the sizes of the formed particles. P407-stabilized LCNs recorded small PS values for the formulae F-2-L, F-5-L, and F-6-L, although the lower stabilizer amounts were included. This warrants the effectiveness of P407 in LCN stabilization. In contrast, the formulations stabilized with TPGS (F-4-L, F-7-L, and F-8-L) revealed higher size results irrespective of the PE type used. The highest PS obtained in the case of F-7-L could be attributed to the lower amount of TPGS included (1.25 mg). All the optimized formulae loaded with TRAVO exhibited a wide range of ZP values ranging from −13.1 ± 1.27 to −72.9 ± 1.97 mV, noting that the higher negative magnitudes were recorded specifically for oleic acid-based LCNs as discussed before. The overall results guaranteed the high stability of the medicated LCN formulae.

Table 4. The compositions and characterization results of TRAVO-loaded optimized LCNs.

Formula Code	A: Stabilizer Amount (mg)	B: PE Type	C: Stabilizer Type	Data * ± SD			
				PS (nm)	PDI	ZP (mV)	EE%
F-1-L	25	Oleic acid	Tween 80	216.20 ± 6.12	0.27 ± 0.03	−72.93 ± 1.97	85.30 ± 4.29
F-2-L	1.25	Oleic acid	P407	167.45 ± 8.54	0.33 ± 0.03	−62.65 ± 3.12	73.36 ± 15.54
F-3-L	25	Captex® 8000	Tween 80	129.40 ± 11.73	0.34 ± 0.03	−17.55 ± 2.10	82.54 ± 7.65
F-4-L	25	Captex® 8000	TPGS	245.85 ± 3.45	0.44 ± 0.05	−13.10 ± 1.27	71.29 ± 8.87
F-5-L	4.252	Captex® 8000	P407	178.08 ± 11.59	0.18 ± 0.02	−19.45 ± 4.38	80.71 ± 3.68
F-6-L	1.25	Captex® 8000	P407	231.35 ± 12.99	0.36 ± 0.01	−27.80 ± 1.27	75.16 ± 6.10
F-7-L	1.25	Capmul® MCM	TPGS	361.57 ± 29.21	0.42 ± 0.04	−43.21 ± 7.22	84.31 ± 5.09
F-8-L	25	Capmul® MCM	TPGS	212.85 ± 16.65	0.43 ± 0.02	−36.60 ± 3.45	77.20 ± 5.43

* All data are mean of triplicates ± SD. All formulae were loaded with Travoprost at a concentration of 40 μg/mL similar to the marketed product Travatan®. PS—particle size; PDI—polydispersity index; ZP—zeta potential; EE—entrapment efficiency; SD—standard deviation.

3.3.2. Entrapment Efficiency %

As noticed, all formulae possessed a high EE% of TRAVO, ranging from 71.29 ± 8.87 to 85.30 ± 4.29%. These results proved the high ability of LCNs to entrap hydrophobic drugs such as TRAVO even in the presence of different stabilizers and PEs. This could be attributed to the composition of the prepared LCNs, which include a high proportion of lipids, providing good compatibility with the hydrophobic drug (log P = 4.6). This is in agreement with the outcome revealed by Mansour et al., 2017 [39], who declared that cubosomes are capable of entrapping high loads of hydrophobic cargo.

3.3.3. LCNs Morphology Examination Using TEM

TEM was employed to examine the morphology of representative TRAVO-loaded LCN formulations (F-1-L, F-3-L, F-4-L, and F-5-L). As illustrated in Figure 4, all formulae exhibited irregular hexagonal to spherical structures. Because of the negative correlation between HLB and CPP, this could be explained by the effect of fatty substances with low HLB values, such as oleic acid, on increasing the curvature of the bicontinuous layer within the liquid crystal. Because of the negative correlation between HLB and CPP, this could be illuminated by the impact of fatty substances with low HLB, such as oleic acid, on increasing the curvature of the bicontinuous layer inside the liquid crystal [51]. Captex molecules with hydrophobic long chains of fatty acids may cause bigger hydrophobic volumes (Vs) in GMO-based cubosomes, resulting in a higher CPP value for the Captex®/GMO combination and encouraging a transition from the inverse cubic phase to the hexagonal phase [52]. This result matched the view stated by Mansour et al. in 2017 [39].

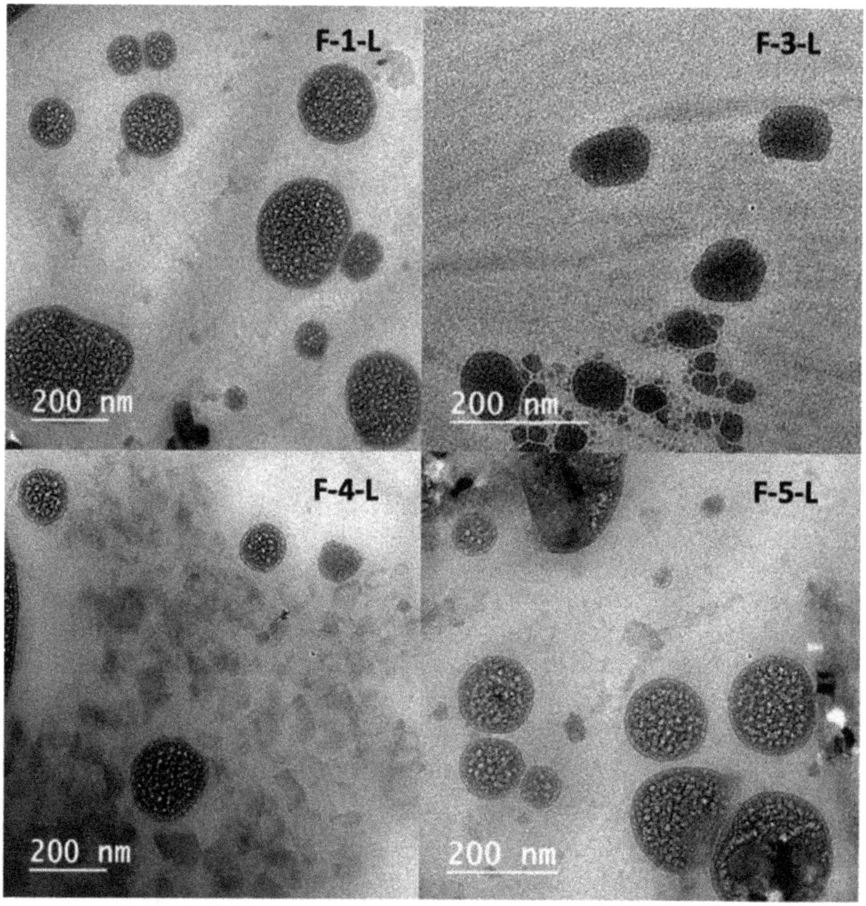

Figure 4. TEM photomicrographs showing the morphology of representative TRAVO-loaded LCNs (F-1-L, F-3-L, F-4-L, and F-5-L).

3.3.4. Crystallinity Study Using X-ray Powder Diffraction (XRPD)

To confirm the crystallinity of different LCNs, XRPD is a useful method. X-ray diffractograms of the representative lyophilized unloaded LCNs (F-1-O, F-3-O, F-4-O, and F-5-O) are presented in Figure 5, compared to the reference formula prepared with GMO and P407 as the lipid and stabilizer, respectively. The X-ray diffractograms of different LCNs showed mutual peaks located at around 32°, 45°, 57°, 76°, and 84° 2θ, as shown in Figure 5. This may be distinctive of the liquid crystals produced, confirming the resemblance of their crystalline structures, as stated by Bei et al., who revealed almost comparable peaks in X-ray patterns [53].

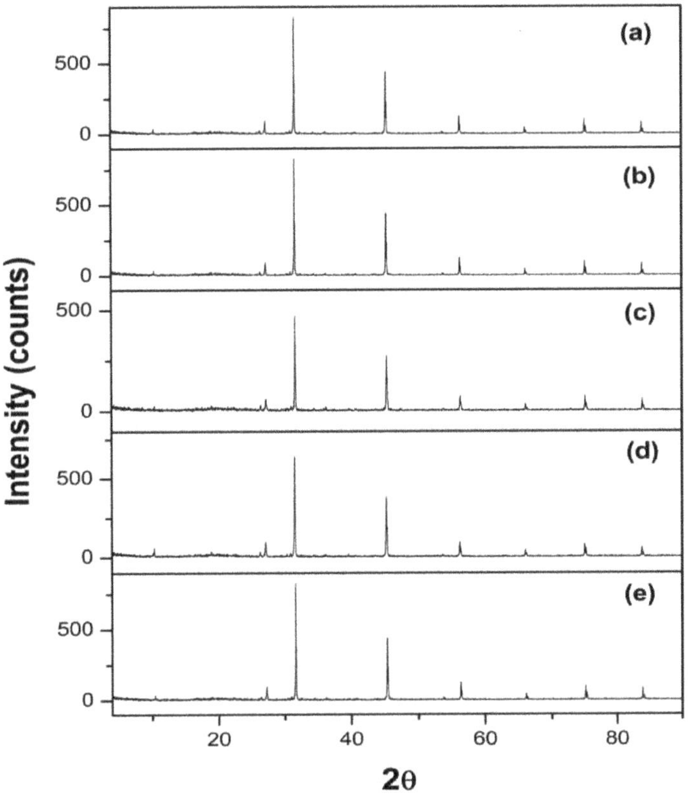

Figure 5. XRPD patterns of (**a**) reference formula, (**b**) F-1-O, (**c**) F-3-O, (**d**) F-4-O, and (**e**) F-5-O.

3.4. Ex Vivo Study for Corneal Permeation of TRAVO-Loaded LCNs

As obvious from Figure 6, the TRAVO-LCN formulae encoded F-1-L, F-3-L, and F-4-L showed the highest cumulative drug amount permeated after 8 h (Q_8), reaching 132.94 ± 4.940, 144.07 ± 1.60 and 132.84 ± 4.55 μg/cm^2, respectively. F-3-L showed a higher significant Q_8 compared to that obtained by both formulas, F-1-L and F-4-L ($p < 0.05$). This was then followed with the LCN formula, F-2-L, which also exhibited a relatively high Q_8 value of 122.54 ± 2.45 μg/cm^2. However, the formulae, coded F-5-L, F-6-L, F-7-L, and F-8-L, revealed slower permeation profiles, as the respective Q_8 data attained 85.40 ± 7.28, 79.00 ± 3.03, 81.28 ± 8.56, and 95.70 ± 9.47 μg/cm^2, respectively. Drug solution (DS) showed the lowest Q_8, reaching only 21.59 ± 7.17 μg/cm^2, with a significant difference compared to the other formulas ($p < 0.05$).

One potential reason that LCNs might enhance corneal permeation is the bio-adhesive property of the liquid crystalline nanoparticles. Their small PS and increased surface area may also promote drug permeation across biological membranes. The nano-sized range and increased surface area of the prepared TRAVO-LCNs could promote adhesion and hence drug penetration through the corneal epithelium, allowing for greater drug delivery to the anterior eye. Furthermore, the structural similarities between the bicontinuous lipid bilayer architectures of cubosomal nanoparticles and corneal epithelial membranes allow membrane fusion and direct transit of the medication into the corneal cells, which may explain the improved penetration of LCN formulations [54]. Furthermore, the cubosomes' main component, GMO, has strong penetration-enhancing properties via ocular membranes [15,55].

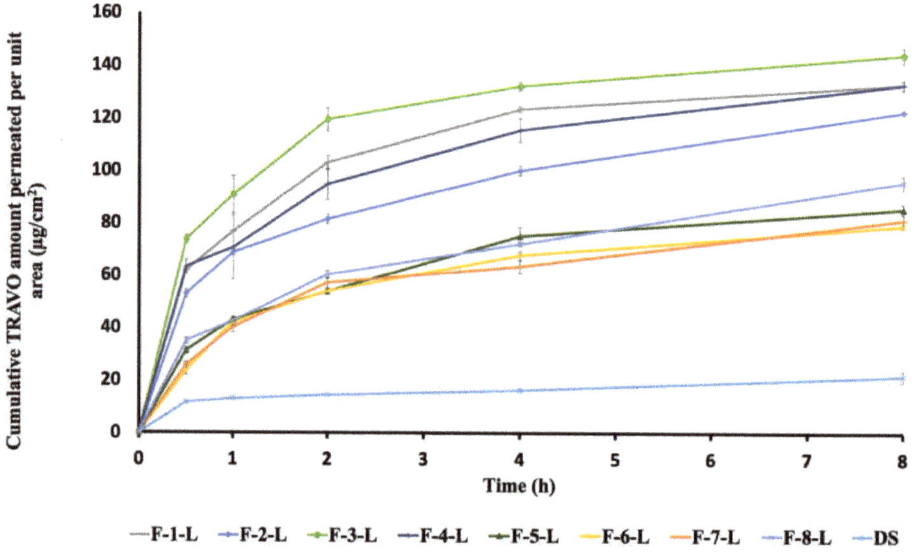

Figure 6. Ex vivo permeation profiles of TRAVO from different loaded LCNs in simulated tear fluid through excised rabbit cornea (mean ± SD, $n = 3$).

Furthermore, the permeation parameters, Jss and Kp, were determined based on the constructed ex vivo permeation profiles, and the results are presented in Table 5. The steady-state flux (Jss) was calculated from the slope of the linear portion of the permeation plots, and the permeation coefficients (Kp) were determined accordingly. As expected, both Tween 80-stabilized formulae, F-1-L and F-3-L, showed the highest fluxes and Kp values, while the LCN formulations stabilized with P407, encoded F-5-L and F-6-L, recorded the least values of permeation parameters, as shown in Table 5. Based on the obtained results, we can deduce the suitability of the optimized TRAVO-LCNs stabilized with Tween 80 coded F-1-L and F-3-L for enhanced ocular delivery. Therefore, these formulations were chosen for further studies.

Table 5. The results of permeation parameters of TRAVO-loaded LCNs.

Formula Code	Data * ± SD	
	Jss (µg/cm²/h)	Kp (cm/h)
F-1-L	25.96 ± 2.05	0.64 ± 0.04
F-2-L	11.92 ± 3.07	0.29 ± 0.09
F-3-L	27.11 ± 3.25	0.67 ± 0.06
F-4-L	12.26 ± 1.54	0.30 ± 0.03
F-5-L	6.85 ± 0.57	0.17 ± 0.01
F-6-L	6.85 ± 0.57	0.14 ± 0.00
F-7-L	8.40 ± 1.05	0.21 ± 0.03
F-8-L	9.85 ± 0.97	0.24 ± 0.04
DS	1.53 ± 0.02	0.03 ± 0.00

* All data are mean of triplicates ± SD. Jss—steady-state flux; Kp—permeability coefficient; DS—drug solution.

3.5. Physical Stability of the Selected TRAVO-Loaded LCNs

The optimized medicated LCN formulae, F-1-L, composed of GMO, oleic acid, and Tween 80 as the lipid, PE, and stabilizer, respectively, and F-3-L, consisting of GMO, Captex® 8000, and Tween 80 as the lipid, PE, and stabilizer, respectively, were stored for 90 days under refrigeration at 5 ± 3 °C. The PS, PDI, ZP, and EE% of the stored samples were determined and compared to the freshly prepared formulations. After storage, the stored LCNs were found to retain their parameters with non-significant variations compared to the fresh preparations ($p > 0.05$), as shown in Table S4 (Supplementary File). The resulting stability might be due to the use of Tween 80, which acts as a stabilizing agent during nanoparticle formation and reduces the surface energy, leading to the inhibition of crystal growth [56].

3.6. Sterilization of TRAVO-Loaded LCNs by Gamma Irradiation

The two potential LCN formulae, F-1-L and F-3-L, were sterilized using gamma irradiation and then tested for their sterility against the presence of any microbial contamination, either bacterial or fungal. Different radiation doses of 5, 10, 15, and 25 kGy were applied to sterilize the selected loaded formulas. After performing the sterilization process, PS, PDI, ZP, and EE% were re-tested, and the data are collected in Table S5 (Supplementary File). All formulae showed non-significant changes in their physical characteristics at all radiation doses ($p > 0.05$). To ensure the sterility of the chosen formulae and to establish the minimal dose (kGy) necessary to achieve their sterility, a confirmatory sterility test was carried out. The absence of any microbial growth in any of the examined samples verifies the formula's sterility and the efficacy of gamma irradiation for sterilization, even at lower doses. Our findings were consistent with those of Youshia et al. (2021) [57].

3.7. In Vivo Ocular Evaluation of the Selected TRAVO-Loaded LCNs

In vivo studies were executed for the estimation of LCNs' ability to deliver TRAVO effectively for glaucoma treatment. Pharmacodynamic and pharmacokinetic studies were performed in rabbits to evaluate the efficacy of the formulae; in addition, the safety of LCN formulae was assessed using the Draize test and histopathological examinations.

3.7.1. Pharmacodynamic Study in Rabbits Using Steroid-Induced Ocular Hypertension Model

The effectiveness of the selected medicated formulae, F-1-L and F-3-L, in lowering the elevated IOP and hence improving glaucoma was assessed in rabbits and then compared to the market product Travatan® eye drops. As shown in Figure 7, the IOP measurements of the right rabbit eyes (non-induced and non-treated) served as negative controls and showed a normal range from 16.43 ± 1.75 to 20.22 ± 1.42 mmHg. After the induction of glaucoma, the initial IOP was measured and recorded at 37.20 mmHg, indicating the glaucomatous eye condition in the left rabbit eyes of all designated groups. After treatment, the eyes of G-I treated with TRAVO-LCNs 'F-1-L' attained their lowest IOP value (15.6 mmHg) at 6 h post-dose application and were shown to maintain the lowering effect for 48 h, after which the IOP starts to rise. However, the medicated formulation F-3-L revealed a much lower mean IOP measurement (13.9 mmHg) after 24 h post-treatment, which lasted during the whole experiment duration (72 h). On the other hand, the marketed product Travatan® demonstrated a gradual reduction in IOP measurements, reaching its peak (14.7 mmHg) at 8 h and persisting for 36 h, after which the IOP significantly increases. As was obvious, the obtained results demonstrated the superiority of the optimized LNC formulations over the commercial product TRAVATAN in lowering IOP for a lasting duration. These results are in alignment with the ex vivo permeation results obtained. The sustained efficacy of the tested LCN formulations could be attributable to the controlled diffusion rate of the drug through the water channels within the nanocrystals [9]. Furthermore, the structural similarity between the bicontinuous lipid bilayer of LCNs and the corneal epithelial cells allows membrane fusion, permitting direct transit of the medication through the corneal cells, which elucidates the improved penetration of LCN formulations [54]. It is important to note that although Travatan® eye drops contain propylene glycol, which acts as a cosolvent with permeation enhancer properties, it was shown to be insufficient to maintain the therapeutic effect of TRAVO for a longer period.

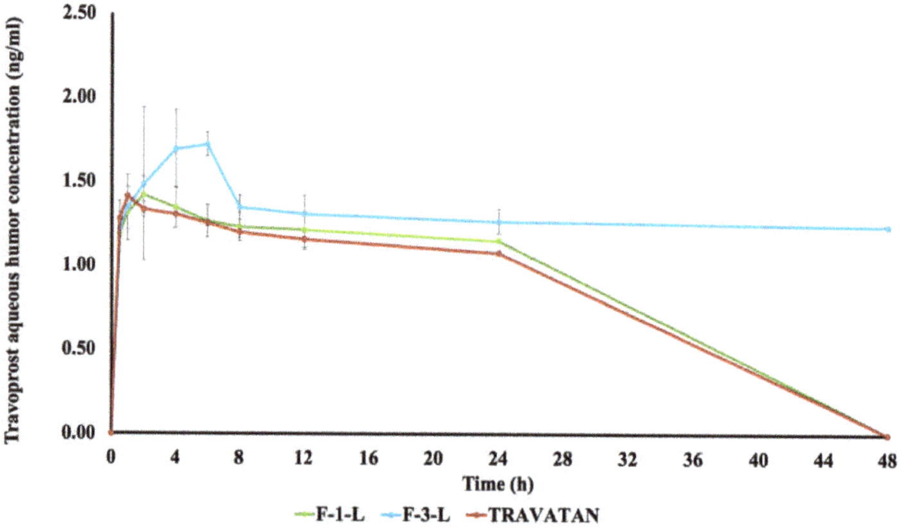

Figure 7. Aqueous humor TRAVO concentrations versus time post-application of F-1-L, F-3-L, and Travatan® in the rabbits' left eyes (mean ± S.D, n = 3).

The percentages of IOP reduction were further calculated for each group at different time intervals based on initial IOP values; the data are presented in Table 6. Both LCN formulations, F-1-L and F-3-L, showed higher IOP reduction for a longer time than the commercial product; this could be due to the synergistic effect of GMO, Tween 80, and oleic acid/Captex® as all LCN components are reported to manifest satisfactory penetration properties [58–60]. The discrepancy in the results of both LCN formulations could emphasize the importance of electrostatic interactions that might occur between the LCN particles and the cornea. As the cornea exhibits negative surface charges, it is reported that the particles with positive charges or less negative charges could be retained for a longer time, allowing for more drug penetration through the cornea [8]. Based on the ZP results obtained previously, F-3-L revealed a significantly lower mean ZP value of −17.55 ± 2.10 mV compared to −72.93 ± 1.97 mV recorded for F-1-L ($p < 0.05$), which in turn can assume a longer residence of the former formula onto the cornea surface, hence an enhanced therapeutic effect. Moreover, the size of the lipid particles is reported to have an influence on corneal permeation, affecting the pharmacological effect of the loaded drug [8]. The sizes of both tested LCN formulae were shown to be significantly different ($p < 0.05$) according to the data stated previously, as F-3-L demonstrated a much lower PS than F-1-L, where the respective sizes were 129.40 ± 11.73 and 216.20 ± 6.12 nm, warranting the enhanced permeation of F-3-L and hence its superiority in lowering IOP.

Table 6. The percent reduction in intraocular pressure in the left rabbit's eye was treated with the different prepared formulae F-1-L, F-3-L, and Travatan® over 72 h.

Time (h)	Mean % IOP Reduction * ± SD		
	G-I: F-1-L	**G-II: F-3-L**	**G-III: TRAVATAN®**
0.5	0.00 ± 0.00	7.53 ± 0.00	14.52 ± 0.00
1	20.79 ± 6.18	14.52 ± 0.00	26.88 ± 0.00
2	37.90 ± 0.00	30.56 ± 6.36	37.90 ± 0.00
4	41.04 ± 5.43	42.65 ± 4.70	55.65 ± 0.00
6	58.06 ± 4.19	52.87 ± 4.81	59.41 ± 0.00
8	52.87 ± 4.81	51.52 ± 4.17	60.48 ± 4.19
10	52.87 ± 4.81	55.56 ± 3.90	59.41 ± 0.00
12	54.30 ± 2.33	58.06 ± 4.19	52.96 ± 2.33
24	51.52 ± 4.17	62.63 ± 6.05	39.52 ± 2.79
36	52.87 ± 4.81	54.30 ± 2.33	34.62 ± 2.88
48	39.34 ± 5.90	50.09 ± 4.81	29.11 ± 3.83
60	20.79 ± 6.18	48.57 ± 6.54	14.52 ± 0.00
72	2.51 ± 4.35	32.62 ± 2.44	0.00 ± 0.00

* All data are mean of triplicates ± SD. IOP—intraocular Pressure; SD—standard deviation. F-1-L is composed of 25 mg GMO, 25 mg oleic acid, and 25 mg Tween 80. F-3-L is composed of 25 mg GMO, 25 mg Captex® 8000 and 25 mg Tween 80.

3.7.2. Pharmacokinetic Study

The results of drug concentration in aqueous humor *versus* time are illustrated in Figure 7, and the calculated pharmacokinetic parameters are collected in Table 7. The LCN formula, F-3-L, showed a significantly higher C_{max} of 1.80 ± 0.15 ng/mL ($p < 0.05$) when compared to 1.46 ± 0.06 and 1.42 ± 0.09 ng/mL obtained in the cases of F-1-L and Travatan®, respectively. It is noted that the difference between the C_{max} of both F-1-L and Travatan® was statistically non-significant ($p > 0.05$). The highest median T_{max} of 6 h attained by F-3-L confirmed more controlled drug permeation behavior than that achieved by Travatan® and F-1-L, recording 1 and 2 h, respectively. Furthermore, the chosen formulation F-3-L showed significantly higher $AUC_{0\text{-}48}$, $AUC_{inf,}$ and MRT in comparison to the respective data obtained from F-1-L and Travatan®, as shown in Table 7. The formula F-1-L showed a relative bioavailability of 106.1%, while F-3-L showed a much higher value of 322.82% with respect to the market product. The obtained results are in good agreement with what was achieved in the pharmacodynamic study, confirming the sustained effect of F-3-L in lowering the IOP compared to F-1-L and Travatan®. The increased ocular bioavailability of LCNs may be due to three factors: the prolonged contact time of LCNs with ocular tissues, the drug's ability to permeate across the cornea, and high drug loading capacity. Liu et al. have investigated pre-ocular retention and revealed that the LCN formulations caused a longer residency on the corneal membrane, potentially lengthening the ocular contact period. This in turn demonstrated a higher flux and permeability of the LCN formulations compared to the drug solution [9]. The unique structural features of LCNs, such as their high packing density and extraordinarily long linear water-filled channels that may hold more medication, may result in increased drug permeability through the cornea [9].

Table 7. The pharmacokinetic parameters of selected TRAVO-loaded LCNs formulae compared to Travatan® measured in rabbits' eye aqueous humor.

PK Parameters	Mean Data * ± SD		
	F-1-L	**F-3-L**	**Travatan®**
T_{max} (h)	2.00	6.00	1.00
C_{max} (ng/mL)	1.46 ± 0.06	1.80 ± 0.15	1.42 ± 0.09
AUC_{0-48} (ng.h/mL)	43.02 ± 2.97	62.77 ± 2.73	41.03 ± 1.63
AUC_{inf} (ng.h/mL)	133.63 ± 11.54	406.69 ± 17.12	125.98 ± 8.54
MRT (h)	11.73 ± 0.22	23.18 ± 0.57	11.58 ± 0.23
%F	106.10	322.82	-

* All data are mean of triplicates ± SD. Tmax: Time of the maximum concentration, Cmax: Maximum concentration, AUC: Area under the curve, MRT: Mean residence time, F = Relative bioavailability.

3.7.3. Ocular Tolerability

Ocular tolerability was performed using the Draize test, which is used for evaluating the toxicity of suspected eye irritants [61]. Ocular irritation (status of the cornea, iris, and conjunctiva) on the treated left eyes, was assessed at 1 h, 24 h, 72 h, and 14 days. As shown in Figure 8, none of the examined LCNs or the marketed product exhibit any symptoms of ocular injury.

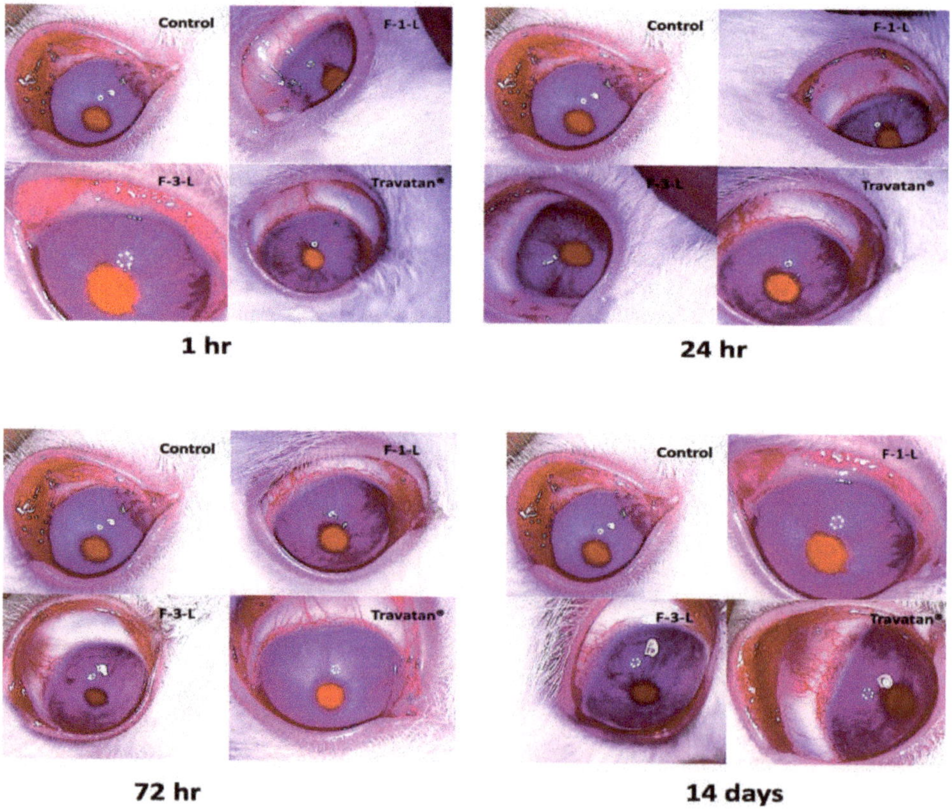

Figure 8. Images of rabbits' eyes post-application of the tested samples. No physiological difference is observed between the eyes treated with the optimized LCNs (F-1-L) and (F-3-L) and the marketed product (Travatan®) compared to the control eye.

3.7.4. Histopathology Examinations

Microscopic examinations of the eye were performed via assessment of the cornea, filtration angle, choroid, retina, and optic nerve. As shown in Figure 9, regarding the cornea, the positive glaucomatous control group showed marked corneal edema manifested by dispersion of the corneal stroma with edematous fluid. Meanwhile, the cornea receiving F-1-L showed mild corneal edema, while F-3-L showed marked improvement, and the cornea appeared apparently normal while the cornea treated with Travatan® was histologically normal. As shown in Figure 9, histopathological changes in the filtration angle were seen in the positive control group, including thickening of the basement membrane with increased collagen deposition and ciliary muscle hyalinosis. Reduced cellular components, increased matrix and fibrillar components, and hyalinization of the trabecular meshwork were found in the meshwork. All other experimental groups revealed apparently normal filtration angles, ciliary bodies, and trabecular meshwork. Figure 9 is concerned with the vascular layer "choroid" of the eyes. The positive control group showed a compressed choroid. Regarding F-1-L, mild choroid compression was observed, while F-3-L and Travatan® exhibited an apparently normal choroid. As shown in Figure 9, a generalized retinal atrophy with loss of inner ganglion cells was seen in the positive control group. The ganglion cells that remained were undersized and hyperchromatic, with pyknotic nuclei. The other experimental groups showed apparently normal retinas. As shown in Figure 9, the optic nerve of the positive control group showed vacuolation, while the optic nerve of the other groups exhibited the absence of histopathological alterations.

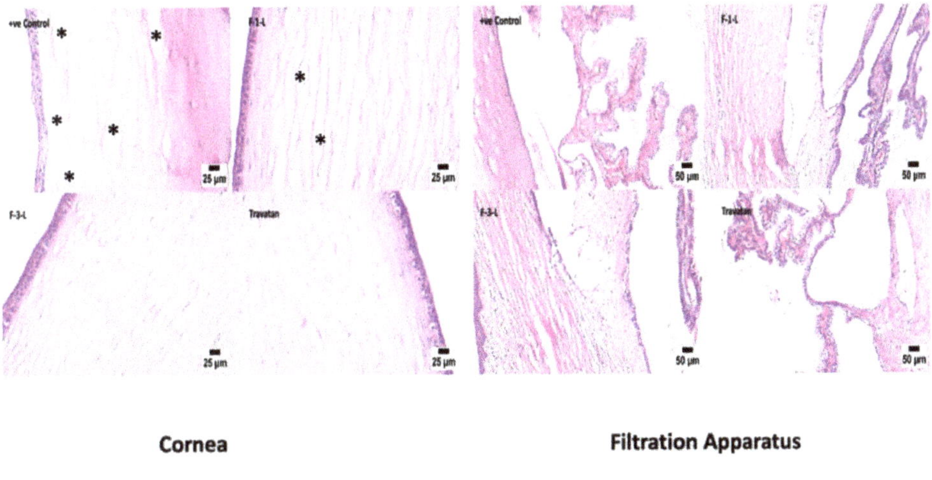

Figure 9. *Cont.*

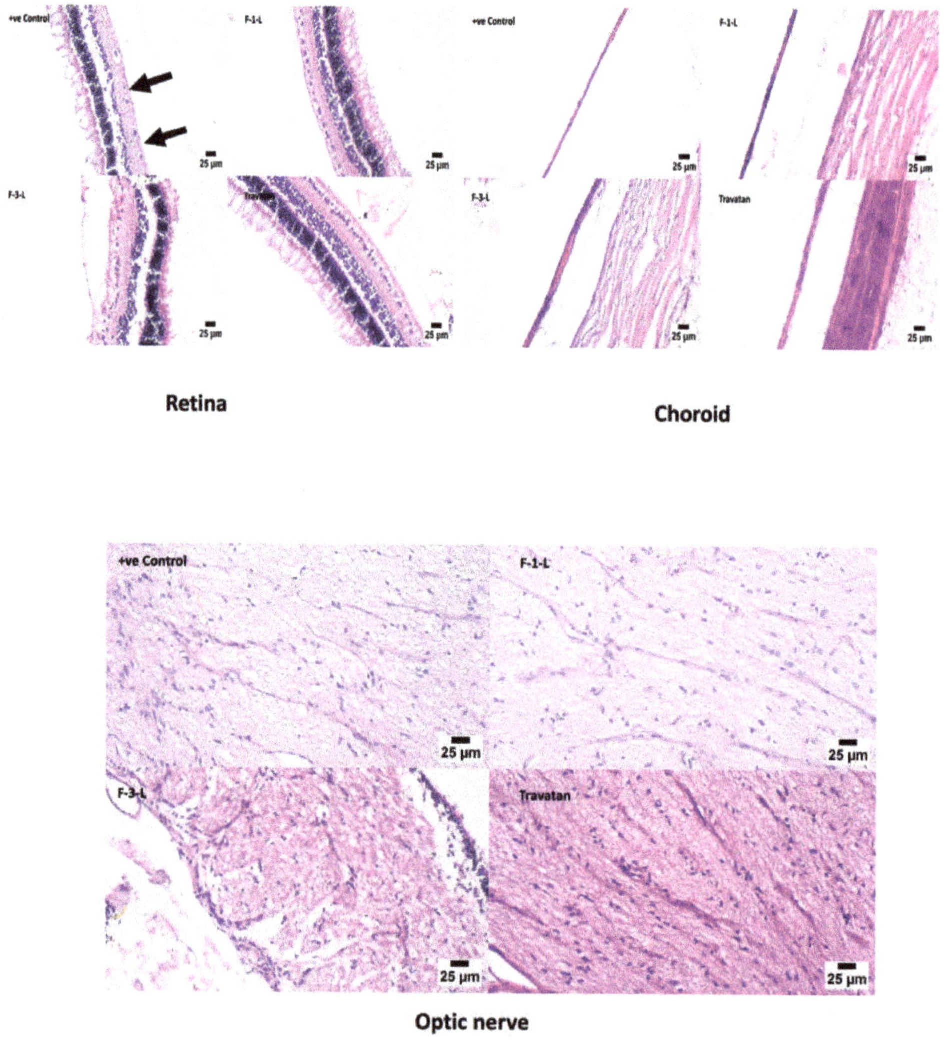

Figure 9. Photomicrographs of the eye of different sections of the tested samples. (*) denotes corneal edema, the black arrows point out undersized hyperchromatic ganglion cells with pyknotic nuclei.

The results revealed that F-3-L, composed of GMO as a lipid, Tween 80 as a stabilizer, and Captex® 8000 as PE, each weighing 25 mg and loaded with TRAVO at a concentration of 40 µg/mL, is the formula of choice as it showed the optimum results in pharmacodynamics and pharmacokinetics studies, accompanied by a high safety profile. The overall results indicate the supreme ability of LCNs to deliver TRAVO by the ocular route and improve glaucoma.

4. Conclusions

The present work describes the successful integration of an innovative ocular penetration enhancer (Captex 8000) into classical liquid crystalline nanostructures. Furthermore, Travoprost loading in these nanostructures resulted in a safe and effective approach to glaucoma treatment. The medicated liquid crystalline nanostructures illustrated favorable drug penetration power throughout the corneal layer, as well as efficient stability and high Travoprost entrapment efficiency. When compared to the amount delivered using the market product, Travatan®, the bioavailability of Travoprost was heightened threefold when delivered from liquid crystalline nanostructures. The pre-clinical in vivo studies in rabbits demonstrated the supremacy of optimized LCNs in alleviating glaucoma following ocular application compared to the marketed product (Travatan®). Such a therapeutic modality represents a worthwhile option to boost the efficacy of anti-glaucoma drugs, awaiting further pre-clinical studies in other animals, such as monkey models, and clinical translation in human beings to validate the effectiveness of these tailored nanoparticles, which would offer a better therapeutic alternative than conventional ophthalmic delivery systems.

Supplementary Materials: The following supporting information can be downloaded at: https://www.mdpi.com/article/10.3390/pharmaceutics15030954/s1, Table S1: Physical characterization of liquid crystalline nanostructure formulae prepared with different lipid types during the preliminary study. Table S2. Physical characterization of liquid crystalline nanostructure formulae prepared using different stabilizers during the preliminary study. Table S3. Physical characterization of liquid crystalline nanostructure formulae prepared using different stabilizer amounts during the preliminary study. Table S4. Physical stability data of the selected TRAVO-loaded LCNs stored under refrigeration at 5 ± 3 °C for 90 days. Table S5. Physical characteristics of the selected TRAVO-loaded LCNs after sterilization by gamma irradiation at different doses (References [62–76] are cited in the Supplementary Materials).

Author Contributions: M.A.E.-G.: Methodology, Investigation, Resources, Data Curation, Writing—Original Draft. M.M.: Conceptualization, Methodology, Resources, Validation, Writing—Review and Editing. M.I.A.E.-A.: Data curation. R.A.H.I.: Conceptualization, Methodology, Validation, Writing—Review and Editing, Visualization. N.D.M.: Writing—Review and Editing, Visualization, Validation, Supervision. All authors have read and agreed to the published version of the manuscript.

Funding: This research received no external funding.

Institutional Review Board Statement: The in vivo study was approved by the Research Ethics Committee of the Faculty of Pharmacy, Ain Shams University (REC approval # REC-ASU 54).

Data Availability Statement: The datasets generated during the current study are available from the corresponding authors upon request.

Conflicts of Interest: The authors declare no conflict of interest.

Abbreviations

AUC—area under the curve; Cmax—maximum concentration; DLS—dynamic light scattering; DS—drug solution; EE%—entrapment efficiency; F%—relative bioavailability; FP receptor—prostaglandin F receptor; G—group; GMO—glyceryl monooleate; H&E—hematoxylin and Eosin; HPLC—high performance liquid chromatography; IOP—intraocular pressure; IS—internal standard; Jss—steady state flux; Kp—permeability coefficient; LCNs—liquid crystalline nanostructures; LDA—laser Doppler Anemometry; LOD—limit of detection; LOQ—limit of quantitation; MO—monoolein; MRM—multiple reactions monitoring; NPs—nanoparticles; NS—nano-sponge; PDI—polydispersity index; PE—penetration enhancer; PS—particle size; PYT—phytantriol; Q8—cumulative drug amount permeated after 8 h; SD—standard deviation; STF—simulated tear fluid; TBME—tertiary butyl-methyl ether; TEM—transmission electron microscopy; Tmax—time to reach maximum concentration; TPGS—tocopherol polyethylene glycol 1000 succinate; TRAVO—Travoprost; XRPD—X-ray powder diffraction; ZP—zeta potential.

References

1. Tran, N.; Mulet, X.; Hawley, M.; Hinton, M.; Mudie, T.; Muir, W.; Giakoumatos, C.; Waddington, J.; Kirby, M.; Drummond, J.C. Nanostructure and Cytotoxicity of Self-Assembled Monoolein–Capric Acid Lyotropic Liquid Crystalline Nanoparticles. *RSC Adv.* **2015**, *5*, 26785–26795. [CrossRef]

2. Elfaky, M.A.; Sirwi, A.; Tolba, H.H.; Shaik, R.A.; Selmi, N.M.; Alattas, A.H.; Albreki, R.S.; Alshreef, N.M.; Gad, H.A. Development, Optimization, and Antifungal Assessment of Ocular Gel Loaded With Ketoconazole Cubic Liquid Crystalline Nanoparticles. *J. Pharm. Sci.* **2021**, *110*, 2210–2220. [CrossRef] [PubMed]
3. Ismail, A.; Nasr, M.; Sammour, O. Nanoemulsion as a Feasible and Biocompatible Carrier for Ocular Delivery of Travoprost: Improved Pharmacokinetic/Pharmacodynamic Properties. *Int. J. Pharm.* **2020**, *583*, 119402. [CrossRef]
4. Nasr, M.; Teiama, M.; Ismail, A.; Ebada, A.; Saber, S. In Vitro and in Vivo Evaluation of Cubosomal Nanoparticles as an Ocular Delivery System for Fluconazole in Treatment of Keratomycosis. *Drug Deliv. Transl. Res.* **2020**, *10*, 1841–1852. [CrossRef]
5. Silva, R.O.; da Costa, B.L.; da Silva, F.R.; da Silva, C.N.; de Paiva, M.B.; Dourado, L.F.N.; Malachias, Â.; de Souza Araújo, A.A.; Nunes, P.S.; Silva-Cunha, A. Treatment for Chemical Burning Using Liquid Crystalline Nanoparticles as an Ophthalmic Delivery System for Pirfenidone. *Int. J. Pharm.* **2019**, *568*, 118466. [CrossRef]
6. Younes, N.F.; Abdel-Halim, S.A.; Elassasy, A.I. Corneal Targeted Sertaconazole Nitrate Loaded Cubosomes: Preparation, Statistical Optimization, in Vitro Characterization, Ex Vivo Permeation and in Vivo Studies. *Int. J. Pharm.* **2018**, *553*, 386–397. [CrossRef]
7. Huang, J.; Peng, T.; Li, Y.; Zhan, Z.; Zeng, Y.; Huang, Y.; Pan, X.; Wu, C.Y.; Wu, C. Ocular Cubosome Drug Delivery System for Timolol Maleate: Preparation, Characterization, Cytotoxicity, Ex Vivo, and In Vivo Evaluation. *AAPS PharmSciTech* **2017**, *18*, 2919–2926. [CrossRef]
8. Ban, J.; Zhang, Y.; Huang, X.; Deng, G.; Hou, D.; Chen, Y.; Lu, Z. Corneal Permeation Properties of a Charged Lipid Nanoparticle Carrier Containing Dexamethasone. *Int. J. Nanomed.* **2017**, *12*, 1329. [CrossRef]
9. Liu, R.; Wang, S.; Fang, S.; Wang, J.; Chen, J.; Huang, X.; He, X.; Liu, C. Liquid Crystalline Nanoparticles as an Ophthalmic Delivery System for Tetrandrine: Development, Characterization, and In Vitro and In Vivo Evaluation. *Nanoscale Res. Lett.* **2016**, *11*, 254. [CrossRef] [PubMed]
10. Verma, P.; Ahuja, M. Cubic Liquid Crystalline Nanoparticles: Optimization and Evaluation for Ocular Delivery of Tropicamide. *Drug Deliv.* **2016**, *23*, 3043–3054. [CrossRef]
11. Achouri, D.; Sergent, M.; Tonetto, A.; Piccerelle, P.; Andrieu, V.; Hornebecq, V. Self-Assembled Liquid Crystalline Nanoparticles as an Ophthalmic Drug Delivery System. Part II: Optimization of Formulation Variables Using Experimental Design. *Drug Dev. Ind. Pharm.* **2015**, *41*, 493–501. [CrossRef]
12. Wu, W.; Li, J.; Wu, L.; Wang, B.; Wang, Z.; Xu, Q.; Xin, H. Ophthalmic Delivery of Brinzolamide by Liquid Crystalline Nanoparticles: In Vitro and in Vivo Evaluation. *AAPS PharmSciTech* **2013**, *14*, 1063–1071. [CrossRef]
13. Li, J.; Wu, L.; Wu, W.; Wang, B.; Wang, Z.; Xin, H.; Xu, Q. A Potential Carrier Based on Liquid Crystal Nanoparticles for Ophthalmic Delivery of Pilocarpine Nitrate. *Int. J. Pharm.* **2013**, *455*, 75–84. [CrossRef] [PubMed]
14. Han, S.; Shen, J.Q.; Gan, Y.; Geng, H.M.; Zhang, X.X.; Zhu, C.L.; Gan, L. Novel Vehicle Based on Cubosomes for Ophthalmic Delivery of Flurbiprofen with Low Irritancy and High Bioavailability. *Acta Pharmacol. Sin.* **2010**, *31*, 990–998. [CrossRef] [PubMed]
15. Gan, L.; Han, S.; Shen, J.; Zhu, J.; Zhu, C.; Zhang, X.; Gan, Y. Self-Assembled Liquid Crystalline Nanoparticles as a Novel Ophthalmic Delivery System for Dexamethasone: Improving Preocular Retention and Ocular Bioavailability. *Int. J. Pharm.* **2010**, *396*, 179–187. [CrossRef] [PubMed]
16. Razak, A.; Iman Mohd Hamdi, N.; Azeera Mohd Ali, N. The Association of Cigarette Smoking on Intraocular Pressure Among Young Adult Male: A Preliminary Study. *Malays. J. Med. Health Sci.* **2021**, *17* (Suppl. 3), 2636–9346.
17. Diaconita, V.; Quinn, M.; Jamal, D.; Dishan, B.; Malvankar-Mehta, M.S.; Hutnik, C. Washout Duration of Prostaglandin Analogues: A Systematic Review and Meta-Analysis. *J. Ophthalmol.* **2018**, *2018*, 3190684. [CrossRef]
18. Aihara, M. Prostanoid Receptor Agonists for Glaucoma Treatment. *Jpn. J. Ophthalmol.* **2021**, *65*, 581–590. [CrossRef]
19. Shukr, M.H.; Ismail, S.; El-Hossary, G.G.; El-Shazly, A.H. Spanlastics Nanovesicular Ocular Insert as a Novel Ocular Delivery of Travoprost: Optimization Using Box–Behnken Design and in Vivo Evaluation. *J. Liposome Res.* **2022**. [CrossRef]
20. Schnichels, S.; Hurst, J.; de Vries, J.W.; Ullah, S.; Gruszka, A.; Kwak, M.; Löscher, M.; Dammeier, S.; Bartz-Schmidt, K.U.; Spitzer, M.S.; et al. Self-Assembled DNA Nanoparticles Loaded with Travoprost for Glaucoma-Treatment. *Nanomedicine* **2020**, *29*, 102260. [CrossRef]
21. Lambert, W.S.; Carlson, B.J.; van der Ende, A.E.; Shih, G.; Dobish, J.N.; Calkins, D.J.; Harth, E. Nanosponge-Mediated Drug Delivery Lowers Intraocular Pressure. *Transl. Vis. Sci. Technol.* **2015**, *4*, 1–16. [CrossRef]
22. Salah, S.; Mahmoud, A.A.; Kamel, A.O. Etodolac Transdermal Cubosomes for the Treatment of Rheumatoid Arthritis: Ex Vivo Permeation and in Vivo Pharmacokinetic Studies. *Drug Deliv.* **2017**, *24*, 846–856. [CrossRef]
23. Hashad, R.A.; Ishak, R.A.H.; Geneidi, A.S.; Mansour, S. Surface Functionalization of Methotrexate-Loaded Chitosan Nanoparticles with Hyaluronic Acid/Human Serum Albumin: Comparative Characterization and in Vitro Cytotoxicity. *Int. J. Pharm.* **2017**, *522*, 128–136. [CrossRef]
24. Salimi, A.; Panahi-Bazaz, M.R.; Panahi-Bazaz, E. A Novel Microemulsion System for Ocular Delivery of Azithromycin: Design, Characterization and Ex-Vivo Rabbit Corneal Permeability. *Jundishapur J. Nat. Pharm. Prod.* **2017**, *12*, e13938. [CrossRef]
25. Asasutjarit, R.; Theerachayanan, T.; Kewsuwan, P.; Veeranondha, S.; Fuongfuchat, A.; Ritthidej, G.C. Gamma Sterilization of Diclofenac Sodium Loaded- N-Trimethyl Chitosan Nanoparticles for Ophthalmic Use. *Carbohydr. Polym.* **2017**, *157*, 603–612. [CrossRef] [PubMed]
26. Elmowafy, E.; Gad, H.; Biondo, F.; Casettari, L.; Soliman, M.E. Exploring Optimized Methoxy Poly(Ethylene Glycol)-Block-Poly(ε-Caprolactone) Crystalline Cored Micelles in Anti-Glaucoma Pharmacotherapy. *Int. J. Pharm.* **2019**, *566*, 573–584. [CrossRef] [PubMed]

27. Ramadan, A.A.; Eladawy, S.A.; El-Enin, A.S.M.A.; Hussein, Z.M. Development and Investigation of Timolol Maleate Niosomal Formulations for the Treatment of Glaucoma. *J. Pharm. Investig.* **2020**, *50*, 59–70. [CrossRef]
28. Ammar, H.O.; Salama, H.A.; Ghorab, M.; Mahmoud, A.A. Nanoemulsion as a Potential Ophthalmic Delivery System for Dorzolamide Hydrochloride. *AAPS PharmSciTech* **2009**, *10*, 808–819. [CrossRef] [PubMed]
29. Fatouh, A.M.; Elshafeey, A.H.; Abdelbary, A. Agomelatine-Based in Situ Gels for Brain Targeting via the Nasal Route: Statistical Optimization, in Vitro, and in Vivo Evaluation. *Drug Deliv.* **2017**, *24*, 1077–1085. [CrossRef]
30. Emad Eldeeb, A.; Salah, S.; Ghorab, M. Proniosomal Gel-Derived Niosomes: An Approach to Sustain and Improve the Ocular Delivery of Brimonidine Tartrate; Formulation, in-Vitro Characterization, and in-Vivo Pharmacodynamic Study. *Drug Deliv.* **2019**, *26*, 509–521. [CrossRef]
31. Luechtefeld, T.; Maertens, A.; Russo, D.P.; Rovida, C.; Zhu, H.; Hartung, T. Analysis of Draize Eye Irritation Testing and Its Prediction by Mining Publicly Available 2008-2014 REACH Data. *ALTEX* **2016**, *33*, 123–134. [CrossRef]
32. Tokuda, K.; Baron, B.; Kuramitsu, Y.; Kitagawa, T.; Tokuda, N.; Morishige, N.; Kobayashi, M.; Kimura, K.; Nakamura, K.; Sonoda, K.H. Optimization of Fixative Solution for Retinal Morphology: A Comparison with Davidson's Fixative and Other Fixation Solutions. *Jpn. J. Ophthalmol.* **2018**, *62*, 481–490. [CrossRef]
33. Bancroft, J.; Gamble, M. *Theory and Practice of Histological Techniques*, 6th ed.; ScienceDirect: Amsterdam, The Netherlands, 2008.
34. Kulkarni, S.A.; Feng, S.S. Effects of Surface Modification on Delivery Efficiency of Biodegradable Nanoparticles across the Blood-Brain Barrier. *Nanomedicine* **2011**, *6*, 377–394. [CrossRef]
35. Yagublu, V.; Karimova, A.; Hajibabazadeh, J.; Reissfelder, C.; Muradov, M.; Bellucci, S.; Allahverdiyev, A. Overview of Physicochemical Properties of Nanoparticles as Drug Carriers for Targeted Cancer Therapy. *J. Funct. Biomater.* **2022**, *13*, 196. [CrossRef] [PubMed]
36. Alkholief, M.; Albasit, H.; Alhowyan, A.; Alshehri, S.; Raish, M.; Abul Kalam, M.; Alshamsan, A. Employing a PLGA-TPGS Based Nanoparticle to Improve the Ocular Delivery of Acyclovir. *Saudi Pharm. J.* **2019**, *27*, 293–302. [CrossRef] [PubMed]
37. Das, S.; Bandyopadhyay, K.; Ghosh, M.M. Effect of Stabilizer Concentration on the Size of Silver Nanoparticles Synthesized through Chemical Route. *Inorg. Chem. Commun.* **2021**, *123*, 108319. [CrossRef]
38. Ishak, R.A.H.; Mostafa, N.M.; Kamel, A.O. Stealth Lipid Polymer Hybrid Nanoparticles Loaded with Rutin for Effective Brain Delivery—Comparative Study with the Gold Standard (Tween 80): Optimization, Characterization and Biodistribution. *Drug Deliv.* **2017**, *24*, 1874–1890. [CrossRef]
39. Mansour, M.; Kamel, A.O.; Mansour, S.; Mortada, N.D. Novel Polyglycerol-Dioleate Based Cubosomal Dispersion with Tailored Physical Characteristics for Controlled Delivery of Ondansetron. *Colloids Surf. B Biointerfaces* **2017**, *156*, 44–54. [CrossRef] [PubMed]
40. Nakano, M.; Sugita, A.; Matsuoka, H.; Handa, T. Small-Angle X-Ray Scattering and 13C NMR Investigation on the Internal Structure of "Cubosomes". *Langmuir* **2001**, *17*, 3917–3922. [CrossRef]
41. Lamer, V.K.; Dinegar, R.H. Theory, Production and Mechanism of Formation of Monodispersed Hydrosols. *J. Am. Chem.Soc.* **1950**, *72*, 4847–4854. [CrossRef]
42. Dibaei, M.; Rouini, M.R.; Sheikholeslami, B.; Gholami, M.; Dinarvand, R. The Effect of Surface Treatment on the Brain Delivery of Curcumin Nanosuspension: In Vitro and in Vivo Studies. *Int. J. Nanomed.* **2019**, *14*, 5477–5490. [CrossRef]
43. Cao, G.; Du, T.; Bai, Y.; Yang, T.; Zuo, J. Effects of Surfactant Molecular Structure on the Stability of Water in Oil Emulsion. *J. Pet. Sci. Eng.* **2021**, *196*, 107695. [CrossRef]
44. Wen, S.N.; Chu, C.H.; Wang, Y.C.; Huang, H.Y.; Wang, Y.J.; Lin, J.Y.; Lu, H.T.; Wang, S.J.; Yang, C.S. Polymer-Stabilized Micelles Reduce the Drug Rapid Clearance in Vivo. *J. Nanomater.* **2018**, *2018*, 5818592. [CrossRef]
45. Patil, R.P.; Pawara, D.D.; Gudewar, C.S.; Tekade, A.R. Nanostructured Cubosomes in an in Situ Nasal Gel System: An Alternative Approach for the Controlled Delivery of Donepezil HCl to Brain. *J. Liposome Res.* **2019**, *29*, 264–273. [CrossRef]
46. Jacobs, C.; Kayser, O.; Müller, R.H. Nanosuspensions as a New Approach for the Formulation for the Poorly Soluble Drug Tarazepide. *Int. J. Pharm.* **2000**, *196*, 161–164. [CrossRef]
47. Sun, W.; Xie, C.; Wang, H.; Hu, Y. Specific Role of Polysorbate 80 Coating on the Targeting of Nanoparticles to the Brain. *Biomaterials* **2004**, *25*, 3065–3071. [CrossRef] [PubMed]
48. Tuomela, A.; Hirvonen, J.; Peltonen, L. Stabilizing Agents for Drug Nanocrystals: Effect on Bioavailability. *Pharmaceutics* **2016**, *8*, 16. [CrossRef]
49. Wu, S.; Wang, G.; Lu, Z.; Li, Y.; Zhou, X.; Chen, L.; Cao, J.; Zhang, L. Effects of Glycerol Monostearate and Tween 80 on the Physical Properties and Stability of Recombined Low-Fat Dairy Cream. *Dairy Sci. Technol.* **2016**, *96*, 377–390. [CrossRef]
50. El-Naggar, N.E.A.; Saber, W.E.I.A.; Zweil, A.M.; Bashir, S.I. An Innovative Green Synthesis Approach of Chitosan Nanoparticles and Their Inhibitory Activity against Phytopathogenic Botrytis Cinerea on Strawberry Leaves. *Sci. Rep.* **2022**, *12*, 3515. [CrossRef]
51. Amar-Yuli, I.; Libster, D.; Aserin, A.; Garti, N. Solubilization of Food Bioactives within Lyotropic Liquid Crystalline Mesophases. *Curr. Opin. Colloid Interface Sci.* **2009**, *14*, 21–32. [CrossRef]
52. Wang, H.; Zetterlund, P.B.; Boyer, C.; Spicer, P.T. Polymerization of Cubosome and Hexosome Templates to Produce Complex Microparticle Shapes. *J. Colloid Interface Sci.* **2019**, *546*, 240–250. [CrossRef]
53. Bei, D.; Zhang, T.; Murowchick, J.B.; Youan, B.-B.C. Formulation of Dacarbazine-Loaded Cubosomes. Part III. Physicochemical Characterization. *AAPS PharmSciTech* **2010**, *11*, 1243–1249. [CrossRef] [PubMed]

54. Chen, Y.; Ma, P.; Gui, S. Cubic and Hexagonal Liquid Crystals as Drug Delivery Systems. *Biomed. Res. Int.* **2014**, *2014*, 815981. [CrossRef]
55. Gaballa, S.A.; el Garhy, O.H.; Moharram, H.; Abdelkader, H. Preparation and Evaluation of Cubosomes/Cubosomal Gels for Ocular Delivery of Beclomethasone Dipropionate for Management of Uveitis. *Pharm. Res.* **2020**, *37*, 198. [CrossRef]
56. Sukmawati, A.; Utami, W.; Yuliani, R.; Da'I, M.; Nafarin, A. Effect of Tween 80 on Nanoparticle Preparation of Modified Chitosan for Targeted Delivery of Combination Doxorubicin and Curcumin Analogue. *IOP Conf. Ser. Mater. Sci. Eng.* **2018**, *311*, 012024. [CrossRef]
57. Youshia, J.; Kamel, A.O.; el Shamy, A.; Mansour, S. Gamma Sterilization and in Vivo Evaluation of Cationic Nanostructured Lipid Carriers as Potential Ocular Delivery Systems for Antiglaucoma Drugs. *Eur. J. Pharm. Sci.* **2021**, *163*, 105887. [CrossRef] [PubMed]
58. Lim, D.G.; Jeong, W.W.; Kim, N.A.; Lim, J.Y.; Lee, S.H.; Shim, W.S.; Kang, N.G.; Jeong, S.H. Effect of the Glyceryl Monooleate-Based Lyotropic Phases on Skin Permeation Using in Vitro Diffusion and Skin Imaging. *Asian J. Pharm. Sci.* **2014**, *9*, 324–329. [CrossRef]
59. Haq, A.; Michniak-Kohn, B. Effects of Solvents and Penetration Enhancers on Transdermal Delivery of Thymoquinone: Permeability and Skin Deposition Study. *Drug Deliv.* **2018**, *25*, 1943. [CrossRef] [PubMed]
60. Ajmeera, D.; Manda, S.; Janapareddi, K.; Kolluri, S. Development of Nanoemulsion to Improve the Ocular Bioavailability and Patient Compliance in Postoperative Treatment Using Indomethacin. *Int. J. Appl. Pharm.* **2020**, *12*, 99–107. [CrossRef]
61. Wilhelmus, K.R. The Draize Eye Test. *Surv. Ophthalmol.* **2001**, *45*, 493–515. [CrossRef]
62. Peng, X.; Zhou, Y.; Han, K.; Qin, L.; Dian, L.; Li, G.; Pan, X.; Wu, C. Characterization of Cubosomes as a Targeted and Sustained Transdermal Delivery System for Capsaicin. *Drug Des. Devel. Ther.* **2015**, *9*, 4209–4218. [CrossRef] [PubMed]
63. Shi, X.; Peng, T.; Huang, Y.; Mei, L.; Gu, Y.; Huang, J.; Han, K.; Li, G.; Hu, C.; Pan, X.; et al. Comparative Studies on Glycerol Monooleate- and Phytantriol-Based Cubosomes Containing Oridonin in Vitro and in Vivo. *Pharm. Dev. Technol.* **2017**, *22*, 322–329. [CrossRef]
64. Hong, L.; Dong, Y.-D.; Boyd, B.J. Preparation of Nanostructured Lipid Drug Delivery Particles Using Microfluidic Mixing. *Pharm. Nanotechnol.* **2019**, *7*, 484–495. [CrossRef]
65. Elmowafy, M.; Samy, A.; Raslan, M.A.; Salama, A.; Said, R.A.; Abdelaziz, A.E.; El-Eraky, W.; el Awdan, S.; Viitala, T. Enhancement of Bioavailability and Pharmacodynamic Effects of Thymoquinone Via Nanostructured Lipid Carrier (NLC) Formulation. *AAPS PharmSciTech* **2016**, *17*, 663–672. [CrossRef]
66. Kassem, M.G.A.; Ahmed, A.M.M.; Abdel-Rahman, H.H.; Moustafa, A.H.E. Use of Span 80 and Tween 80 for Blending Gasoline and Alcohol in Spark Ignition Engines. *Energy Rep.* **2019**, *5*, 221–230. [CrossRef]
67. Kumar, G.P.; Rajeshwarrao, P. Nonionic Surfactant Vesicular Systems for Effective Drug Delivery—An Overview. *Acta Pharm. Sin. B* **2011**, *1*, 208–219. [CrossRef]
68. Young, T.J.; Johnston, K.P.; Pace, G.W.; Mishra, A.K. Phospholipid-Stabilized Nanoparticles of Cyclosporine a by Rapid Expansion from Supercritical to Aqueous Solution. *AAPS PharmSciTech* **2004**, *5*, 70–85. [CrossRef] [PubMed]
69. Helgason, T.; Awad, T.S.; Kristbergsson, K.; McClements, D.J.; Weiss, J. Effect of Surfactant Surface Coverage on Formation of Solid Lipid Nanoparticles (SLN). *J. Colloid Interface Sci.* **2009**, *334*, 75–81. [CrossRef]
70. Kulkarni, S.A.; Feng, S.S. Effects of Particle Size and Surface Modification on Cellular Uptake and Biodistribution of Polymeric Nanoparticles for Drug Delivery. *Pharm. Res.* **2013**, *30*, 2512–2522. [CrossRef]
71. Yegin, Y.; Oh, J.K.; Akbulut, M.; Taylor, T. Cetylpyridinium Chloride Produces Increased Zeta-Potential on Salmonella Typhimurium Cells, a Mechanism of the Pathogen's Inactivation. *NPJ Sci. Food* **2019**, *3*, 1–7. [CrossRef]
72. Tlijani, M.; Lassoued, M.A.; Bahloul, B.; Sfar, S. Development of a BCS Class II Drug Microemulsion for Oral Delivery: Design, Optimization, and Evaluation. *J. Nanomater.* **2021**, *2021*. [CrossRef]
73. Spicer, P.T.; Hayden, K.L.; Lynch, M.L.; Ofori-Boateng, A.; Burns, J.L. Novel Process for Producing Cubic Liquid Crystalline Nanoparticles (Cubosomes). *Langmuir* **2001**, *17*, 5748–5756. [CrossRef]
74. Choulis, N.H. Miscellaneous Drugs, Materials, Medical Devices, and Techniques. *Side Eff. Drugs Annu.* **2011**, *33*, 1009–1029. [CrossRef]
75. Prajapati, H.N.; Dalrymple, D.M.; Serajuddin, A.T.M. A Comparative Evaluation of Mono-, Di- and Triglyceride of Medium Chain Fatty Acids by Lipid/Surfactant/Water Phase Diagram, Solubility Determination and Dispersion Testing for Application in Pharmaceutical Dosage Form Development. *Pharm. Res.* **2012**, *29*, 285–305. [CrossRef]
76. McClements, D.J. Crystals and Crystallization in Oil-in-Water Emulsions: Implications for Emulsion-Based Delivery Systems. *Adv. Colloid Interface Sci.* **2012**, *174*, 1–30. [CrossRef] [PubMed]

MDPI AG
Grosspeteranlage 5
4052 Basel
Switzerland
Tel.: +41 61 683 77 34

MDPI Books Editorial Office
E-mail: books@mdpi.com
www.mdpi.com/books

www.ingramcontent.com/pod-product-compliance
Lightning Source LLC
LaVergne TN
LVHW070207100526
838202LV00015B/2012